100 Interesting Case Studies in Neurointervention: Tips and Tricks

Vipul Gupta • Ajit S. Puri
Rajsrinivas Parthasarathy
Editors

100 Interesting Case Studies in Neurointervention: Tips and Tricks

BYWORD BOOKS™

Springer

Editors
Vipul Gupta
Neurointerventional Surgery, Stroke Unit
Artemis Agrim Institute of Neuroscience
Gurgaon
India

Rajsrinivas Parthasarathy
Department of Vascular Neurology and
Neurointerventional Surgery
Artemis Agrim Institute of Neuroscience
Gurgaon
India

Ajit S. Puri
Division of Neurointerventional Surgery
University of Massachusetts Medical
Center
Worcester
MA
USA

ISBN 978-981-13-1345-5 ISBN 978-981-13-1346-2 (eBook)
https://doi.org/10.1007/978-981-13-1346-2

Library of Congress Control Number: 2018965218

Co-publishing partnership between Byword Books Private Limited and Springer Nature India Private Limited
This Springer imprint is published by the registered company Springer Nature Singapore Pte Ltd.
The registered company address is: 152 Beach Road, #21-01/04 Gateway East, Singapore 189721, Singapore

Dedicated to my family
My inspiration, G
My children Nainika and Nilay

—Dr. Vipul Gupta

Preface

Neurointervention has come a long way in last two decades. Recent positive trials in acute stroke (to me the "holy grail" of neurointervention) and device evolution in aneurysmal management have brought this field to the fore with increasing role in neurosurgical as well as neurological disorders.

However, the training programs have not kept pace in spite of increasing need for more neurointerventionists. There is dearth of evolved centers (with adequate volume, quality, and teaching) running training programs in South and Southeast Asia. Not just this at times training done in West may not suit the clinical and financial profile of the patients in this region.

During my career, I have worked in close association with neurosurgeons and neurologists of high repute and on many occasions explained "Tips and Tricks" I use to manage particularly difficult cases. I was encouraged by my colleagues to collate these discussions succinctly into a book for the benefit of young aspiring neurointerventionists. This book is the result of their persistent prompting and unstinting support.

Book is designed as a practical teaching atlas, a quick reference for neurointerventionists when handling challenging situations. Format we have used explains the technique employed – "the how I do it," the decision-making process, alternate clinical management options, and pre- and post-procedure images. At the end of each case, there is a "Tip and Trick" section wherein I share my personal experience in an attempt to shorten the learning curve for my young colleagues in the field of neurointervention.

I sincerely hope that you find this book a useful tool in your armamentarium and more importantly it enables you to better your technical and clinical outcomes.

Gurgaon, India

Dr. Vipul Gupta

Acknowledgments

From the bottom of my heart, I thank my coeditors Dr. Rajsrinivas Parthasarthy and Dr. Ajit S. Puri who were pivotal not only in writing cases but also in reviewing the case material provided by other authors. I am indebted to my coauthors who took time out of their busy schedules to contribute cases for the book. A special mention of my colleagues and dear friends Dr. Aditya Gupta and Dr. Sumit Singh for their support during this period; I am profoundly grateful to Dr. Swati Chinchure, Dr. Milind Sawant, and Dr. Anshul Mahajan who helped in reviewing the cases. Our patients played a big role in our learning and gave consent for the images to be used for academic purpose. And lastly, full credit to my editors Dinesh Sinha and Naren Aggarwal for their patience and support.

Contents

About the Editors

Vipul Gupta is the director of Neurointerventional Surgery and co-director of Stroke Unit at Artemis Agrim Institute of Neurosciences, Artemis Hospitals, India. He trained in interventional neuroradiology from All India Institute of Medical Sciences, Delhi. He is a pioneer in the field in India, and his main focus has been on designing new techniques to suit individual patient management challenges. Besides, he is a passionate teacher and has taught and trained young neurointerventionalists from across the country through curriculum-based fellowship program, national conferences, and focused workshops. He has published in acclaimed journals and written book chapters. He is the current secretary of the Society of Therapeutic Neurointervention, India.

Rajsrinivas Parthasarathy is one of the few neurologists trained in vascular neurology and neurointerventional surgery. He is a "Royal college of Physicians" of "UK" certified neurologist and has completed his training from prestigious institutes in Yorkshire deanery, UK. His fellowship training included cerebrovascular diseases (1 year) and interventional neuroradiology (2 years). He is an avid researcher who has published "original research" in highly commended journals.

Ajit S. Puri is the director of the Integrated Cerebrovascular Program and Neurointerventional Radiology at the University of Massachusetts Medical School. Dr. Puri received advanced fellowship training in diagnostic neuroradiology and neurointerventional surgery from Harvard Medical School—Brigham and Women's Hospital, Boston Children's Hospital, and Beth Israel Deaconess Medical Center. He is highly published, written numerous articles in prestigious journals, authored several book chapters, and is a frequent speaker at national and international neurointerventional surgery meetings.

Contributors

Mohammed A. Almekhlafi, MSc, FRCPC Department of Neurology, Faculty of Medicine, King Abdulaziz University, Jeddah, Saudi Arabia

Swati D. Chinchure, DMRD, DNB, DAM (Neuroradiology) Medanta Institute of Neurosciences, Medanta Hospital, Vijay Nagar, Indore, India

Helen Cliffe, MA(Cantab) MBBChir FRCR Leeds Teaching Hospitals NHS Trust, Leeds, UK

Aviraj Deshmukh, MD, DM Neurointerventional Surgery, Artemis Agrim Institute of Neuroscience, Gurgaon, India

Mayank Goyal, MD, FRCPC Department of Radiology, Seaman Family MR Research Centre, Foothills Medical Centre, Calgary, AB, Canada

Vipul Gupta, MD Neurointerventional Surgery, Stroke Unit, Artemis Agrim Institute of Neuroscience, Gurgaon, India

Hans Henkes Neuroradiological Clinic, Klinikum Stuttgart, Stuttgart, Germany

Srinivasan Paramasivam, M Ch., MRCS Ed., FINR (USA) Neuro Endovascular Surgery, Apollo Hospitals, T. Nagar, Chennai, India

Rajsrinivas Parthasarathy, CCT(UK) Neuro, Fellow Stroke-INR Vascular Neurology and Neurointerventional Surgery, Artemis Agrim Institute of Neuroscience, Gurgaon, India

Tufail Patankar, PhD, FRCR Leeds Teaching Hospitals NHS Trust, Leeds, UK

Marta Aguilar Pérez Neuroradiological Clinic, Klinikum Stuttgart, Stuttgart, Germany

Ajit S. Puri, MD, DM Radiology, and Neurosurgery, Division of Neurointerventional Surgery, Neurointerventional Fellowship Program, University of Massachusetts Medical Center, Worcester, MA, USA

Abbreviations

2D	Two-dimensional
3D	Three-dimensional
ACA	Anterior cerebral artery
ACOM	Anterior communicating artery
AICA	Anterior inferior cerebellar artery
BA	Basilar artery
CCA	Common carotid artery
ECA	External carotid artery
EVD	External ventricular drain
FD	Flow diverter
ICA	Internal carotid artery
LVA	Left vertebral artery
MCA	Middle cerebral artery
MRI	Magnetic resonance imaging
PCA	Posterior cerebral artery
PCOM	Posterior communicating artery
PICA	Posterior inferior cerebellar artery
RVA	Right vertebral artery

Part I

Aneurysms

Basilar Top Aneurysm with Extreme Tortuosity: Triaxial Technique

1

Vipul Gupta

Case

An Eighty four year old lady presented with subarachnoid haemorrhage (Hunt & Hess Grade II; Fisher Grade 3). Angiogram (Fig. 1.1) revealed a small basilar top aneurysm with a broad neck. The aneurysm was lobulated, and the neck was more towards the origin of left PCA. Both vertebral arteries were extremely tortuous with loops just beyond the origin and at the V2 segments.

Issue

- A stable microcatheter position is desirable to safely coil small ruptured aneurysms. When guiding catheter is too proximal or not stable, microcatheter movements cannot be controlled and can result in rupture during catheterisation or coiling. Therefore, the key challenge is to safely navigate the guiding catheter as distally as possible beyond the loops.

Management

The procedure was performed under general anaesthesia. A bolus of 3000 IU of heparin was given at the start of procedure. A long sheath (6F, raphe) was placed in left subclavian artery to provide support and stability to the guiding catheter. A flexible guiding catheter Neuron (Penumbra, Alameda, California, USA) was then navigated into the left vertebral artery. To take it across the loops, a soft inner catheter (Penumbra 0.041″, Alameda, California, USA) was taken up to the V3 segment over a microcatheter Prowler 21 (Codman & Sheurtleff, Inc. USA) and Traxcess 0.014 (MicroVention, Tustin, California, USA) microwire as shown in Fig. 1.2. The placement of Penumbra catheter provided support for the Neuron guiding catheter to take it across the proximal loops and was placed in desired position of distal segment of the V2 vertebral artery. Thereafter, a balloon catheter (Scepter XC 4 × 11 mm, MicroVention, Tustin, California, USA) was placed in the left PCA following which the sac was catheterised using an Echelon 10 microcatheter (ev3 Inc., Irvine, California, USA). The aneurysm was embolised with multiple soft coils resulting in complete aneurysm occlusion. The final check angiogram revealed complete occlusion with coil loops in all of the lobules of the sac (Fig. 1.2e).

Tips and Tricks

1. It is absolutely critical to obtain a stable and distal guiding catheter location in patients with proximal tortuosity. This is particularly

V. Gupta
Neurointerventional Surgery, Stroke unit, Artemis Agrim Institute of Neuroscience, Gurgaon, India
e-mail: vipul.gupta@artemishospitals.com

V. Gupta et al. (eds.), *100 Interesting Case Studies in Neurointervention: Tips and Tricks*, https://doi.org/10.1007/978-981-13-1346-2_1

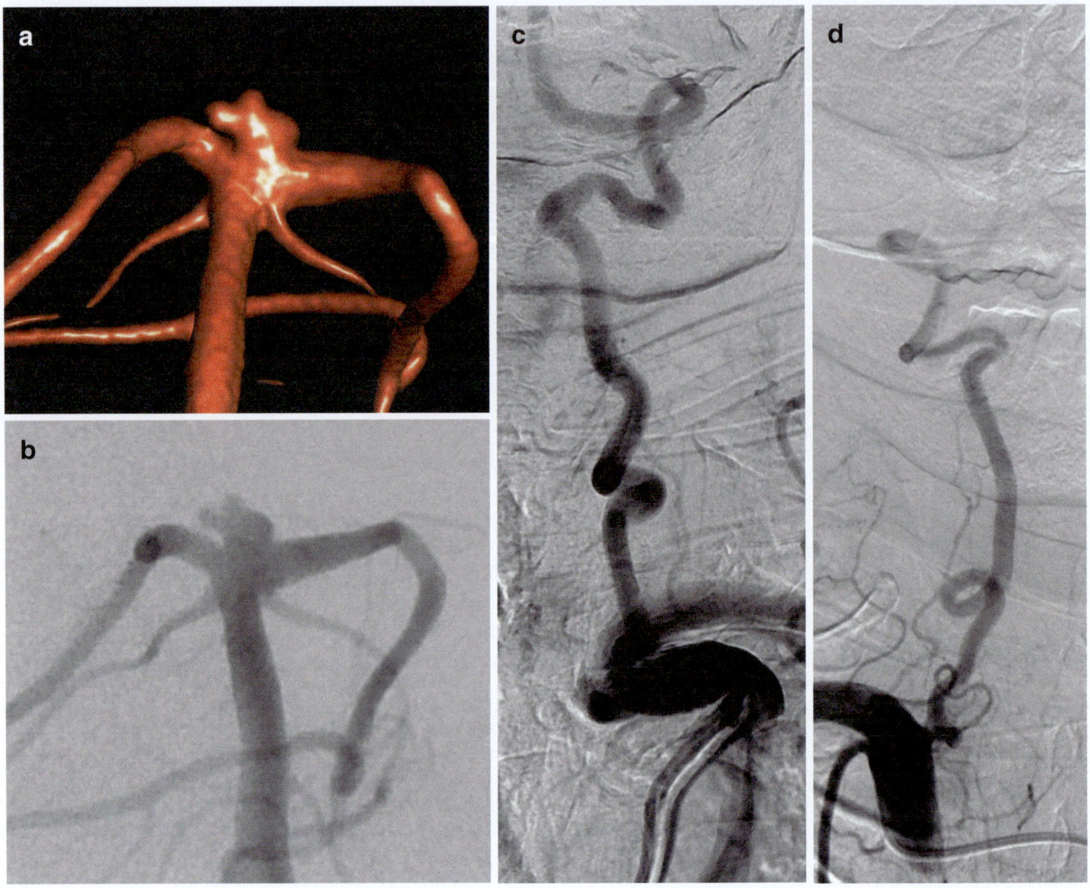

Fig. 1.1 (**a** and **b**) 3D reconstructed and DSA angiogram images showing small, lobulated and broad neck basilar top aneurysm. (**c** and **d**) Subclavian artery injections showing marked tortuosity and loops in both vertebral arteries

important in cases with small and friable aneurysms.

2. The long sheath in our case provided the necessary support to aid distal placement of guiding catheter.
3. A soft-tipped guiding catheter is preferred as it can be taken across the loops without injuring the vessel wall. It usually is navigated over an inner snugly fitting coaxial catheter to both provide the necessary support and eliminate the space between the outer and inner catheter to avoid wall injury particularly at bends. The inner catheter was in turn placed over a microcatheter.
4. In old patients with tortuous anatomy, the difficulty encountered during placing the catheter systems predisposes to thromboembolism, and therefore adequate heparin levels should be maintained during the procedure.

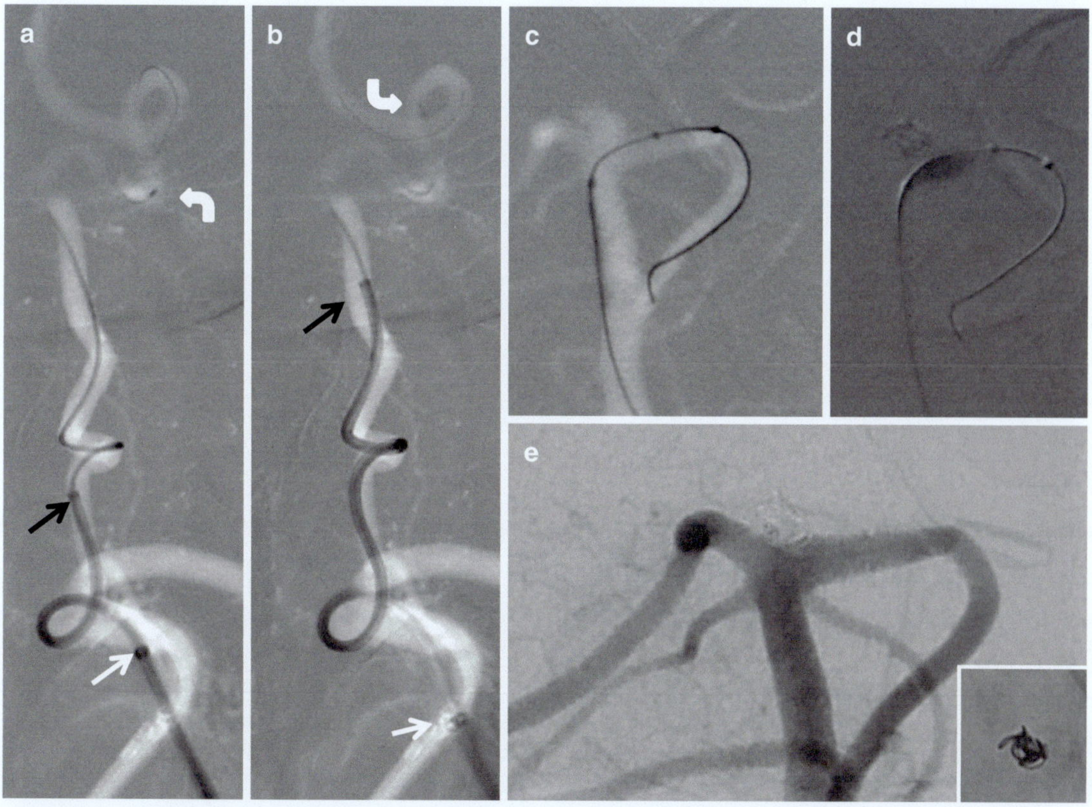

Fig. 1.2 (**a** and **b**) Road map images depicting placement of guiding catheter. A long sheath (white arrows) was placed in the left subclavian artery, and a Neuron 6F guiding catheter (black arrows) was navigated over a Penumbra 0.041 catheter (curved arrows). (**c**) Balloon microcatheter placement in left PCA. (**d**) Showing balloon-assisted coiling. (**e**) Final DSA image showing complete occlusion of aneurysm. Coil mass in in situ showing coil loops in all the lobules of aneurysm

Suggested Reading

Chaudhary N, Pandey AS, Thompson BG, et al. Utilization of the Neuron 6 French 0.053 inch inner luminal diameter guide catheter for treatment of cerebral vascular pathology: continued experience with ultra distal access into the cerebral vasculature. J Neurointerv Surg. 2012;4:301–6.

Park MS, Stiefel MF, Fiorella D, et al. Intracranial placement of a new, compliant guide catheter: technical note. Neurosurgery. 2008;63:E616–7.

Simon SD, Ulm AJ, Russo A, et al. Distal intracranial catheterization of patients with tortuous vascular anatomy using a new hybrid guide catheter. Surg Neurol. 2009;72:737–40.

2 Aneurysm Embolization in Patient with Tortuous Aorta

Vipul Gupta

Case

A 68-year-old female presented with sudden onset right third nerve palsy. MRI revealed a right internal carotid artery (ICA) aneurysm. DSA revealed a lobulated broad-neck ICA aneurysm (Fig. 2.1a). The patient had congenital kyphoscoliosis with excessive tortuosity of the aorta (Fig. 2.1b, c). The management plan was to perform a stent-assisted coil embolization.

Issue

1. Difficulty in placement of guiding catheter due to excessive tortuosity.
2. Guide catheter can become unstable during the procedure.

Management

The patient was loaded with antiplatelet agent (ecosprin 300 mg and clopidogrel 300 mg) the evening before the procedure. An 8F short sheath was placed in the right femoral artery. Following that, a 6F long sheath (arrow) was placed in the right common carotid artery (Fig. 2.2a) using a coaxial catheter (Slipcath 5.5 F, Cook). Once the long sheath was placed, a guiding catheter (Envoy 6F) (Codman & Shurtleff, Inc. USA) was placed in the right ICA (Fig. 2.2b). Thereafter, stent-assisted coil embolization was performed after trapping the microcatheter in the aneurysm (Fig. 2.2c). Almost complete occlusion of the aneurysm was achieved (Fig. 2.2d, e).

Tips and Tricks

1. In patients with excessively tortuous access, it is advisable to place a long sheath so that the guiding catheter is stable.
2. In cases with excessive angulations, a flexible long sheath such as Arrow may be easier to navigate than a stiffer one.
3. Using a coaxial catheter helps in these cases. Once a flexible coaxial catheter is in place, it is easier to navigate the long sheath.

V. Gupta
Neurointerventional Surgery, Stroke unit,
Artemis Agrim Institute of Neuroscience,
Gurgaon, India
e-mail: vipul.gupta@artemishospitals.com

V. Gupta et al. (eds.), *100 Interesting Case Studies in Neurointervention: Tips and Tricks*,
https://doi.org/10.1007/978-981-13-1346-2_2

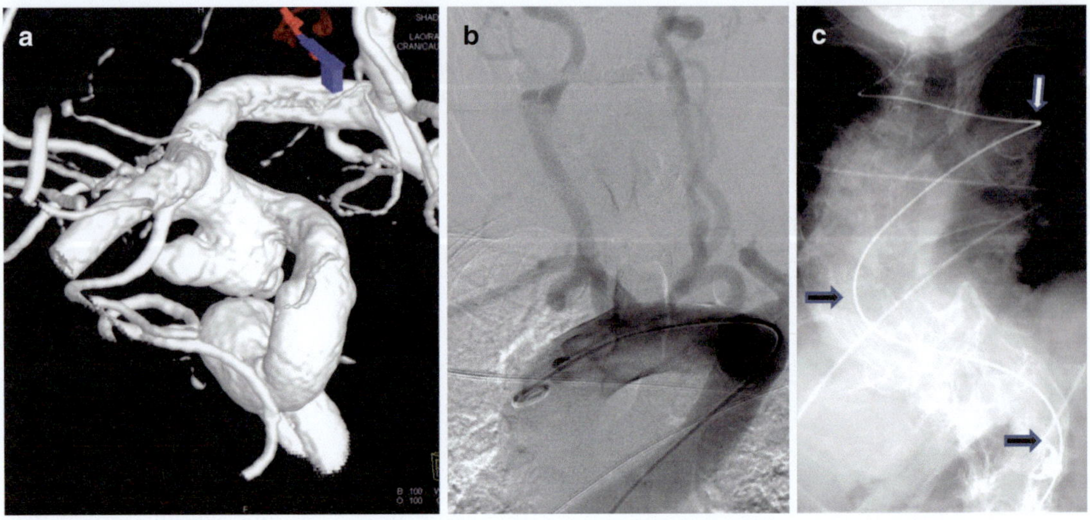

Fig. 2.1 DSA was done along with 3D angiogram. A broad-neck lobulated ICA aneurysm was seen (**a**). Marked tortuosity of the aorta and arch vessels was noticed on pig tail run (**b**). Arrows in (**c**) outline the course of diagnostic catheter

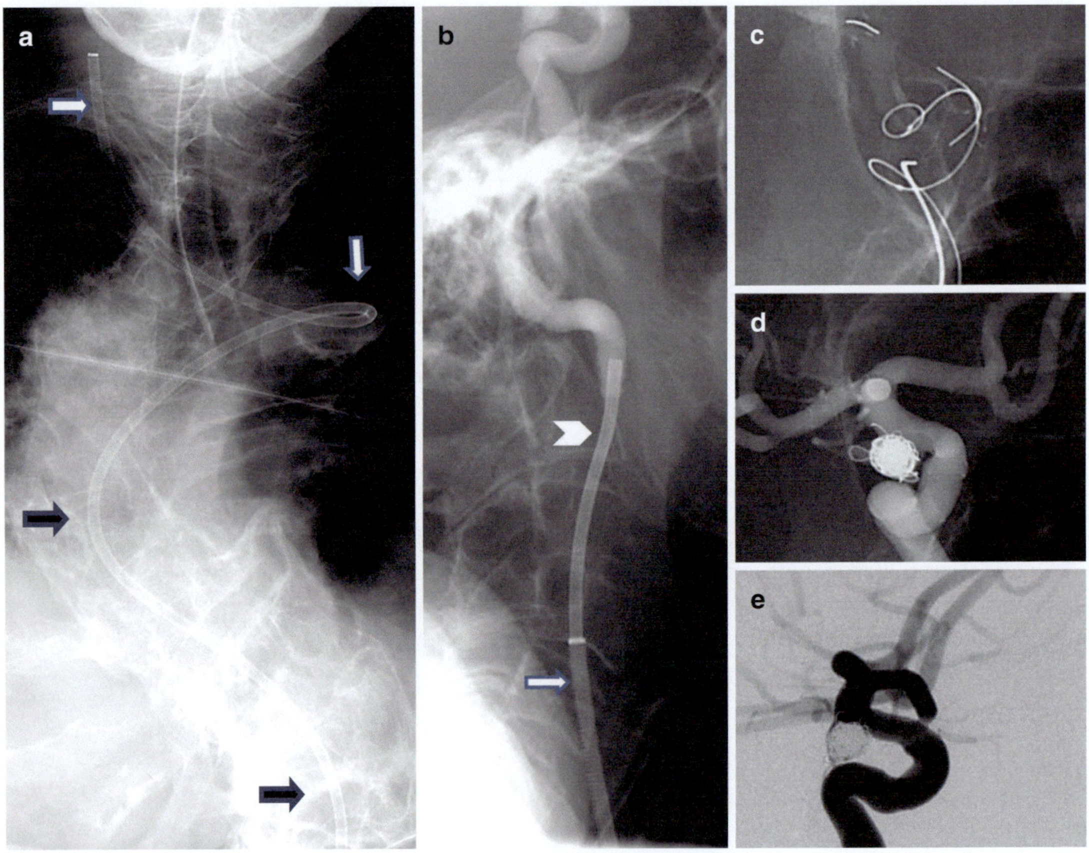

Fig. 2.2 A long sheath (arrows, **a**) was placed in right common carotid artery with coaxial catheter. A guiding catheter (arrowhead, **b**) was placed through the sheath (arrow, **b**). Stent-assisted coiling was performed (**c**) with complete occlusion of aneurysm (**d**, **e**)

Suggested Reading

Chaudhary N, Pandey AS, Thompson BG, et al. Utilization of the Neuron 6 French 0.053 inch inner luminal diameter guide catheter for treatment of cerebral vascular pathology: continued experience with ultra-distal access into the cerebral vasculature. J Neurointerv Surg. 2012;4:301–6.

Park MS, Stiefel MF, Fiorella D, et al. Intracranial placement of a new, compliant guide catheter: technical note. Neurosurgery. 2008;63:E616–7.

Simon SD, Ulm AJ, Russo A, et al. Distal intracranial catheterization of patients with tortuous vascular anatomy using a new hybrid guide catheter. Surg Neurol. 2009;72:737–40.

3 Cerebral Aneurysm with Tortuous Access: Distal Access Catheter Placement Using Coaxial Technique

Rajsrinivas Parthasarathy and Vipul Gupta

Case

A 56-year-old lady presented with a sudden onset of headache and loss of consciousness. Plain CT brain scan on admission revealed diffuse SAH with intraventricular extension. Cerebral angiography revealed a saccular wide-neck paraclinoid aneurysm of left ICA measuring 4.2 × 3.6 mm. Left ICA was tortuous with a loop in the cervical segment. Balloon-assisted coiling was planned.

Issues

1. Tortuous course of access artery posing a challenge for placement of guide catheter in the distal ICA.
2. Small aneurysms are difficult to catheterize with a higher chance of rupture during the procedure particularly in the presence of proximal tortuosity.

R. Parthasarathy (✉)
Vascular Neurology and Neurointerventional Surgery, Artemis Agrim Institute of Neuroscience, Gurgaon, India

V. Gupta
Neurointerventional Surgery, Stroke unit, Artemis Agrim Institute of Neuroscience, Gurgaon, India
e-mail: vipul.gupta@artemishospitals.com

Management

Endovascular embolization of the aneurysm was done via right transfemoral route under general anesthesia. A 6F long sheath (Flexor Check-Flo Introducer, Cook Medical, Bloomington, USA) was introduced into the left CCA. DAC 070/105 cm (Concentric Medical, Inc., Mountain View, CA) was navigated over DAC 044/115 cm (Concentric Medical, Inc., Mountain View, CA) and 0.035″ Terumo guide wire (Terumo Corporation, Tokyo, Japan) across the tortuous ICA. It was done by progressive advancement of DAC 044 over Terumo wire for a distance followed by navigation of DAC 070 over DAC 044. The snugly fitting smaller profile inner catheter provided the necessary support and eliminated the dead space between the inner and outer thereby allowing for smooth advancement across bends without injuring the arterial wall (Fig. 3.1).

With distal tip of DAC 070 in the proximal cavernous ICA, DAC 044 and Terumo guide wire were removed. A 4 × 11 mm Scepter XC balloon (Microvention, Inc., Tustin, CA) was placed across the neck of aneurysm, and aneurysm was embolized with detachable coils using Echelon-10 microcatheter (Micro therapeutics, Inc., ev3 Neurovascular, Irvine, California). Post-procedure angiogram shows complete obliteration of the aneurysm (Fig. 3.2).

V. Gupta et al. (eds.), *100 Interesting Case Studies in Neurointervention: Tips and Tricks*,
https://doi.org/10.1007/978-981-13-1346-2_3

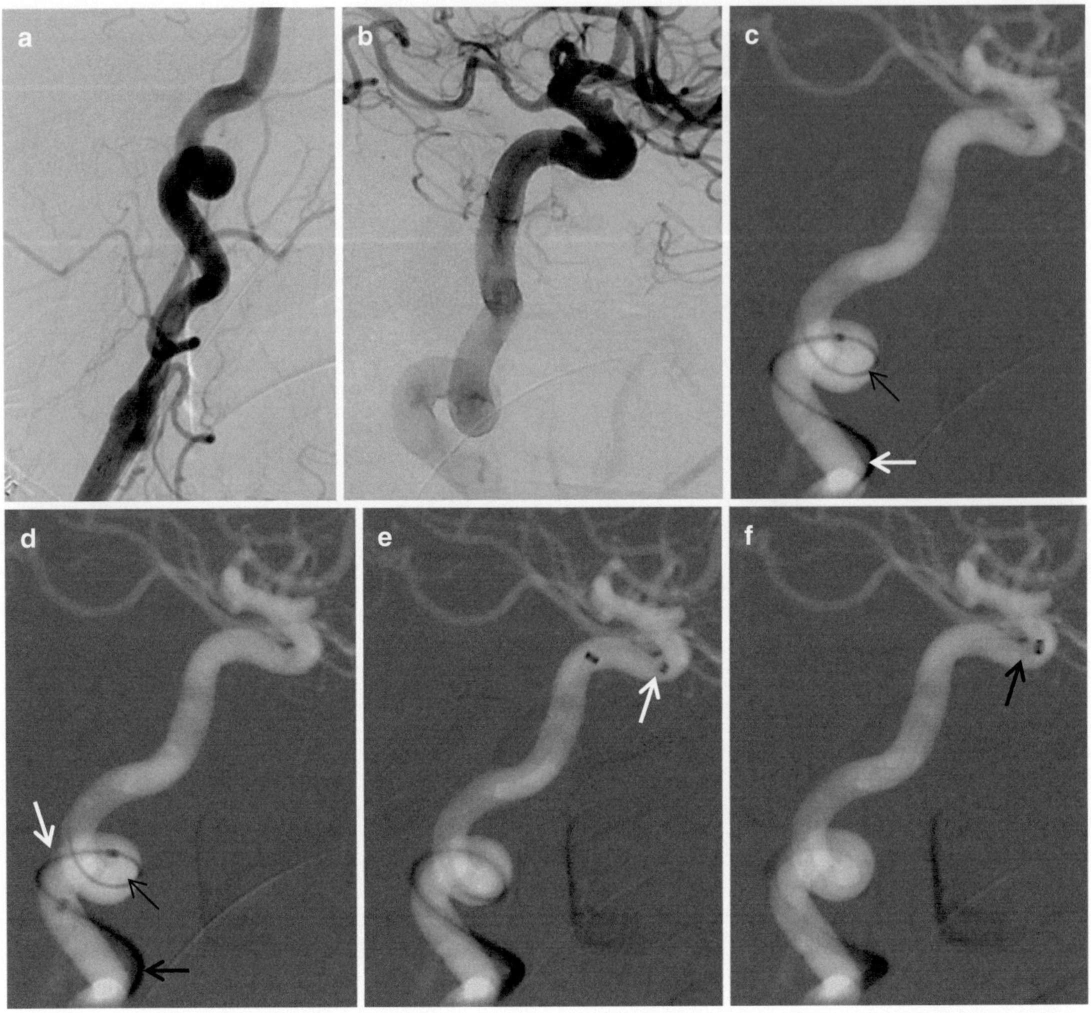

Fig. 3.1 Left CCA angiogram (**a**) reveals extreme tortuous course of left ICA, and left ICA angiogram (**b**) reveals small wide-neck paraclinoid aneurysm. With road map (**c**–**e**), DAC 044 (white bold arrow) was advanced into ICA over Terumo wire (black arrow) followed by advancement of DAC 070 (black bold arrow) over DAC 044 in a stepwise manner. On reaching cavernous ICA (**f**), DAC 044 and Terumo wire were removed. Coaxial system of distal access catheters helped to navigate tortuous loop in the cervical ICA

Tips and Tricks

1. Placement of guide catheter in the distal ICA helps to provide stability which is particularly important in the coiling of small aneurysms.
2. Triaxial system of navigation across tortuous artery helps to minimize the trauma to the vessel.
3. Using DAC 070/105 cm with inner longer DAC 044/115 cm coaxially helps in the navigation through tortuous arteries.
4. Because of braided wall design, these distal access catheters offer flexibility to navigate difficult access arteries and provide enough stability to support microcatheters.

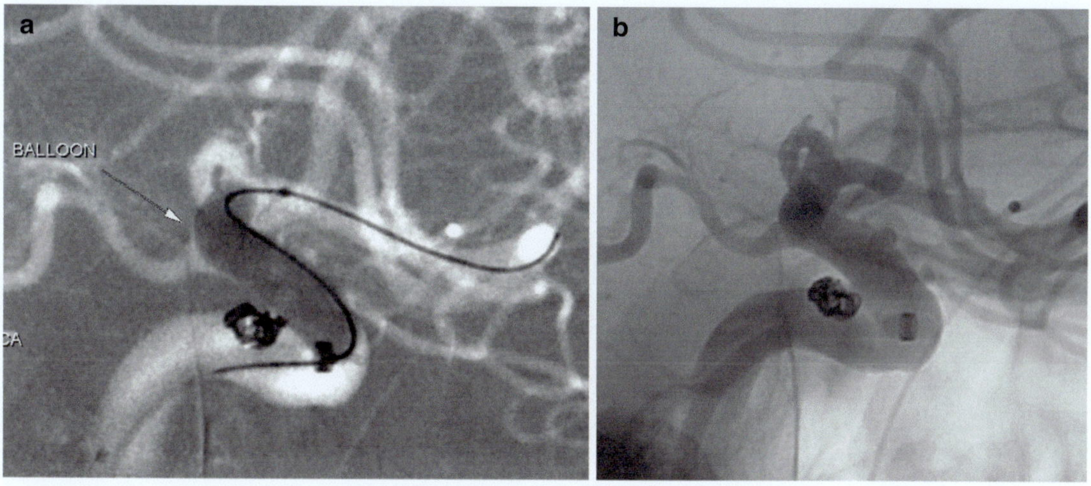

Fig. 3.2 Road map image (**a**) shows balloon inflated across the neck of aneurysm and coils within the aneurysm. Subtracted image (**b**) shows complete obliteration of the aneurysm. Distal position of the DAC 070 helped to provide stable support for microcatheter during aneurysm coiling

Suggested Reading

Hauck EF, et al. Use of the outreach distal access catheter as an intracranial platform facilitates coil embolization of select intracranial aneurysms: technical note. J Neurointerv Surg. 2011;3(2):172–6.

Lin L-M, et al. Pentaxial access platform for ultra-distal intracranial delivery of a large-bore hyperflexible DIC (distal intracranial catheter): a technical note. Neurosurgery. 2016;6:29–34.

Interrupted Aortic Arch: Access—Direct Carotid Puncture

4

Rajsrinivas Parthasarathy and Vipul Gupta

Case

A 40-year-old male presented with subarachnoid haemorrhage from a ruptured ACOM aneurysm. He was diagnosed with an interrupted aortic arch while being investigated for refractory hypertension.

Issue

- Access to the right ICA in a patient with interrupted arch
- Blood pressure management

Management

Balloon-assisted coiling was planned to treat this large broad-based ACOM aneurysm (Fig. 4.1). Both brachial approaches were deemed not suitable due to the acute angle origin of the right CCA from the right approach and reverse origin from the left approach. Therefore, for access, a direct carotid puncture was undertaken.

Steps for Carotid Puncture

- 21 G Venflon was used to puncture the right common carotid artery under ultrasound guidance.
- Following that, the inner stylet was removed and an injection taken to define the anatomy of the bifurcation (Fig. 4.2a).
- Then a guidewire from a 5F micropuncture (Cook Medical, Bloomington, USA) set was introduced through the Venflon into the ECA.
- The Venflon was exchanged with a 4F dilator into the ECA.
- A 0.035 Terumo wire was then introduced through the dilator, and the dilator was exchanged with a 5F dilator followed by a 6F 11 cm short sheath (Fig. 4.2b, c).
- Following that, Envoy 6F guiding catheter was taken through the carotid sheath and parked in the petrous right ICA (Fig. 4.2d).

A Scepter XC 4 × 11 balloon was parked across the neck of the aneurysm, and the sac was catheterized using Echelon-10 microcatheter. The sac was embolized with multiple detachable coils. Post-procedure Xper CT revealed no haemorrhage.

R. Parthasarathy (✉)
Vascular Neurology and Neurointerventional Surgery, Artemis Agrim Institute of Neuroscience, Gurgaon, India

V. Gupta
Neurointerventional Surgery, Stroke unit, Artemis Agrim Institute of Neuroscience, Gurgaon, India
e-mail: vipul.gupta@artemishospitals.com

V. Gupta et al. (eds.), *100 Interesting Case Studies in Neurointervention: Tips and Tricks*,
https://doi.org/10.1007/978-981-13-1346-2_4

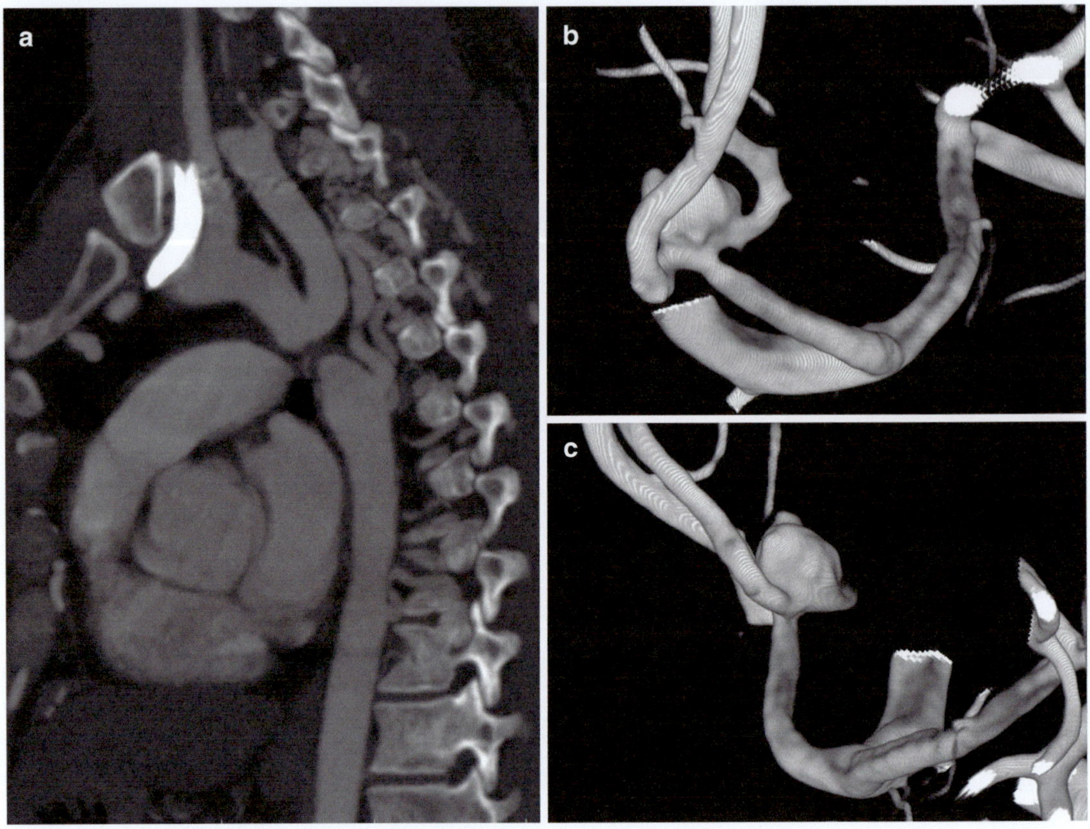

Fig. 4.1 (**a**) Interrupted aortic arch; (**b**, **c**) ACOM aneurysm neck view and end on view

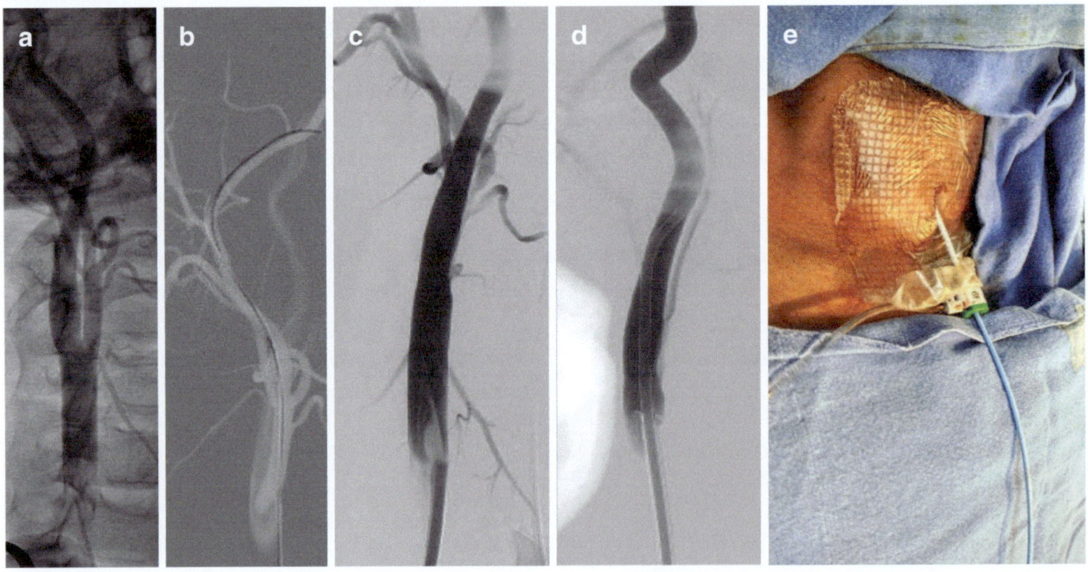

Fig. 4.2 (**a**) Injection through 21 G venflon; (**b**) 0.035′ Terumo wire in the ECA; (**c**) Injection through the 6F sheath; (**d**) 6F envoy guiding catheter in the Internal Carotid artery. (**e**) The set up on the surface showing a 6F sheath and the Envoy guiding catheter

Tips and Tricks

1. Use a 0.018′ atraumatic wire through the Venflon to avoid intimal damage.
2. Ensure that the dilator (4F/5F/6F) does not enter the internal carotid artery to avoid intimal damage.
3. Avoidance of haematoma during sheath removal can be crucial task for the success of the procedure.
4. Manual compression in most cases is a simple and effective means to achieve haemostasis.
5. In patients with interrupted arch, achieving haemostasis can be a challenging task due to the high blood pressures. One can lower the blood pressure pharmacologically for brief period during the carotid compression to achieve haemostasis.
6. These patients have a higher blood pressure to maintain renal and cord perfusion below the level of the interrupted arch. Care should be taken to avoid prolonged periods of lower BP to prevent renal/spinal cord hypoperfusion that can result in acute renal failure or cord ischaemia.
7. Closure devices including Angio-Seal and StarClose have been used; however, no specific recommendations can be given as very few patients have had a closure device used to achieve haemostasis.

Suggested Reading

Mokin M, et al. Direct carotid artery puncture access for endovascular treatment of acute ischemic stroke: technical aspects, advantages, and limitations. J Neurointerv Surg. https://doi.org/10.1136/neurintsurg-2013-011007.

Giant Cavernous Aneurysm: Parent Vessel Occlusion After Balloon Occlusion Test

5

Vipul Gupta

Case

A 28-year-old female presented with headaches and diplopia. Examination revealed right third and sixth cranial nerve palsy. MRI revealed a giant aneurysm in right cavernous sinus. DSA showed giant broad-neck aneurysm involving cavernous segment of right ICA (Fig. 5.1a, b). Good-sized ACOM and PCOM arteries were seen (Fig. 5.1c, d). Parent vessel occlusion after balloon test occlusion was planned.

Issues

- Giant cavernous ICA aneurysm—assessing suitability for parent artery occlusion.

Management

Patient was given tab. Ecosprin 150 mg a day before the procedure. The balloon occlusion test was performed under local anaesthesia. Loading dose of heparin (5000 IU) was given. A guiding catheter (Envoy, Codman & Shurtleff, Inc., USA) was placed in right ICA. Another diagnostic catheter (Picard, Cook Medical, Bloomington, USA) was placed in left ICA. A compliant balloon (Hyperglide, ev3 Inc., Irvine, California, USA) was placed in petrous segment and inflated to achieve complete occlusion of the right ICA and was documented by guiding catheter injection. With balloon being inflated, injection of left ICA (Fig. 5.2a–c) was performed which revealed good collateral flow with synchronous filling of both hemispheres. Venous phase timing was performed where one looks for any delay in contrast enhancement of veins on the side of temporary ICA occlusion (Fig. 5.2b). As there was no delay, complete occlusion of right ICA was performed using pushable coils (Nester, Cook Medical, Bloomington, USA) as shown in Fig. 5.2d. Repeat angiograms of left VA (Fig. 5.2e) and left ICA (Fig. 5.2f) revealed complete filling of right ICA territory. Patient remained neurologically intact during and after the procedure. She was given LMWH (Inj. Clexane 0.4 ml twice a day) for 2 days. She was on bed rest for 2 days and then slowly mobilized. Care was taken to maintain good hydration. Tab ecosprin was continued for 3 months. Her symptoms resolved over the next 3-month and 6-month follow-up, and MRI revealed complete regression of the aneurysm with no signs of ischaemia in right hemisphere.

V. Gupta
Neurointerventional Surgery, Stroke unit, Artemis Agrim Institute of Neuroscience, Gurgaon, India
e-mail: vipul.gupta@artemishospitals.com

V. Gupta et al. (eds.), *100 Interesting Case Studies in Neurointervention: Tips and Tricks*,
https://doi.org/10.1007/978-981-13-1346-2_5

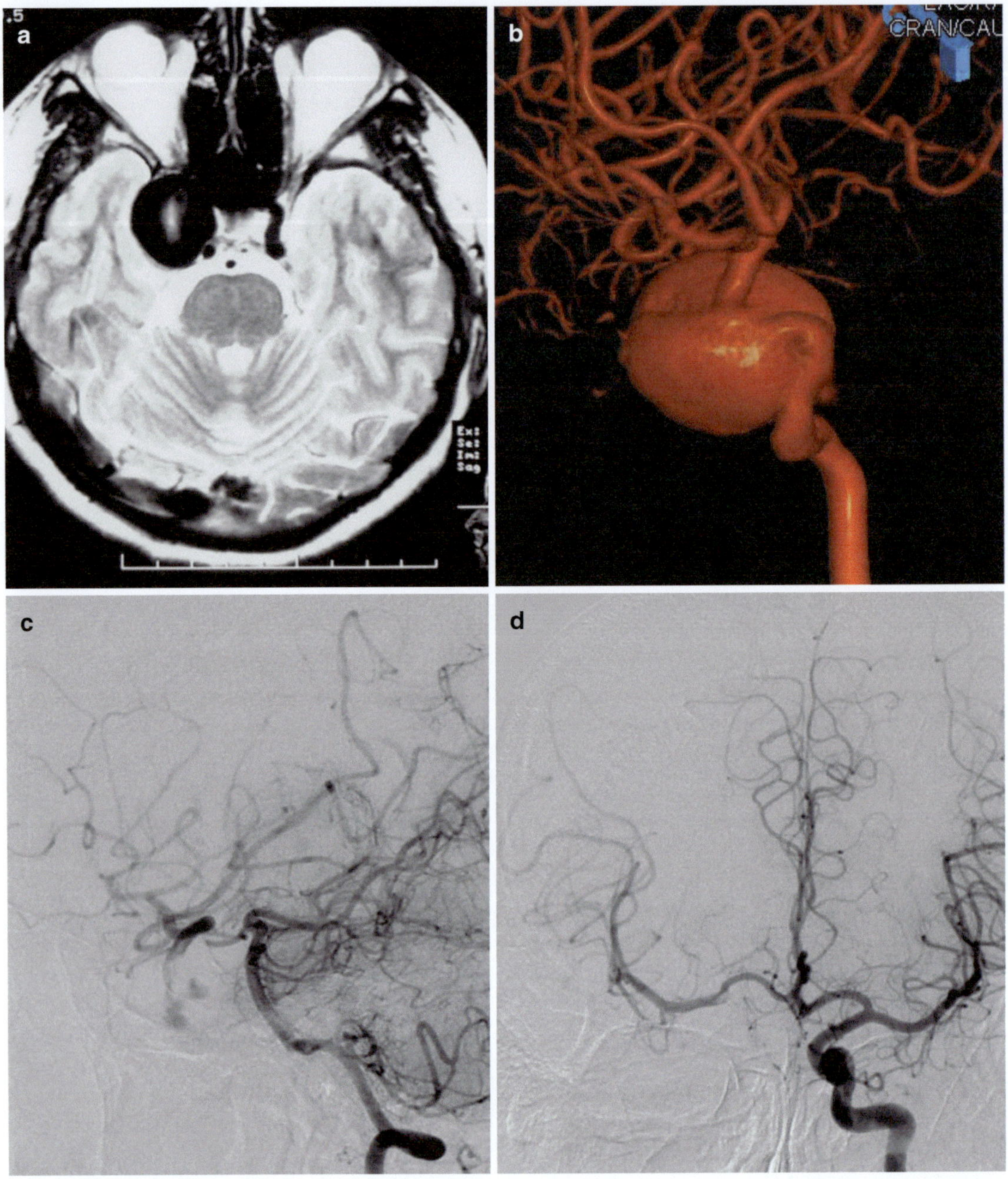

Fig. 5.1 (**a**) MR image showing giant aneurysm in cavernous sinus; (**b**) 3D reconstructed image showing giant broad neck aneurysm in cavernous segment of right ICA; (**c** and **d**) Left vertebral (**c**) and left ICA (**d**) injections with manual compression of right CCA reveal good sized PCOM and ACOM arteries

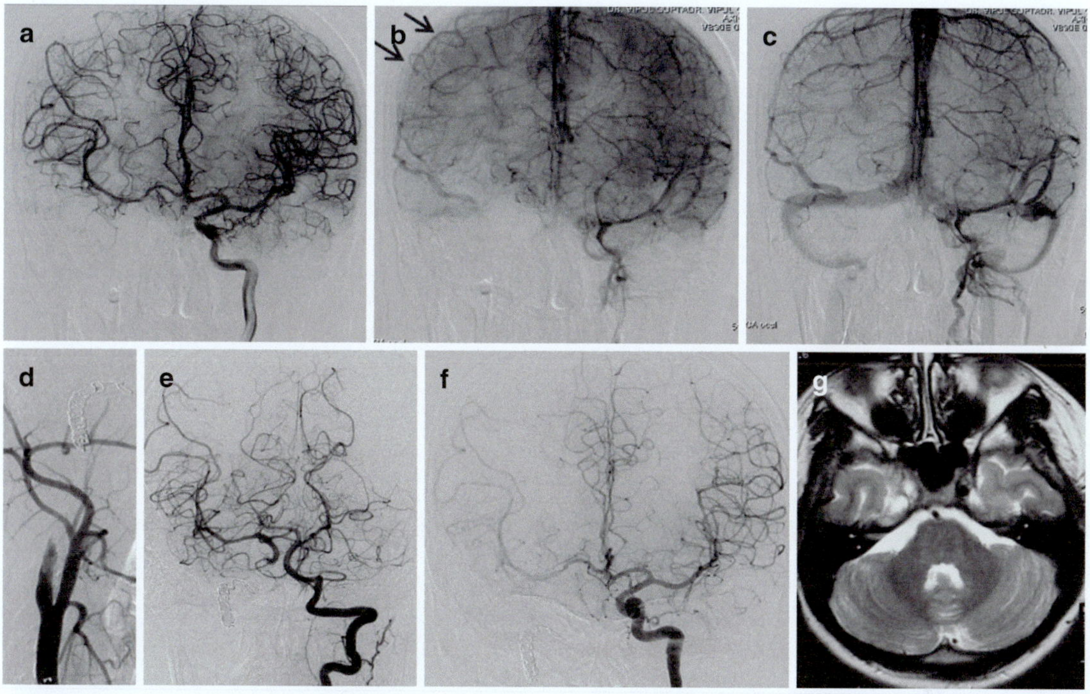

Fig. 5.2 (**a**–**c**) Left ICA injection with balloon occlusion of right ICA reveal symmetrical arterial filling (**a**) venous opacification (**b** and **c**); (**d**) DSA after complete occlusion of right ICA; (**e** and **f**) Post-embolization angiograms of left VA (**e**) and left ICA (**f**) revealing good flow through the ACOM and PCOM arteries; (**g**) Follow-up MRA with complete regression of the aneurysm

Tips and Tricks

1. Parent vessel occlusion remains an acceptable safe technique in cases of giant aneurysms of cavernous ICA with adequate collateral flow.
2. Various techniques and criteria have been described in literature for balloon test occlusion such as prolonged occlusion, hypotensive challenge, and perfusion imaging. There are studies showing "venous phase timing" as a very reliable method to assess the adequacy of collateral flow.
3. In the study by Moret J et al., occlusion was considered to be feasible when the delay between the venous drainage of the injected and the occluded hemisphere was not >2 s. Venous drainage delay >4 s was considered as contraindication to ICA permanent occlusion. In patients with venous drainage delay of 2–4 s, the occlusion was performed only in selected cases.
4. In the study by van Rooij WJ et al., synchronous filling (a <0.5-s delay of opacification between the cortical veins of the occluded and collateral vascular territories) was considered a predictor for tolerance to permanent occlusion.
5. We prefer to give antiplatelet agents for a few months to prevent thromboembolism in such cases. LMWH may be useful to prevent excessive clot formation.

Suggested Reading

Abud DG, Spelle L, Piotin M, Mounayer C, Vanzin JR, Moret J. Venous phase timing during balloon test occlusion as a criterion for permanent internal carotid artery sacrifice. AJNR Am J Neuroradiol. 2005;26(10):2602–9.

Lesley WS, Rangaswamy R. Balloon test occlusion and endosurgical parent artery sacrifice for the evaluation and management of complex intracranial aneurysmal disease. J Neurointerv Surg. 2009;1(2):112–20.

van Rooij WJ, Sluzewski M, Slob MJ, Rinkel GJ. Predictive value of angiographic testing for tolerance to therapeutic occlusion of the carotid artery. AJNR Am J Neuroradiol. 2005;26(1):175–8.

6 Dual Microcatheter Technique

Ajit S. Puri and Rajsrinivas Parthasarathy

Case

A 48-year-old female had undergone endovascular coiling for a ruptured PCOM aneurysm (SAH Hunt & Hess 1 & Fisher grade 2). She was admitted at an interval for treatment of the broad-neck right MCA bifurcation aneurysm (Fig. 6.1).

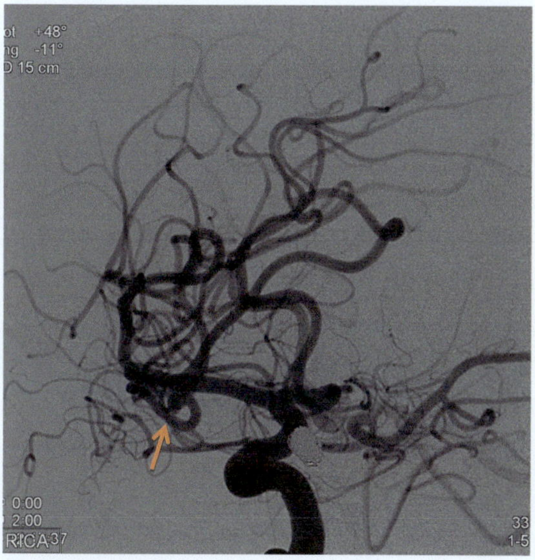

Fig. 6.1 Small wide necked right MCA bifurcation aneurysm (orange arrow)

Issue

A broad-neck MCA bifurcation aneurysm; therefore, the risk for coil prolapse into the parent artery and distal migration

Management

A dual microcatheter technique was undertaken under general anaesthesia. After placing the guiding catheter in the ICA, the first microcatheter (SL 10, Stryker Neurovascular, CA, USA) was placed within the aneurysm pouch (Fig. 6.2a). A framing coil was then partly/completely deployed inside the aneurysm sac until it formed a suitable cage; however, the coil was not detached. The second microcatheter (SL 10, Stryker Neurovascular, CA, USA) was then placed with the aneurysm sac near the neck, and another coil was deployed within the prior coil frame (Fig. 6.2b, orange arrow). This coil was detached, and sequential coiling was continued from the second microcatheter. Once the coil frame was

A. S. Puri (✉)
Radiology, and Neurosurgery,
Division of Neurointerventional Surgery,
Neurointerventional Fellowship Program,
University of Massachusetts Medical Center,
Worcester, MA, USA
e-mail: ajit.puri@umassmemorial.org

R. Parthasarathy
Vascular Neurology and Neurointerventional Surgery,
Artemis Agrim Institute of Neuroscience,
Gurgaon, India

V. Gupta et al. (eds.), *100 Interesting Case Studies in Neurointervention: Tips and Tricks*,
https://doi.org/10.1007/978-981-13-1346-2_6

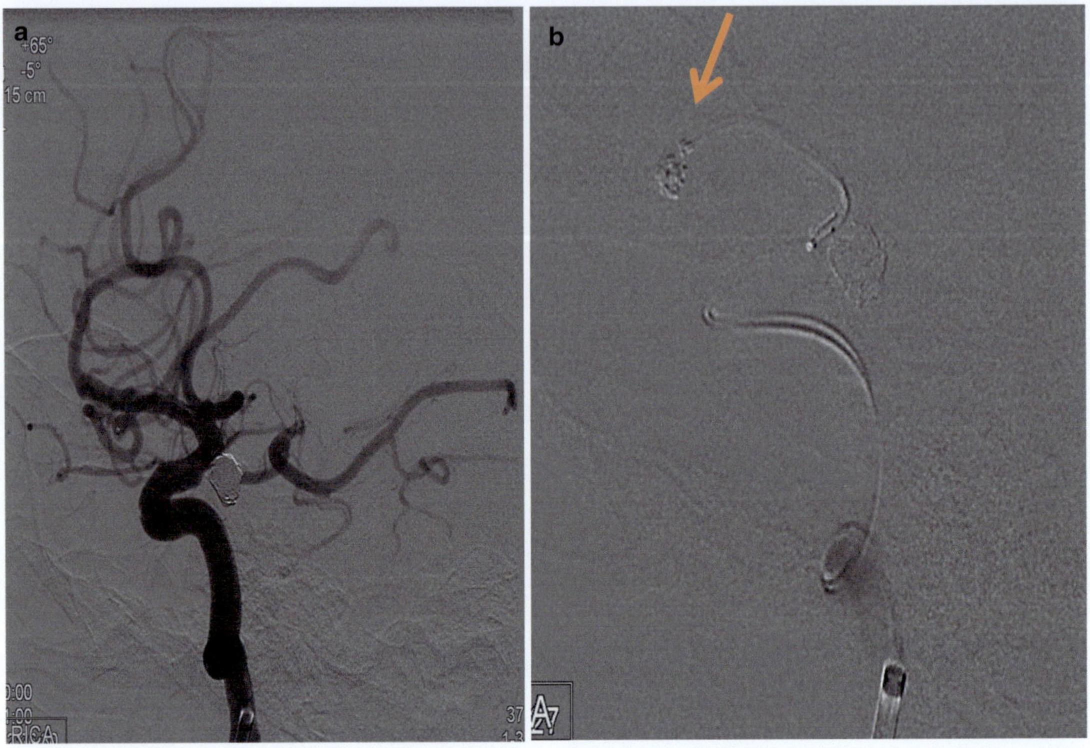

Fig. 6.2 (**a**) The first microcatheter is placed within the aneurysm pouch. Framing coil is then partly or completely placed inside the aneurysm pouch WITHOUT DETACHING THE COIL. (**b**) The second microcatheter is then placed with the aneurysm and another coil is now placed and deployed within the prior coil frame (orange arrow). This coil is usually detached and sequential coiling can be continued from the second microcatheter. Once the coil frame is stable the "first" coil with the "first" microcatheter can be detached

stable, the "first" coil within the "first" microcatheter was detached. Final angiogram showed complete occlusion of the aneurysm (Fig. 6.3) with adequate packing density and patent inferior division. Patient recovered, and follow-up angiogram showed complete occlusion.

Tips and Tricks

1. Coil prolapse and distal migration are not uncommon if a temporary scaffold at the neck is not available in broad-necked aneurysms.
2. A dual microcatheter technique is particularly helpful when the risk of prolapse and migration exists after detachment of the first coil as in the case of a small broad-necked aneurysm based on a high-flow artery.
3. The fist coil is deployed either partly or completely to form a good cage. This is crucial to avoid coil bulge into the parent artery during deployment of subsequent coils. Do not detach this coil.
4. Initial coil size selection is the key to achieving complete occlusion. The coil should be sized such that the cage should oppose all the walls of the sac to avoid eccentric filling that can result in instability of the coil mass.
5. Multiple coils are then deployed through a second microcatheter to form a stable coil mass. Once complete occlusion is achieved, the coil in the first microcatheter that was used to form the initial frame is detached.
6. In small aneurysms, one may have to place the tip of the second microcatheter at the neck to avoid displacement of the previously deployed loops.

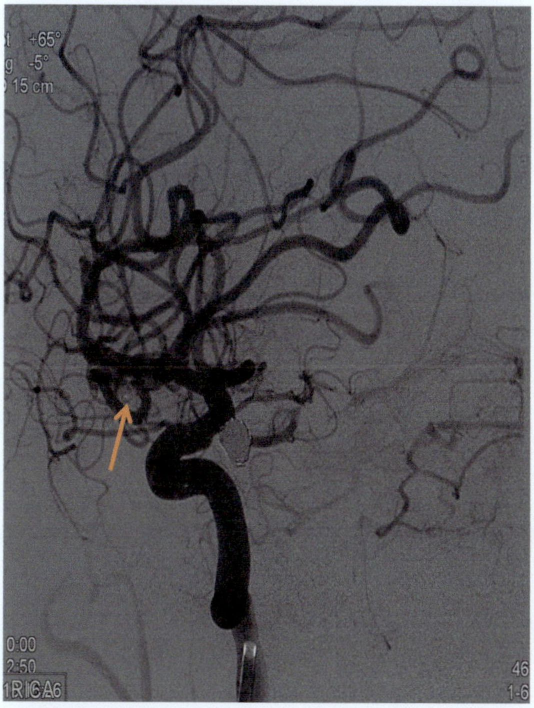

Fig. 6.3 Post-coiling no residual aneurysm and patent inferior division of the right MCA

Suggested Reading

Griessenauer CJ, et al. Dual diagnostic catheter technique in the endovascular management of anterior communicating artery complex aneurysms. Surg Neurol Int. 2016;7:87.

Horowitz M, et al. The dual catheter technique for coiling of wide-necked cerebral aneurysms. Interv Neuroradiol. 2005 Jun;11(2):155–60.

Balloon-Assisted and Dual Microcatheter Technique (Geometry Assessment and Catheter Shaping)

7

Ajit S. Puri and Rajsrinivas Parthasarathy

Case

A 67-year-old lady presented with subarachnoid haemorrhage (Hunt and Hess Grade 2; Fisher Grade 3). Frontal and lateral angiograms from the left vertebral artery demonstrate a wide-necked bilobed basilar tip aneurysm with a pseudo-lobule on the superior aspect (orange arrow) (Fig. 7.1).

Issues

1. Both lobules should be adequately packed; in particular, the pseudo-lobule arising from the anterior sac is likely to represent the ruptured site (Fig. 7.2).
2. Assessment of the neck of the aneurysm. Careful study of the 3d rotational angiography and lateral projections reveal circumferential involvement of the top of the basilar artery suggestive of a wide neck; therefore, the need for adjunctive coiling should be considered (Fig. 7.2).
3. Determining microcatheter shapes to adequately access both the lobules.

Management

The procedure was performed under general anaesthesia. To adequately pack both the lobules, a dual microcatheter technique along with balloon assistance was considered the most appropriate strategy. Access was obtained in both vertebral arteries; a 6F guide catheter through the larger VA and a 5F guide catheter through the smaller VA. A compliant HyperGlide balloon (ev3, Irvine, USA) was placed into the distal basilar artery (Fig. 7.3, bold arrow). SL-10 microcatheters (Stryker Neurovascular, CA, USA) were used to access separate lobes of the aneurysm, and coiling was done with intermittent balloon inflation (Fig. 7.3, double black arrows). Note position of inflated balloon in the distal basilar covering the neck of the aneurysm and partially the right PCA (Fig. 7.3, single black arrow). On the frontal view, there appears to be coil loops bulging into the parent artery; however, a lateral end-hole view clearly demonstrates that the loops are within the aneurysm sac and, therefore, was not repositioned. Complete

A. S. Puri (✉)
Radiology, and Neurosurgery,
Division of Neurointerventional Surgery,
Neurointerventional Fellowship Program,
University of Massachusetts Medical Center,
Worcester, MA, USA
e-mail: ajit.puri@umassmemorial.org

R. Parthasarathy
Vascular Neurology and Neurointerventional Surgery,
Artemis Agrim Institute of Neuroscience,
Gurgaon, India

V. Gupta et al. (eds.), *100 Interesting Case Studies in Neurointervention: Tips and Tricks*,
https://doi.org/10.1007/978-981-13-1346-2_7

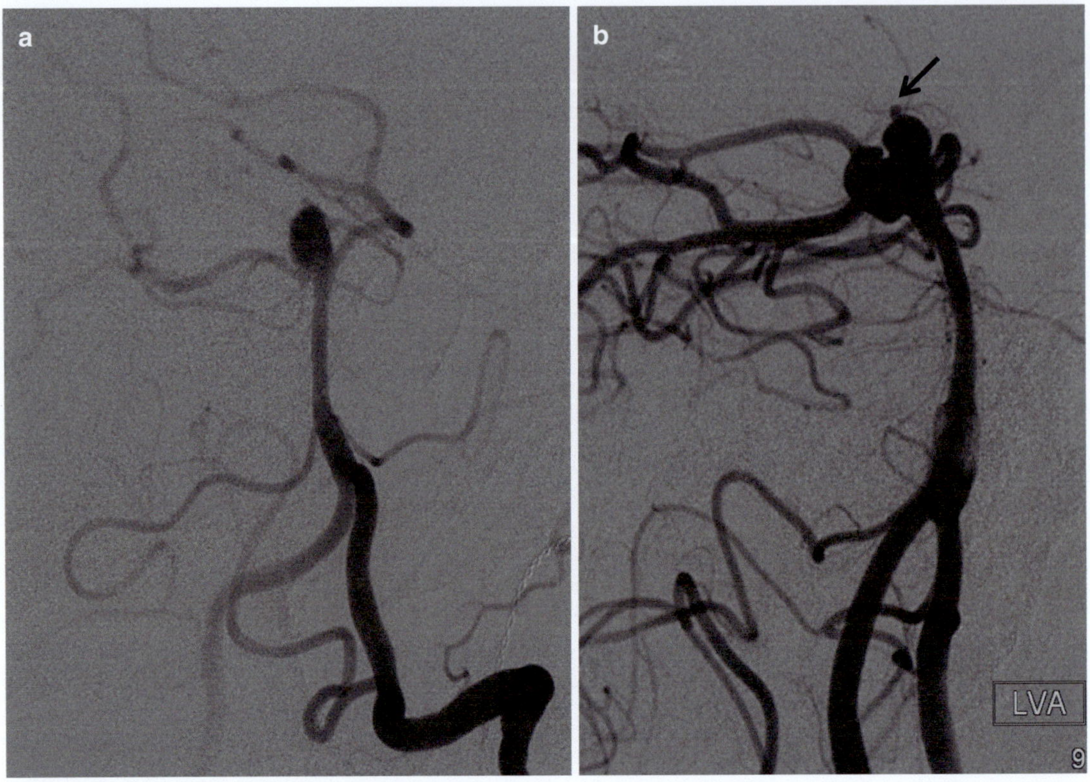

Fig. 7.1 Frontal (**a**) and Lateral (**b**) from the left vertebral demonstrate wide necked bi-lobed basilar tip aneurysm with a pseudo lobule on the superior aspect (black arrow)

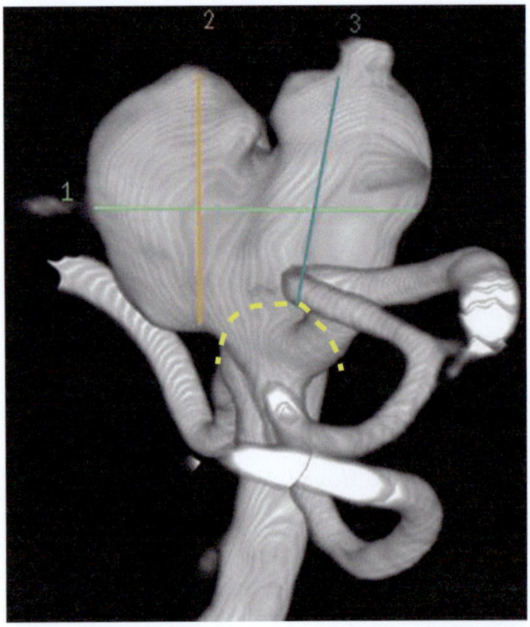

Fig. 7.2 Bilobed aneurysm with Circumferential involvement of the basilar top (dotted yellow line)

occlusion of both the lobes of the aneurysm sac was achieved. Post-procedure, lateral angiogram reveals circumferential reconstruction of the basilar top (Fig. 7.4). Patient made full recovery on follow-up. Interval cerebral angiography showed stable result with no recanalization.

Tips and Tricks

1. Adequate packing of bilobed/partitioned aneurysms may not be possible with a single microcatheter. More often than not, one may have to reshape the catheter to access the other lobule. A difficult geometry, as in a reverse origin of one of the lobules, may be difficult to access after partial coiling has been undertaken. Therefore, one may decide to use two microcatheters and catheterize both the lobules from the start.
2. The curvature of the basilar trunk in relation to the long axis of the lobules is the key to

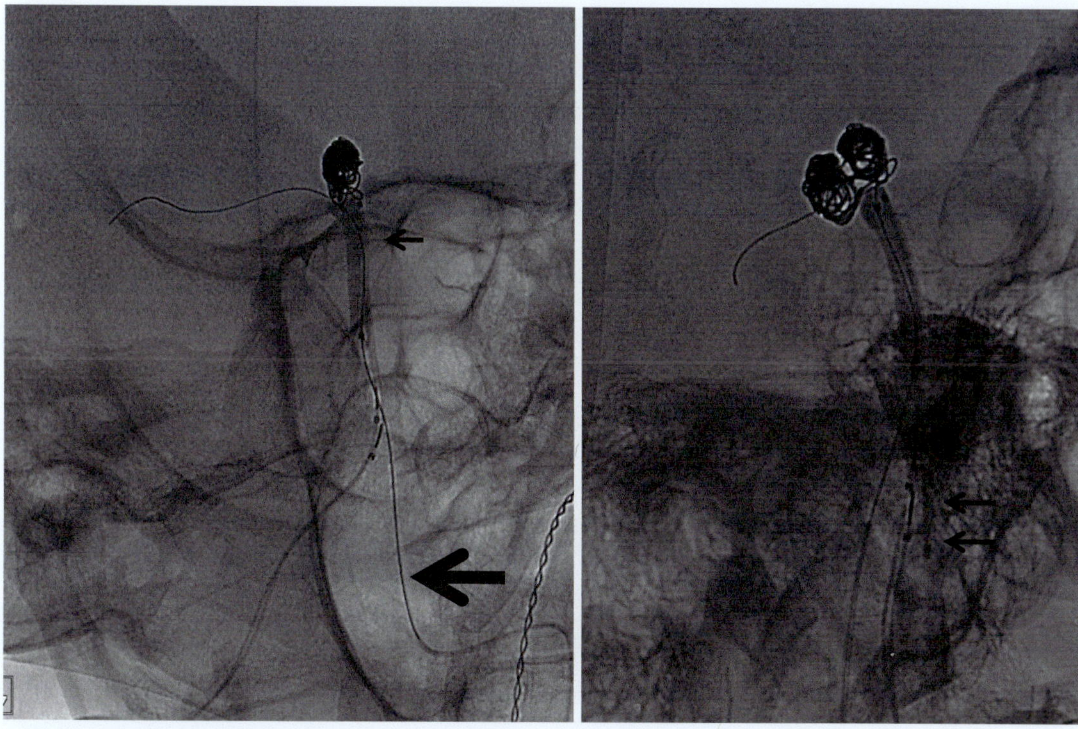

Fig. 7.3 A Hyperglide balloon was placed into the distal basilar artery. SL-10 microcatheters were used to assess separate lobes of the aneurysm (double black arrows) and coiling was done with intermittent balloon inflation (bold arrow). Note position of inflated balloon in the distal basilar covering the neck of the aneurysm and partially the right PCA (single arrow)

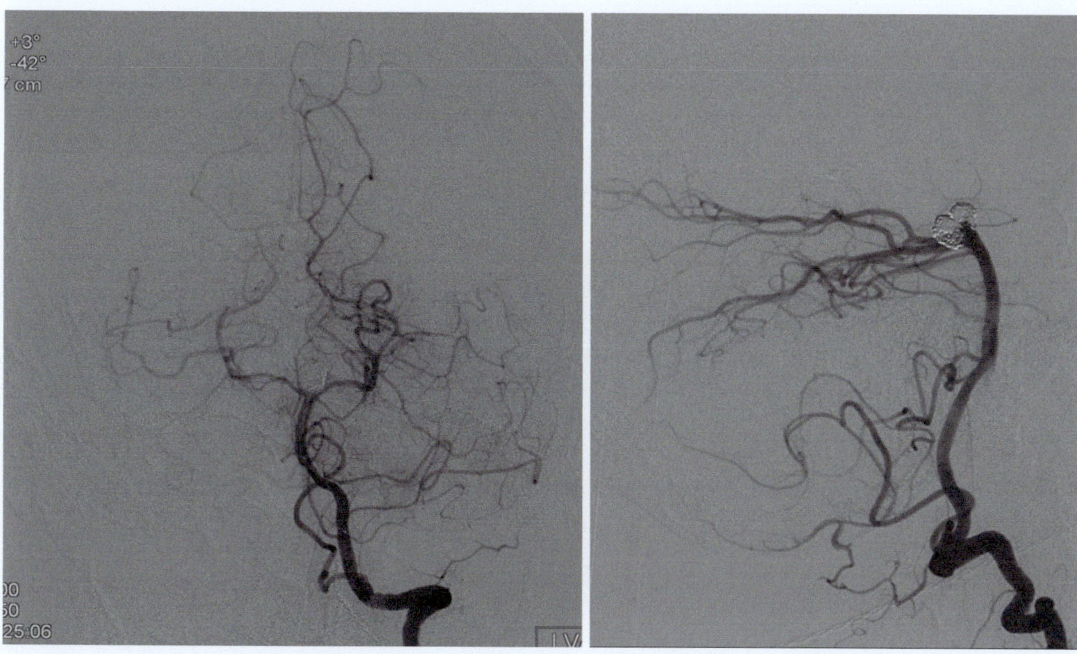

Fig. 7.4 Post intervention angiograms show complete aneurysm occlusion

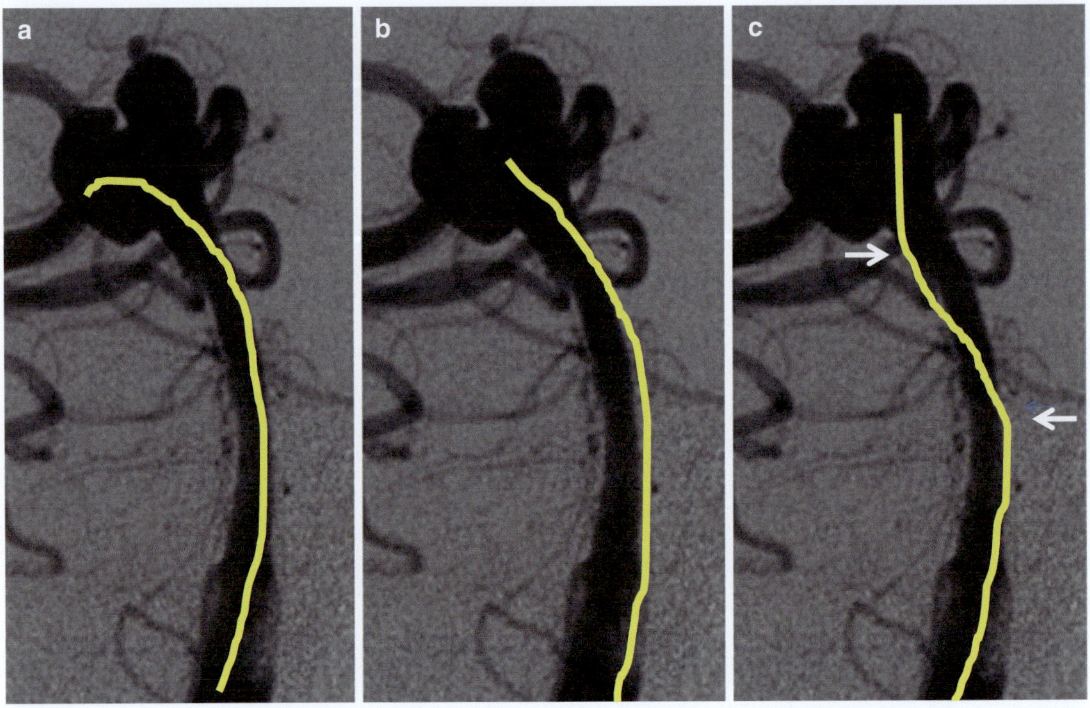

Fig. 7.5 (**a**) A gentle curve at the tip pointing at the posterior sac; (**b**) a straight tip catheter pointing midway; (**c**) a reverse curve catheter pointing well into the anterior sac

determining the shape of the distal tip of the microcatheter. A gentle curve at the tip is likely to point at the posterior sac as the curvature of the basilar trunk is convex anterior (Fig. 7.5a). A straight tip catheter is likely to point at the mid part (Fig. 7.5b), and a reverse curve at the tip is likely to point well into the anterior sac (Fig. 7.5c). Packing the anterior sac adequately was considered crucial as a pseudo-lobule was noted arising from this sac.

3. Balloon was considered essential as the neck assessment revealed a wide-neck aneurysm as there was circumferential involvement of the basilar top. This was evident on geometry assessment on 3d rotational angiography. See illustrative diagram (Fig. 7.2).
4. A hyper-compliant balloon can be used to allow for some bulge into the neck and in turn reconstruct the neck adequately.
5. When three microcatheter systems are used, one must have two guiding catheters. Use a smaller diameter second guiding catheter as only a single microcatheter system will pass through it. This will allow for adequate flow in the basilar artery. Adequate heparinization must be maintained, and flush lines should be monitored to avoid fluid overload particularly in patients with depressed cardiac function.

Suggested Reading

Griessenauer CJ, et al. Dual diagnostic catheter technique in the endovascular management of anterior communicating artery complex aneurysms. Surg Neurol Int. 2016;7:87.

Horowitz M, et al. The dual catheter technique for coiling of wide-necked cerebral aneurysms. Interv Neuroradiol. 2005;11(2):155–60.

Embolization of Internal Carotid Artery (ICA) Aneurysm Incorporating Origin of Posterior Communicating Artery

8

Vipul Gupta

Case

A 58-year-old female patient presented with subarachnoid haemorrhage due to rupture of right ICA aneurysm. DSA revealed a broad-neck aneurysm arising from right ICA (Fig. 8.1a, b). The right posterior communicating artery was arising from the aneurysm. P1 segment of right PCA was present (Fig. 8.1c).

Issue

The aneurysm is broad neck with an artery arising from it; any attempt at coil occlusion is likely to compromise the origin of PCOM.

Management

Balloon-assisted coil embolization was planned in view of broad neck of the aneurysm. After placing the balloon across the aneurysm neck, a microcatheter was navigated in to the aneurysm. The first loop of the coil was deployed prior to balloon inflation, so that any sudden movement of microcatheter tip during inflation doesn't cause injury to the aneurysm wall (Fig. 8.2a). The coil mass was seen to overlap the origin of PCOM. Since a reasonable calibre right P1 PCA was present, it is likely that it would support the right PCA territory and fill the PCOM retrogradely. Therefore, coil overlap was allowed (Fig. 8.2b). Balloon was deflated to check for stability of the first coil. Further coils were placed in single inflation of the balloon, and complete occlusion of aneurysm was achieved (Fig. 8.2c–e). Final angiogram showed flow in PCOM through the coil mass. Patient was placed on LMWH for 48 h followed by oral aspirin (150 mg/day). Follow-up DSA after 6 months revealed well-occluded aneurysm with continued flow in PCOM (Fig. 8.2f).

Tips and Tricks

1. In cases with PCOM arising from the aneurysm, coils can be allowed to overlap the origin of the artery if good-sized P1 PCA is present. Even if PCOM is completely occluded, it is likely to fill retrogradely through the PCA. However care should be taken to prevent protrusion of coil loops into the PCOM so as to avoid compromising the perforators arising from this arterial segment.
2. When coils overlap the arterial origin, it can result in thrombus formation and embolism from coil mass. It is advisable to start the patient on anticoagulant and anti-platelet agents as described so as to prevent thromboembolism.

V. Gupta
Neurointerventional Surgery, Stroke unit, Artemis Agrim Institute of Neuroscience, Gurgaon, India
e-mail: vipul.gupta@artemishospitals.com

V. Gupta et al. (eds.), *100 Interesting Case Studies in Neurointervention: Tips and Tricks*,
https://doi.org/10.1007/978-981-13-1346-2_8

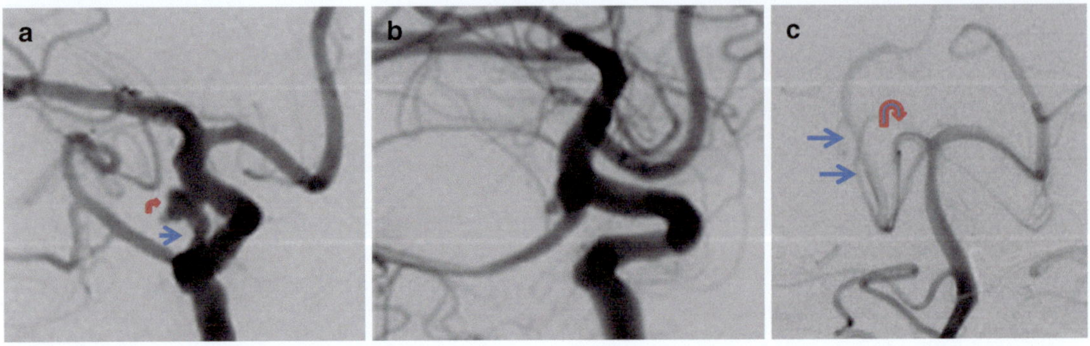

Fig. 8.1 (**a** and **b**) Right internal carotid angiogram revealing broad-neck aneurysm (curved red arrow, **a**) arising at origin of right posterior communicating artery (PCOM). A large PCOM is seen to arise from aneurysm neck. (**c**) Vertebral artery angiogram reveals good-sized right P1 segment of right posterior cerebral artery (curved arrow) which fills the PCA (arrows)

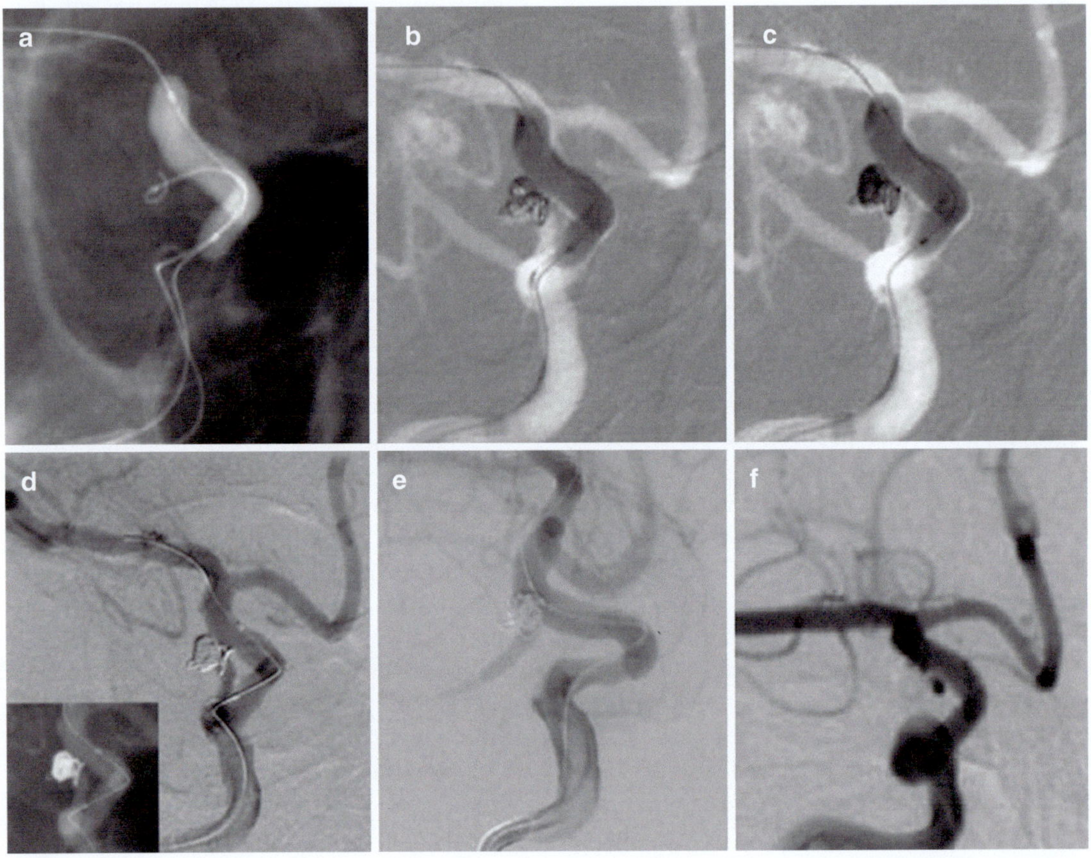

Fig. 8.2 (**a**) Balloon-assisted coiling was performed. (**b**) To achieve stable coil mass in this broad-neck aneurysm, it was decided to sacrifice the origin of the PCOM (considered to be safe due to presence of P1 PCA). (**c**) In a single balloon inflation, multiple coils were placed to achieve a stable coil mass. (**d** and **e**) Final angiograms showing complete occlusion of the aneurysm. Although coil loops are present at the origin of PCOM, forward flow is still present. (**f**) Follow-up angiogram revealed stable result as well as filling of PCOM

3. While using balloon assistance, a coil loop should be deployed in the aneurysm through the microcatheter before inflating the balloon. The coil loop is much softer than the catheter tip and is less likely to cause rupture in case of movement of catheter tip during balloon inflation. This is particularly important in cases of small ruptured aneurysms.

Suggested Reading

Kim BM, Park SI, Kim DJ, Kim DI, Suh SH, Kwon TH, et al. Endovascular coil embolization of aneurysms with a branch incorporated into the sac. AJNR Am J Neuroradiol. 2010;31:145–51.

Lubicz B, Lefranc F, Levivier M, Dewitte O, Pirotte B, Brotchi J, et al. Endovascular treatment of intracranial aneurysms with a branch arising from the sac. AJNR Am J Neuroradiol. 2006;27:142–7.

Aneurysm with Probable Near the Neck Rupture: Endovascular Management

9

Vipul Gupta

Case

A 48-year-old female presented with a subarachnoid haemorrhage (Hunt & Hess II and Fisher grade III). Angiogram revealed a broad-neck anterior communicating artery aneurysm (Fig. 9.1a). A lobule was seen projecting from base of aneurysm, near the neck, indicating the probable site of rupture.

Issue

1. Endovascular management of a broad-neck aneurysm while preserving both the ACAs.
2. Achieving occlusion of the lobule near the neck is critical to prevent a rebleed.
3. Rupture during the procedure may be difficult to control exclusively because of near the neck location.

Management (Fig. 9.1b–f)

A balloon-assisted coiling was planned and undertaken. After placing the guiding catheter in the ICA, a balloon catheter (Eclipse, Balt, France) was placed in right ACA, the side on which the neck was wider and the lobule was projecting to achieve the control of the neck in that region. After placing a microcatheter (SL 10, Stryker Neurovascular), coiling was performed (Fig. 9.1c). In an attempt to place coil loops in the lobule, microcatheter was slightly withdrawn towards the neck. Further placement of a small (2.5 mm diameter) coil resulted in coils entering the lobule (Fig. 9.1d). Another coil was placed in the same inflation of balloon to completely pack the probable rupture spot and adjacent aneurysm. Final angiogram showed complete occlusion of the aneurysm (Fig. 9.1e) with reasonable packing density (Fig. 9.1f). Patient recovered and follow-up angiogram showed complete occlusion.

Tips and Tricks

1. It is important to recognize irregularity or lobules near the neck in a ruptured aneurysm. These geometrical changes may indicate the rupture site. Rotational angiography with 3D reconstruction is extremely useful for this purpose.
2. Surgical clipping can be challenging, and intraoperative rupture that is difficult to control can occur.
3. During embolization one should ensure that near the neck lobule is well occluded. This can be difficult because it is adjacent to parent

V. Gupta
Neurointerventional Surgery, Stroke unit, Artemis Agrim Institute of Neuroscience, Gurgaon, India
e-mail: vipul.gupta@artemishospitals.com

V. Gupta et al. (eds.), *100 Interesting Case Studies in Neurointervention: Tips and Tricks*,
https://doi.org/10.1007/978-981-13-1346-2_9

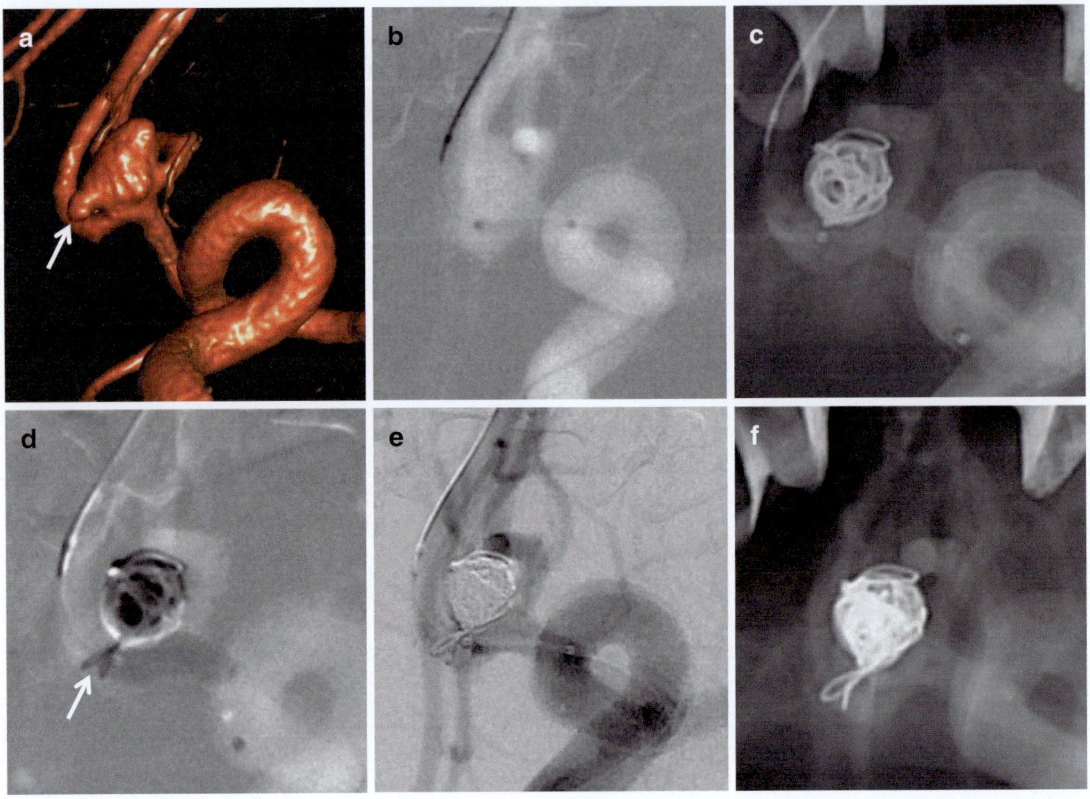

Fig. 9.1 (**a**) 3D reconstruction showing a broad-neck anterior communicating artery aneurysm with a lobule projecting near the neck region (arrow). (**b**) Road map image showing balloon placement in right ACA. (**c**) Initial coil mass; note there are no coil loops in the lobule. (**d**) Road map image showing further coil placement with few loops in the lobule near the neck (arrow); balloon is inflated so that coil doesn't prolapse in to parent vessel. (**e**) Final angiogram showing good result. (**f**) Coil mass

vessel, and any overzealous manipulation can result in rupture.

4. Rupture during embolization in such cases can be difficult to control because the leakage site is near the neck. This limits aggressive coil placement in the near the neck lobule.
5. We prefer to place a balloon into the branch on the side where the near the neck weak spot is located.
6. One may have to change catheter position to ensure that coil goes in to the lobule. When coil loops enter the lobule, we prefer to place multiple small and soft coils without deflation of balloon. This is done to ensure complete occlusion in the same catheter position. This also ensures immediate occlusion in the event of possible injury to the wall of lobule or rupture.

Suggested Reading

Fiehler J, Byrne JV. Factors affecting outcome after endovascular treatment of intracranial aneurysms. Curr Opin Neurol. 2009;22(1):103–8.

Songsaeng D, Geibprasert S, terBrugge KG, Willinsky R, Tymianski M, Krings T. Impact of individual intracranial arterial aneurysm morphology on initial obliteration and recurrence rates of endovascular treatments: a multivariate analysis. J Neurosurg. 2011;114:994–1002.

Small Lobulated Aneurysm: Balloon-Assisted Coiling

10

Vipul Gupta

Case

A 37-year-old lady presented with subarachnoid haemorrhage (Hunt and Hess Grade III; Fisher Grade IV). The angiogram revealed a small but broad-neck anterior communicating artery aneurysm filling from left internal carotid artery injection. Both anterior cerebral arteries were filling from left side with absence of A1 segment of right ACA. The aneurysm had a lobule projecting from the fundus (Fig. 10.1) as well a small lobule near the neck. Balloon-assisted coiling was planned.

Issues

1. Small broad-neck aneurysm with both ACAs arising from the base of aneurysm.
2. Two lobules, one from fundus and one from the neck region, were noted; it was critical to occlude these projections to secure the aneurysm.
3. The side on which balloon is to be placed should be chosen carefully.

Management

Balloon-assisted coiling was planned under general anaesthesia. The 6F guiding catheter was placed in left ICA. The balloon catheter, Scepter XC (MicroVention, Inc.), was placed in the left ACA (Fig. 10.1c) as the lobule near the base of aneurysm was towards that side. Thereafter, coiling was performed resulting in almost complete aneurysm occlusion in one of the working angles (Fig. 10.1d). However, in the other plane (Fig. 10.1e), the lobule near the neck was patent. Further attempts at coil placement were unsuccessful because the catheter was not pointing towards this lobule. Therefore, the coiling microcatheter was withdrawn, and another straight microcatheter was used which pointed into the lobule. A very small ultrasoft coil (1 mm × 2 cm) was placed in the lobule (Fig. 10.1f). A new road map was used to clearly visualize the coil in relation to the previous coil mass as depicted in the images (Fig. 10.1f). Final angiogram revealed complete occlusion of aneurysm including both the lobules. Coils could be clearly seen in the main body of aneurysm as well as in the lobule at the fundus (Fig. 10.2c) and at the base (Fig. 10.2d). Patient made uneventful recovery.

V. Gupta
Neurointerventional Surgery, Stroke unit, Artemis Agrim Institute of Neuroscience, Gurgaon, India
e-mail: vipul.gupta@artemishospitals.com

V. Gupta et al. (eds.), *100 Interesting Case Studies in Neurointervention: Tips and Tricks*,
https://doi.org/10.1007/978-981-13-1346-2_10

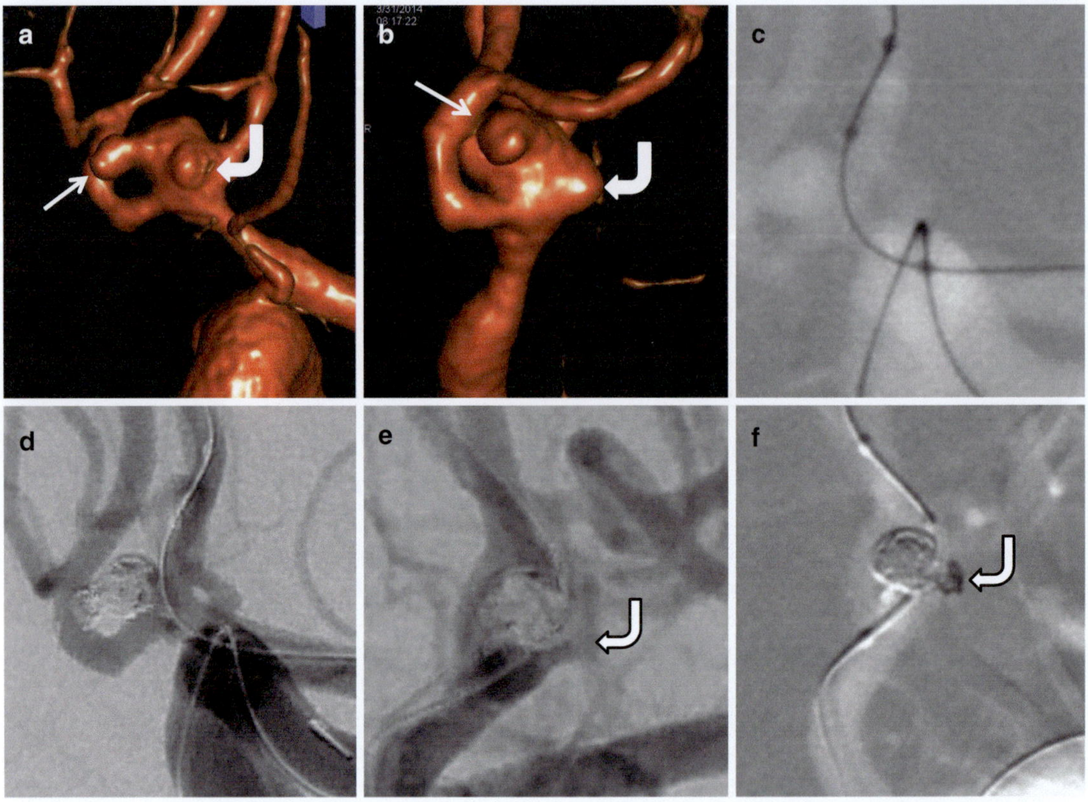

Fig. 10.1 (**a** and **b**) Three-dimensional reconstructed images showing a small broad-neck anterior communicating artery aneurysm. A lobule can be seen at the fundus (straight arrow) and at the base near the neck (curved arrow). Coiling was performed in these two angles with the second one (as **b**) profiling the lobule near the neck. (**c**) Balloon catheter placed in left ACA. (**d** and **e**) DSA revealed near complete occlusion of the aneurysm in **d**; however, in the image **e**, one can observe that the lobules near the neck is patient (curved arrow). (**f**) Road map image showing coil in the lobule near the neck

Tips and Tricks

1. For lobule near the neck, balloon is immensely useful and should be placed in the branch arising in proximity to the lobule.
2. Coiling of some of the lobules requires separate catheterization with different shape. It is pertinent to profile near the neck lobule in one of the working angles to aid catheterization and coil embolization of the lobule. In our case, all the lobules of aneurysm were not visible in the main working angle. However, a second view was chosen such that the other lobule can be profiled.
3. Use of very small coil is useful in such cases; however, sufficient length should be used for stability of the coil. The coil is detached in such cases with balloon inflated, and microcatheter is withdrawn with balloon partially inflated.

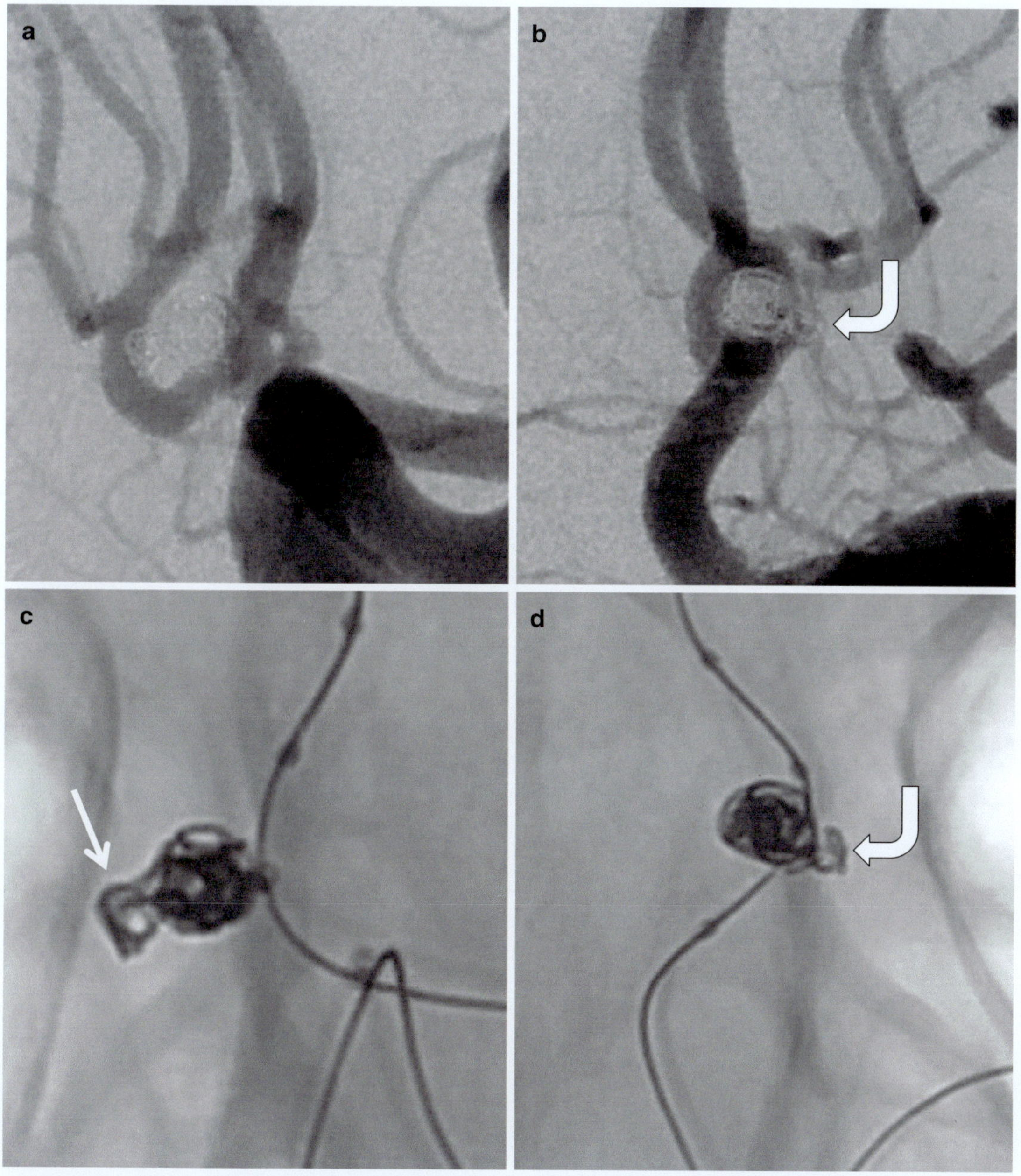

Fig. 10.2 (**a** and **b**) DSA images show complete occlusion of the aneurysm. (**c** and **d**) Fluoroscopic image in the two angles of coiling reveals well-coiled aneurysm with coils in the lobule at the fundus (straight arrow) as well as one near the neck (curved arrow)

Suggested Reading

Aletich VA, Debrun GM, Misra M, Charbel F, Ausman JI. The remodeling technique of balloon-assisted Guglielmi detachable coil placement in wide-necked aneurysms: experience at the University of Illinois at Chicago. J Neurosurg. 2000;93:388–96.

Shapiro M, Babb J, Becske T, Nelson PK. Safety and efficacy of adjunctive balloon remodeling during endovascular treatment of intracranial aneurysms: a literature review. AJNR Am J Neuroradiol. 2008;29:1777–81.

11 Balloon-Assisted Coiling of Large Internal Carotid Artery (ICA) Bifurcation Aneurysm: Assessment of Neck

Vipul Gupta

Case

A 52-year-old male was shifted from another hospital with a diagnosis of subarachnoid haemorrhage. His clinical condition was poor with a Hunt and Hess grade of IV. CT scan showed Fisher grade IV haemorrhage with haematoma in left basal ganglia. Ventricular dilatation was seen, and emergency placement for external ventricular drain was performed to reduce the intracranial pressure. DSA (Fig. 11.1) revealed a large left ICA bifurcation aneurysm. Balloon-assisted coiling was planned.

Issues

1. Large broad-neck aneurysm.
2. Branch vessel (MCA) arising at a relatively acute angle to parent vessel.

Management

Procedure was performed under general anaesthesia. A 6F guiding catheter was placed in the left ICA. A balloon catheter (Scepter XC, MicroVention, Tustin, California, USA) was navigated across the aneurysm neck using a 0.014 guidewire (Synchro, Stryker Neurovascular, CA, USA), and the coiling microcatheter was placed into the aneurysm sac. Thereafter, coiling was performed using balloon remodelling. The balloon was allowed to bulge into the neck (Fig. 11.1d) of the aneurysm in order to spare the pathway for the MCA and ACA that were arising at a relatively acute angle to the ICA. Some coils were seen to project into the neck after coil embolization. The balloon was inflated, and a new blank road map (without dye injection) was acquired. Balloon deflation did not reveal displacement of coil loops (Fig. 11.2a). This indicated that the coils were in aneurysm sac either anterior or posterior to neck. Final angiogram revealed complete occlusion of the aneurysm with preservation of all arteries. Patient made a slow but progressive recovery and was independent (mRS 2) on interval follow-up. Interval cerebral angiography showed stable result with no recanalization.

Tips and Tricks

1. Understanding the neck anatomy is crucial to achieving satisfactory coil occlusion of the aneurysm sac while preserving the patency of the artery harbouring the aneurysm.
2. In bifurcation aneurysms where the branch vessel (such as MCA in this case) is arising at

V. Gupta
Neurointerventional Surgery, Stroke unit, Artemis Agrim Institute of Neuroscience, Gurgaon, India
e-mail: vipul.gupta@artemishospitals.com

V. Gupta et al. (eds.), *100 Interesting Case Studies in Neurointervention: Tips and Tricks*,
https://doi.org/10.1007/978-981-13-1346-2_11

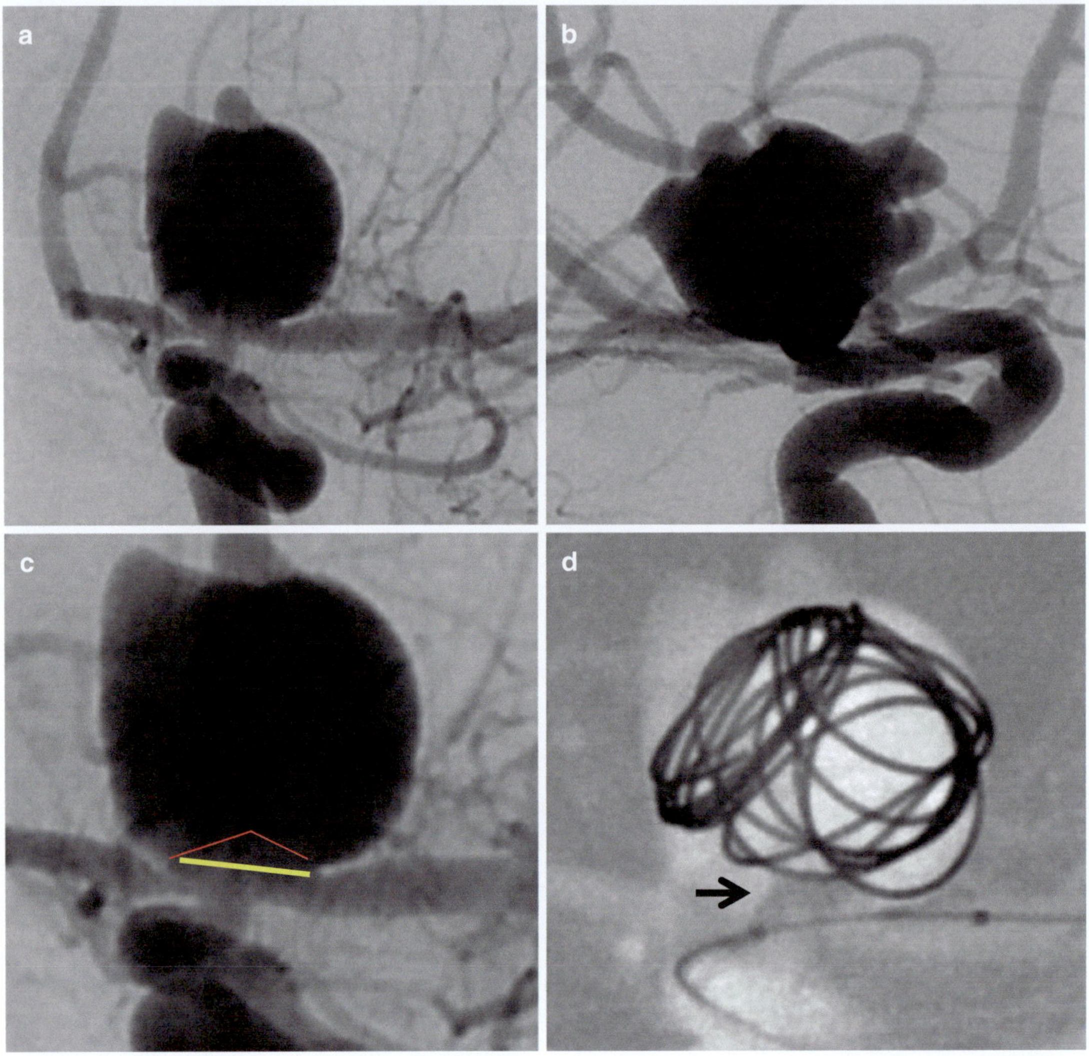

Fig. 11.1 (**a** and **b**) Left ICA angiogram shows large irregular ICA bifurcation aneurysm. (**c**) Yellow line indicates the conventional opinion about the neck. However in view of angle of origin of MCA, the red line should be regarded as the desirable neck. Otherwise, there will be coil bulge in neck region and possible thrombus formation. (**d**) Balloon-assisted coiling being done, with balloon bulging into the neck so as to create the neck outline shown in **c**

an acute angle, one should aim to spare part of the aneurysm neck to maintain the flow pattern.

3. Balloon inflation with slight bulge into the neck will help in reconstruction of the neck.
4. Extra/hypersoft balloon such as Scepter XC or HyperForm are useful as these extra compliant balloons can be made to bulge into the aneurysm sac with ease as compared to regular balloons (HyperGlide). We are inclined to use balloons (Scepter XC) with which one can use 0.014 wires as they are easier to manipulate in comparison to 0.010 wires. Thicker wires make the balloon stable during the procedure.
5. In patients who have a ventricular drain in place, all precaution should be taken to prevent coil prolapse as this may necessitate anticoagulant or anti-platelet use.
6. When coil prolapse into the neck is suspected, one can inflate the balloon and take a

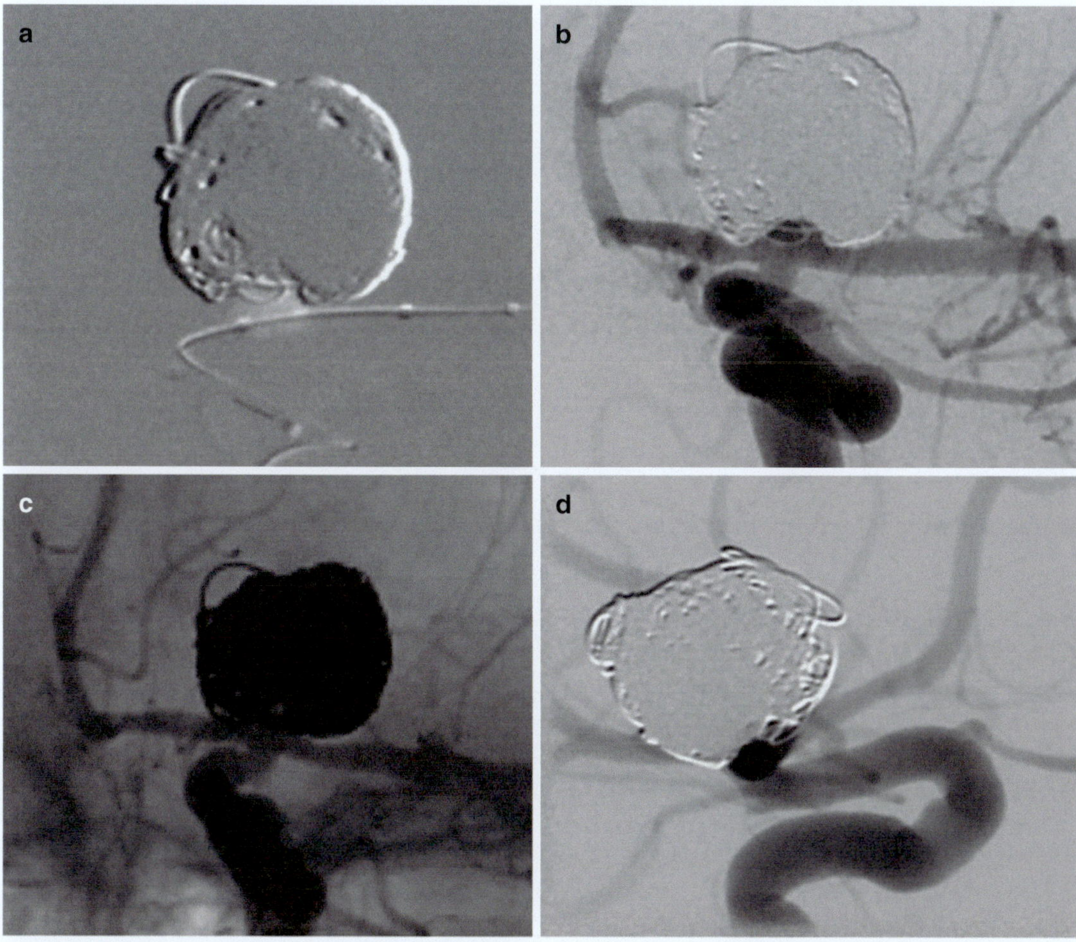

Fig. 11.2 (**a**) Road map shows the space occupied by the balloon relative to the coil mass. (**b**) Final DSA image showing complete occlusion of the aneurysm. Few coil loops seen in the neck regions are along posterior wall of aneurysm because no movement of these loops were seen during balloon inflation and deflation (**a**). (**c**) Coil mass. (**d**) Lateral view shows well-occluded aneurysm with circumferential reconstruction of the artery

new blank road map. On deflation of balloon (as shown in Fig. 11.2a), one will notice coil movement if coil prolapse was present. If coil loops do not move, then coils are in the aneurysm sac either anterior or posterior to the neck.

Suggested Reading

Fiorella D, Woo HH. How I treat: balloon assisted treatment of intracranial aneurysms: the conglomerate coil mass technique. J Neurointerv Surg. 2009;1(2):121–31.

12 Aneurysm with a Branch Arising from the Sac: Balloon over Inflation Technique

Vipul Gupta

Case

A 68-year-old female presented with subarachnoid haemorrhage 2 weeks back. Selective right internal carotid angiogram (Fig. 12.1) revealed right posterior communicating artery aneurysm with posterior cerebral artery (PCA) arising from the aneurysm. The PCA was filling solely from the internal carotid artery (ICA) injections. Vertebral artery angiogram did not reveal any opacification of right PCA due to absent P1 segment of right PCA. The aneurysm was broad neck along with a small projection from the fundus, probably the rupture point.

Issue

The issue in this case was to occlude the broad-neck aneurysm while preserving the PCA arising from the aneurysm.

Management

DSA in working projections were obtained (Fig. 12.1c, d). In Fig. 12.1d, the relationship of the PCA with the aneurysm is quite clear. It is important to have a working projection to profile the branch vessel to be preserved. A 4 mm × 20 mm HyperGlide balloon (ev3, Irvine, USA) was inflated in the ICA across the neck of the aneurysm. Gradual control over inflation resulted in a slight bulge into the neck of the aneurysm (Fig. 12.2a, b).

First coil placement is critical in these cases. Angiogram (Fig. 12.2d) after deployment of first coil showed that there were no loops at origin of PCA. Once first coil placement is done, further small coil placement is usually possible, and the final angiogram (Fig. 12.3) showed complete occlusion of the aneurysm with preservation of the PCA. It is advisable to observe for few minutes for any possible thrombus formation after the procedure. Whenever we use balloon in an old patient, we prefer to give low molecular weight heparin or IV heparin for the initial 48 h.

Tips and Tricks

1. In cases with a branch vessel arising near the neck of the aneurysm, one of the "tricks" can be to inflate a balloon in the parent vessel to a degree that results in a slight bulge into the aneurysm sac to preserve the artery arising from the neck of the aneurysm.
2. The balloon inflation should be done gradually under high-resolution fluoroscopy so as to avoid excessive bulge in to the aneurysm.

V. Gupta
Neurointerventional Surgery, Stroke unit, Artemis Agrim Institute of Neuroscience, Gurgaon, India
e-mail: vipul.gupta@artemishospitals.com

V. Gupta et al. (eds.), *100 Interesting Case Studies in Neurointervention: Tips and Tricks*, https://doi.org/10.1007/978-981-13-1346-2_12

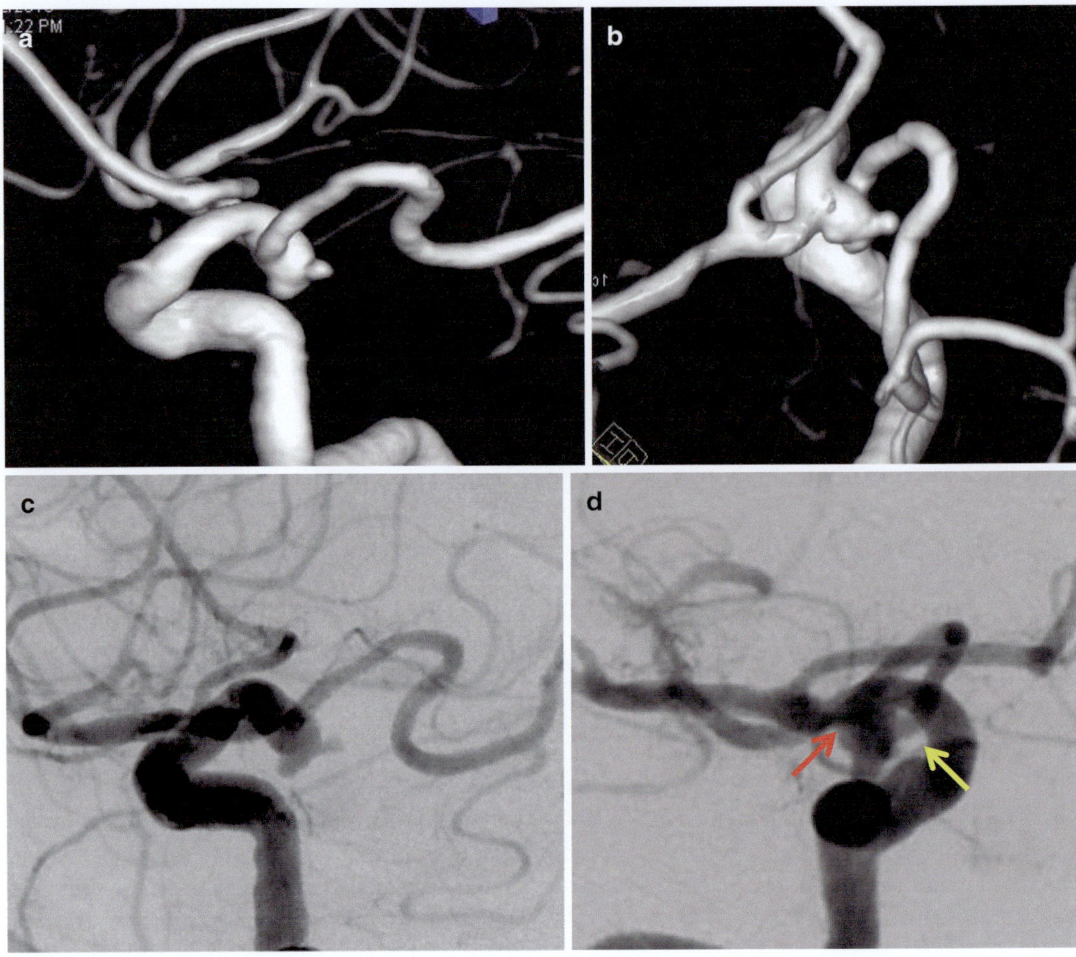

Fig. 12.1 (**a**, **b**) Three-dimensional selective right internal carotid artery angiogram shows a broad-neck posterior communicating artery aneurysm with the posterior cerebral artery arising from the aneurysm. Note the projection from the fundus, which is the probable rupture point. (**c**, **d**) Selective right internal carotid artery angiogram. In (**d**), the relationship between the PCA (yellow arrow) and aneurysm neck (red arrow) is well profiled

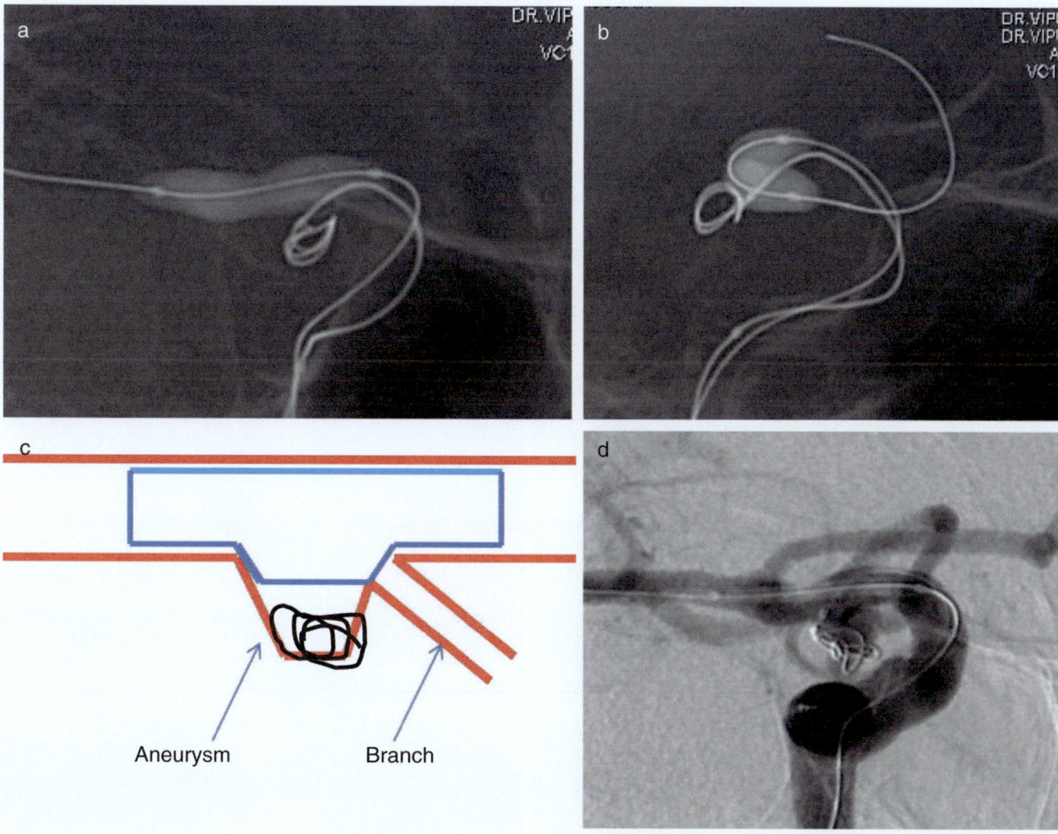

Fig. 12.2 (**a**, **b**) Fluoroscopic images of balloon-assisted coiling. Balloon is bulging slightly into the aneurysm, resulting in remodelling of the coils at the neck. (**c**) Diagrammatic representation depicting the technique. Red outline is of artery, blue denotes the balloon, and black is the coil. (**d**) Right internal carotid artery angiogram after placement of the coil shows that the origin of PCA is spared

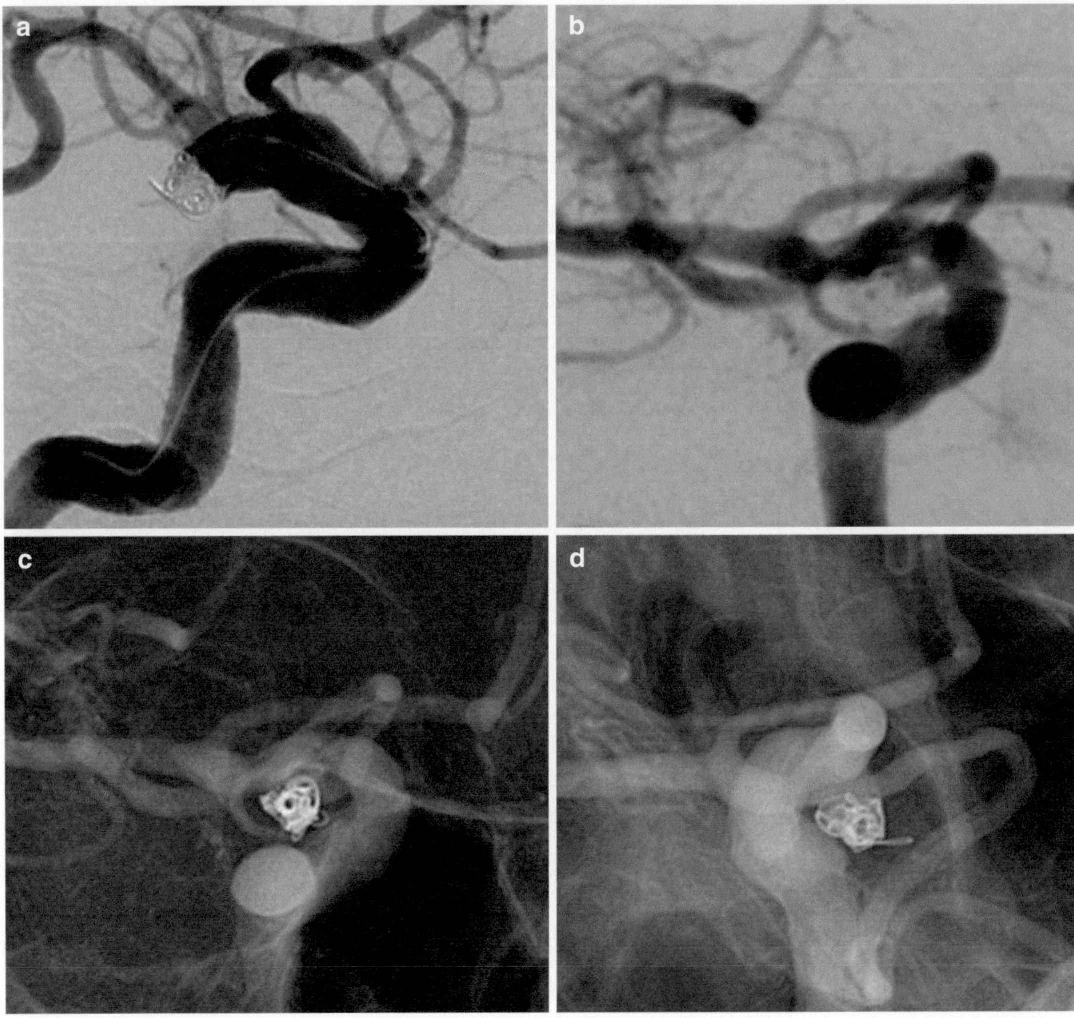

Fig. 12.3 (**a**, **b**) Post-embolization angiogram showing complete occlusion of the aneurysm with preservation of the PCA. (**c**, **d**) Un-subtracted images in working projection show the coil mass. Relationship between coil mass and PCA is particularly well seen in (**d**)

Suggested Reading

Kim BM, Park SI, Kim DJ, et al. Endovascular coil embolization of aneurysms with a branch incorporated into the sac. AJNR Am J Neuroradiol. 2010;31: 145–51.

Lubicz B, Lefranc F, Levivier M, et al. Endovascular treatment of intracranial aneurysms with a branch arising from the sac. AJNR Am J Neuroradiol. 2006;27:142–7.

Multilobulated Broad-Neck Aneurysm: End-Hole Technique

13

Vipul Gupta

Case

A 58-year-old male presented with subarachnoid haemorrhage (Hunt and Hess grade II, Fisher grade III). DSA (Fig. 13.1a, b) revealed a broad-neck, multilobulated aneurysm arising from basilar bifurcation and extending to involve left posterior cerebral artery.

Issues

1. A broad-neck aneurysm with overlap of the lobules of aneurysm over the PCA may give an appearance of prolapse of coils into the parent artery; however, this is a result of overlap of coils in the lobules of the sac on the parent vessel. Therefore, selecting a working view that clearly delineates the parent artery from the aneurysm sac is essential to achieve complete aneurysm occlusion.
2. Multilobular shape may cause issues in complete packing of the aneurysm.

Management

Balloon-assisted coiling under general anaesthesia was undertaken. A 6F guiding (Neuron, Penumbra, USA) was placed in the left vertebral artery. A balloon catheter (Scepter, MicroVention, USA) was placed in left PCA over microguidewire (Synchro, Stryker Neurovascular, USA). Another microcatheter (Echelon, Covidien, USA) was placed in aneurysm. An end-hole working view for the left PCA and the neck of the aneurysm was obtained from 3D rotational angiography (Fig. 13.1c). This was confirmed by inflating the balloon and looking for end-on appearance. After the first coil placement (Fig. 13.1c), a new road map was obtained before balloon deflation. This is very useful in visualizing any coil loop movement after deflation of the balloon (Fig. 13.1d). Further coiling was performed in this view; however, partial filling of aneurysm was seen in peripheral areas (Fig. 13.2a). Selective catheterization of these lobules was performed, and small soft coils were

V. Gupta
Neurointerventional Surgery, Stroke unit, Artemis Agrim Institute of Neuroscience, Gurgaon, India
e-mail: vipul.gupta@artemishospitals.com

V. Gupta et al. (eds.), *100 Interesting Case Studies in Neurointervention: Tips and Tricks*,
https://doi.org/10.1007/978-981-13-1346-2_13

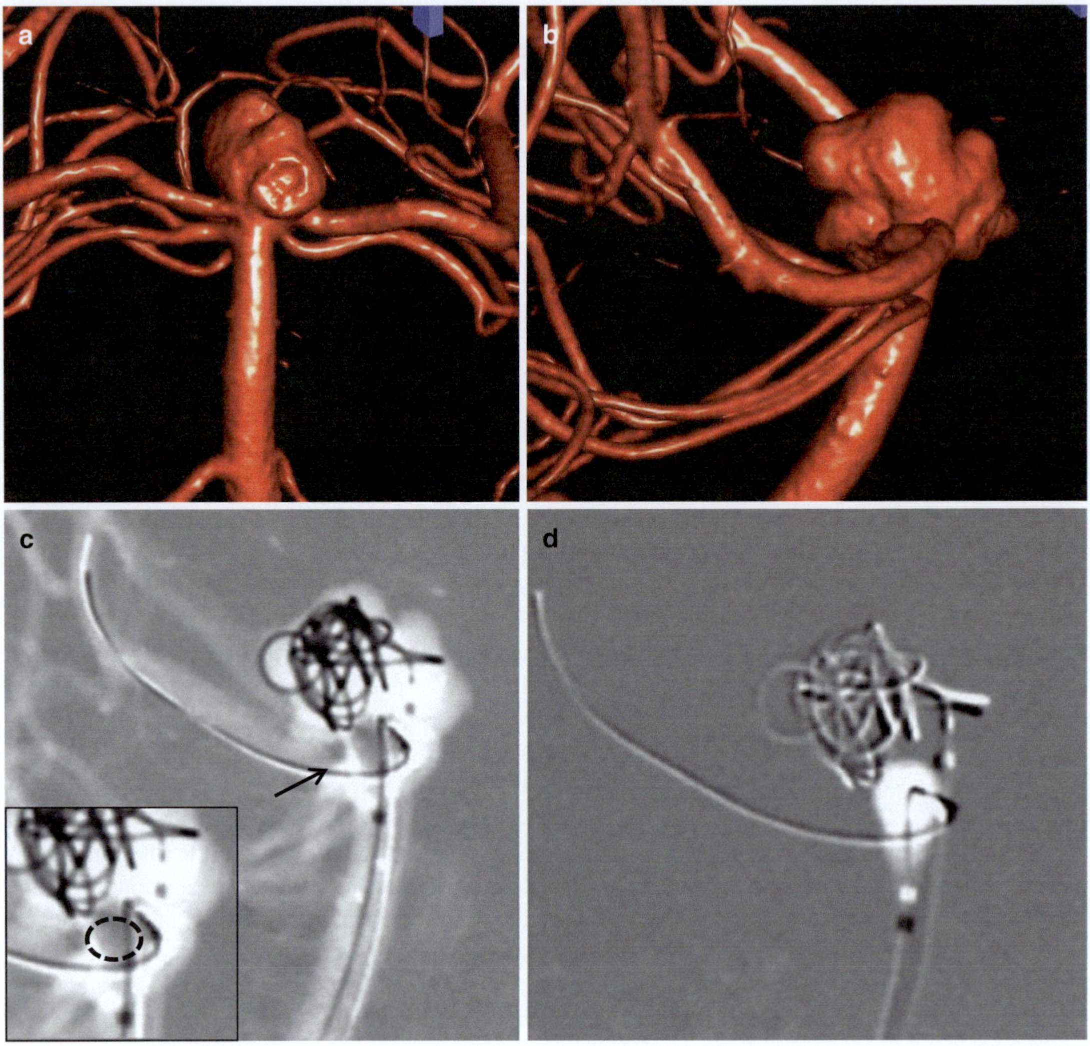

Fig. 13.1 (**a**, **b**)—Rotational angiography with reconstruction images in AP and lateral views shows a broad-neck lobulated aneurysm at basilar bifurcation extending along left posterior cerebral artery. (**c**)—Road map image in lateral view shows inflated balloon with placement of first coil. The balloon provides end-hole view of posterior cerebral artery (as shown by outline in inset). (**d**)—A new road map was taken, and balloon was deflated. No significant coil movement was observed. The bright area indicated space occupied by balloon

placed to achieve complete occlusion of aneurysm (Fig. 13.2c–f). Repeat runs were taken after 20 min to look for any thrombus formation. He was extubated in intact clinical condition and was given low molecular weight heparin for 48 h followed by ecosprin (75 mg) for 6 weeks.

Tips and Tricks

1. In multilobulated broad-neck aneurysms, it may be difficult to have clear visualization of the neck. In these cases, a balloon is immensely useful to preserve the artery.

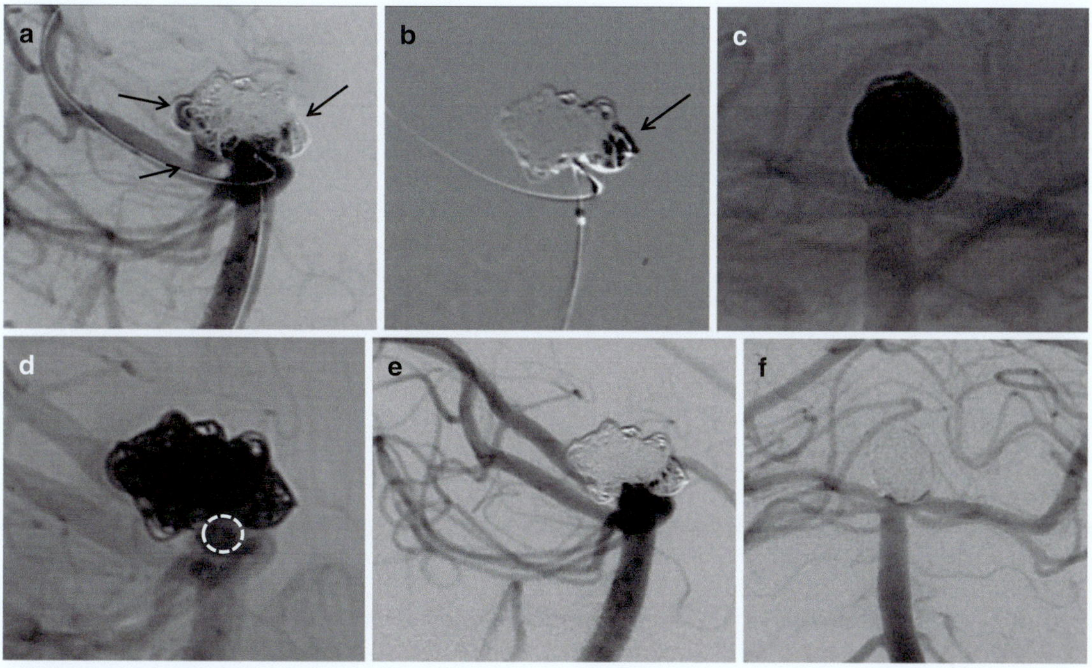

Fig. 13.2 (**a**)—DSA image shows partial coiling of aneurysm with small areas of residual filling (arrows). (**b**)—Selective catheterization was performed in these areas and further coiling was done. (**c**, **d**)—Final angiogram showing the coil mass, although there is overlap of coils and PCA in the AP view (**c**); lateral view (**d**) clearly shows that there is no prolapse of coils in to the parent vessel (outlined). (**e**, **f**)—DSA showing complete occlusion of aneurysm

2. Try to visualize the balloon in an end-hole manner; one can appreciate the relationship of parent artery to aneurysm neck better in this working view.
3. In multilobulated aneurysm as presented in the case, one may not achieve complete occlusion from initial location of the catheter. In such cases, one may have to do selective catheterization of partially coiled sections of aneurysm.
4. In view of overlapping coils, it may be difficult to visualize thrombus formation in these cases. End-hole view may not reveal a small clot formation because of density of contrast. One should watch for 20–25 min for any clot formation. If aneurysm is well occluded, it is advisable to give anticoagulants/anti-platelet agents in the postoperative period.

Suggested Reading

Fiorella D, Woo HH. How I treat: balloon assisted treatment of intracranial aneurysms: the conglomerate coil mass technique. J NeuroIntervent Surg. 2009;1(2):121–31.

Layton KF, et al. Balloon-assisted coiling of intracranial aneurysms: evaluation of local thrombus formation and symptomatic thromboembolic complications. AJNR Am J Neuroradiol. 2007;28(6):1172–5.

Piotin M, et al. Balloons and stents in the endovascular treatment of cerebral aneurysms: vascular anatomy remodeled. Front Neurol. 2014;5:41.

ICA Bifurcation Aneurysm: Balloon Placement Through Anterior Communicating Artery

14

Vipul Gupta

Case

A 48-year-old female presented with subarachnoid haemorrhage due to rupture of a giant ICA bifurcation aneurysm. Angiography revealed a giant broad-neck aneurysm involving origins of both middle and anterior cerebral arteries (Fig. 14.1a–c). The case was planned for balloon-assisted coiling.

Issues

1. Placement of balloon from right ICA into either MCA or ACA is unlikely to protect the origin of the other artery.
2. The aneurysm neck was extending along the posterior aspect of ICA bifurcation.
3. Giant aneurysms have high incidence of recurrence, and therefore adequate packing at the neck is desirable.

Management

A good calibre ACOM was noted (Fig. 14.1c); therefore, it was decided to place the balloon through ACOM across the aneurysm sac at the right ICA bifurcation (Fig. 14.1d). This enabled complete coverage of the aneurysm neck protecting both the MCA and ACA (Fig. 14.1e, f). At later stage of coiling, overlap of few coil loops over the parent vessel was noted. It was difficult to determine whether the loops were in the aneurysm neck along the posterior wall of ICA bifurcation or were protruding in to the artery. A new road map was taken, and the balloon was inflated; lack of coil movement confirmed preservation of parent vessel (Fig. 14.2a, b). Final angiogram revealed complete aneurysm occlusion (Fig. 14.2c–f). Follow-up angiogram after 6 months revealed stable result (Fig. 14.3a, b).

Tips and Trick

1. In ICA bifurcation aneurysms, there is the possibility of placing balloons or stents from contralateral route across the ACOM so as to secure origin of MCA and ACA.
2. Balloons are very useful to confirm location of overlapping coil loops. A new road map can be taken while inflating or deflating the balloon to detect any coil movement.
3. Attempt should be made in large and giant aneurysms to achieve dense packing and neck reconstruction to prevent recurrences.

V. Gupta
Neurointerventional Surgery, Stroke unit, Artemis Agrim Institute of Neuroscience, Gurgaon, India
e-mail: vipul.gupta@artemishospitals.com

V. Gupta et al. (eds.), *100 Interesting Case Studies in Neurointervention: Tips and Tricks*,
https://doi.org/10.1007/978-981-13-1346-2_14

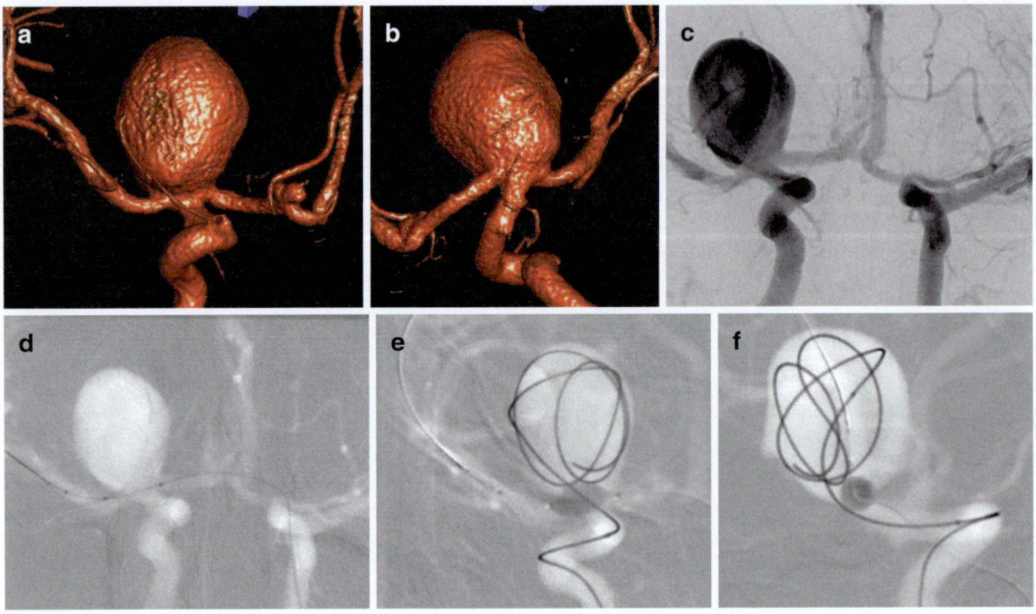

Fig. 14.1 (**a**)—A 3D image shows a giant right ICA bifurcation aneurysm with a broad neck. An unruptured small anterior communicating artery (ACOM) aneurysm is also seen. (**b**)—3D image from posterior aspect shows that aneurysm is extending to involve the ICA bifurcation. (**c**)—DSA image showing good size of ACOM. (**d**)—Balloon catheter was placed from left ICA through the ACOM across the right ICA bifurcation. (**e**, **f**)—AP and lateral views showing coil placement with balloon remodelling

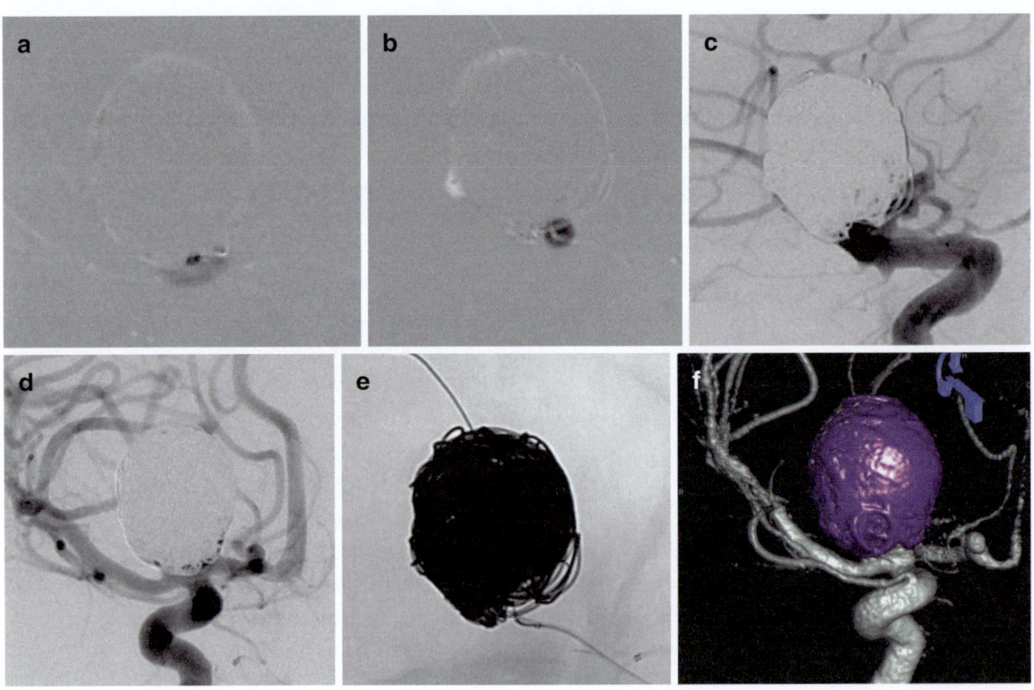

Fig. 14.2 (**a**, **b**)—During coiling there was doubt of few coil loops protruding in to the parent vessel. A fresh road map was taken, and the balloon was inflated; since no coil movement was seen, it confirmed that the overlapping loops were in aneurysm neck. (**c**, **d**)—Final angiogram showing complete aneurysm occlusion. The coil loops overlapping the ICA bifurcation in (**d**) are in the aneurysm neck along the posterior wall of ICA. (**e**)—Coil mass. (**f**)—Post-embolization 3D image

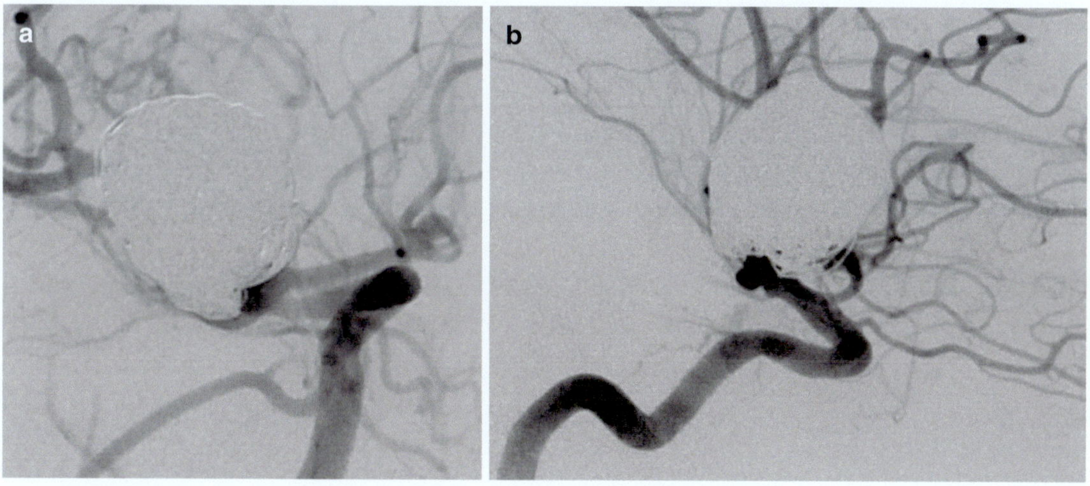

Fig. 14.3 (**a**, **b**)—Follow-up DSA images showing well-occluded ICA aneurysm

Suggested Reading

Fiorella D, Woo HH. How I treat: balloon assisted treatment of intracranial aneurysms: the conglomerate coil mass technique. J NeuroIntervent Surg. 2009;1(2):121–31.

Sebastian B, Mounayera C, Moreta J. Balloon-assisted coil placement in wide-neck bifurcation aneurysms by use of a new, compliant balloon microcatheter. AJNR Am J Neuroradiol. 2003;24:1222–5.

Shapiro M, Babb J, Becske T, et al. Safety and efficacy of adjunctive balloon remodeling during endovascular treatment of intracranial aneurysms: a literature review. AJNR Am J Neuroradiol. 2008;29:1777–81.

Double Balloon Technique for Wide-Neck Aneurysms

15

Rajsrinivas Parthasarathy and Vipul Gupta

Case

A 42-year-old female presented with subarachnoid hemorrhage (Hunt and Hess grade 2, Fischer grade 2). Cerebral angiography revealed a multilobulated dysplastic right MCA bifurcation aneurysm. The superior division was noted arising from the base of the aneurysm sac; the inferior division was also incorporated. Balloon-assisted coiling was planned.

Issues

Broad-based MCA bifurcation aneurysm incorporating both divisions. Both divisions should be protected; one can attempt coiling by placing balloons in both divisions, while the other option is to attempt Y-stenting with coiling (Fig. 15.1).

R. Parthasarathy (✉)
Vascular Neurology and Neurointerventional Surgery, Artemis Agrim Institute of Neuroscience, Gurgaon, India

V. Gupta
Neurointerventional Surgery, Stroke unit, Artemis Agrim Institute of Neuroscience, Gurgaon, India
e-mail: vipul.gupta@artemishospitals.com

Management

The procedure was performed under general anesthesia. A 6F guiding catheter was placed in the left ICA. A balloon catheter (Scepter XC, MicroVention, Tustin, California, USA) was navigated across the aneurysm neck using a 0.014 guidewire (Synchro, Stryker Neurovascular, CA, USA) first into the superior division. Another balloon was then navigated into the inferior division. Following that, the coiling microcatheter was placed into the aneurysm sac. Thereafter, coiling was performed using balloon remodeling (Fig. 15.2a). The balloon was inflated, and a new blank road map (without dye injection) was acquired. Balloon deflation did not reveal displacement of coil loops (Fig. 15.2b). Final angiogram revealed complete occlusion of the aneurysm with preservation of all arteries (Fig. 15.2c, d). The patient made complete recovery and was independent on interval follow-up. Interval cerebral angiography showed stable result with no recanalization.

Tips and Tricks

1. Broad-neck aneurysm incorporating both branches at a bifurcation may require double balloon to protect the parent arteries.
2. Superior division is smaller and arising at an acute reverse angle from the M1 MCA making

V. Gupta et al. (eds.), *100 Interesting Case Studies in Neurointervention: Tips and Tricks*,
https://doi.org/10.1007/978-981-13-1346-2_15

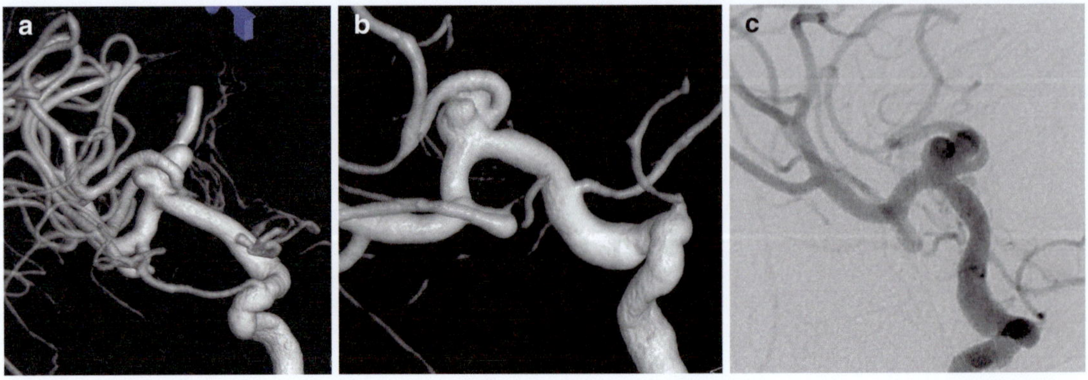

Fig. 15.1 (**a**, **b**)—3D reconstructed images showing multi-lobulated aneurysm at right MCA bifurcation with the superior division arising form the aneurysm. (**c**)—DSA image in working projection

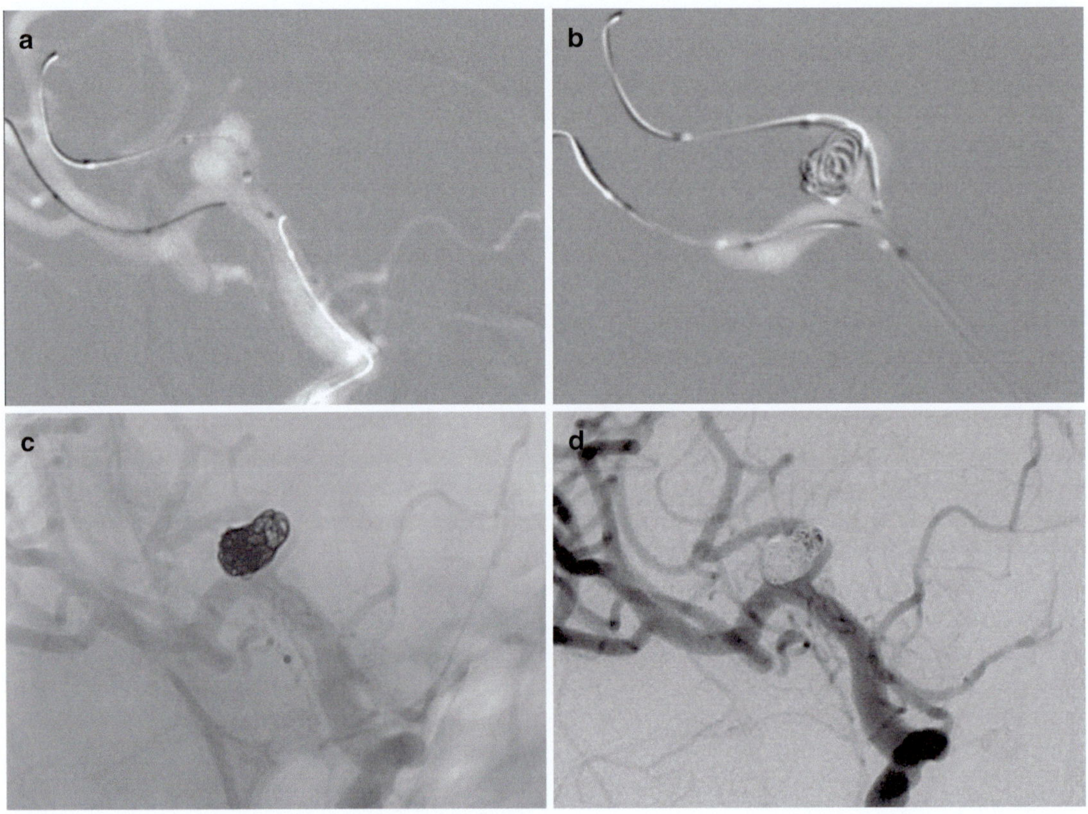

Fig. 15.2 (**a**)—Road map image showing placement of the balloons in both the MCA divisions. Notice that the balloon in upper division is slightly further ahead of the other balloon. (**b**)—Balloon deflation after placement of first coil. This was performed under blank roadmap. (**c**)—Final coil mass (**d**)—Post-embolization DSA showing complete occlusion with preservation of normal vessels

it challenging to cannulate as compared to the inferior division. Therefore, it is advisable to navigate the first balloon into the superior division.

3. Usually one balloon is placed ahead of the other balloon such that proximal end of one balloon overlaps the body of the other balloon.
4. The branch that is more incorporated by the aneurysm is the one in which the balloon is placed slightly ahead to offer complete protection to that parent artery.
5. Thromboembolism is common when more catheters are placed. Therefore, adequate heparinization should be maintained at all times to avoid this complication.

Suggested Reading

Shima H, et al. Embolization of a wide-necked basilar bifurcation aneurysm by double-balloon remodeling using HyperForm compliant balloon catheters. J Clin Neurosci. 2009;16(4):560–2.

16 Dissecting Aneurysm of MCA: Stent-Assisted Coiling

Vipul Gupta

Case

A 54-year-old hypertensive female presented with subarachnoid hemorrhage (Fisher grade III). She was clinically well preserved (Hunt and Hess grade II). DSA revealed a fusiform aneurysm at left MCA bifurcation. The aneurysm was extending into the lower division, which showed fusiform dilatation. A small lobule was projecting laterally from the aneurysm (Fig. 16.1a, b).

Issues

- Dissecting aneurysms have friable walls and tend to show progressive growth. These aneurysms require stent assistance for coiling and reconstruction of the vessel wall.
- Difficulty in navigation of stent microcatheter into the lower division of MCA.

Management

The aneurysm was considered to be dissecting in nature due to the fusiform morphology and circumferential involvement of MCA. Stent-assisted coiling was proposed as the appropriate management strategy. The plan was to place the stent in the lower division of MCA. Under general anesthesia a guiding catheter (Envoy, Codman & Shurtleff, Inc. USA) was placed in left ICA. An attempt was made to place the stent microcatheter (Renegade, Stryker Neurovascular, CA, USA) into the lower division. However, because of the acute angle of origin of the inferior division, repeated prolapse of the wire into the aneurysm sac was noted while attempting to navigate the wire distal to the sac in the inferior division. Therefore, a smaller profile microcatheter (Echelon 10, ev3 Inc, Irvine, California, USA) was used to catheterize the MCA inferior division (Fig. 16.1c, d). The microcatheter was steam shaped to give a sharp curve at the tip. This enabled hooking of the lower division (Fig. 16.1c) with relative ease and provided the required support to navigate the microwire distally. The microcatheter was taken distally over the wire to enable performing an exchange maneuver with the stent microcatheter. Patient was initially administered with heparin to raise the ACT to more than 300 s and was then given a loading dose of anti-platelet drugs (Tab Ecosprin 300 mg and Tab clopidogrel 450 mg) through nasogastric tube. A Neuroform stent was delivered uneventfully into the lower division across the aneurysm neck (Fig. 16.1e). A coiling microcatheter (Echelon 10, ev3 Inc, Irvine, California, USA) was navigated through the struts into the neck of aneurysm, and a coil was placed in the aneurysm sac. Final angiogram showed near complete occlusion with minimal filling of the lobule arising from the

V. Gupta
Neurointerventional Surgery, Stroke unit, Artemis Agrim Institute of Neuroscience, Gurgaon, India
e-mail: vipul.gupta@artemishospitals.com

V. Gupta et al. (eds.), *100 Interesting Case Studies in Neurointervention: Tips and Tricks*,
https://doi.org/10.1007/978-981-13-1346-2_16

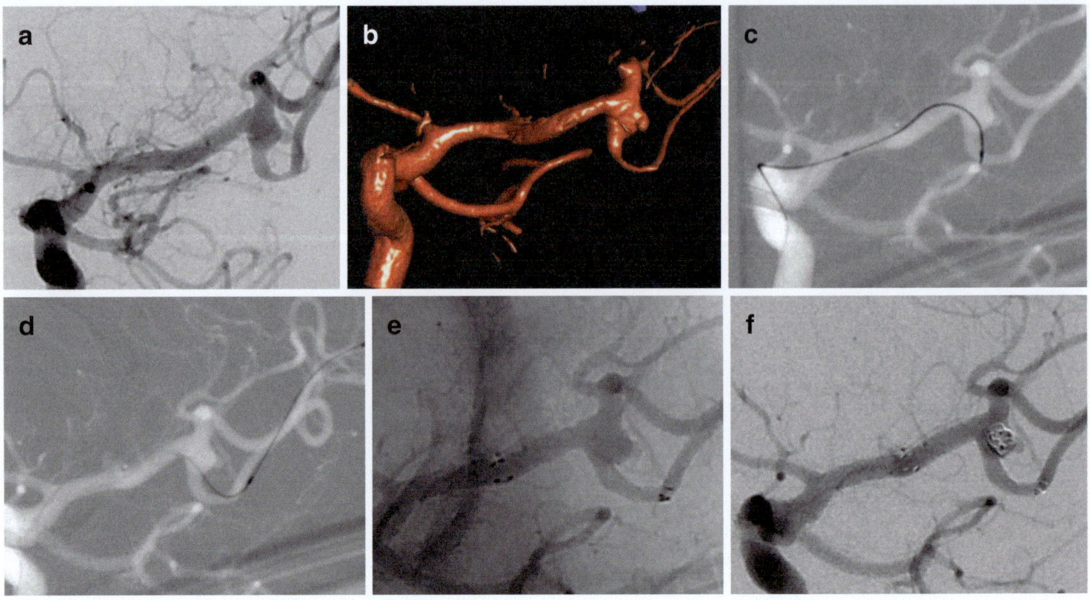

Fig. 16.1 (**a**, **b**)—DSA (**a**) with 3D reconstruction (**b**) shows a fusiform aneurysm involving left MCA bifurcation particularly the lower division. (**c**, **d**)—Road map images showing a microcatheter being navigated to lower division of MCA. (**e**)—Stent deployment in lower division of MCA. (**f**)—DSA after coil placement showing almost complete occlusion

aneurysm (Fig. 16.1f). Patient made uneventful recovery. A check angiogram performed 6 months after the procedure revealed significant increase in size of the aneurysm lobule (Fig. 16.2a–c). Repeat embolization was performed under general anesthesia. Three-dimensional images (Fig. 16.2b, c) were used to profile the neck of the recurrent aneurysm relative to the coil mass. A microcatheter (Echelon 10, ev3 Inc, Irvine, California, USA) could be placed at the aneurysm neck (Fig. 16.2d), and the residual/recurrent aneurysm was completely occluded using HyperSoft 1.5 mm × 3 cm coils. Follow-up angiogram at 3 months revealed complete occlusion of the aneurysm with moderate stenosis in the stented segment of MCA. Double anti-platelet therapy was continued, and follow-up angiogram (12 months after the first procedure) revealed mild decrease in the stenosis. After 1 year the clopidogrel was stopped, and patient continued on tab Ecosprin 150 mg once daily.

Tips and Tricks

1. It is critical to suspect dissecting nature of acutely ruptured cerebral aneurysms. These aneurysms frequently require stent assistance and have higher chance of recurrence as compared to berry aneurysms.
2. We prefer to perform early check angiograms in these cases to evaluate for recurrence.
3. An exchange maneuver may have to be performed to place the stent microcatheter in acutely angulated arteries arising from the dissected segments.
4. A 3D angiogram with different colors of coil mass and parent vessel can help in understanding the anatomy in recurrent aneurysms.
5. Stenosis after placement of self-expanding stents is usually benign and self-limiting. We prefer to continue double anti-platelet therapy in such cases for a longer period.

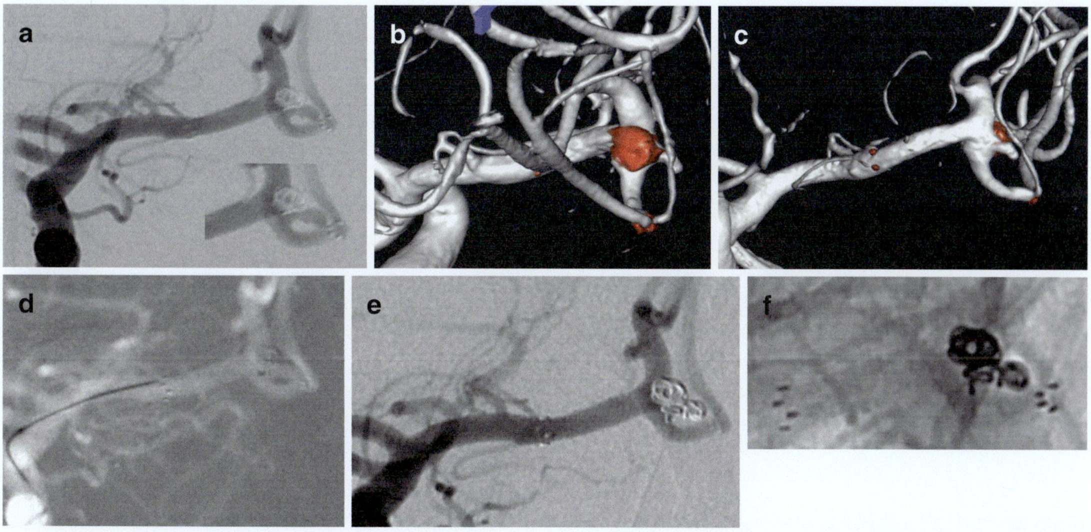

Fig. 16.2 (**a**)—Follow-up angiogram revealing growth of residual aneurysm. (**b**, **c**)—3D angiography; (**b**)—overlap of coil mass (orange) and the recurrent aneurysm seen. (**c**)—By changing the angulation, the neck of the recurrent aneurysm could be profiled. (**d**)—Road map image showing tip of coiling microcatheter at the neck of the aneurysm. (**e**)—Post-coiling angiogram showing complete occlusion. (**f**)—Native image showing the coil mass

Suggested Reading

Bodily KD, Cloft HJ, Lanzino G, et al. Stent-assisted coiling in acutely ruptured intracranial aneurysms: a qualitative, systematic review of the literature. AJNR Am J Neuroradiol. 2011;32(7): 1232–6.

Consoli A, Vignoli C, Renieri L, et al. Assisted coiling of saccular wide-necked unruptured intracranial aneurysms: stent versus balloon. J Neurointerv Surg. 2014;8:52.

Nishido H, Piotin M, Bartolini B, et al. Analysis of complications and recurrences of aneurysm coiling with special emphasis on the stent-assisted technique. AJNR Am J Neuroradiol. 2014;35(2):339–44.

Raymond J, Darsaut TE, Bing F, et al. Stent-assisted coiling of bifurcation aneurysms may improve endovascular treatment: a critical evaluation in an experimental model. AJNR Am J Neuroradiol. 2013;34(3):570–6.

Stent-Assisted Coiling of Dissecting Aneurysm of Posterior Cerebral Artery

17

Vipul Gupta

Case

A 54-year-old lady presented with headache. CT head revealed subarachnoid haemorrhage in the basal cisterns. DSA revealed a small broad-neck aneurysm of left posterior cerebral artery (PCA). Adjacent arterial segment was irregular and slightly attenuated (Fig. 17.1a). These features suggested dissection of parent artery. Stent-assisted coiling was planned.

Issue

Dissecting aneurysms are generally friable, have a broad neck and evolve with time. Stent-assistance acts as a scaffold for coil deployment and allows for healing of the parent artery over time.

Catheterization of small friable aneurysm can be technically challenging after stent placement. Henceforth, jailing the coil delivery microcatheter appears to be a relatively easier strategy. However, the key drawbacks are that the coiling microcatheter can frequently be displaced during stent delivery and navigating the microcatheter can be difficult once stent has been deployed.

V. Gupta
Neurointerventional Surgery, Stroke unit, Artemis Agrim Institute of Neuroscience, Gurgaon, India
e-mail: vipul.gupta@artemishospitals.com

Management

The procedure was performed under general anaesthesia. Stent delivery microcatheter (Prowler 21, Codman, USA) was placed in PCA distal to the aneurysm. Thereafter, coil delivery microcatheter was navigated into the aneurysm using a microguidewire. A partially retrievable stent (Enterprise, 28 mm, Cordis Neurovascular/Johnson & Johnson, Bridgewater, NJ, USA) was used (Fig. 17.1b–d). The stent was partly deployed across the neck of the aneurysm; this allowed for manipulation of the coil delivery microcatheter if required. The initial coil cage was partly herniating into the parent artery (Fig. 17.1b). Subtle microcatheter repositioning was done, and thereafter coil cage could be formed within the aneurysm sac (Fig. 17.1c). Another small coil (2 mm × 2 cm) was deployed, and complete occlusion of the aneurysm sac was achieved. Thereafter, the coil delivery microcatheter was removed, and the stent was completely deployed. Final angiogram revealed completely occluded aneurysm with patent parent artery (Fig. 17.1e, f). Patient was loaded with anti-platelet agents (Ecosprin 300 mg and clopidogrel 450 mg) through Ryles tube soon after stent delivery. Intravenous infusion of heparin was continued for 5 h after the procedure to maintain ACT of above 300 s. Patient recovered completely, and 4-year follow-up MRA revealed stable result.

V. Gupta et al. (eds.), *100 Interesting Case Studies in Neurointervention: Tips and Tricks*,
https://doi.org/10.1007/978-981-13-1346-2_17

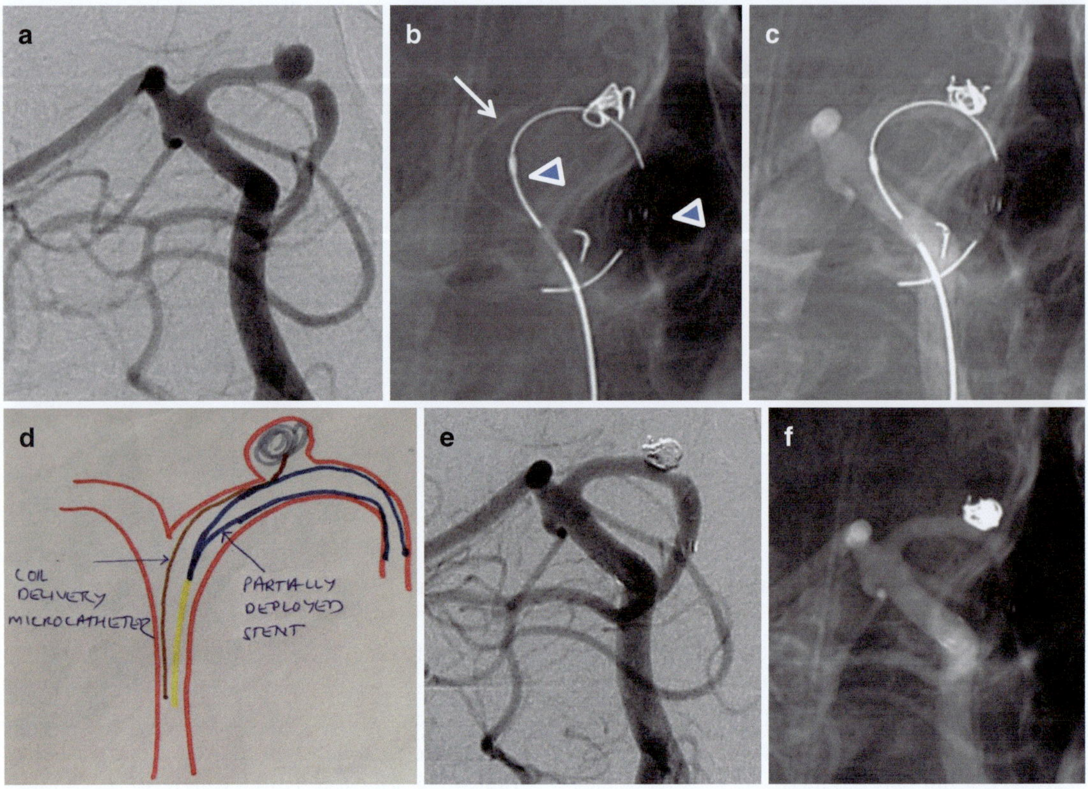

Fig 17.1 DSA (**a**) shows a broad-neck aneurysm of left PCA. Stent-assisted coiling was performed. Coil delivery microcatheter (arrow) was trapped in the aneurysm, and stent was partially deployed across the aneurysm (arrowhead) (**b–d**). Initial coil cage was partially herniating into the aneurysm (**b**). After slight repositioning of the microcatheter, satisfactory coil placement could be achieved (**c**). Afterward, stent delivery was completed. Final angiogram revealed complete occlusion of the aneurysm (**e**, **f**). In (**d**), the cartoon depicts coiling with partial deployment of stent

Tip and Tricks

1. Jailing the coil delivery microcatheter during stent-assisted coiling is a relatively simpler strategy; however, one should be watchful of forward/backward migration of the coil delivery microcatheter during stent deployment.
2. Partial deployment of a stent is a useful technique to help in microcatheter manipulation during stent-assisted coiling of very small aneurysm. Using a partial/completely retrievable stent gives the interventionist flexibility to reposition the microcatheter if needed.

Suggested Reading

Anxionnat R, de MeloNeto JF, Bracard S, et al. Treatment of hemorrhagic intracranial dissections. Neurosurgery. 2003;53:289–301.

Berger MS, Wilson CB. Intracranial dissecting aneurysms of the posterior circulation: report of six cases and review of the literature. J Neurosurg. 1984;61:882–94. https://doi.org/10.3171/jns.1984.61.5.0882.

Coert BA, Chang SD, Do HM, Marks MP, Steinberg GK. Surgical and endovascular management of symptomatic posterior circulation fusiform aneurysms. J Neurosurg. 2007;106:855–65.

Taqi MA, Lazzaro MA, Pandya DJ, Badruddin A, Zaidat OO. Dissecting aneurysms of posterior cerebral artery: clinical presentation, angiographic findings, treatment, and outcome. Front Neurol. 2011;2:38.

Use of Open-Cell Nitinol Stents for Aneurysms with Branch at Base (Ophthalmic and Anterior Choroidal Artery Aneurysms, etc.)

18

Ajit S. Puri and Rajsrinivas Parthasarathy

Case

A 54-year-old lady presented with headache. MRI revealed an incidental para-ophthalmic ICA aneurysm. DSA revealed a small broad-neck para-ophthalmic ICA aneurysm. The ophthalmic artery was noted arising from the base of the sac (Fig. 18.1a). Owing to the broad-neck stent-assisted coiling was planned.

Issue

Preserving the origin of the ophthalmic artery while securing the aneurysm

Catheterising the aneurysm sac that is arising from the superior wall of the ICA

Antiplatelet regimen

A. S. Puri (✉)
Radiology, and Neurosurgery,
Division of Neurointerventional Surgery,
Neurointerventional Fellowship Program,
University of Massachusetts Medical Center,
Worcester, MA, USA
e-mail: ajit.puri@umassmemorial.org

R. Parthasarathy
Vascular Neurology and Neurointerventional Surgery,
Artemis Agrim Institute of Neuroscience,
Gurgaon, India

Management

Stent-assisted coiling was undertaken under general anaesthesia. A 6F long sheath was parked in the right common carotid artery. Thereafter, a 6 F guiding catheter (DAC 0.070, Stryker Neurovascular, CA, USA) was navigated to the cavernous ICA. A XT 27 (Stryker Neurovascular, CA, USA) microcatheter was then navigated beyond the ophthalmic segment. A Neuroform stent 4 × 20 mm (Stryker Neurovascular, CA, USA) was deployed across the aneurysm sac. XPER CTA revealed gator backing and strut protrusion into the aneurysm sac (Fig. 18.1b, c). A through the cell wire based catheterisation of the aneurysm sac was undertaken with SL 10 (Stryker Neurovascular, CA, USA) microcatheter, and the sac was occluded with multiple detachable coils (Fig. 18.1d). Ophthalmic artery was briskly filling post procedure. Post procedure Xper CT revealed no haemorrhage. The postoperative period was uneventful, and the patient recovered.

Tips and Tricks

1. Gator backing, i.e. the stents' tendency to flare its struts outward, forming protrusions when the stent is deployed around a bend, is noted only with open-cell design. This feature of open-cell design stent can be considered beneficial particularly in instances where an artery is arising from the base of the aneu-

V. Gupta et al. (eds.), *100 Interesting Case Studies in Neurointervention: Tips and Tricks*,
https://doi.org/10.1007/978-981-13-1346-2_18

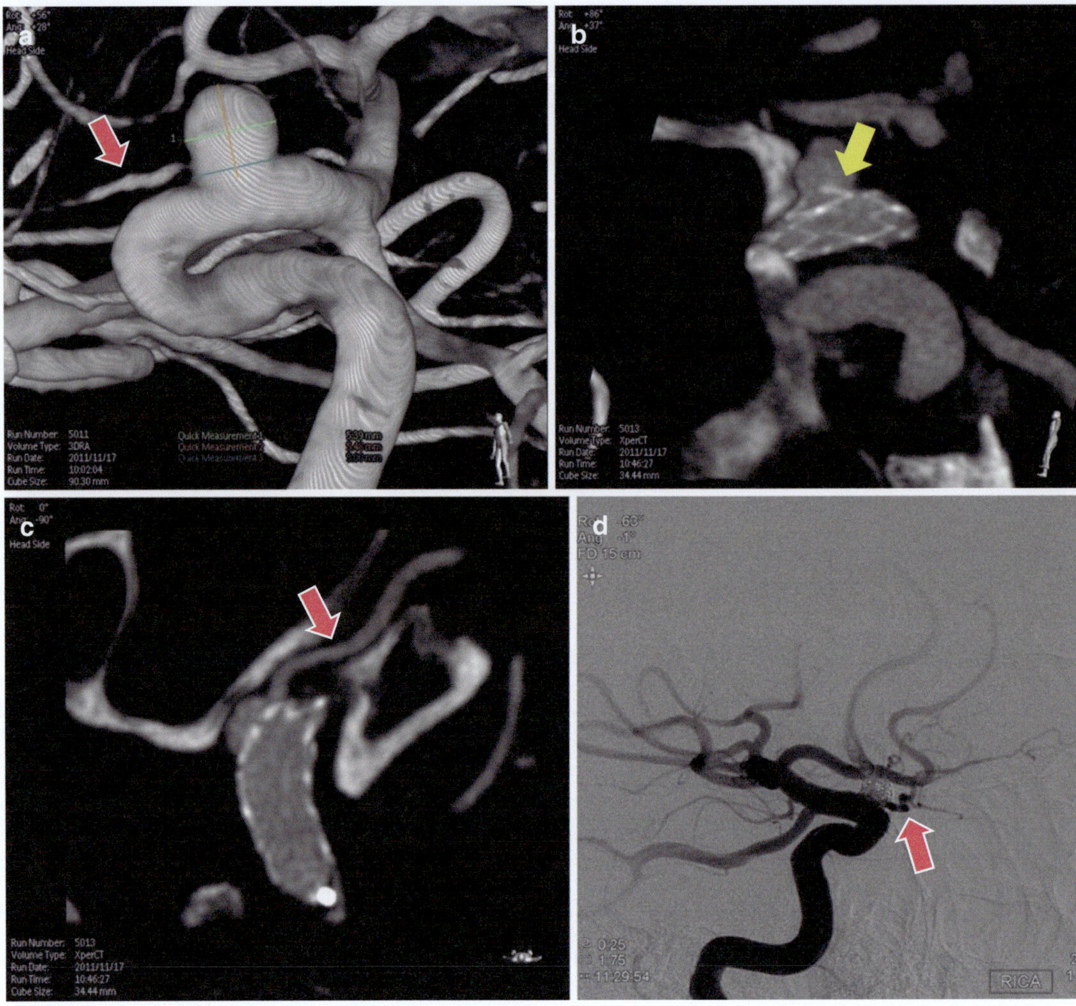

Fig. 18.1 (**a**)—3D angiogram demonstrates the ophthalmic artery arising from the base of the aneurysm (pink arrow). (**b**)—"Out-pouching" of the stent struts into the aneurysm neck (yellow arrow). (**c**)—Ophthalmic artery (pink arrow on the cone beam CT). (**d**)—These struts provide a base for the coils and prevent occlusion of the branch arising from the aneurysm (pink arrow)

rysm sac that is located on the convex outer wall; the crown protrusion allows for preservation of the ophthalmic artery by preventing coil mass from reaching the base of the sac. This feature is not noted with closed-cell designs.

2. It is preferable to under-pack the base of the aneurysm sac; this allows for flow in the ophthalmic artery even if some coils are noted at the origin of the ophthalmic artery.
3. In unruptured aneurysms, flow diverters are suitable alternatives.
4. Catheterising the sac on the superior wall of the ICA can be challenging; in particular, jailing a microcatheter can be difficult unless a stable microcatheter position is achieved.
5. Catheter tip shape can be the key to achieving stable catheter position and thereafter adequate packing.
6. Geometry assessment on 3D RTA is the key to determining the appropriate microcatheter tip shape.
7. A simple curve at the tip tends to point away from the sac due to the anterior cavernous bend. A straight tip is likely to behave better as it tends to point towards the base of the sac; however, a stable microcatheter position may not be achieved (Fig. 18.2a, b).

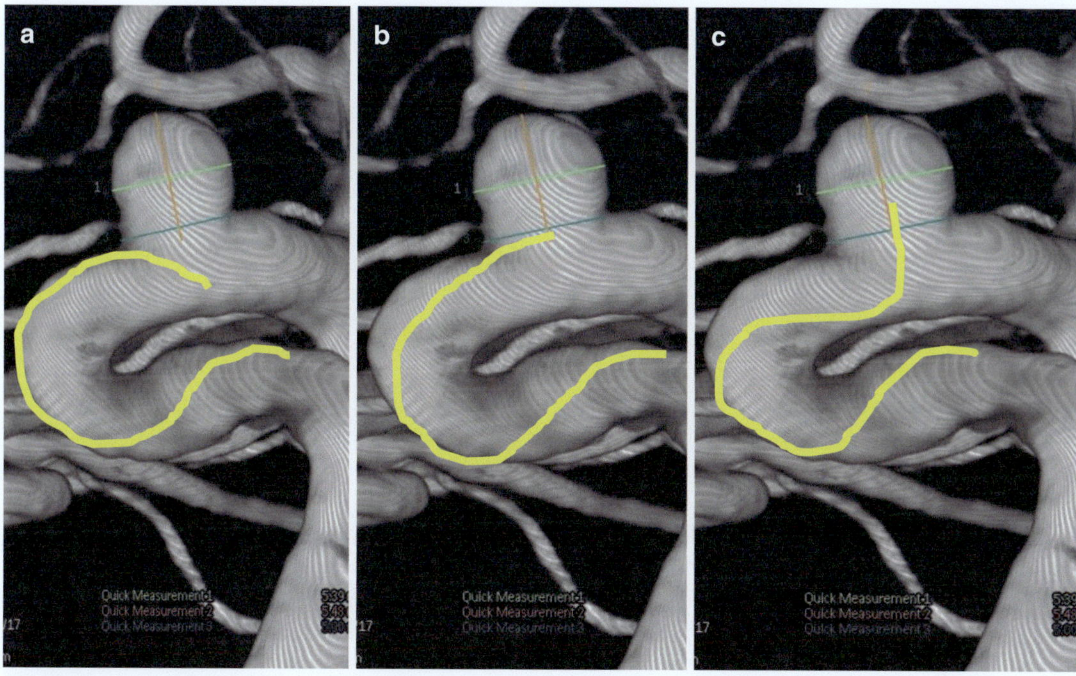

Fig. 18.2 (**a**)—Catheter with a J-shaped curve at the tip. (**b**)—Straight catheter shape. (**c**)—Reverse catheter shape

8. A reverse curve is likely to offer a stable microcatheter position. It is important to appreciate that the reverse curve will kick in only when the part of the catheter distal to the distal bend is within the aneurysm sac. This is illustrated in (Fig. 18.2c).
9. A wire based through the strut catheterisation is relatively easier with open cell as opposed to close-cell design.

Suggested Reading

Kadkhodayan Y, et al. Comparison of Enterprise with Neuroform stent-assisted coiling of intracranial aneurysms. AJR Am J Roentgenol. 2013;200(4):872–8.

Maldonado IL, et al. Neuroform stent−assisted coiling of unruptured intracranial aneurysms: short- and midterm results from a single-center experience with 68 patients. AJNR Am J Neuroradiol. 2011;32(1): 131–6.

19 Microstent-Assisted Aneurysm Sac Catheterization

Rajsrinivas Parthasarathy and Vipul Gupta

Case

A 48-year-old male patient presented with subarachnoid haemorrhage. Cerebral angiography showed small, sessile, broad-based, blister-like superiorly pointing anterior communicating artery (ACOM) aneurysm (Fig. 19.1a, b). Plan was to do stent-assisted coiling, with Leo + Baby stent.

Issues

1. The sheer geometry of the blister-like aneurysm poses a challenge to sac catheterization.
   The difficulty in sac catheterization is compounded by the fact that its orientation is superiorly pointing.
2. The preferred catheter shape in superiorly pointing aneurysms.

R. Parthasarathy (✉)
Vascular Neurology and Neurointerventional Surgery, Artemis Agrim Institute of Neuroscience, Gurgaon, India

V. Gupta
Neurointerventional Surgery, Stroke unit, Artemis Agrim Institute of Neuroscience, Gurgaon, India
e-mail: vipul.gupta@artemishospitals.com

Management

Procedure was performed under general anaesthesia. A 6F guiding catheter was placed in the left ICA. Stent microcatheter (Vasco 10, BALT extrusion, Montmorency, France) with microwire was placed in right A2 ACA from left A1 ACA. Due to small size of the aneurysm, catheterization was difficult. A pull-back technique using a catheter with a reverse curve at the tip was tried. This failed. The sac geometry analysis revealed that the axis of the aneurysm sac was perpendicular to the plane of the A 1 ACA–ACOM complex. Therefore, a catheter with a curve in perpendicular planes was used. It tended to point towards the sac, but catheterization was not possible. Henceforth, the Baby Leo (2.5 × 25) (BALT extrusion, Montmorency, France) was partly deployed to the ACOM segment, and then the coiling microcatheter was pulled back. This partly deployed stent provided the necessary support to enable catheterization of the aneurysm sac. Part of the first coil was deployed into the sac and was followed with stent deployment to provide the necessary scaffold to complete coil delivery (Fig. 19.2e–g). Post-stenting Vaso CT showed well-opposed stent along the right ACA with coil in the aneurysm (Fig. 19.2h). Final angiogram revealed complete occlusion of the aneurysm with preservation of all arteries. Patient made complete recovery. Interval cerebral angiography showed stable result with no recanalization.

V. Gupta et al. (eds.), *100 Interesting Case Studies in Neurointervention: Tips and Tricks*,
https://doi.org/10.1007/978-981-13-1346-2_19

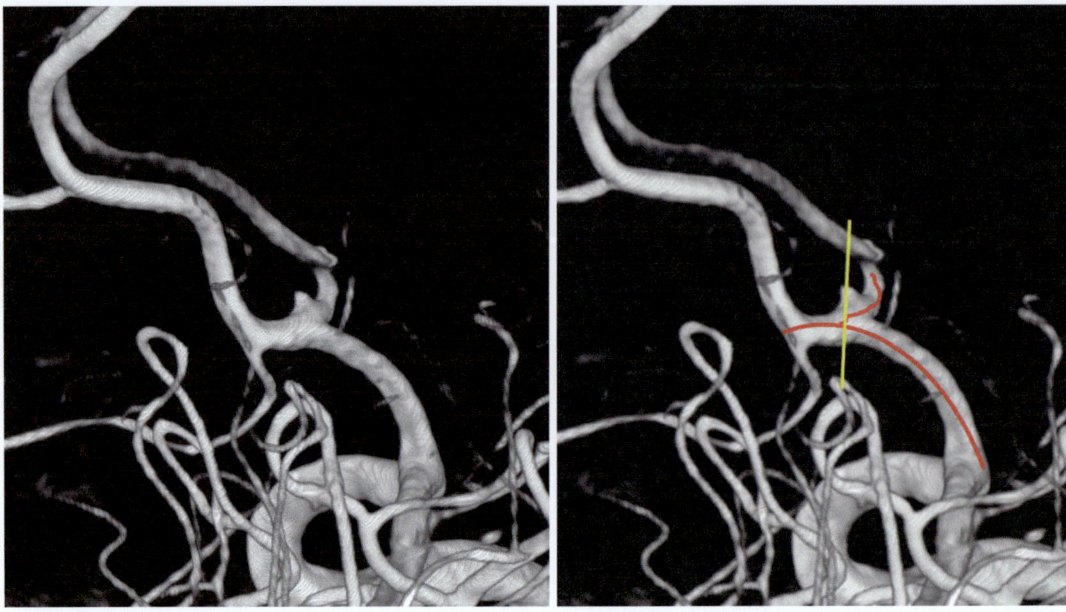

Fig. 19.1 (**a**) Superiorly pointing ACOM aneurysm (**b**) axis of aneurysm sac (yellow) perpendicular to axis of A1 ACA and ACOM (red line)

Tips and Tricks

1. The aneurysm morphology poses considerable challenge to endovascular management of such blister-like aneurysms (Fig. 19.2).
2. Note the axis of the A1 ACA–ACOM complex (Fig. 19.1; red line) is perpendicular to the axis of the aneurysm (Fig. 19.1, yellow line). Therefore, two curves in perpendicular plane were used.
3. Catheterization was not possible despite an appropriately shaped catheter. The tip of the catheter was tending to point in the horizontal plane in the ACOM. To provide support to the catheter, the stent was partly deployed up to the aneurysm segment in the ACOM. The coiling catheter was then pulled back; the partly deployed stent prevented the catheter from tending to point in the horizontal direction and provided the necessary support to keep it pointing superiorly thereby enabling the catheterization of the aneurysm sac. Part of the first coil was deployed, and then, the rest of the stent distal to the point of no return was deployed.
4. Shelfing technique was employed to provide an adequate scaffold at the base and avoid coil migration into the ipsilateral ACA.

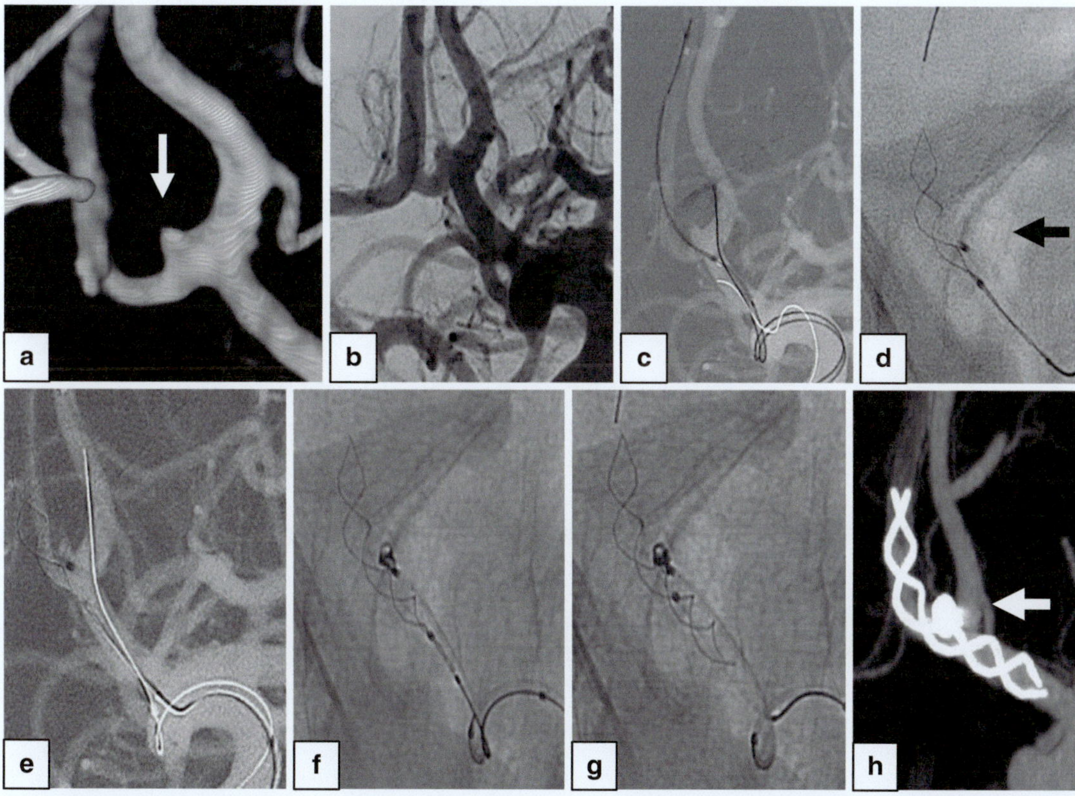

Fig. 19.2 Angiography showed small, sessile, broad-based anterior communicating artery (ACOM) aneurysm (may be a blister aneurysm) (**a**, **b**). Plan was to do stent-assisted coiling, with Leo + Baby stent. Stent microcatheter (Vasco 10) with microwire was placed in right A2 ACA from left A1 ACA. Due to small size of the aneurysm, it was difficult to have stable catherization; hence it was planned to partially deploy the stent with microcatheter in left A2 ACA (**c**). Aneurysm was later catheterized with the help of partially opened Leo stent (2.5 × 25), which acts as a scaffolding to support coiling microcatheter at the neck of the aneurysm (**d**). Aneurysm was then embolized using a 1.5 mm × 4 cm coil (**e**). Stent was then fully deployed, and coiling was completed (**f**, **g**). Post-stenting Vaso CT showed well-opposed stent along the right ACA with coil in the aneurysm (**h**)

Suggested Reading

Alvarado MV. Study of conformability of the new leo plus stent to a curved vascular model using flat-panel detector computed tomography (DynaCT). Neurosurgery. 2009;64(3 Suppl):ons130.

Negrotto M, et al. Assisted coiling using LEO Baby or LVIS Jr stents: report of six cases. Interv Neuroradiol. 2015;21(5):566–74.

20 Microstent-Assisted Coiling of Dissecting Aneurysm of the Left MCA Bifurcation

Rajsrinivas Parthasarathy and Vipul Gupta

Case

A 63-year-old female presented with subarachnoid haemorrhage. Three-dimensional rotational angiography revealed fusiform dilatation along superior division of the middle cerebral artery (MCA), with small blister-like aneurysm (Fig. 20.1). Stent-assisted coiling was planned.

Issues

1. A pyramidal shape dilatation noted along with a pseudolobule arising from the apex. The etiological mechanism for the aneurysm is debatable as this site is common for saccular aneurysm; however, the morphology favoured a focal dissecting aneurysm.
2. Do we opt for a single stent with coil or Y stenting with coil?
3. Aneurysm sac catheterisation – the preferred catheter shape.
4. Shelfing technique – the preferred stent type.
5. Antiplatelet option in ruptured aneurysms.

Management

Procedure was performed under general anaesthesia. A 6F guiding catheter was placed in the left ICA. A Vasco 10 microcatheter (BALT extrusion, Montmorency, France) was navigated into the superior division over a 0.014 micro-guidewire (Synchro, Stryker Neurovascular, CA, USA). Thereafter, the coiling catheter was navigated over a Traxcess 0.014′ microwire into the pyramid shape aneurysm base. A Baby Leo stent 2.5 × 18 (BALT extrusion, Montmorency, France) was partly deployed from the superior division and across the aneurysm base to the M1 MCA. A shelf was created by pushing on the stent and microcatheter at the angle between the M1 MCA and the superior division, and coils were deployed. Two loops of the second coil entered the pseudolobule. Adequate packing of the pseudolobule and the base of the aneurysm was achieved. The stent was deployed, and prior to withdrawing the coiling microcatheter, a wire was navigated through the struts into the inferior division. In the event of coil instability, a second microcatheter can be navigated into this division and another stent be deployed from this division to complete the Y configuration. However, no instability was noted on withdrawal of the coiling microcatheter. Final angiogram revealed complete occlusion of the aneurysm with preservation of all arteries. Patient made complete recovery. Interval cerebral angiography showed stable result with no recanalisation.

R. Parthasarathy (✉)
Vascular Neurology and Neurointerventional Surgery, Artemis Agrim Institute of Neuroscience, Gurgaon, India

V. Gupta
Neurointerventional Surgery, Stroke unit, Artemis Agrim Institute of Neuroscience, Gurgaon, India
e-mail: vipul.gupta@artemishospitals.com

V. Gupta et al. (eds.), *100 Interesting Case Studies in Neurointervention: Tips and Tricks*,
https://doi.org/10.1007/978-981-13-1346-2_20

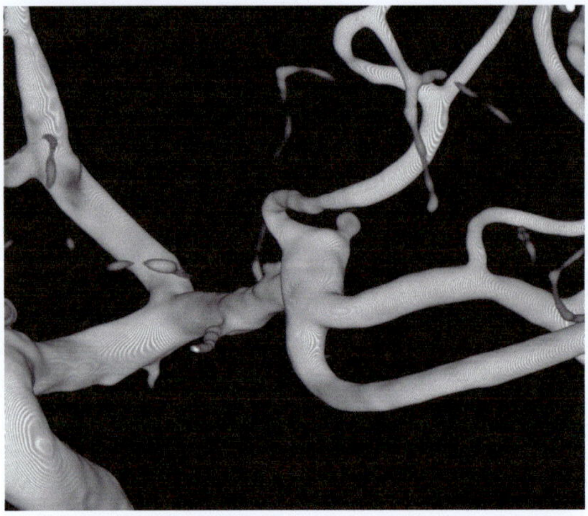

Fig. 20.1 Blister like aneurysm arising from dysplastic bifurcation of left MCA

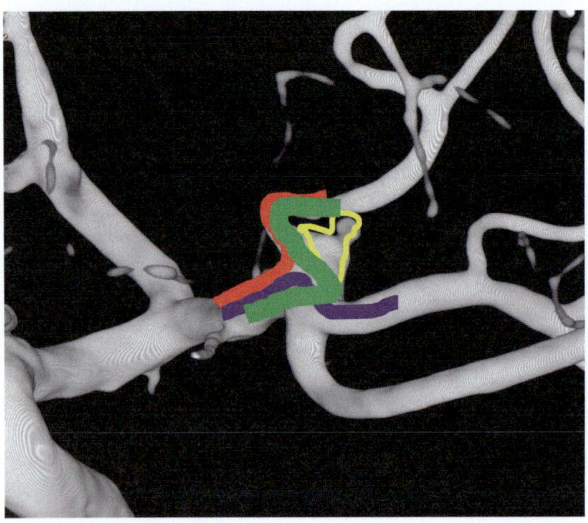

Fig. 20.2 The yellow outline depicts the aneurysm morphology; the green line depicts the shelfing techniques with a single stent (c.f. red line which is the usual stent deployment strategy); red and violet lines depict Y stent configuration

Tips and Tricks

1. The aneurysm morphology poses considerable challenge to endovascular management of blister-like aneurysms (Fig. 20.2, yellow line).
2. Options of single stent with coil and Y stenting with coil were considered. Y stenting with coil placement is technically challenging Fig. 20.2 (red and violet configuration). If one is able to provide the necessary scaffold for retaining coils in place with a single stent, then it arguably is a better strategy in such circumstances. The pyramidal shape swelling is predominantly centred over the superior division; therefore we planned a single stent with coil (Fig. 20.2) green configuration.
3. The superior division was catheterised using a Vasco 10 microcatheter. A double curve was given at the tip of the microwire to enable navigation into the superior division (Fig. 20.3c inset).
4. Prior to stent delivery, the aneurysm sac was catheterised with a coiling microcatheter. The shape of the distal end of microcatheter was crucial to avoid catheter movement during stent deployment and adequate positioning to enable coil entry into the pseudo-aneurysm.
5. The MCA had a concave anterior curve in the axial plane (Fig. 20.4a). In the end on view of the M1 MCA, the aneurysm is located in the postero-superior aspect, i.e. perpendicular to plane of the M1 MCA curve. Therefore two curves in perpendicular planes were used to catheterise the aneurysm sac as depicted in Fig. 20.4c, d.
6. Shelfing technique was employed (Fig. 20.2, deployment indicated by green line). The stent is deployed across the neck of the aneurysm. To provide an adequate scaffold at the base and avoid coil migration into the inferior division, the microcatheter along with the stent is pushed forward at the angle between the M1 and M2 MCA to achieve a configuration as depicted in Fig. 20.2 (green line). Braided stents better conform to the vascular anatomy as compared to laser cut stents.
7. The stent was partly deployed to just distal to the point of no return. This provides with the flexibility of retrieving and re-deploying if required.

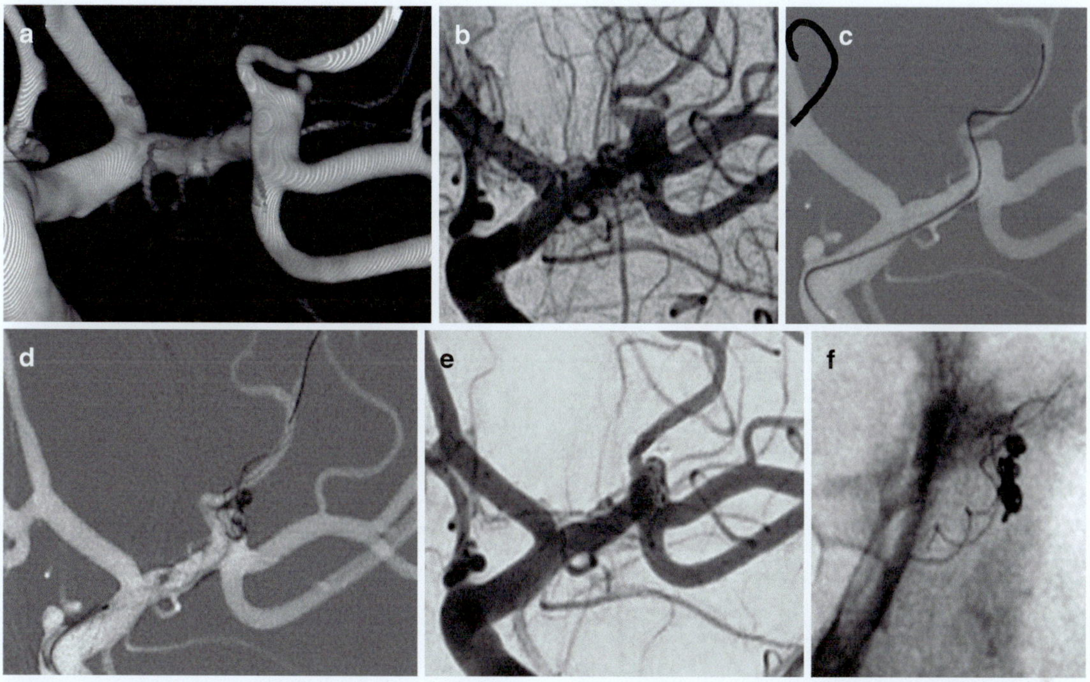

Fig. 20.3 (**a**) 2D image showed same finding along with acute angulation along the superior division MCA (**b**). Plan was to put Leo + Baby stent and to coil the aneurysm using "shelfing technique." Wire placement (Synchro 14) in the superior division of MCA was done, and microcatheter (Vasco 10) was navigated over it (**c**). Inset in figure C shows the shape of the microwire used to catheterise the superior division. Coiling microcatheter was placed in aneurysm, and partial coiling of aneurysm was done followed by partial stent deployment (Baby Leo 2.5 × 18) (**d**). Opposition of stent at the neck of the aneurysm was achieved by **shelfing technique**, in which once the stent was partially deployed at the neck, it was pushed further to change the angle of the stent and to form the shelf at the base of the aneurysm followed by coiling of the aneurysm. Post-procedure run showed well-opposed stent along superior MCA division without any filling of the blister aneurysm (**e**). Native image showing well-opened stent with coil mass (**f**)

Leo Stent Pearls (Strength and Weakness)

Leo is a braided stent, tends not to kink at bends, and provides better scaffold with shelfing technique.

Braid has 16 wires; cell size is small and approximately 0.9 mm.

The stent can be re-sheathed up to 90% of its deployment length and can be repositioned.

Don't rely on the proximal opening of the stent to confirm detachment. Add torquer, and with slight forward tension on the pusher wire, rotate no more than 90°clockwise and anti-clockwise and back. Allow time for the distal end to rotate

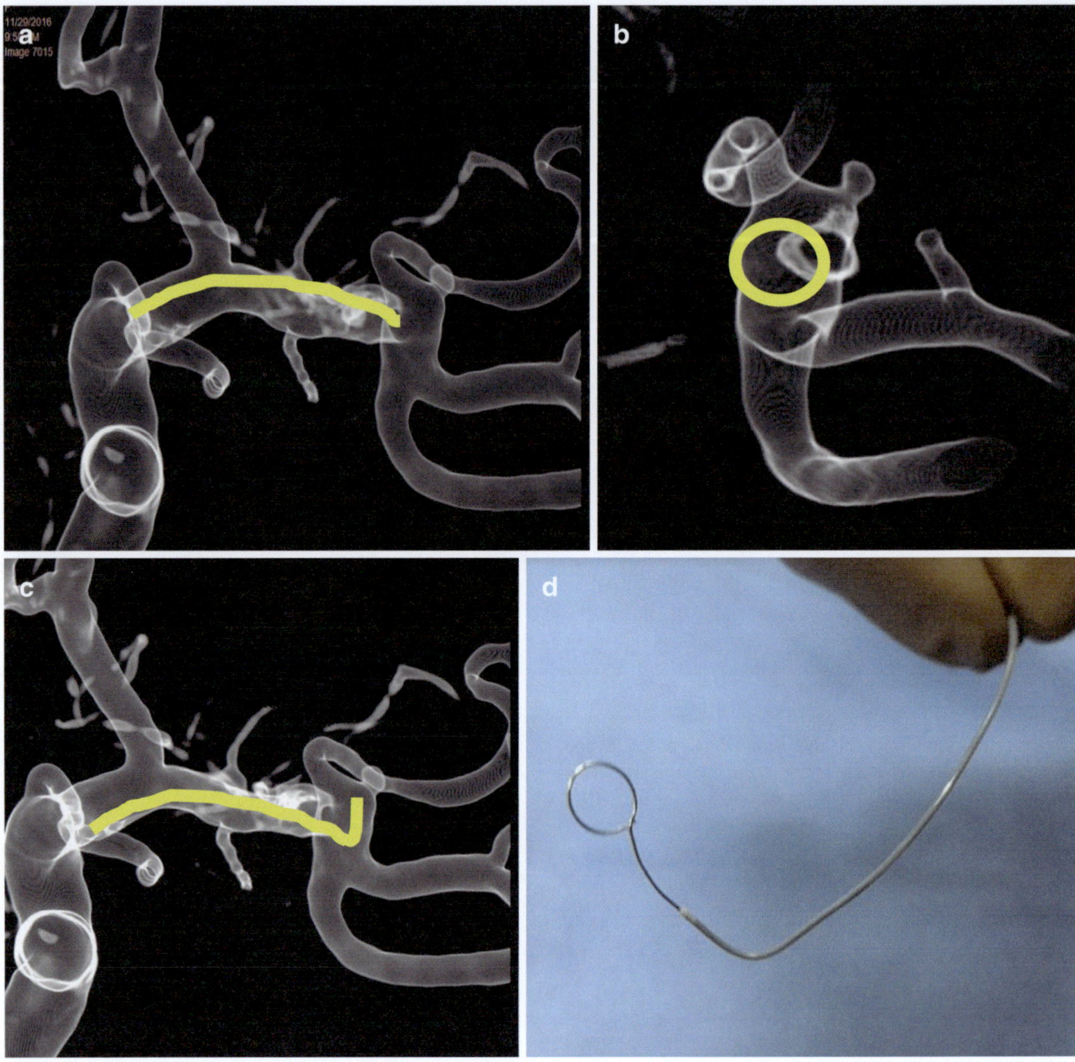

Fig. 20.4 (**a**) concave anterior curve in the terminal ICA and M1 MCA in the axial plane; (**b**) end on view of M1 MCA depicted the postero-superior relation of the aneurysm to the M1 MCA; (**c**, **d**) required shape of the microcatheter to catheterise the aneurysm, i.e. curves in perpendicular planes

Suggested Reading

Alvarado MV. Study of conformability of the new Leo plus stent to a curved vascular model using flat-panel detector computed tomography (DynaCT). Neurosurgery. 2009;64(3 Suppl):ons130.

Negrotto M, et al. Assisted coiling using LEO Baby or LVIS Jr stents: Report of six cases. Interv Neuroradiol. 2015;21(5):566–74.

Yen Du EH, et al. LVIS Jr 'shelf' technique: an alternative to Y stent-assisted aneurysm coiling. J Neurointerv Surg. 2016; https://doi.org/10.1136/neurintsurg-2015-012246.

Shelfing Technique for Stent-Assisted Coiling of Bifurcation Aneurysms

21

Vipul Gupta

Case

A 54-year-old lady presented with transient ischemic attack of right middle cerebral artery territory. Investigations revealed unruptured distal anterior cerebral artery aneurysm (Fig. 21.1a, b). It was a dominant ACA, and bilateral callosomarginal trunks and peri-callosal arteries were arising from the aneurysm. The case was planned for stent-assisted coiling.

Issue

The aneurysm was broad neck with both the distal ACAs arising from the base of aneurysm. Options were of Y stenting; however, authors do not prefer to place two stents in distal vessels. The case was planned for single stent-assisted coiling with "shelf" technique.

Management

After general anaesthesia, a 6 F guiding catheter (DAC, Stryker Neurovascular, Fremont, CA, USA) was placed in the left internal carotid artery. Stent delivery microcatheter (Vasco 10, BALT extrusion, Montmorency, France) was placed in the right ACA beyond the aneurysm (Fig. 21.1c) with the help of microguidewire (Traxcess, MicroVention, Tustin, California, USA). Thereafter, coiling microcatheter (Echelon 10, ev3 Inc., Irvine, California, USA) was navigated over the microguidewire into the aneurysm. Few loops of coil (TargetUltrasoft 3 × 6, Stryker Neurovascular, Fremont, CA, USA) were formed in the aneurysm (Fig. 21.1c). The microstent (Leo + Baby stent, BALT extrusion, Montmorency, France) was partially deployed across the neck, and then subtle pressure was applied on stent microcatheter so as to expand the stent across the neck so as to form a shelf and cover part of the neck giving rise to the left ACA (Fig. 21.1d). Thereafter the first coil was fully deployed (Fig. 21.1e), and after achieving a stable cage formation sparing both the ACAs, the stent was fully deployed. Further coils were placed to achieve complete occlusion of the aneurysm. Patient was stable on follow-up (Fig. 21.2).

Tips and Tricks

1. In patients with broad neck bifurcation aneurysms, "shelf" technique can be used in an attempt to cover maximal part of the neck. This can help to protect both the vessels and avoid using double stent technique.

V. Gupta
Neurointerventional Surgery, Stroke unit, Artemis Agrim Institute of Neuroscience, Gurgaon, India
e-mail: vipul.gupta@artemishospitals.com

V. Gupta et al. (eds.), *100 Interesting Case Studies in Neurointervention: Tips and Tricks*,
https://doi.org/10.1007/978-981-13-1346-2_21

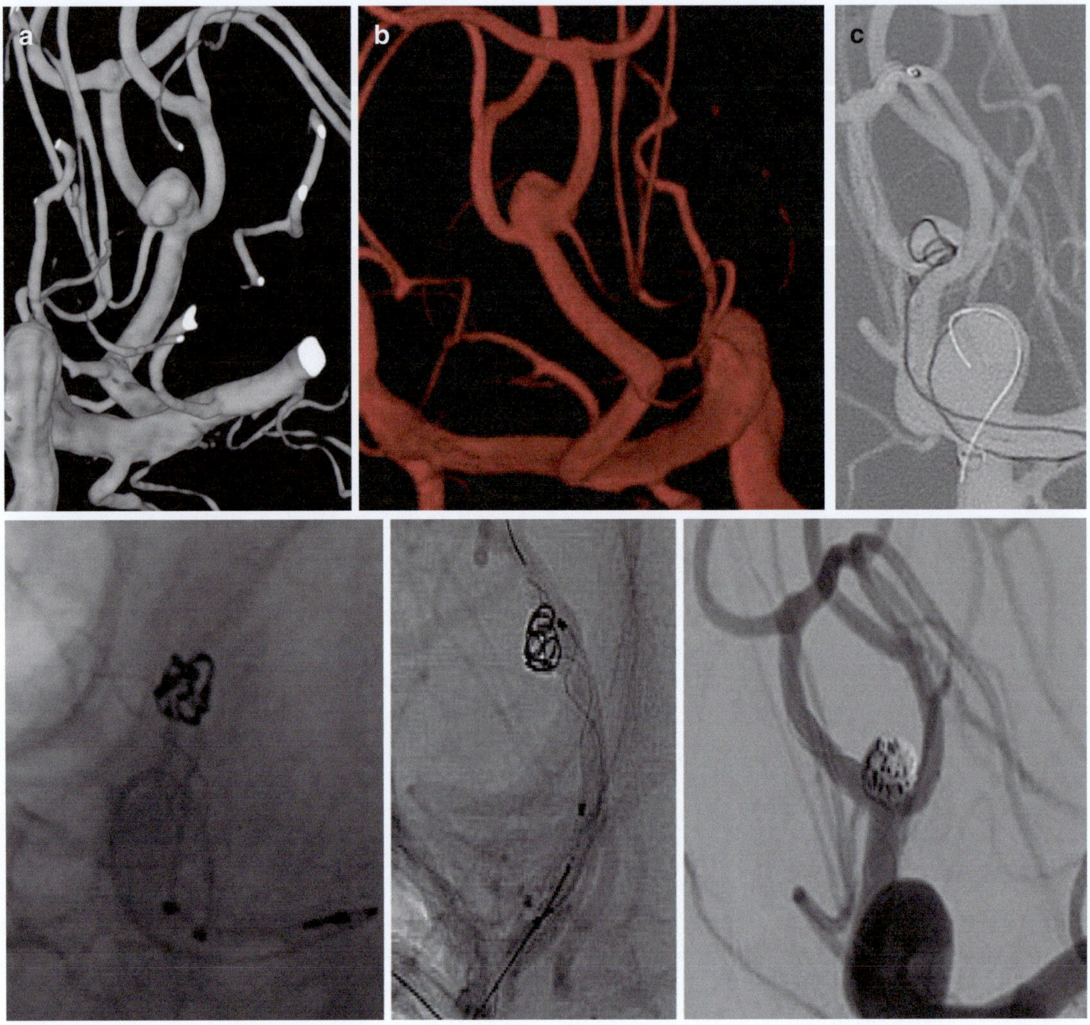

Fig. 21.1 A 54-year-old female patient with unruptured distal ACA (anterior cerebral artery) aneurysm. (**a**, **b**)—3D angiography showed broad-neck aneurysm with a small lobule pointing anteriorly; bilateral ACA was arising from the base of the aneurysm. Plan was to do stent-assisted coiling with a Leo + Baby stent along the right ACA and use shelfing technique to cover the neck of the aneurysm. (**c**)—Stent microcatheter was navigated in the right ACA, and coiling microcatheter was positioned in the aneurysm. (**d**, **e**)—Leo + Baby stent (2.5 × 18) was then deployed with shelfing at the neck of the aneurysm, followed by coiling of aneurysm sac. (**f**)—Post-procedure run showed well-opened and opposed stent, with patent right ACA, without any filling of aneurysm sac

2. One can give subtle forward pressure on the microcatheter after partially deploying the stent to achieve a "shelf".
3. In authors' experience, braided stents are more suitable for this technique.
4. We like to form few loops of coil in the aneurysm before deploying the stent, so as to stabilize the coiling microcatheter and to prevent any aneurismal wall injury due to tip movement during stent deployment.
5. Only after forming a stable cage of the coil the stent is deployed completely. It gives us the flexibility to reposition the coiling microcatheter in these small aneurysms.

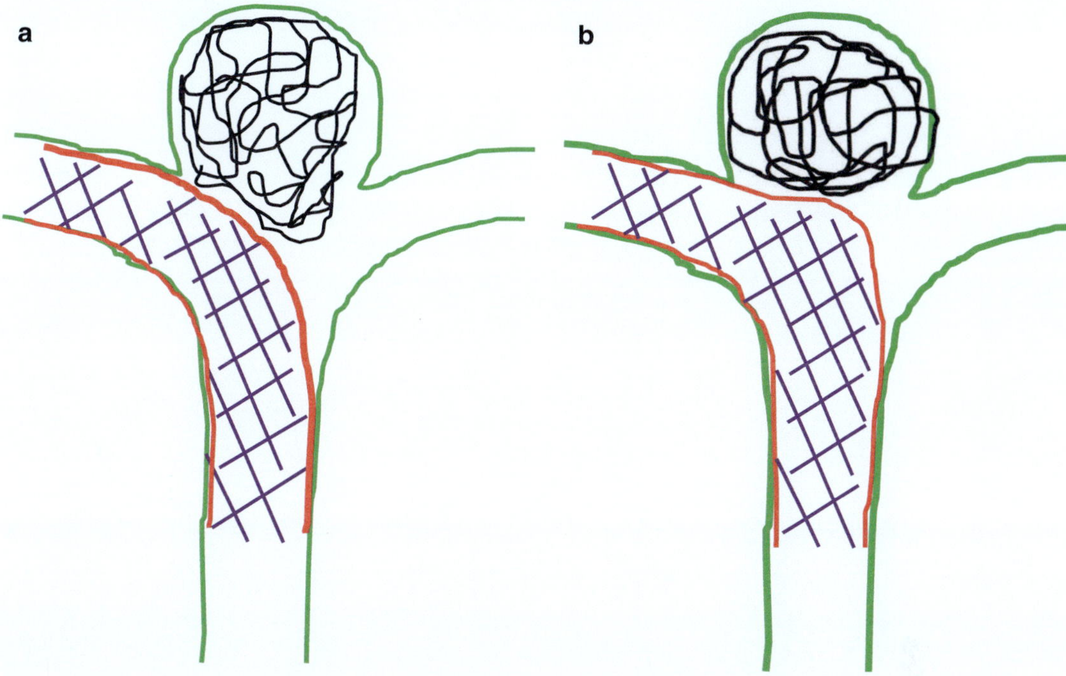

Fig. 21.2 (**a**)—Cartoon image showing stent delivered in regular manner by withdrawing the catheter. (**b**)—Stent delivered by "shelfing" technique. After partial deployment of stent across the neck, microcatheter and the stent delivery wire were advanced to further open the stent at the level of the neck, achieving considerable more coverage of the aneurysmal neck

Suggested Reading

Yen Du EH, et al. LVIS Jr 'shelf' technique: an alternative to Y stent-assisted aneurysm coiling. J Neurointerv Surg. https://doi.org/10.1136/neurintsurg-2015-012246.

Y Stenting and Coil Embolisation of Broad-Based Aneurysm Using LVIS Jr. Stents

22

Ajit S. Puri and Rajsrinivas Parthasarathy

Case

A young lady with a broad-neck left MCA aneurysm. Frontal and lateral angiograms demonstrate the aneurysm. Three-dimensional images show the aneurysm size and the size of the MCA branches (Figs. 22.1 and 22.2). Plan is to do Y stenting and coil embolisation of the aneurysm sac.

Issue

- The aneurysm neck is incorporating the bifurcation and both divisions, more so the superior division. Therefore, simple coiling cannot be attempted.
- Treatment options include a single stent and coil and Y stent and coiling. Can single stent and coil be attempted? One can deploy the stent in the superior division and try to provide an effective scaffold by attempting a 'shelfing' technique. However, it may not be possible to achieve an effective scaffold and coil prolapse into the inferior division can occur.
- Y – Stent can be technically challenging; in particular, crossing through the struts to deploy the second stent may not always be possible.
- The superior division is circumferentially involved; therefore, coil overlap onto the stent is to be expected. Henceforth, the choice of stent and coil should be such that coil prolapse into the parent artery through the cell does not occur.

Management

Y stenting with coil placement was attempted under general anaesthesia. Two guide catheters were parked in the ICA: a 6F at the cavernous ICA and 5F at the distal cervical ICA. The distally placed 6 F guiding catheter was used for the coiling microcatheter as it provided stability and better one-to-one response. The superior MCA division was catheterised with a Headway 17 microcatheter over a Synchro2 microwire (Fig. 22.3). The SL10 microcatheter was then placed into the aneurysm sac; loop of the framing coil was advanced into the aneurysm. Following that, the LVIS Jr. stent was then deployed spanning from the superior division MCA to the M1 MCA. Once deployed, the

A. S. Puri (✉)
Radiology, and Neurosurgery,
Division of Neurointerventional Surgery,
Neurointerventional Fellowship Program,
University of Massachusetts Medical Center,
Worcester, MA, USA
e-mail: ajit.puri@umassmemorial.org

R. Parthasarathy
Vascular Neurology and Neurointerventional Surgery,
Artemis Agrim Institute of Neuroscience,
Gurgaon, India

V. Gupta et al. (eds.), *100 Interesting Case Studies in Neurointervention: Tips and Tricks*,
https://doi.org/10.1007/978-981-13-1346-2_22

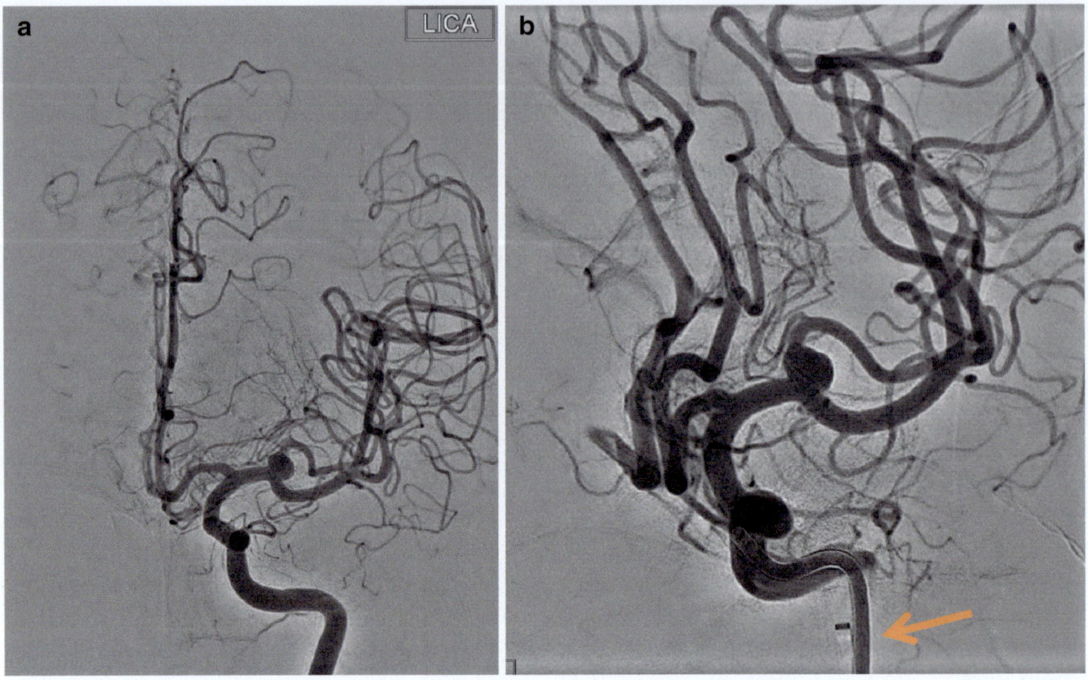

Fig. 22.1 (**a**) Showing the left MCA bifurcation aneurysm. (**b**) Note the two guide catheters in the ICA for the intervention. Usually one is a 6F and one is a 5F guide catheter. The one which is more distal/stable is used for the coiling microcatheter (provides stability and better one-to-one response)

same Headway 17 was advanced into the proximal stent over the deployment wire. The Synchro2 wire was used to access the inferior division of the MCA. Then 'Y stenting' was performed by deploying another LVIS Jr. stent from the inferior division to the M1 MCA (Fig. 22.4). The coiling was then completed (Fig. 22.5).

Tips and Tricks

1. Separate guiding catheters offer advantage in that the jailed microcatheter movement during stent deployment is less likely during the 'push and pull' movement needed to deploy the stent.
2. Stent delivery microcatheter is first placed in the most difficult to catheterise branch. The superior division of the MCA tends to originate at reverse angle from the main MCA trunk and is often the difficult branch to catheterise.
3. The coiling microcatheter is then navigated through the most distally placed guiding catheter to have a better 'one-to-one' control over the microcatheter. Following that, the initial loops of the framing coils are deployed as measure to avoid inadvertent catheter perforation due to forward movement during stent deployment.
4. The delivery wire should be visualised at all times to avoid wire perforation.
5. The microcatheter should be advanced over the delivery wire after stent deployment into

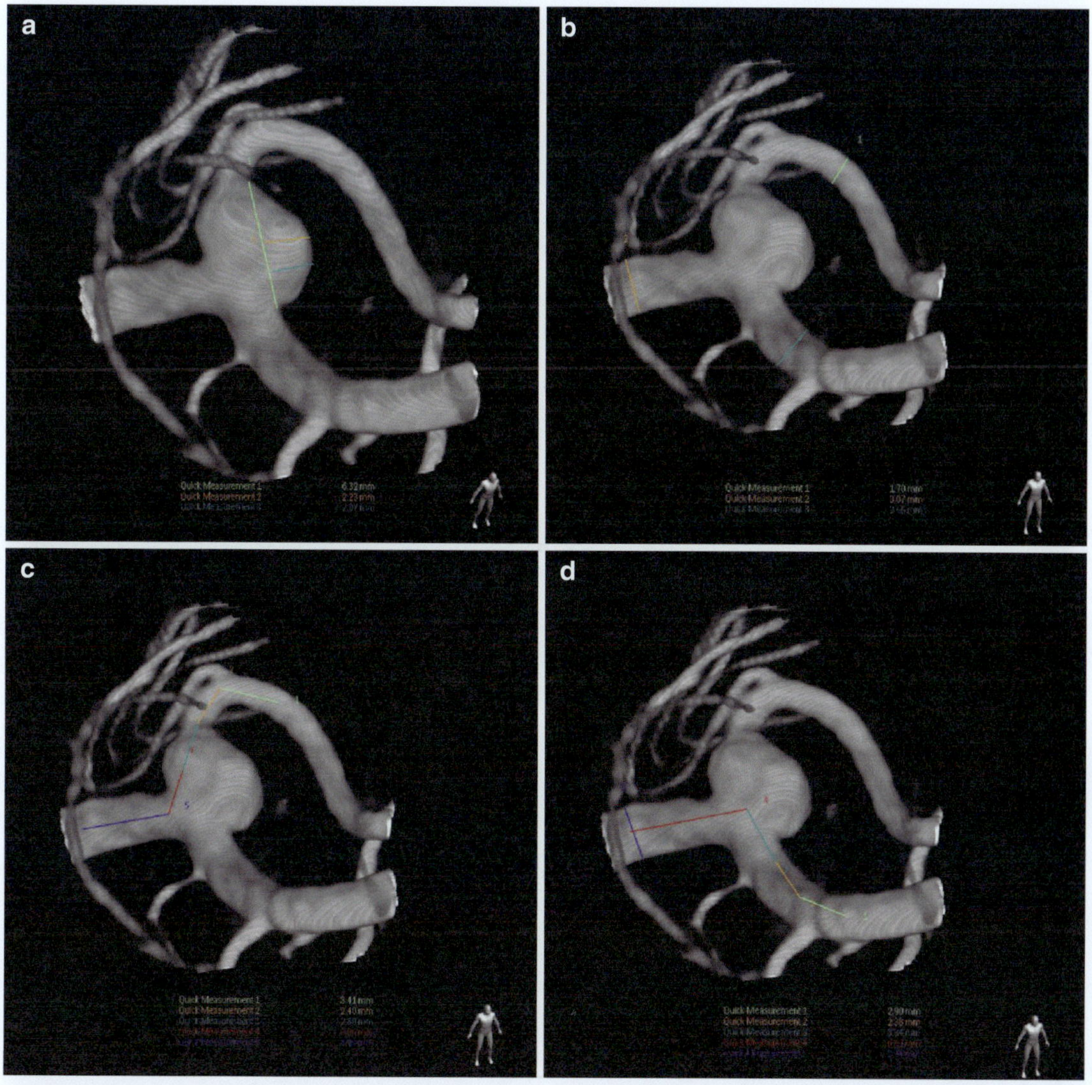

Fig. 22.2 (**a–d**)—Showing the geometry of the aneurysm and measurements

the proximal aspect of the deployed stent. This negates the need for recrossing the proximal end of the stent with the delivery microcatheter over a microwire.

6. Crossing through the struts can be challenging. Use a 0.014′ microwire to avoid the 'edge' effect, i.e. if a thinner wire is used it may not support the catheter and the tip of catheter can get stuck against the strut due to the dead space between the wire and the microcatheter.
7. The second stent should be sized such that the minimum possible diameter should be equivalent to the diameter of the initial stent.
8. Micro-stents are delivered through a 0.017′ catheter and therefore relatively easier to navigate through struts.

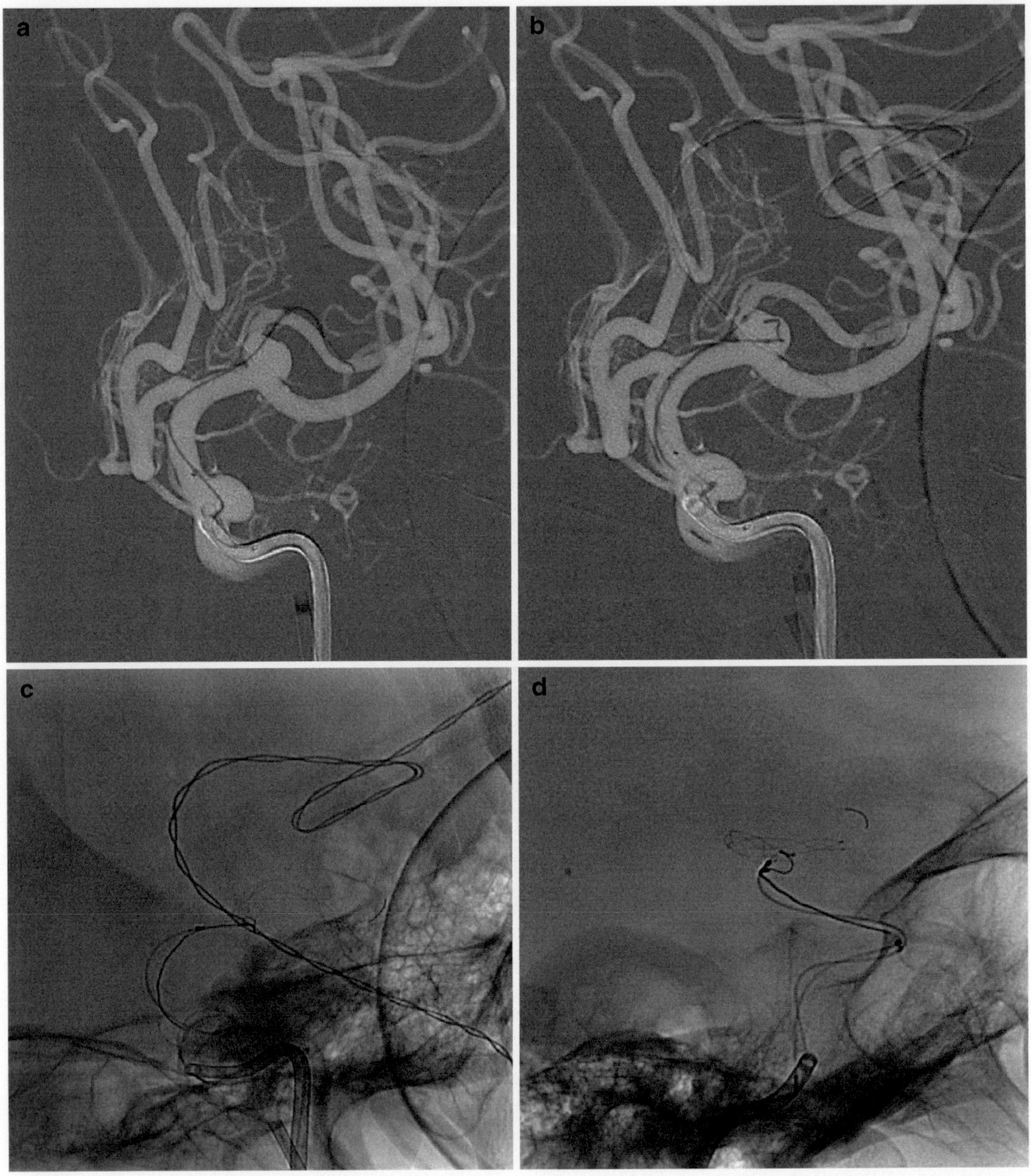

Fig. 22.3 (**a**)—The superior MCA division was catheterized with a Headway 17 microcatheter over a Synchro2 microwire. (**b**)—The SL10 microcatheter was then placed into the aneurysm sac; loop of the framing coil was advanced into the aneurysm. (**c**, **d**)—Due to the wide neck, the LVIS Jr. stent was then deployed spanning from the superior division MCA to the M1 MCA

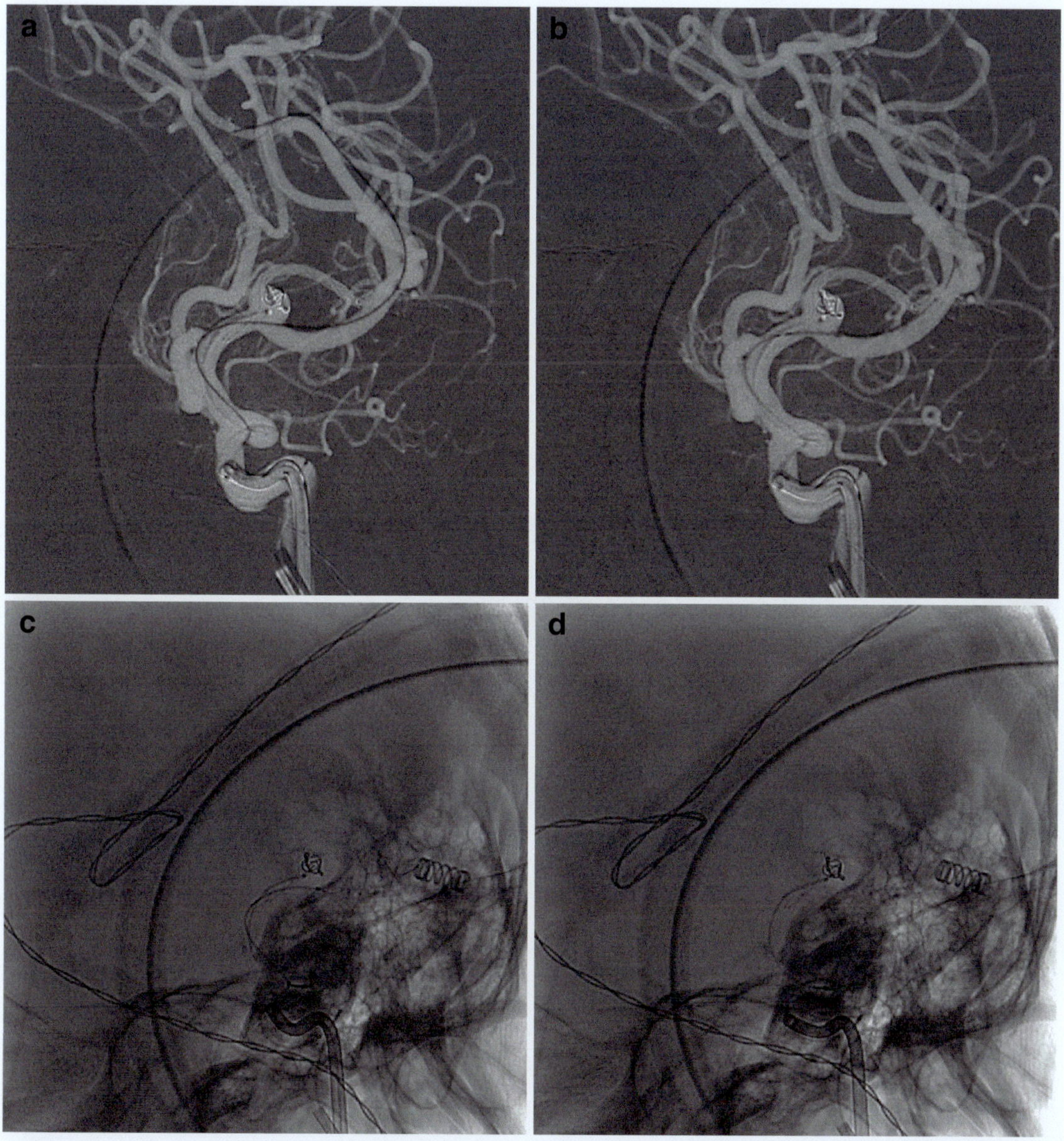

Fig. 22.4 (**a**, **b**)—The Headway 17 is advanced into the proximal stent over the deployment wire. Then Synchro2 wire is again used to access the inferior division of the MCA. (**c**, **d**)—The "Y stenting" is then performed using another LVIS Jr. stent. Then coiling is then finished

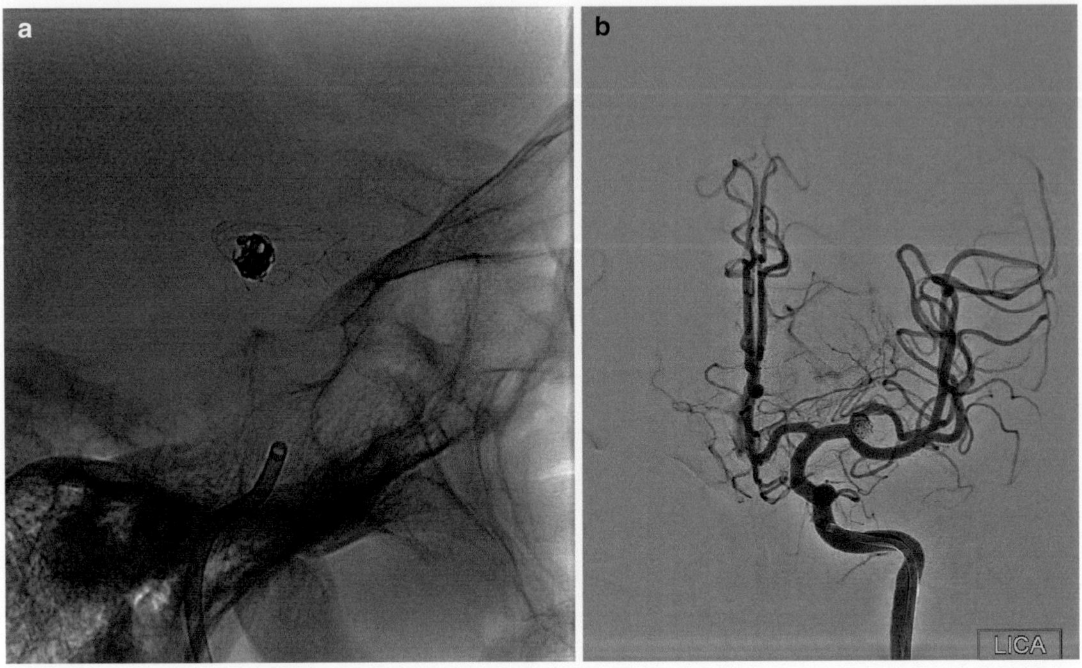

Fig. 22.5 (**a**, **b**)—Unsubtracted and subtracted images showing the final result

Suggested Reading

Conrad MD, et al. Y stenting assisted coiling using a new low profile visible intraluminal support device for wide necked basilar tip aneurysms: a technical report. J Neurointerv Surg. 2014;6(4):296–300.

Balloon-Assisted Catheter Access in Large and Giant Aneurysms

23

Ajit S. Puri and Rajsrinivas Parthasarathy

Case

A 45-year-old female was noted to have an incidental large broad-based supraclinoid ICA aneurysm. Flow diverter placement was contemplated as it was a dysplastic broad-based fusi-saccular supraclinoid ICA aneurysm.

Issue

The aneurysm sac is noted arising from the supraclinoid ICA; it is located in the segment of the ICA where there is an acute bend resulting in the inflow jet being directed away from the distal vasculature. Crossing the aneurysm sac and accessing the distal vasculature can be challenging as the sac has a broad neck; is arising from the posteromedial wall, the wall that would give the support while navigating the catheter; and is circumferentially involving the wall of the ICA wall (Figs. 23.1 and 23.2).

A. S. Puri (✉)
Radiology, and Neurosurgery,
Division of Neurointerventional Surgery,
Neurointerventional Fellowship Program,
University of Massachusetts Medical Center,
Worcester, MA, USA
e-mail: ajit.puri@umassmemorial.org

R. Parthasarathy
Vascular Neurology and Neurointerventional Surgery,
Artemis Agrim Institute of Neuroscience,
Gurgaon, India

Management

Flow diverter placement was planned under general anaesthesia. A 6F guiding catheter was placed in the proximal cavernous ICA. It was anticipated that crossing the sac can be challenging based on the assessment of the geometry of the aneurysm. Therefore, the microwire was looped through the sac and was followed with the microcatheter. Once the microcatheter was taken distally, an exchange length Excelerator—10 (ev3, Irvine, USA) microwire was used to take the Hyperform balloon (ev3, Irvine, USA) into the MCA (Fig. 23.3). The balloon was inflated, and the whole system was gently pulled back to straighten the loop. A 0.010′ wire may not provide the necessary support to navigate a 0.027′ microcatheter; therefore, a SL 10 microcatheter (Stryker Neurovascular, CA, USA) was taken across the sac, and the 0.010′ microwire exchanged for a 0.014′ exchange length Synchro 0.014′ wire (Stryker Neurovascular, CA, USA). Following that an XT 27 (Stryker Neurovascular, CA, USA) microcatheter was taken across the sac over the Synchro exchange wire (Fig. 23.4). After that a pipeline embolisation device was deployed across the neck of the sac (Fig. 23.5).

V. Gupta et al. (eds.), *100 Interesting Case Studies in Neurointervention: Tips and Tricks*,
https://doi.org/10.1007/978-981-13-1346-2_23

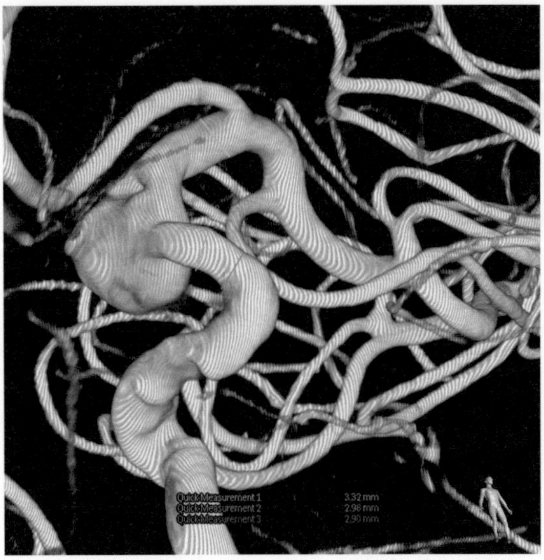

Fig. 23.1 3D angiogram demonstrates a large supraclinoid ICA aneurysm

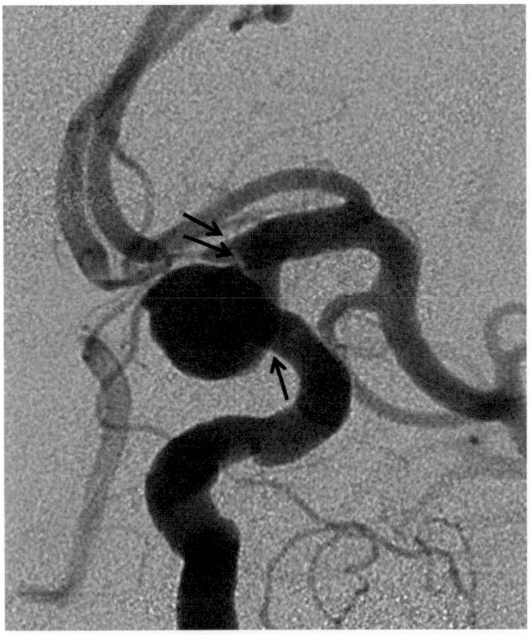

Fig. 23.2 Note the inflow (*single black arrow*) and the outflow (*double black arrows*) make direct catheterisation of the distal vasculature difficult

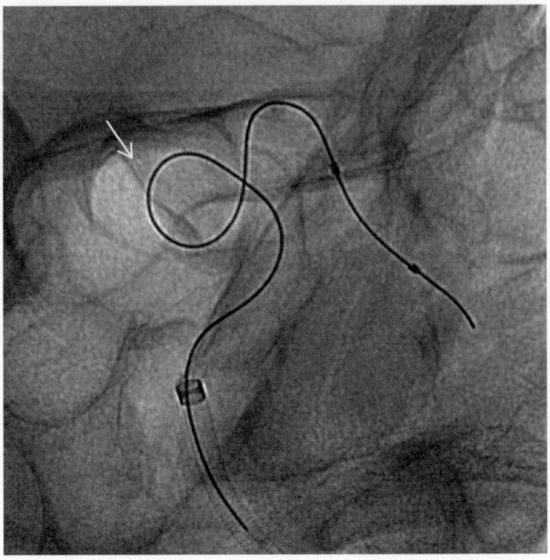

Fig. 23.3 HyperForm balloon looped inside the catheter, balloon in the left MCA (*white arrow*)

Tips and Tricks

1. In large and giant aneurysms with a broad neck and unfavourable geometry, accessing the distal vasculature can be extremely difficult. In unruptured aneurysm, one can try to loop the microwire within the sac of the aneurysm and gain access to the distal artery. The inflow jet would direct the microwire into the sac and the flow dynamics in the sac is likely to guide the wire to the outflow. A trick would be trying the superior wall of the sac initially; if this does not provide the mechanical advantage to access the distal artery, one can try the lateral wall.
2. Use a soft and curved tip thin (0.014′) microwire to do the looping manoeuvre to avoid injury to the wall of the sac.
3. A small calibre microcatheter (Echelon 10/SL 10) with a curve at the tip is generally preferred as it tends to navigate over the loop with relative ease.

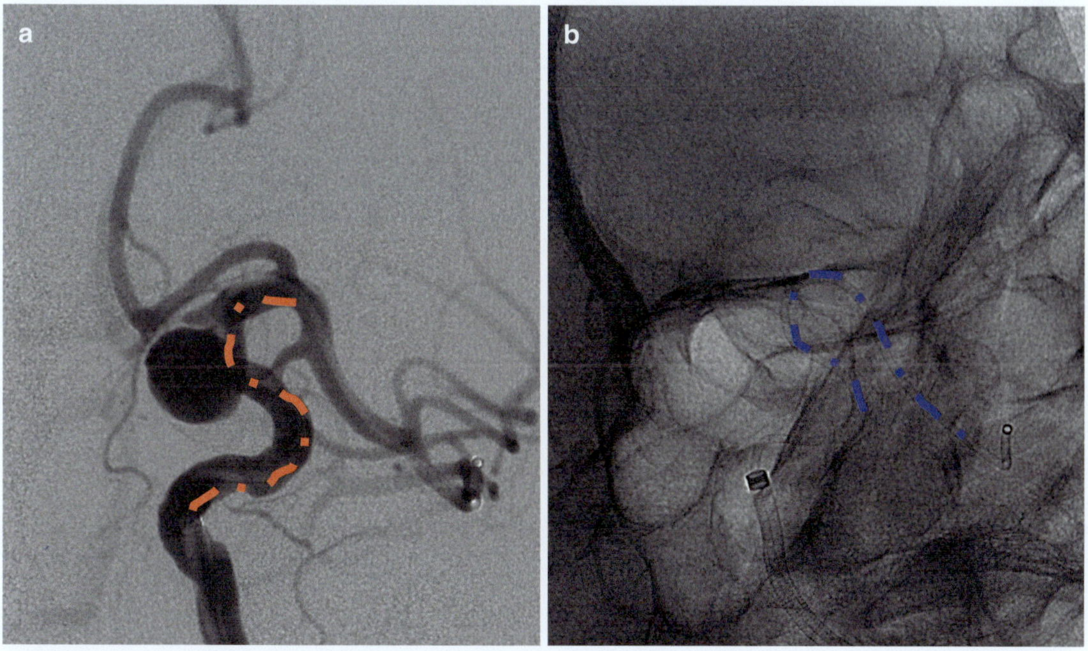

Fig. 23.4 (**a**, **b**) XT27 now in the distal left MCA without a loop inside the catheter

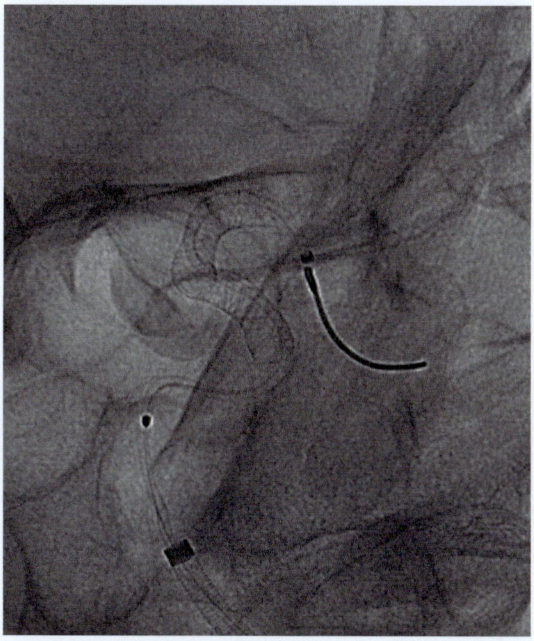

Fig. 23.5 Pipeline embolisation device has been deployed across the aneurysm

4. A 0.010′ exchange length wire was used in our case as it was compatible with Hyperform (ev3, Irvine, USA) balloon; however, a 0.010′ wire may not offer the necessary support to navigate a larger bore microcatheter that is needed to deploy a flow diverter. To avoid multiple exchanges, one can use a dual-lumen balloon (Scepter XC 4-11, Microvention, Tustin, California, USA) that is compatible with a 0.014′ wire.
5. Distal wire access (as distal as possible) is maintained during exchanges as it allows for the stiffer part of the wire to be across the neck of the aneurysm sac. This offers the necessary support while navigating the microcatheter across and prevents inadvertent proximal migration of the wire.

Suggested Reading

Peeling L, et al. Balloon-assisted guide catheter positioning to overcome extreme cervical carotid tortuosity: technique and case experience. J Neurointerv Surg. 2014;6(2):129.

Stent Retriever-Assisted Access

24

Ajit S. Puri and Rajsrinivas Parthasarathy

Case

A 45-year-old male with chronic headache was diagnosed with an unruptured large left supraclinoid aneurysm. Flow diverter placement to treat the large supraclinoid ICA aneurysm was planned.

Issue

The aneurysm sac is noted arising from the supraclinoid ICA; it is located in the segment of the ICA where there is an acute bend resulting in the inflow jet being directed away from the distal vasculature. Crossing the aneurysm sac and accessing the distal vasculature can be extremely challenging as the sac has a broad neck; is arising from the posteromedial wall, the wall that would give the support while navigating the catheter; and is circumferentially involving the wall of the ICA wall (Figs. 24.1 and 24.2).

A. S. Puri (✉)
Radiology, and Neurosurgery,
Division of Neurointerventional Surgery,
Neurointerventional Fellowship Program,
University of Massachusetts Medical Center,
Worcester, MA, USA
e-mail: ajit.puri@umassmemorial.org

R. Parthasarathy
Vascular Neurology and Neurointerventional Surgery,
Artemis Agrim Institute of Neuroscience,
Gurgaon, India

Management

Flow diverter placement under general anaesthesia was undertaken. A 6 F guiding catheter was placed in the petrous ICA. It was anticipated that crossing the sac can be challenging based on the assessment of the geometry of the aneurysm. Therefore, the 0.014′ microwire was looped through the sac and was followed with the microcatheter (SL 10, Stryker Neurovascular, CA, USA) into the distal vasculature (Fig. 24.3). Once the microcatheter was taken distally, an exchange length 0.014′ microwire was used to take Prowler Select microcatheter (ev3, Irvine, USA) into the MCA. Following that, a Solitaire 4 × 20 mm stent (ev3, Irvine, USA) was navigated to the MCA (Fig. 24.4). The stent was partly deployed in the MCA to provide for the necessary anchorage to allow for the straightening of the microcatheter by gently pulling back on the system. The Solitaire stent was removed, and a 0.014′ exchange length microwire was used to navigate Marksman 0.027′ microcatheter (ev3, Irvine, USA). A SL 10 microcatheter (Stryker Neurovascular, CA, USA) was used to catheterise the sac. The sac was partly filled with coils, and the Pipeline embolisation device was deployed across the aneurysm sac (Fig. 24.5). No complications were encountered, and the patient recovered.

V. Gupta et al. (eds.), *100 Interesting Case Studies in Neurointervention: Tips and Tricks*,
https://doi.org/10.1007/978-981-13-1346-2_24

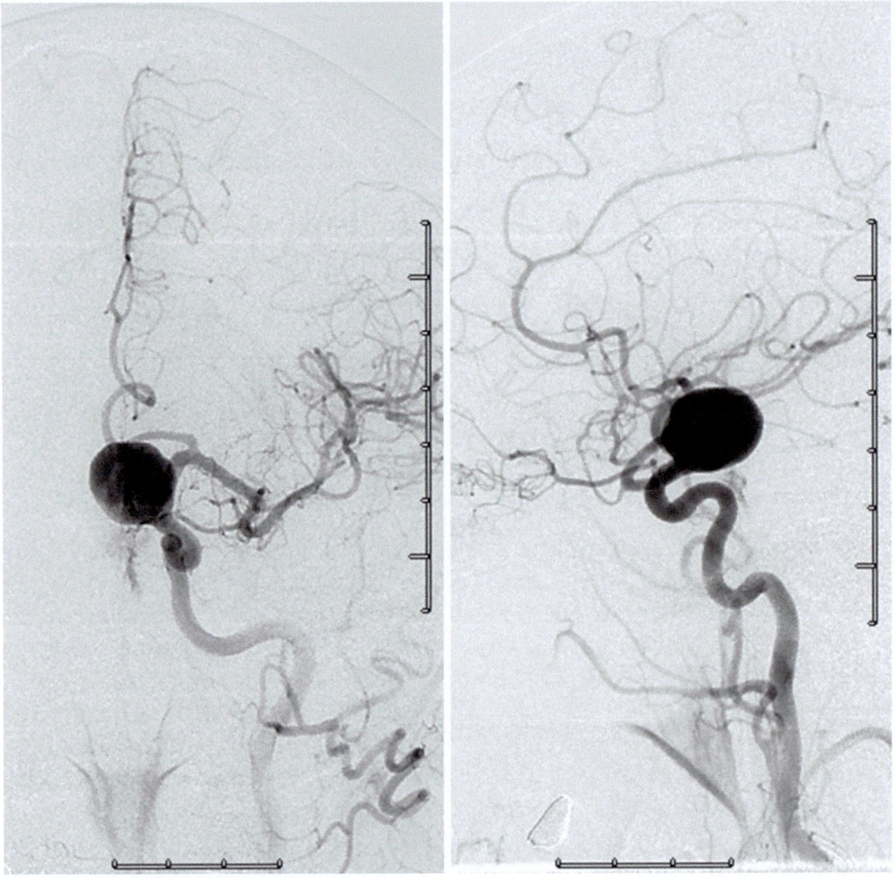

Fig. 24.1 Frontal and lateral angiograms show a large left supraclinoid ICA aneurysm (Case courtesy: Dr. Jasmeet Singh, Wake Forest University, NC, USA)

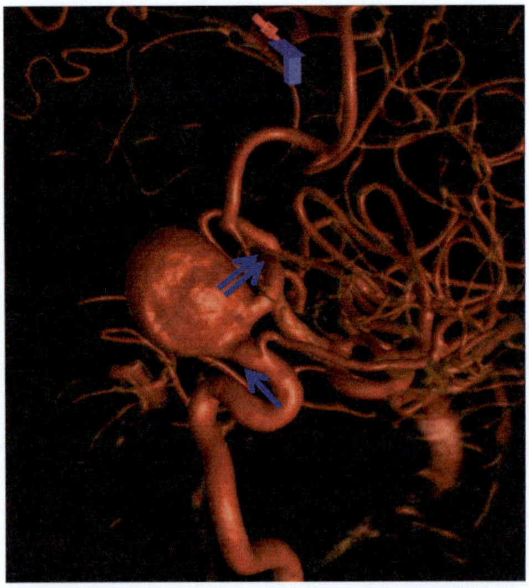

Fig. 24.2 3D angiogram shows the inflow (*single arrow*) and the outflow (*double arrows*) close by making direct catheterisation of the distal MCA vasculature difficult (Case courtesy: Dr. Jasmeet Singh, Wake Forest University, NC, USA)

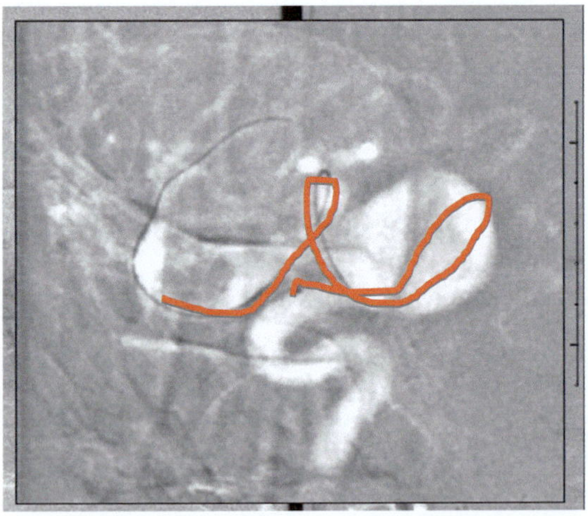

Fig. 24.3 Road map images show the course of the microcatheter-microwire loped inside the aneurysm with the distal wire in the M2 MCA (Case courtesy: Dr. Jasmeet Singh, Wake Forest University, NC, USA)

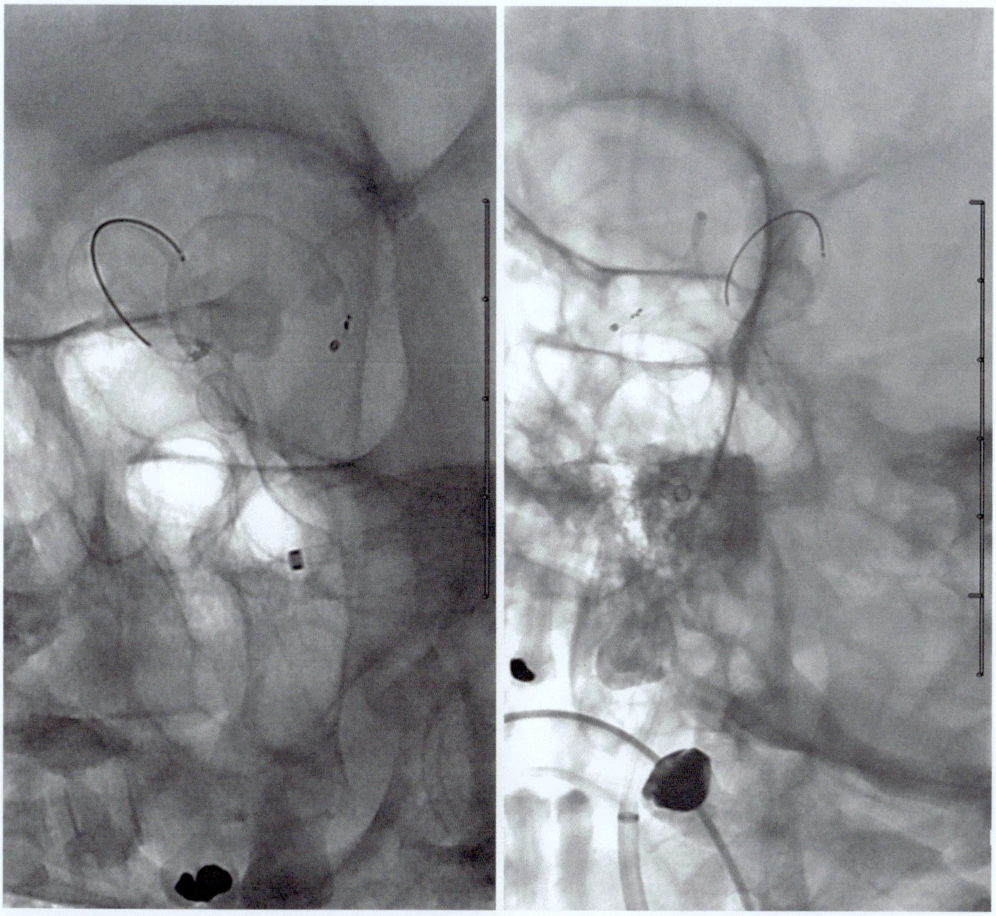

Fig. 24.4 The Solitaire 4 × 20 mm stent noted within the stent delivery microcatheter (Case courtesy: Dr. Jasmeet Singh, Wake Forest University, NC, USA)

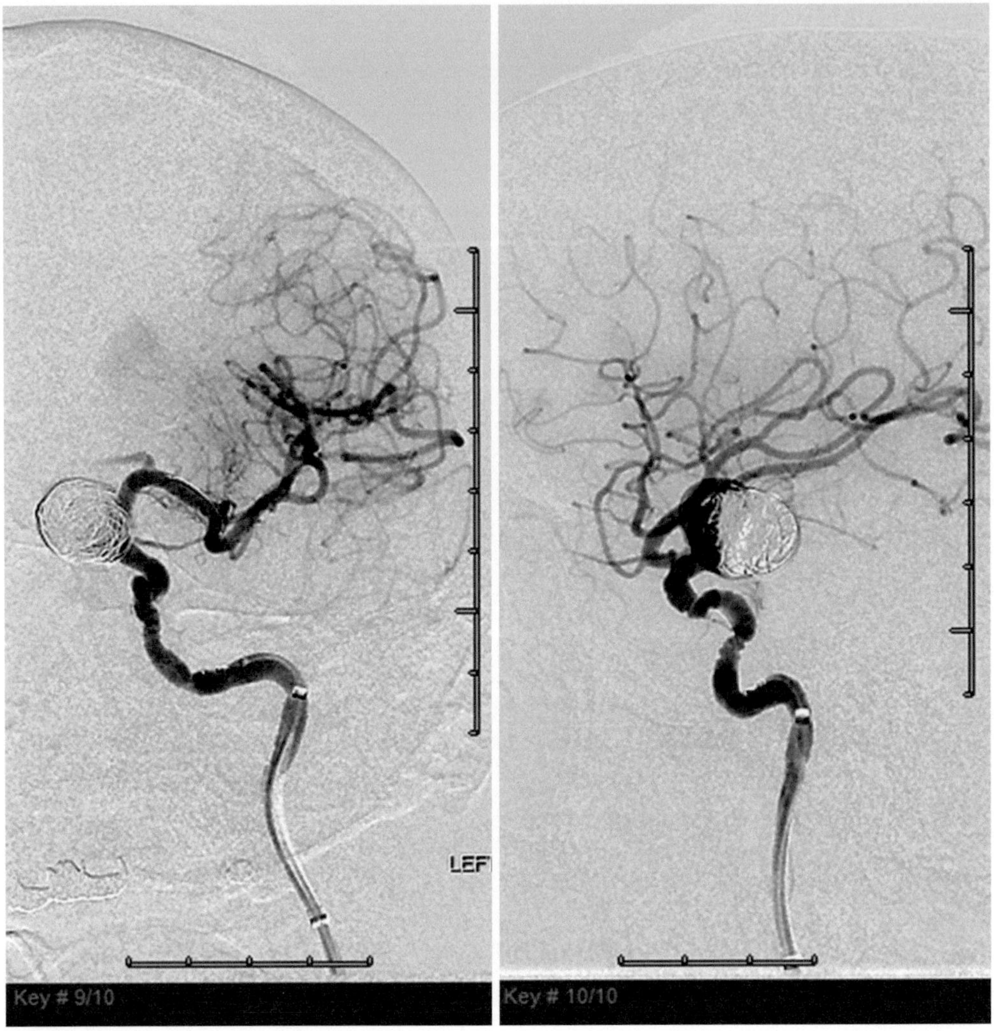

Fig. 24.5 In this case a PED was deployed covering the aneurysm neck along with some coils inside the aneurysm (Case courtesy: Dr. Jasmeet Singh, Wake Forest University, NC, USA)

Tips and Trick

1. In unruptured large aneurysm, one can try to loop the microwire within the sac of the aneurysm and gain access to the distal artery. The inflow jet usually directs the microwire into the sac, and the flow dynamics in the sac is likely to guide the wire to the outflow.
2. A trick would be trying the superior wall of the sac initially; if this does not provide the mechanical advantage to access the distal artery, one can try the lateral wall.
3. Use a soft and curved tip thin (0.014′) microwire to do the looping manoeuvre to avoid injury to the wall of the sac.
4. A small calibre microcatheter (0.017′) with a curve at the tip is generally preferred as it tends to navigate over the loop with relative ease.
5. A 0.014′ exchange length microwire is used to take the stent microcatheter distally into the MCA. An exchange length platinum tip transcend 0.014′ wire offers the necessary support proximally at the aneurysmal segment and at the same time has distal soft atraumatic tip.

6. An exchange length Synchro 0.014′ microwire may not offer the necessary support and therefore is advisable to take the wire as distally possible so that the stiffer part is across the aneurysm segment.
7. The stent microcatheter, usually a Prowler Select 0.021′ (Codman Neurovascular) or Rebar 18 (ev3, Irvine, USA), is navigated to the MCA.
8. The Solitaire stent is deployed in a straight segment in the M1 MCA. A nondetachable Solitaire stent is preferred as it offers reasonable radial force and good wall opposition; it is likely to provide the necessary distal anchorage required to unloop the microcatheter by pulling back on the system.

Suggested Reading

Singh J, et al. Anchor technique: Use of stent retrievers as an anchor to advance thrombectomy catheters in internal carotid artery occlusions. Interv Neuroradiol. 2015;21(6):707–9.

Quadri-axial Technique to Gain Access for Flow Diverter Deployment

25

Rajsrinivas Parthasarathy and Vipul Gupta

Case

A 64-year-old lady presented with headaches, facial pain, and left ptosis. Investigation revealed giant left internal carotid artery (ICA) aneurysm (Fig. 25.1). DSA and 3D angiography showed a wide-neck aneurysm. Inadequate flow across anterior and posterior communicating arteries was seen, and the case was planned for flow diverter stent placement (Surpass, Stryker).

Issues

1. Aortic ectasia and tortuosity.
2. Loop in proximal ICA.
3. To deliver Surpass catheter, one may require to cross the aneurysm with the distal access catheter.

Management

The procedure was performed under general anaesthesia. Access to the left CCA was difficult as the guiding catheter would not navigate into the distal left CCA. A SIM2 catheter was used to access the left CCA. Following that, an Amplatz extra stiff exchange wire was used to exchange the SIM2 catheter with a coaxially advanced 5F Vert and 8F Neuron Max (Penumbra .041″ Alameda, California, USA) (Fig. 25.2). The 0.057 DAC was coaxially navigated across the loop in the proximal ICA over a 0.038 DAC to the petrous ICA (Fig. 25.3a–d). The efferent artery was accessed by looping a Traxcess wire within the aneurysm sac. Following that an Echelon 10 microcatheter (ev3 Inc., Irvine, California, USA) was navigated into the distal artery (Fig. 25.4a). A docking wire was used, and the Echelon 10 exchanged with a dual lumen balloon catheter Scepter XC 4 × 11 mm (Microvention, Tustin, California, USA) (Fig. 25.4b). The balloon was navigated to the middle cerebral artery. The balloon was inflated at the M1 segment of MCA, and the loop within the sac straightened (Fig. 25.4c). Thereafter, the attempt to navigate a 0.057 DAC across the aneurysm neck over a XT 27 microcatheter failed due to the dead space between the catheters resulting in the edge of the 0.057 DAC (Concentric Medical) getting stuck at the aneurysm neck. Henceforth, the 0.057 DAC was taken coaxially across the neck over a 0.038 DAC and 0.021 Prowler select microcatheter. Following that the Surpass flow diverter was deployed across the aneurysm sac. Post-deployment there was significant flow reduction into the aneurysm sac (Fig. 25.4d–f).

R. Parthasarathy (✉)
Vascular Neurology and Neurointerventional Surgery, Artemis Agrim Institute of Neuroscience, Gurgaon, India

V. Gupta
Neurointerventional Surgery, Stroke unit, Artemis Agrim Institute of Neuroscience, Gurgaon, India
e-mail: vipul.gupta@artemishospitals.com

V. Gupta et al. (eds.), *100 Interesting Case Studies in Neurointervention: Tips and Tricks*,
https://doi.org/10.1007/978-981-13-1346-2_25

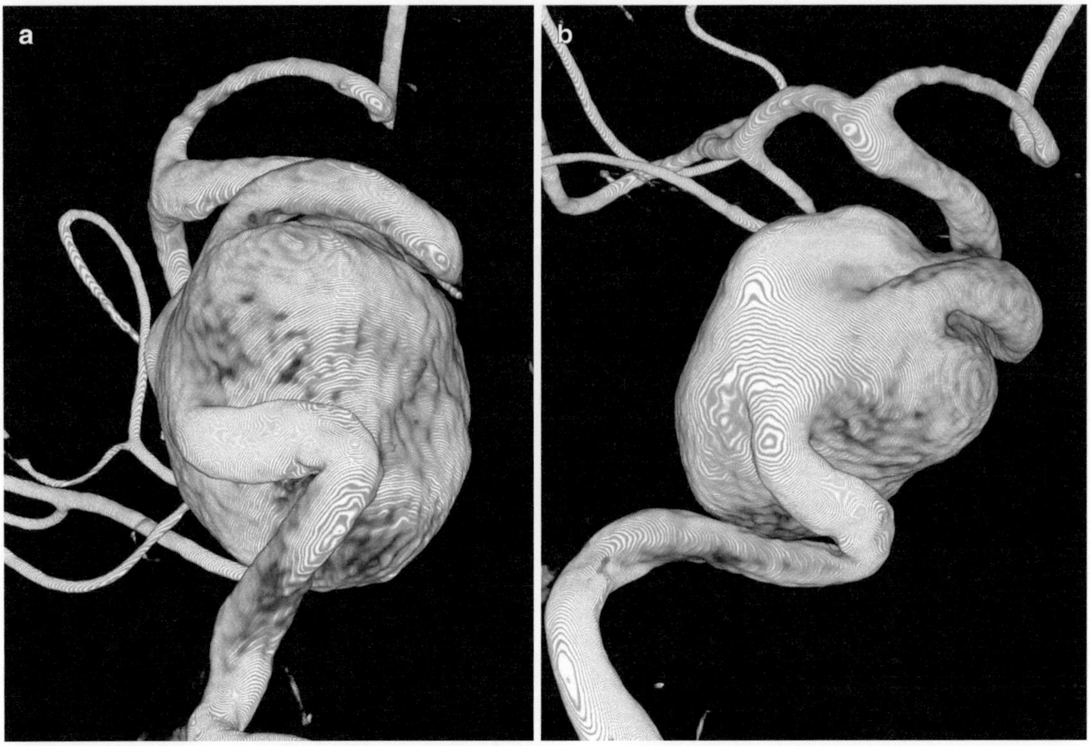

Fig. 25.1 (**a**, **b**)—3D angiography images showing a broad-neck giant aneurysm of cavernous ICA

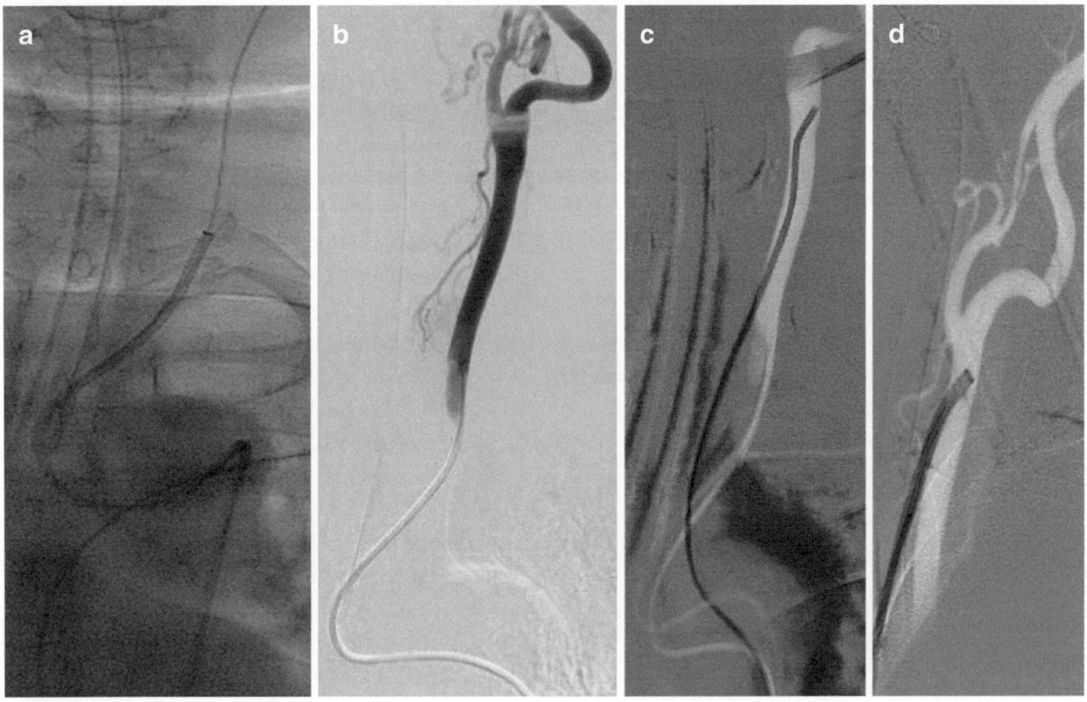

Fig. 25.2 Manoeuvres for placement of long sheath on common carotid artery. (**a**)—Image showing attempt of placing the guiding catheter, which was unsuccessful because of aortic tortuosity. (**b**)—SIM 2 catheter used to hook the left common carotid artery. (**c**)—The catheter navigated into distal CCA. (**d**)—Exchanged with long sheath (Neuron MAX, 6F)

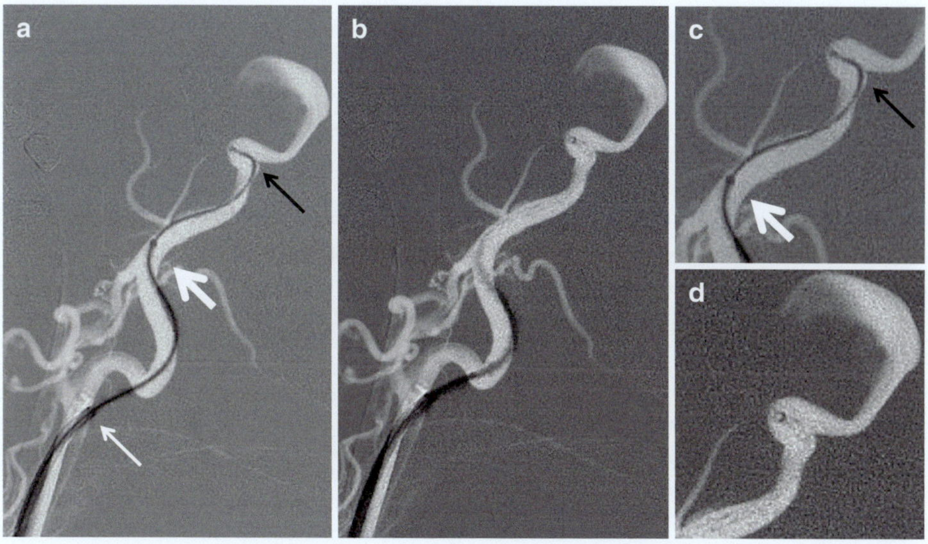

Fig. 25.3 (**a**)—Navigation of 5F DAC in left ICA. (**a**)—A DAC 057 (*thick white arrow*) was placed through the sheath (*thin white arrow*). It was navigated through the loop in the ICA in a coaxial manner using a DAC 038 (*black arrow*). (**b**)—Distal position of DAC 057. (**c**, **e**)—magnified images of (**a**) and (**b**)

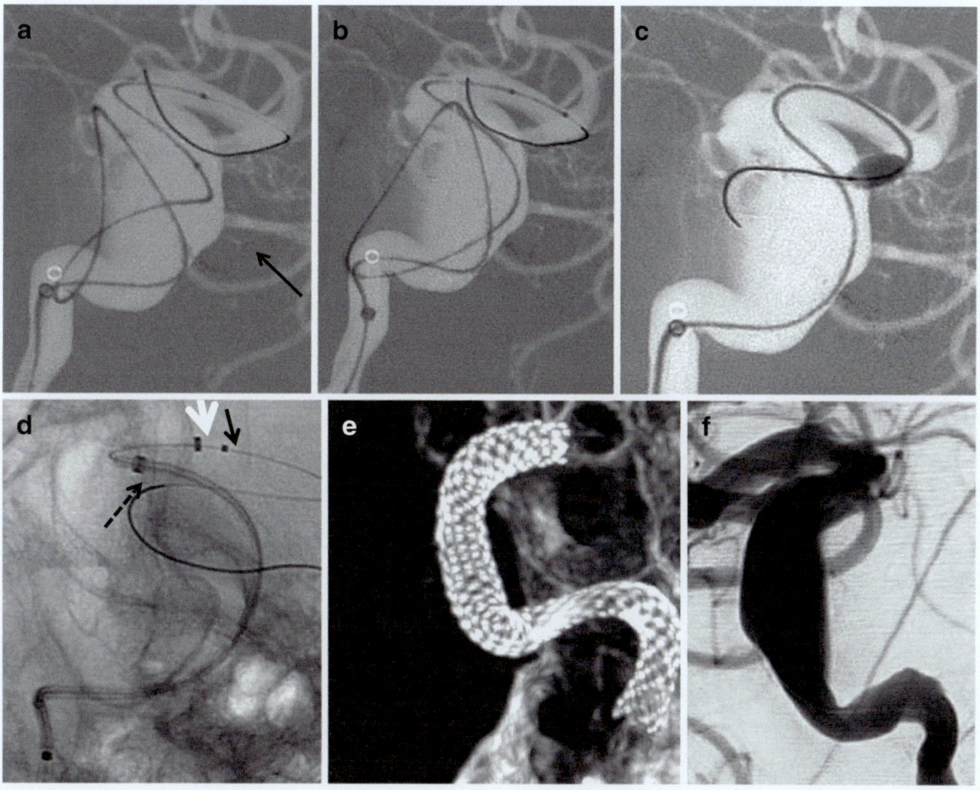

Fig. 25.4 Navigation of catheter beyond the aneurysm and delivery of stent. (**a**)—Microcatheter navigated into the left middle cerebral artery after forming a loop in the aneurysm. (**b**)—Exchanged with a balloon catheter. (**c**)—Straightening of balloon catheter with inflated balloon stabilizing the distal position. (**d**)—Navigation of DAC 057 (*dashed arrow*) over a DAC 038 (*white arrow*) which was placed in left MCA over a Prowler 21 microcatheter (*black arrow*) using a microguidewire. (**e**, **f**)—Flow diverter across the aneurysm. (**f**)—DSA showing significant slowing of flow in aneurysm

Tips and Tricks

1. Accessing the left CCA in a type 3 aortic arch can be extremely challenging. Use a SIM2 catheter to access the left CCA. Forward movement of the SIM2 catheter is possible only if there is a wire stiff enough to allow forward movement of the proximal curve into the left CCA. An Amplatz extra stiff wire usually gives the necessary support to perform an exchange with the sheath.
2. A coaxial snugly fitting catheter will eliminate the dead space between the catheters and allows for easy navigation of large-bore catheters across the aneurysm neck into the efferent artery.
   (a) A suggested quadri-axial system to access distal ICA/ MCA would be:
   - 0.014′ micro wire, 0.021′ Prowler Select/ Rebar 18, 0.038 DAC, 0.057 DAC

   (b) A suggested quadri-axial system to navigate proximal tight loops in the ICA:
   - 0.014′ microwire, 0.027′ XT 27/Rebar 27, 0.044 DAC, 0.070 DAC

Suggested Reading

Hauck EF, et al. Use of the outreach distal access catheter as an intracranial platform facilitates coil embolization of select intracranial aneurysms: technical note. J Neurointerv Surg. 2011;3(2):172–6.

Lin L-M, et al. Pentaxial access platform for ultra-distal intracranial delivery of a large-bore hyperflexible DIC (distal intracranial catheter): A technical note. Neurosurgery. 2016;6:29–34.

Multiple Blister Aneurysm of ICA: Management by Pipeline Device

26

Vipul Gupta

Case

A 52-year-old female presented with subarachnoid haemorrhage (Hunt and Hess grade II; Fisher grade III). DSA (Fig. 26.1a–c) revealed a fusiform aneurysm of left ICA at the level of PCOM artery with a prominent bulge on ventral aspect of ICA. There was another small ICA aneurysm in the paraclinoidal segment. A third, very small aneurysmal bulge was seen arising from posterior aspect of left ACA.

Issue

- Treating a blister-like aneurysm with fusiform dilatation of the parent vessel that is not easily amenable to usual endovascular techniques such as balloon- or stent-assisted coiling.
- Although the largest of the aneurysms had most likely bled, in view of uncertainty it was advisable to treat other aneurysms as well.

Management

We planned to deploy the flow diverter (FD) device extending from the proximal left M1 MCA to the cavernous ICA in order to cover both the ICA aneurysms and the origin of the ACA. As there was a good-sized ACOM artery, covering the origin of the left ACA is likely to result in significant flow reduction in the ipsilateral A1 ACA and consequent regression of the ACA aneurysm. Two hours before the procedure, loading dose of antiplatelet agents was given (Tab Ecosprin 150 mg and Tab Prasugrel 50 mg). A long sheath (Cook medical, Bloomington, USA) was placed in the left common carotid artery. A 6F guiding catheter (Chaperon, Microvention, Tustin, California, USA) was placed in petrous segment of ICA. Pipeline delivery microcatheter was taken to M2 segment of left MCA over microguidewire (Traxcess, Microvention, Tustin, California, USA). A relatively shorter curve given to the tip of the wire avoided wire entry into the aneurysm sac. This was followed by pipeline deployment (Fig. 26.1d). Post-stenting angiogram did not reveal any gross change in filling of the aneurysms (Fig. 26.1e, f). Repeat check angiogram was performed up to 20 min after the procedure to look for thromboembolism. AngioCT (DynaCT, Siemens, Erlangen) didn't reveal fresh bleed. Patient was extubated in intact clinical condition and made complete recovery. A follow-up angiogram (Fig. 26.2) was performed after 2 months, which revealed complete occlusion of both of the ICA aneurysms. Minimal filling of left ACA was seen with regression of the aneurysm. Left ACA was seen to fill from right ICA injections.

V. Gupta
Neurointerventional Surgery, Stroke unit, Artemis Agrim Institute of Neuroscience, Gurgaon, India
e-mail: vipul.gupta@artemishospitals.com

V. Gupta et al. (eds.), *100 Interesting Case Studies in Neurointervention: Tips and Tricks*,
https://doi.org/10.1007/978-981-13-1346-2_26

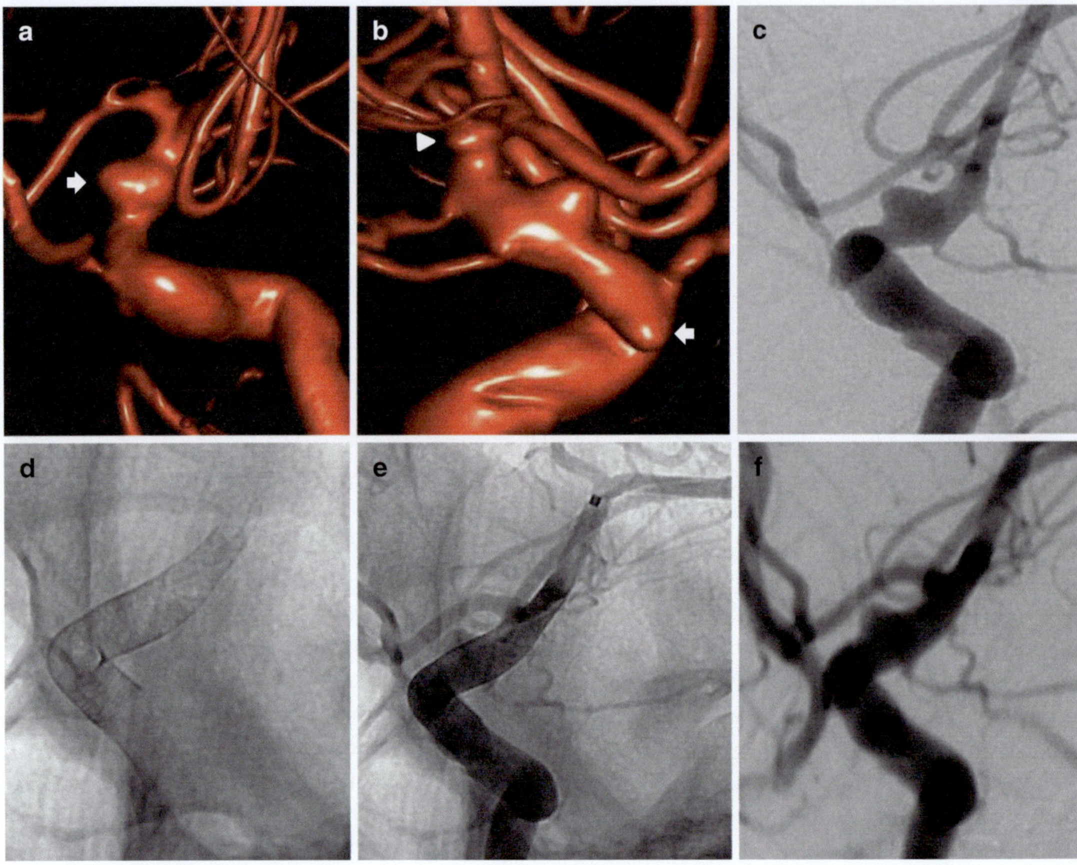

Fig. 26.1 (**a**, **b**) 3D reconstructed images show a fusiform aneurysm of supraclinoid ICA at the level of PCOM with a prominent ventral bulge (*arrow*, **a**). Another very small aneurysmal bulge seen from A1 segment of right ACA (*arrowhead* **b**). Small aneurysm also seen in right ICA paraclinoidal segment pointing medially (*arrow*, **b**). (**c**) DSA in working projection. (**d**) Pipeline reconstruction device. (**e**) Native image showing good opposition of the flow diverter to the arterial wall. (**f**) Post-stenting DSA shows persistent filling of the aneurysm

Tips and Tricks

1. Ruptured blisters are difficult to treat surgically. They are difficult to clip with high rates of intraoperative rupture.
2. Endovascular management in the past required single/overlapping stent or stent with coil placement. Despite treatment, continued growth and re-rupture was seen.
3. Recent reports indicate good clinical and morphological outcomes with parent artery reconstruction with flow diverter devices.
4. Placement of FD required antiplatelet therapy. The need for an external ventricular drain should be evaluated prior to loading with antiplatelet. We prefer to time administration of antiplatelet agents in such a way that the maximal platelet inhibition occurs at the time of FD device deployment. This avoids the risk of premature antiplatelet-related aneurysmal bleed. For the newer ADP antagonists (prasugrel and ticagrelor), we administer the drugs 2 h prior to expected device deployment.
5. There is an option of treating difficult aneurysms of A1 segment of ACA by flow diversion technique provided the ACOM artery is patent
6. We prefer to do an early check angiogram in these cases to document the status of aneurysm.

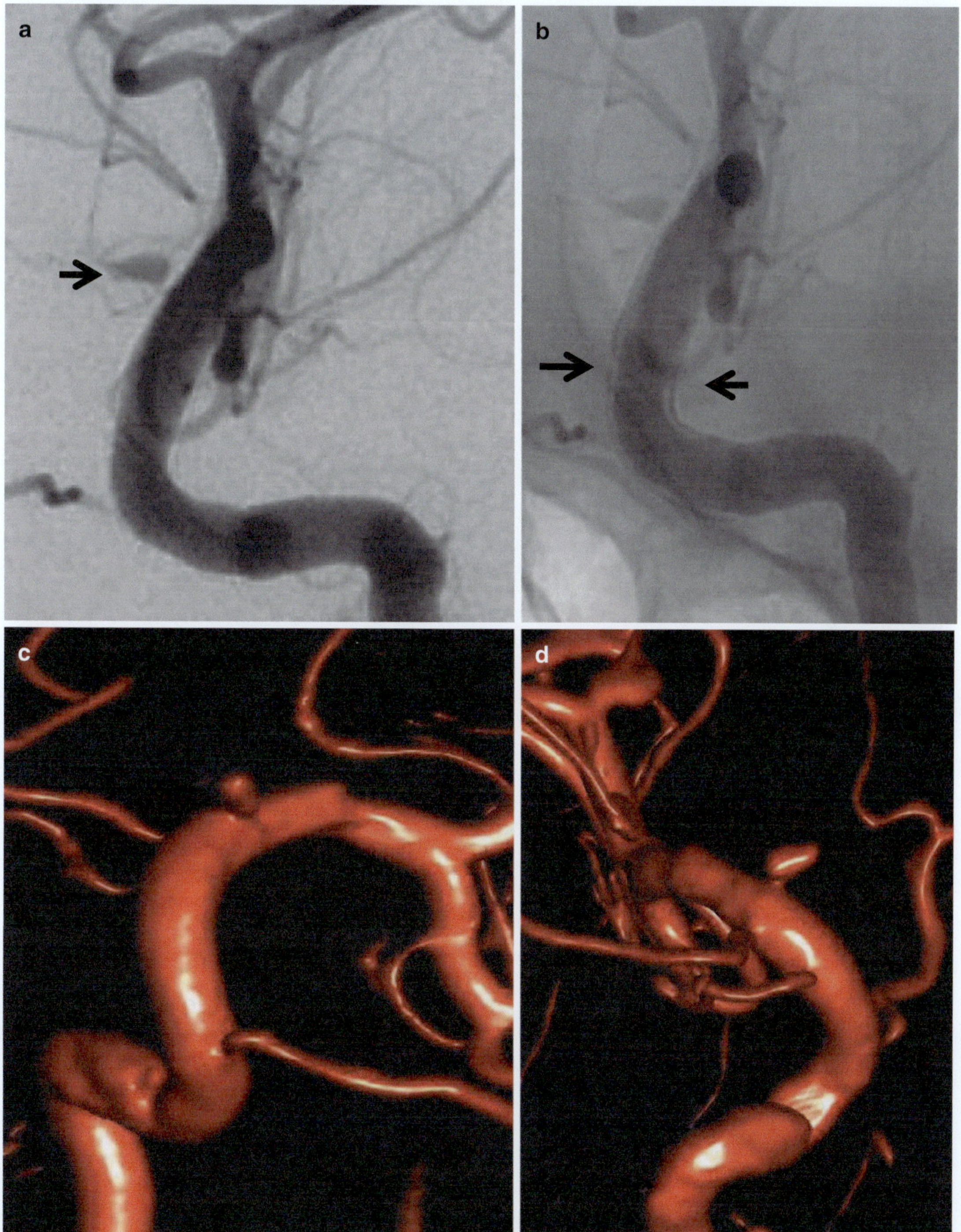

Fig. 26.2 Follow-up angiogram. (**a**) DSA shows complete occlusion of the fusiform aneurysm. Minimal filling of left ACA seen. (**b**) Native image of DSA shows intimal growth over the stent. (**c**, **d**) 3D reconstructed images show complete occlusion of the ICA aneurysms with minimal opacification of ACA

Suggested Reading

Burrows AM, Cloft H, Kallmes DF, Lanzino G. Periprocedural and mid-term technical and clinical events after flow diversion for intracranial aneurysms. J Neurointerv Surg. 2015;7(9):646–51.

Fargen KM, Hoh BL. Flow diversion technologies in evolution: a review of the first 4 generations of flow diversion devices. World Neurosurg. 2014;81(3–4):452–3.

Tse MM, Yan B, Dowling RJ, Mitchell PJ. Current status of pipeline embolization device in the treatment of intracranial aneurysms: a review. World Neurosurg. 2013;80(6):829–35.

27 Long Flow Diverter (FD) in Partly Thrombosed Basilar Trunk Aneurysms

Aviraj Deshmukh, Rajsrinivas Parthasarathy, and Vipul Gupta

Case

A 21-year-old male presented with headache for 5 years and recent episodes of short-lasting right-sided weakness. MRI was suggestive of acute lacunar infarct in the right medulla along with partly thrombosed fusiform proximal basilar artery aneurysm (Fig. 27.1a). DSA showed a long-segment, fusiform basilar artery aneurysm (Fig. 27.1b).

Issues

- The perils with flow diversion in fusiform basilar trunk aneurysm are (a) progressive sac thrombosis with perforator occlusion and (b) wall weakening and rupture caused by wall thrombus triggering the inflammatory cascade.
- Long-segment aneurysm needing either a single long or overlapping FD.
- Timing of intervention in acutely symptomatic lesion, early vs. late.

Management

Antiplatelet loading was done a day before the procedure with Ecosprin (325 mg) and ticagrelor (180 mg). Procedure was done in general anaesthesia. An 8F Neuron Max (Penumbra Inc.) was advanced to the distal V2 segment of right vertebral artery. Following this 5F catalyst catheter (Stryker Neurovascular) was coaxially advanced over Traxcess wire (014) and XT-27 microcatheter (Stryker Neurovascular) into right PCA (Fig. 27.1c). Surpass 4 × 50 mm stent (Stryker Neurovascular) was deployed, with slowly withdrawing the FD outer catheter, the distal end of FD positioned in the distal basilar and proximal end in the distal right vertebral artery (Fig. 27.1d). Post-procedure run showed well-opened stent along with stasis in the aneurysm sac (Fig. 27.1e, f). Early post-procedure angiography revealed near complete exclusion of the aneurysm.

A. Deshmukh · V. Gupta
Neurointerventional Surgery, Stroke unit, Artemis Agrim Institute of Neuroscience, Gurgaon, India
e-mail: vipul.gupta@artemishospitals.com

R. Parthasarathy (✉)
Vascular Neurology and Neurointerventional Surgery, Artemis Agrim Institute of Neuroscience, Gurgaon, India

V. Gupta et al. (eds.), *100 Interesting Case Studies in Neurointervention: Tips and Tricks*,
https://doi.org/10.1007/978-981-13-1346-2_27

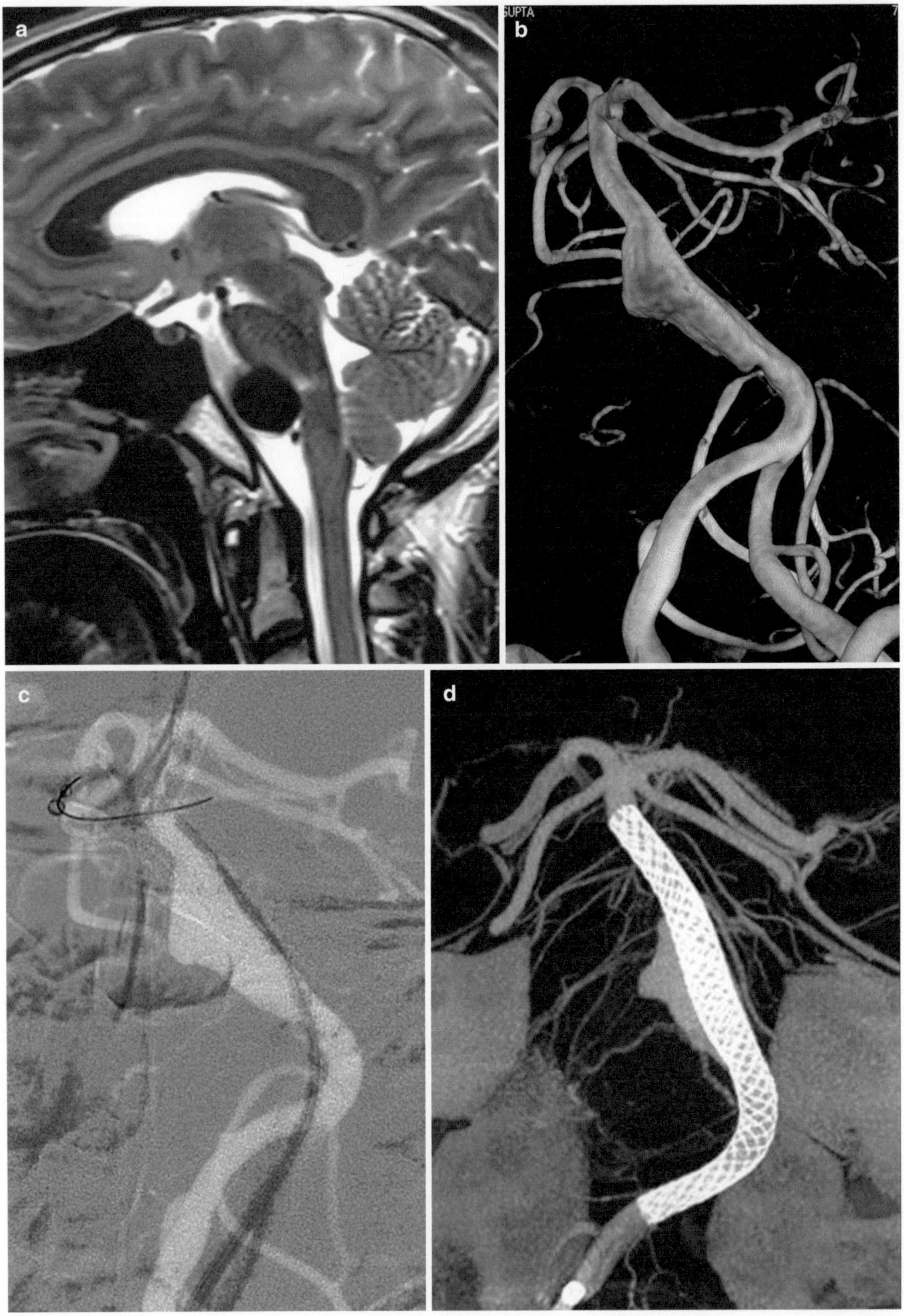

Fig. 27.1 (**a**) Partly thrombosed large basilar trunk aneurysm; (**b**) 3d rotation angiography showing a long-segment fusiform basilar aneurysm; (**c**) 5F catalyst across the aneurysm; (**d**) stent CT showing the deployed FD from the distal vertebral artery to the distal basilar artery. (**e**, **f**) Note stasis in the aneurysm sac post-stent deployment

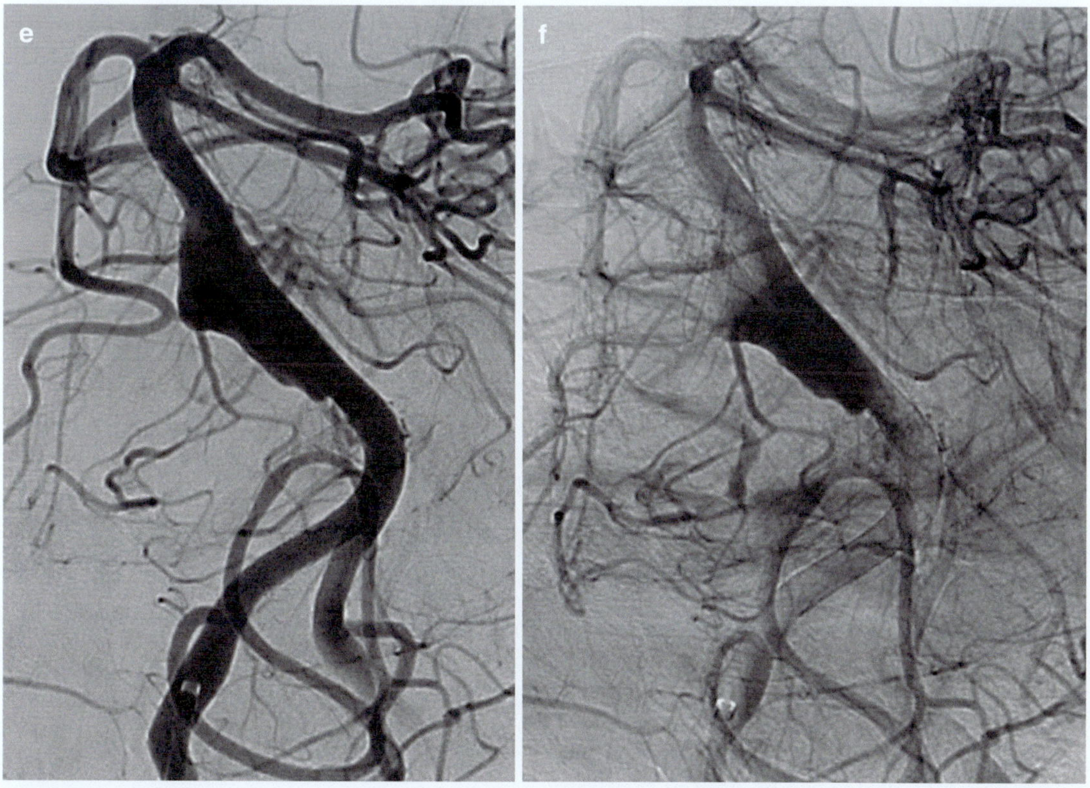

Fig. 27.1 (continued)

Tips and Tricks

1. Early intervention in acutely symptomatic lesion may be safe and therefore can be considered.
2. A single long FD is preferred over multiple devices deployed in a telescopic manner as it is technically less challenging, and there is less risk of perforator occlusion.
3. Surpass was favoured over the other devices for the following reasons:
   (a) A single 50 mm device can span across the entire length of the aneurysm.
   (b) More wires (72 wires in 4 mm device) provide a stable braid and therefore offer twist and kink resistance compared with the other devices which tend to kink and twist when the device diameter and/or the length increases.
   (c) Free wire access negates the risk of wire perforation.
4. Use of 5F catalyst catheter is necessary with Surpass FD due to stiff architecture of the device. Distal access with the 5F catalyst can be achieved by advancing it coaxially over microwire and 0.027′ microcatheter.
5. Three types of dissecting aneurysms have been described:
   (a) Type 1—acute disruption of internal elastic lamina (IEL); presents with SAH.
   (b) Type 2—fragmented IEL resulting in segmental ectasias and intimal thickening; no thrombus formation
   (c) Type 3—fragmentation of the internal elastic lamina, multiple dissections of thickened intima, and organized thrombus in the lumen
6. A type 3 aneurysm, as is the case in this patient, is usually symptomatic and tends to progress with time. Timely treatment with a carefully selected device can be lifesaving in such cases.
7. Delayed aneurysm rupture: Studies suggest a potential role of intra-aneurysmal thrombus in

the pathophysiologic mechanism of aneurysm rupture as the intra-luminal thrombus is a source of various proteases with high proteolytic activity which could participate in the degradation of the arterial wall and lead to aneurysm rupture.
8. Perforator occlusion: The diseased arterial segment generally tends to lack functional perforators. As long as the braid is well apposed to the wall of the normal arterial segment, perforator occlusion is less likely.
9. Ticagrelor was preferred over prasugrel as the risk haemorrhage was higher with prasugrel in a patient with ischemic stroke.

Surpass Flow Diverter (Strengths and Weakness)

- The number of braid wire increases with the increase in the diameter of the device; this offers twist and kink resistance across bends when larger diameter device is used.
- A single long device can be used in fusiform aneurysms involving long segments.
- The wire is backloaded onto the device; this offers the advantage of positioning the wire in a safe segment of the artery throughout the procedure.
- To deploy the device, a 5F intermediate catheter needs to be taken across the aneurysm sac. The availability of more easily navigable intermediate catheters has made this possible. This offers better control over stent delivery. However, in tortuous anatomy this can pose a problem as navigating a large bore catheter to the M1/M2 MCA can be challenging at times.

Suggested Reading

Rouchaud A, et al. Delayed haemorrhagic complications after flow diversion for intracranial aneurysms: a literature overview. Neuroradiology. 2016;58(2):171–7.

Taschner CA, et al. Surpass flow diverter for treatment of posterior circulation aneurysms. Am J Neuroradiol. 2017;38(3):582–9.

Wakhloo AK, et al. Surpass flow diverter in the treatment of intracranial aneurysms: a prospective multicentre study. Am J Neuroradiol. 2015;36(1):98–107.

28 Pipeline Flex Embolization Device for Treatment of Pericallosal Artery Aneurysm

Ajit S. Puri and Rajsrinivas Parthasarathy

Case

A 59-year-old female with incidental discovery of multiple cerebral aneurysms while undergoing workup for eye pain and headache. The patient is an active smoker. On angiogram, she was found to have a posterior communicating artery aneurysm of a fetal posterior cerebral artery, an anterior communicating artery, and a bilobed pericallosal aneurysm (Fig. 28.1a–c). The PCoM aneurysm was treated using dual microcatheter and balloon remodeling technique, and the ACoM aneurysm was coiled using standard single microcatheter technique. The anterior cerebral artery is of azygous variation (Fig. 28.1a).

Issue

It is paramount to protect the normal branch arising from the base of the aneurysm of the azygous anterior cerebral artery (ACA). There is no contralateral ACA. Hence, there is no possibility of supply to distal ACA via contralateral supply. There is the option to under-coil the aneurysm, leaving the base to keep the branch patent. However, that is a recipe for recurrence.

Management

Under general anesthesia, in a triaxial fashion, a Marksman microcatheter (150 cm) (ev3, Irvine, USA) was advanced in the distal ACA over a synchro 2 micro-guidewire. The angiogram and roadmap that shows the distal and proximal landing zone of the flow diverter device is used (Fig. 28.2a). Under high-quality biplane fluoroscopy, the Pipeline Flex device is advanced to the optimal site (Fig. 28.2b–d). The device was deployed via slow unsheathing only (different than normal Pipeline device deployment). After device deployment, the wire is slowly pulled back while paying special attention to see if there is interaction between the core wire and the distal braids of the device (usually seen better under un-subtracted fluoroscopy) (Figs. 28.3).

A. S. Puri (✉)
Radiology, and Neurosurgery,
Division of Neurointerventional Surgery,
Neurointerventional Fellowship Program,
University of Massachusetts Medical Center,
Worcester, MA, USA
e-mail: ajit.puri@umassmemorial.org

R. Parthasarathy
Vascular Neurology and Neurointerventional Surgery,
Artemis Agrim Institute of Neuroscience,
Gurgaon, India

V. Gupta et al. (eds.), *100 Interesting Case Studies in Neurointervention: Tips and Tricks*,
https://doi.org/10.1007/978-981-13-1346-2_28

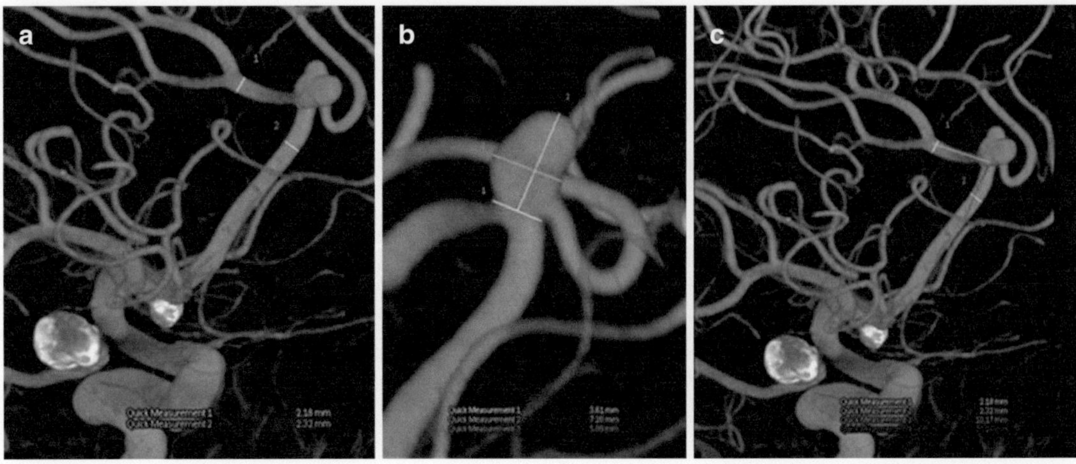

Fig. 28.1 (**a**) 3D angiogram shows the wide-necked pericallosal aneurysm with the callosomarginal artery arising from the aneurysm (like "bagpipe appearance"). (**b**, **c**) Shows the measurements of the parent vasculature

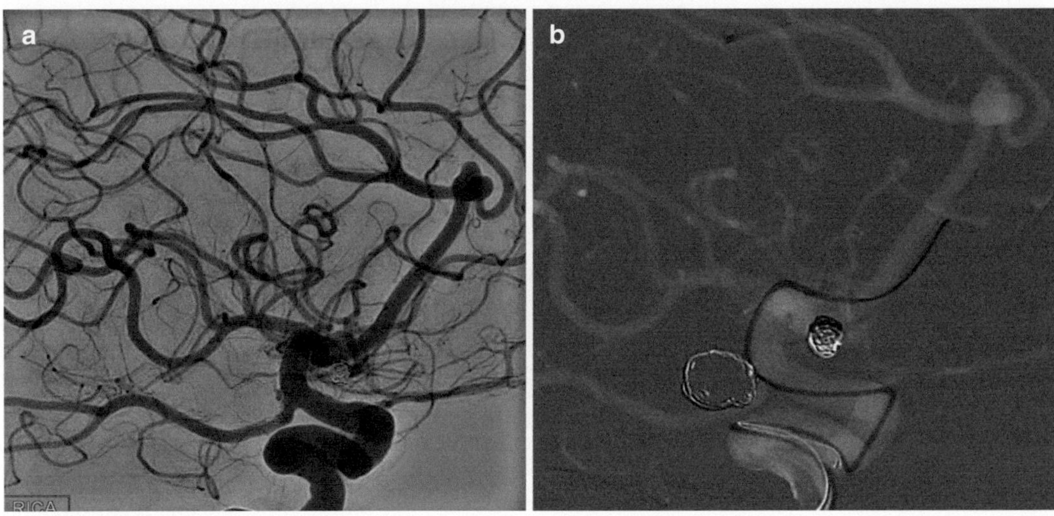

Fig. 28.2 (**a**) Is lateral angiogram, which shows the distal and proximal landing zone of the device. (**b**, **c**) Shows the sequential advancement of the PED flex to the site of future deployment. (**c**) Shows the distal tip of the microcatheter (*single arrow*), the distal boundary of the device (*double arrows*). Pay attention to the anatomy change from the device, seen by straightening of the vessel and change in the coil mass from the ACoM aneurysm (*yellow arrow*). (**d**) Shows the different segments of the PED flex device, distal wire (*single arrow*), distal boundary of the device (*double arrows*, remember the PTFE wings holding the distal edge are not radiographically visible), point to which re-sheathing is possible (*yellow arrow*), and proximal boundary of the device (*red arrow*)

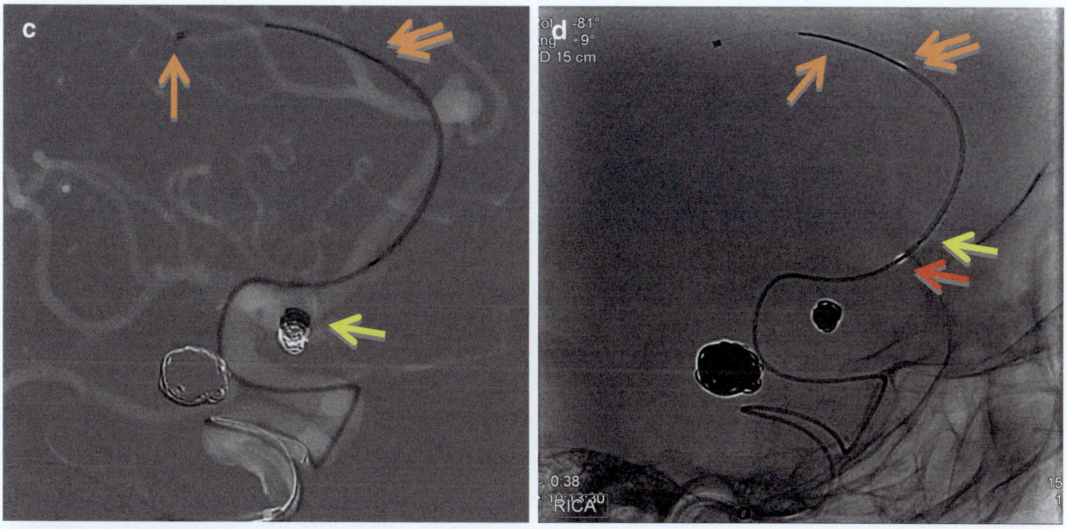

Fig. 28.2 (continued)

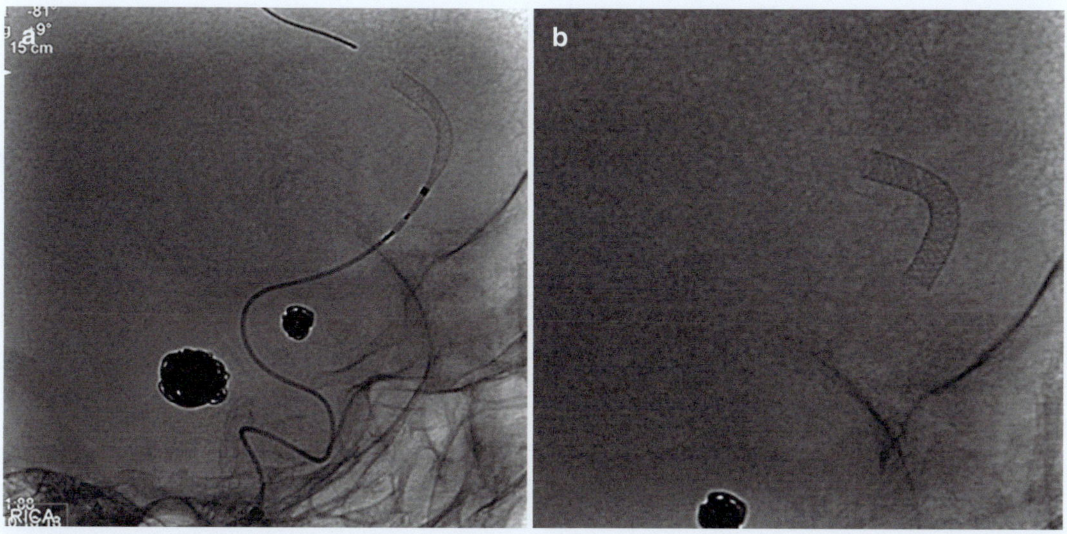

Fig. 28.3 (**a**) Shows the partial deployment (note the device can still be re-sheathed and repositioned). (**b**) Shows the final deployment. (**c**) Is lateral angiogram showing patency of all ACA branches and contrast stagnation within the aneurysm. (**d**) Is cone beam CT using dilute contrast medium demonstrating the placement of the device. This is very helpful to assess for wall apposition of the device (less of a concern in these smaller distal cerebral vessels)

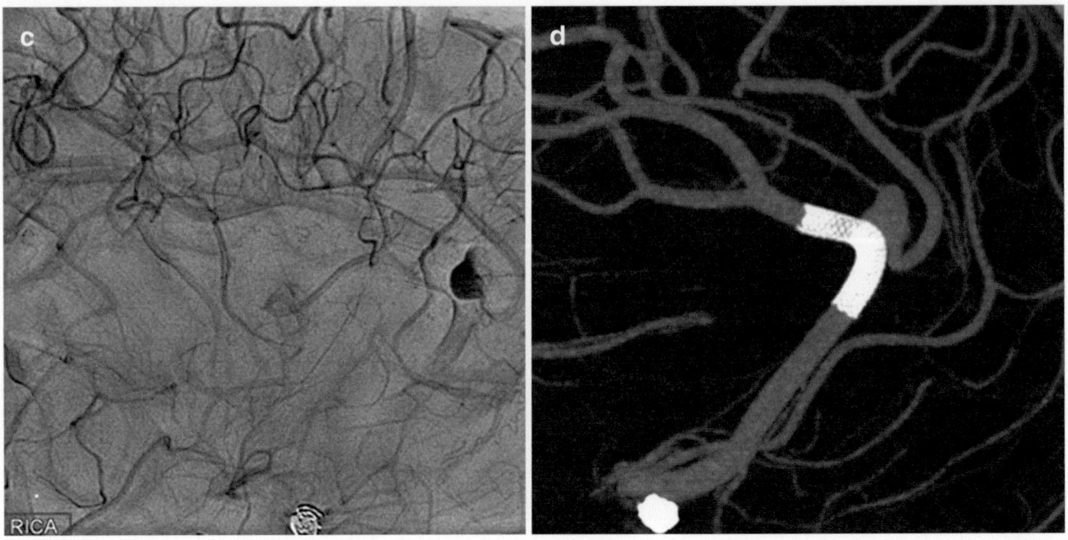

Fig. 28.3 (continued)

Tips and Tricks

1. Use strong proximal support, like a triaxial assembly, like 6F Cook shuttle sheath (this case) or 6F Neuron Max or 5/6 F Intermediate catheter (5F Navien 115 cm in this case).
2. Pay special attention to the vascular anatomy change after advancing the device distally, which can change the roadmap, which was used for navigation of the microcatheter.
3. Use un-subtracted images with bony landmarks to deploy the device.
4. Deploy flow diverters slowly. They are not stents!

Pipeline Flex Device Pearls (Strengths and Weaknesses)

Distal guidewire is 15 mm long, and the distal tip is curved to avoid inadvertent entry into a small vessel during device deployment. *Tip of the distal wire can be shaped further if required.*

Be aware that 7–14 mm of the device may need to be exposed before full expansion of the distal end.

Torquing the delivery wire is strictly not allowed.

PTFE sleeves overlap the distal edge of the stent and offer protection to the leading edge of the stent during the initial deployment. In case one has to re-sheath the device, do not re-sheath the distal end/edge of the stent. The PTFE sleeves tend to flare out after the initial deployment, and therefore do not offer protection to the distal end of the stent during repeat deployment.

The re-sheath marker is approximately 3 mm distal to the proximal marker band. Always aim to re-sheath by withdrawing the delivery wire into the delivery catheter, rather than pushing (advancing) the catheter over the wire.

Suggested Reading

Pereira VM, Kelly M, et al. New pipeline flex device: initial experience and technical nuances. J Neurointerv Surg. 2015;7:920–5. https://doi.org/10.1136/neurintsurg-2014-011347.

Puri A, et al. E-042 use of flow diverters in vessels less than 2.5 mm during intracranial aneurysm treatment. J Neurointerv Surg. 2014;6(Suppl 1):A57.

29 Feeding Artery Recurrent Aneurysm Treated with a p64 Flow Diverter

Hans Henkes and Marta Aguilar Pérez

Case

This 38-year-old woman had a history of occasional partial and complex seizures associated with a large brain AVM of the left frontal and temporal lobe. In October 2015, MRI showed a minor SAH as the reason of severe headache (Figs. 29.1 and 29.2). An aneurysm of the left ICA at the origin of the left AchoA, which among other vessels supplied the AVM, was occluded with coils (Figs. 29.3 and 29.4). A reperfusion of this aneurysm was found only 2 months later (Fig. 29.5). A second coil occlusion of the aneurysm was carried out another 3 months later (Fig. 29.6). The brain AVM was partially embolized and was irradiated with a CyberKnife in May 2016. Six weeks later, severe headache and an increased frequency of seizures occurred. MRI and DSA revealed a hematoma in the left frontal lobe, an early obliteration of a significant part of the AVM and again a recurrent perfusion of the AchoA aneurysm (Fig. 29.7). The aneurysm was obliterated in third coil procedure (Fig. 29.8). Follow-up DSA after only 4 weeks again showed a reperfusion of the aneurysm (Fig. 29.9a). The origin of the left AchoA and the aneurysm were now covered by a p64 flow diverter (Fig. 29.9b–d). After 3 months the aneurysm was still partly perfused, and within the p64 a minor in-stent stenosis was visible (Fig. 29.10). The 9-month follow-up DSA confirmed the complete occlusion of the AchoA aneurysm, the resolution of the in-stent stenosis, and only a minor residual AV-shunt with the most part of the AVM being obliterated after embolization and radiosurgery (Fig. 29.11).

Issue

The main issue encountered in this case was the rapid and repeated recurrence of an AchoA aneurysm which was ruptured in the beginning. The degree of aneurysm reperfusion was certainly carrying a risk of re-hemorrhage. Coil occlusion, while technically straightforward, did not result in a permanent separation of the aneurysm from blood circulation.

The association of a brain AVM and a ruptured aneurysm under the hemodynamic influence of said AVM increased the complexity of the case. Without the AVM the second treatment step for the AchoA aneurysm would have been flow diversion. Under the given circumstances, we were hesitant to implant a flow diverter as long as the AVM was not obliterated. We eventually decided to use a flow diverter since we thought the risk from the recurrent aneurysm might be larger than the risk from the irradiated and at least partly obliterated AVM.

H. Henkes (✉) · M. A. Pérez
Neuroradiological Clinic, Klinikum Stuttgart, Stuttgart, Germany

V. Gupta et al. (eds.), *100 Interesting Case Studies in Neurointervention: Tips and Tricks*, https://doi.org/10.1007/978-981-13-1346-2_29

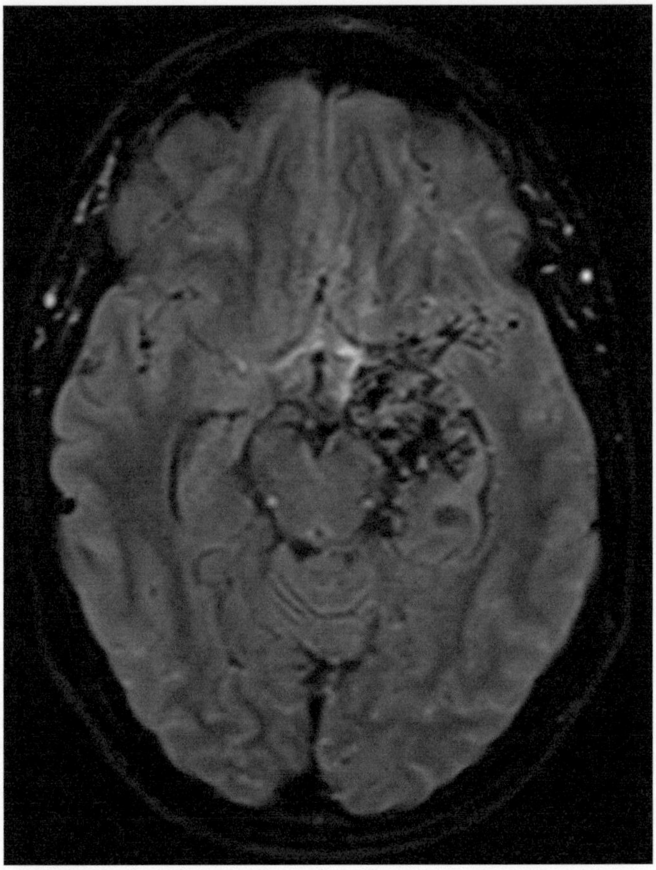

Fig. 29.1 T2WI MRI (FLAIR) of a 38-year-old woman with occasional seizures and severe headache and left oculomotor palsy since 1 week. MRI shows an AVM of the left hippocampus and a small amount of blood in the subarachnoid space adjacent to the left ICA

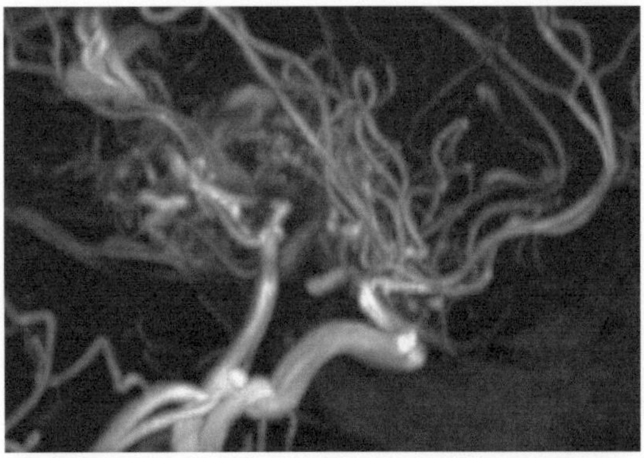

Fig. 29.2 On MRA (TOF), apart from the AVM, an aneurysm of the left ICA at the AchoA is visible

Procedures and Follow-Up

Aneurysm treatment #1 (10/2015): General anesthesia, 6F Heartrail II as guide catheter, Excelsior SL10 straight as microcatheter, 7 coils inserted into the AchoA aneurysm: Microplex10, 1× 4/8, 1× 3/6, 1× 2/4; Target Helical nano, 3/8, both not inserted, 1× 2/6, 1× 1.5/2

AVM embolization #1 (12/2015): 1× Magic 1.2 FM, Glubran2/lipiodol

AVM embolization #2 (1/2016): 2× Marathon/Mirage, Glubran2/lipiodol

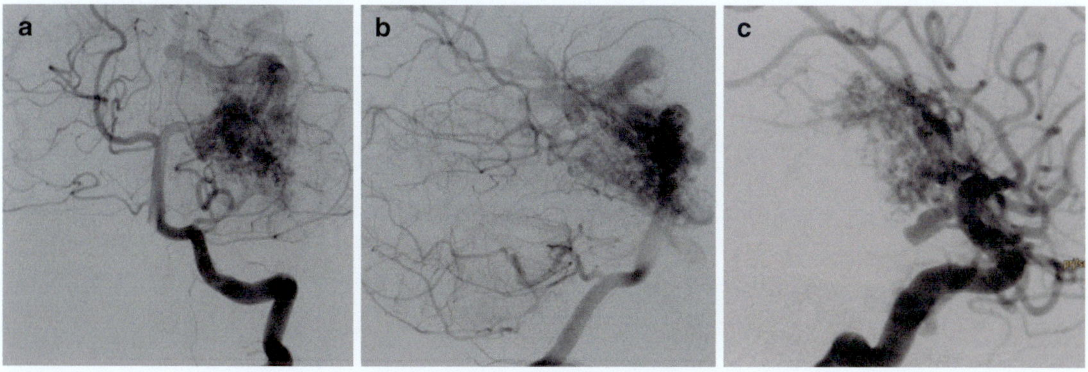

Fig. 29.3 DSA in October 2015 showed the supply of the AVM from the left PCA (**a**, **b**) and from the left MCA (**c**), as well as the ruptured left AchoA aneurysm with a diameter of the aneurysm sac of about 5 mm

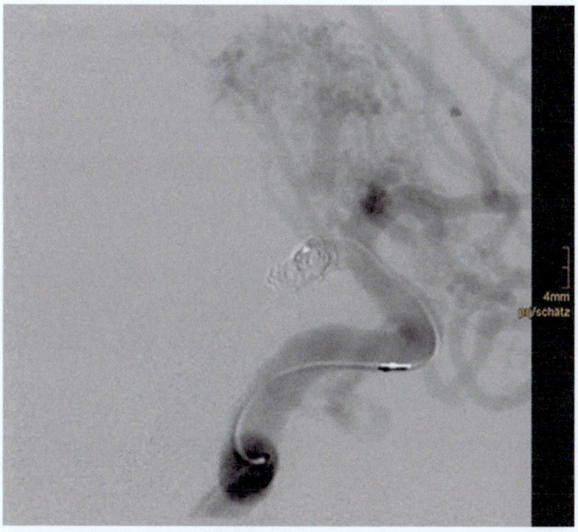

Fig. 29.4 This aneurysm was catheterized and occluded with coils

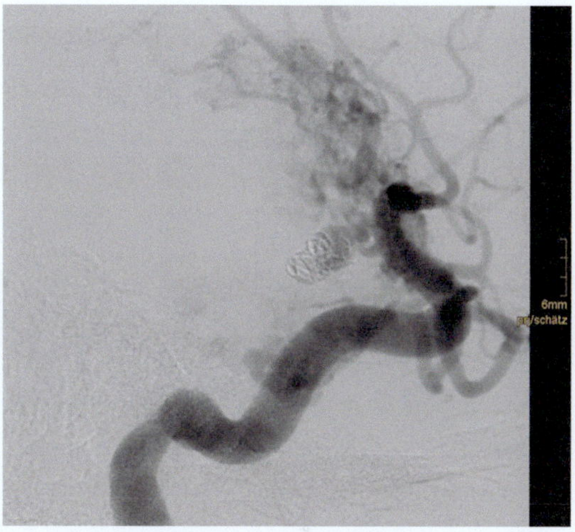

Fig. 29.5 An early follow-up DSA only 2 months after this treatment revealed a significant reperfusion of the AchoA aneurysm, mainly due to coil compaction

Aneurysm treatment #2 (2/2016): General anesthesia, 6F Heartrail II as guide catheter, Excelsior SL10 straight as microcatheter, five coils inserted into the AchoA aneurysm: Axium 1× 3D 6/15, 4× Helix 4/12, 4/12, 4/8, 2.5/8

AVM embolization #3 (2/2016): 1× Magic 1.2, Glubran2/lipiodol

AVM embolization #4 (2/2016): 2× Magic 1.2, Glubran2/lipiodol

AVM radiosurgery (5/2016): CyberKnife

Aneurysm treatment #3 (6/2016): General anesthesia, 6F Heartrail II as guide catheter, Excelsior SL10 straight as microcatheter, seven coils inserted into the AchoA aneurysm: Axium

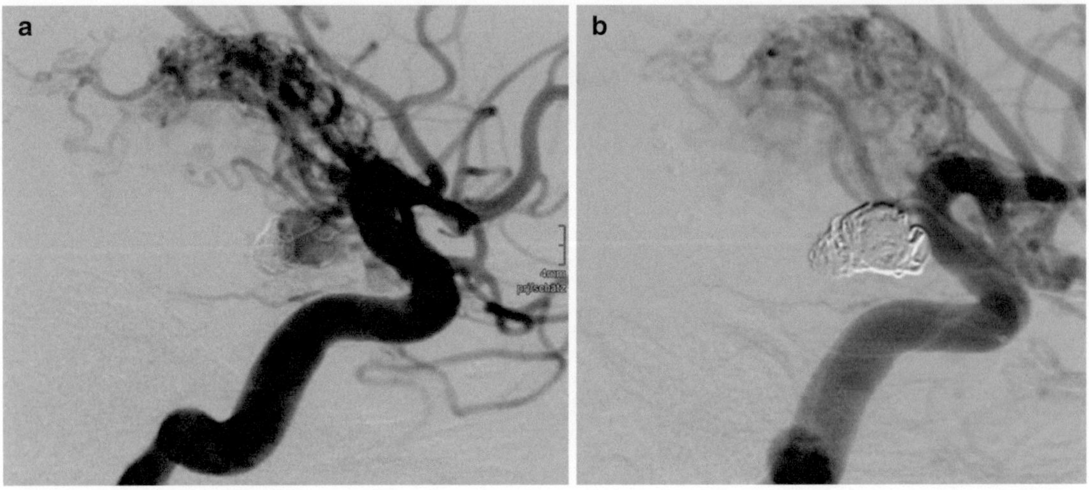

Fig. 29.6 Another 3 months later, the reperfused aneurysm was even larger (**a**) and therefore again occluded with coils (**b**). The brain AVM was meanwhile partially embolized. The patient underwent stereotactic irradiation of the residual AVM (CyberKnife) in May 2016

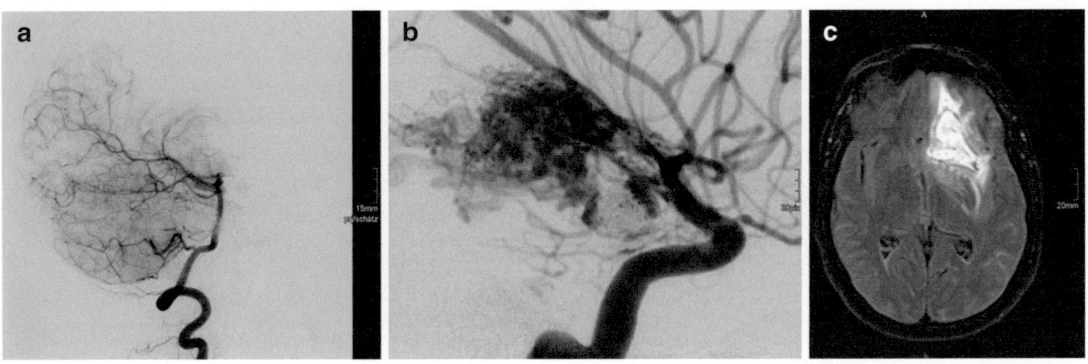

Fig. 29.7 Six weeks after the radiosurgical treatment, the patient presented with an increased frequency of partial and complex seizures. The AVM was significantly devascularized (**a**), the left AchoA aneurysm was again reperfused (**b**), and adjacent to the AVM was a large intracerebral hematoma of the left frontal lobe seen on MRI (**c**)

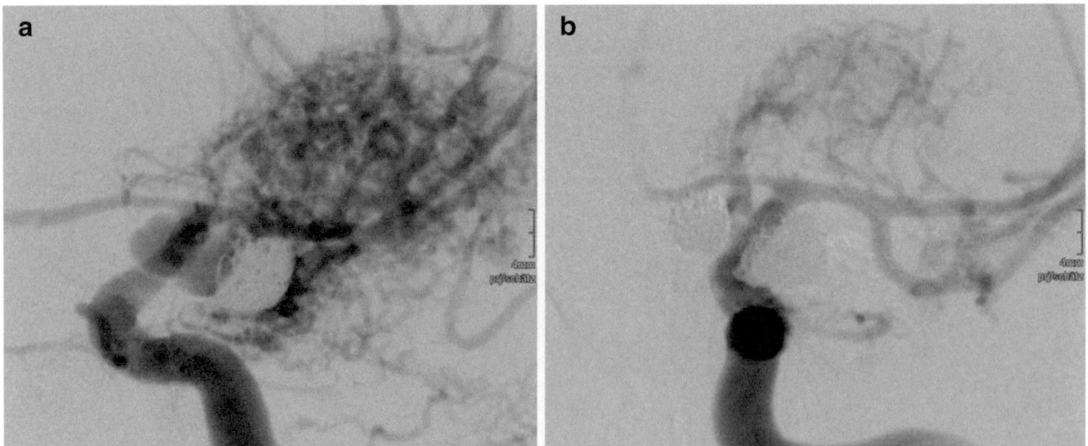

Fig. 29.8 The recurrent left AchoA aneurysm (**a**) was again occluded with coils (**b**)

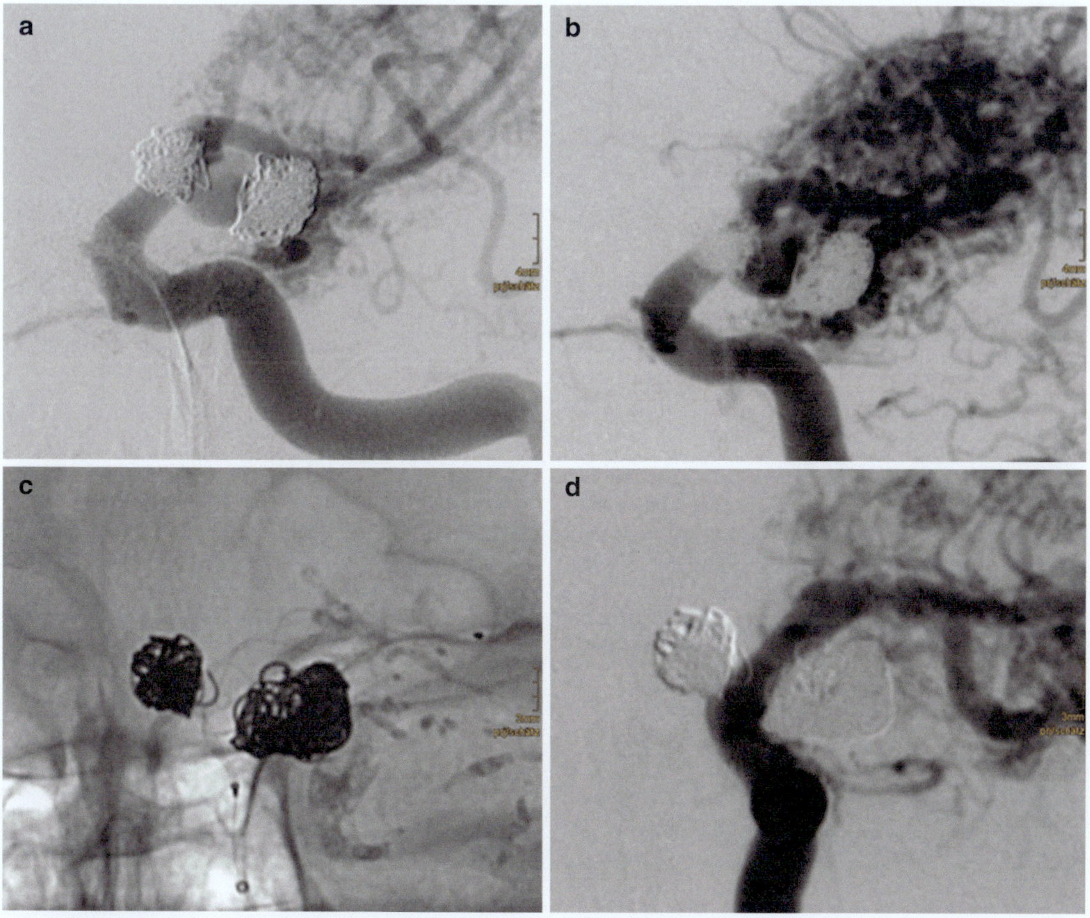

Fig. 29.9 The follow-up DSA only 4 weeks later demonstrated again a significant reperfusion of the aneurysm (**a**). Within the aneurysm sac, the coils appeared separated into two lobules (**b**). A p64 flow diverter was deployed from the left M1 segment to the distal segment of the left ICA (**c**). The flow inside the recurrent AchoA aneurysm was instantaneously reduced (**d**)

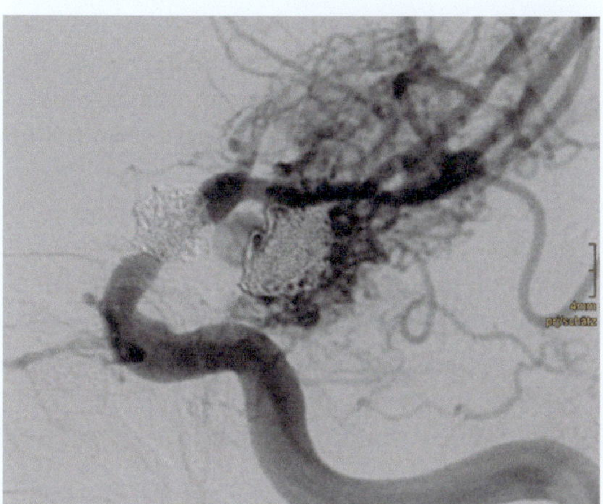

Fig. 29.10 On the first follow-up DSA after 3 months, a minor in-stent stenosis and residual flow inside the aneurysm was seen

prime 1× 3D 5/10, 1× 3D 4/6; Target Helical nano 2× 3/8; Target 360 ultra 1× 2.5/4; Kaneka ED10 ES 1× 2.5/6, 1× 2/8

Aneurysm treatment #4 (7/2016): Loading dose, 1× 500 mg ASA, 1× 180 mg ticagrelor on the day prior to the treatment; multiplate prior to the procedure, dual platelet function inhibition; general anesthesia, 3000 U heparin IV, 6F Heartrail II as guide catheter, Excelsior XT27 preshaped as microcatheter; flow diverter, p64 4/15; post medication, 1× 100 mg ASA PO daily forever, 2× 90 mg ticagrelor PO daily for 1 year

Follow-up DSA #1 (after 3 months): Reduced aneurysm perfusion, minor in-stent stenosis

Follow-up DSA #2 (after 9 months): Aneurysm occluded, AchoA patent, in-stenosis resolved, AVM partly obliterated.

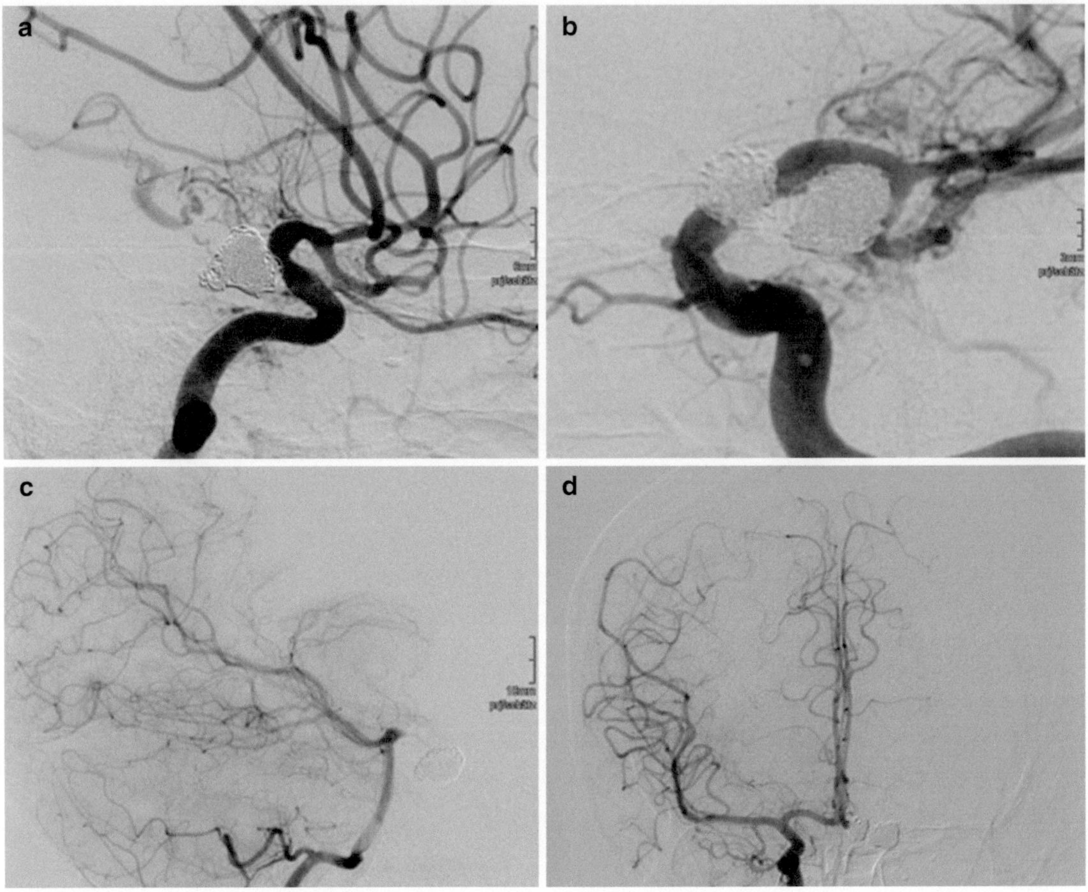

Fig. 29.11 The second follow-up DSA after 9 months confirmed the complete occlusion of the aneurysm with the AchoA patent (**a**, **b**). The supply of the AVM from the right PCA was obliterated (**c**). Since the p64 had intentionally been deployed over the origin of the left A1 segment, the supply of the left ACA had been taken over by the right ICA via the AcomA (**d**). The patient was neurologically asymptomatic; her seizures had ceased under anticonvulsive medication

Tips and Tricks

1. Intracranial aneurysms under the hemodynamic influence of a brain AVM show sometimes a behavior different from regular aneurysms. An increased rate of rapid recurrence after coil occlusion is one of the features.
2. While AVM-associated aneurysms sometimes disappear after the AVM is obliterated, they are not necessarily benign lesions. We frequently start with the treatment of the aneurysm(s) and continue later with the AVM treatment, in contrary to the concept of Lasjaunias et al.
3. A failure to permanently exclude an intracranial aneurysm by coil occlusion as in this patient is fortunately rare, but this case illustrates the importance of rigorous follow-up examinations. The extent of aneurysm reperfusion as encountered in this case can be associated with a massive re-hemorrhage.
4. The timing and extent of the AVM obliteration in this patient after radiosurgery is unusual and subject to speculations. Plexiform AVMs with a compact nidus and small caliber feeding arteries seem to respond better, as it was the case in this woman.
5. Residual aneurysm perfusion and a minor in-stent stenosis after 3 months are frequently

seen. The in-stent stenosis resolves in the far majority of patients spontaneously. The AVM supply via the AchoA in this patient with a direct hemodynamic effect on the aneurysm contributed to the delayed obliteration of the aneurysm after flow diversion.

6. AchoA aneurysms in general are well suitable for flow diversion. The obliteration rate of these aneurysms is high, and the rate of symptomatic occlusion of the AchoA is low.

Suggested Reading

Aguilar Pérez M, Bhogal P, Henkes E, Ganslandt O, Bäzner H, Henkes H. In-stent stenosis after p64 flow diverter treatment. Clin Neuroradiol. 2017; https://doi.org/10.1007/s00062-017-0591-y.

André A, Boch AL, Di Maria F, Nouet A, Sourour N, Clémenceau S, Gabrieli J, Degos V, Zeghal C, Chiras J, Cornu P, Clarençon F. Complication risk factors in anterior choroidal artery aneurysm treatment. Clin Neuroradiol. 2017; https://doi.org/10.1007/s00062-017-0575-y.

Aoki T, Hirohata M, Noguchi K, Komaki S, Orito K, Morioka M. Comparative outcome analysis of anterior choroidal artery aneurysms treated with endovascular coiling or surgical clipping. Surg Neurol Int. 2016;7(Suppl 18):S504–9. https://doi.org/10.4103/2152-7806.187492.

Bhogal P, Ganslandt O, Bäzner H, Henkes H, Perez MA. The fate of side branches covered by flow diverters—results from 140 patients. World Neurosurg. 2017;103:789–98. https://doi.org/10.1016/j.wneu.2017.04.092.

Ding D, Xu Z, Starke RM, Yen CP, Shih HH, Buell TJ, Sheehan JP. Radiosurgery for cerebral arteriovenous malformations with associated arterial aneurysms. World Neurosurg. 2016;87:77–90. https://doi.org/10.1016/j.wneu.2015.11.080.

Fischer S, Aguilar-Pérez M, Henkes E, Kurre W, Ganslandt O, Bäzner H, Henkes H. Initial experience with p64: a novel mechanically detachable flow diverter for the treatment of intracranial saccular sidewall aneurysms. Am J Neuroradiol. 2015;36(11):2082–9. https://doi.org/10.3174/ajnr.A4420.

Flores BC, Klinger DR, Rickert KL, Barnett SL, Welch BG, White JA, Batjer HH, Samson DS. Management of intracranial aneurysms associated with arteriovenous malformations. Neurosurg Focus. 2014;37(3):E11. https://doi.org/10.3171/2014.6.FOCUS14165.

He L, Gao J, Thomas AJ, Fusco MR, Ogilvy CS. Disappearance of a ruptured distal flow-related aneurysm after ateriovenous malformation nidal embolization. World Neurosurg. 2015;84(5):1496.e1–6. https://doi.org/10.1016/j.wneu.2015.05.065.

Henkes H, Fischer S, Liebig T, Weber W, Reinartz J, Miloslavski E, Kühne D. Repeated endovascular coil occlusion in 350 of 2759 intracranial aneurysms: safety and effectiveness aspects. Neurosurgery. 2008;62(6 Suppl 3):1532–7. https://doi.org/10.1227/01.neu.0000333815.79777.3b.

Jha V, Behari S, Jaiswal AK, Bhaisora KS, Shende YP, Phadke RV. The “focus on aneurysm” principle: classification and surgical principles of management of concurrent arterial aneurysm with arteriovenous malformation causing intracranial hemorrhage. Asian J Neurosurg. 2016;11(3):240–54. https://doi.org/10.4103/1793-5482.145340.

Lv X, Wu Z, He H, Ge H, Li Y. Proposal of classification of aneurysms coexisting with AVM and possible treatment strategies. Turk Neurosurg. 2016;26(2):229–33. https://doi.org/10.5137/1019-5149.JTN.8600-13.1.

Neki H, Caroff J, Jittapiromsak P, Benachour N, Mihalea C, Ikka L, Moret J, Spelle L. Patency of the anterior choroidal artery covered with a flow-diverter stent. J Neurosurg. 2015;123(6):1540–5. https://doi.org/10.3171/2014.11.JNS141603.

Omodaka S, Endo H, Fujimura M, Niizuma K, Sato K, Matsumoto Y, Tominaga T. High-grade cerebral arteriovenous malformation treated with targeted embolization of a ruptured site: wall enhancement of an intranidal aneurysm as a sign of ruptured site. Neurol Med Chir (Tokyo). 2015;55(10):813–7. https://doi.org/10.2176/nmc.cr.2015-0052. Epub 2015 Sep 15

Platz J, Berkefeld J, Singer OC, Wolff R, Seifert V, Konczalla J, Güresir E. Frequency, risk of hemorrhage and treatment considerations for cerebral arteriovenous malformations with associated aneurysms. Acta Neurochir. 2014;156(11):2025–34. https://doi.org/10.1007/s00701-014-2225-3.

Rangel-Castilla L, Munich SA, Jaleel N, Cress MC, Krishna C, Sonig A, Snyder KV, Siddiqui AH, Levy EI. Patency of anterior circulation branch vessels after pipeline embolization: longer-term results from 82 aneurysm cases. J Neurosurg. 2017;126(4):1064–9. https://doi.org/10.3171/2016.4.JNS16147.

Raz E, Shapiro M, Becske T, Zumofen DW, Tanweer O, Potts MB, Riina HA, Nelson PK. Anterior choroidal artery patency and clinical follow-up after coverage with the pipeline embolization device. Am J Neuroradiol. 2015;36(5):937–42. https://doi.org/10.3174/ajnr.A4217.

Reynolds MR, Arias EJ, Chatterjee AR, Chicoine MR, Cross DT 3rd. Acute rupture of a feeding artery aneurysm after embolization of a brain arteriovenous malformation. Interv Neuroradiol. 2015;21(5):613–9. https://doi.org/10.1177/1591019915591740.

Stein KP, Wanke I, Forsting M, Zhu Y, Moldovan AS, Dammann P, Sandalcioglu IE, Sure U. Associated aneurysms in supratentorial arteriovenous malformations: impact of aneurysm size on haemorrhage. Cerebrovasc Dis. 2015;39(2):122–9. https://doi.org/10.1159/000369958.

"Catheter Push" Technique to Open Flow Diverter

30

Vipul Gupta

Case

A 55-year-old female presented with left side facial pain and recent onset left sixth and partial third nerve palsies. Cross-sectional imaging revealed a giant cavernous aneurysm. DSA and 3D angiography revealed a giant partially thrombosed internal carotid artery (ICA) aneurysm along with a small ophthalmic aneurysm (Fig. 30.1a, b). Balloon test occlusion revealed inadequate collateral flow. Patient was planned for flow diverter placement.

Issue

Inadequate opening of flow diverter device during the procedure.

Management

Procedure was performed under general anesthesia. A 6 F long sheath (Cook Corp) was placed in the left common carotid artery and thereafter a 6 F guiding catheter in the left ICA (6F DAC, Stryker Neurovascular, Fremont, CA, USA). A Pipeline embolization device (Medtronic, Minneapolis, Minnesota, USA) was placed across the aneurysms. Post stent angiogram (Fig. 30.1c, d) revealed incomplete opening of the device. Stent delivery catheter, Marksman (Medtronic, Minneapolis, Minnesota, USA), was navigated across the stent over the delivery wire, without any change in the proximal partially open stent. Thereafter, a distal access catheter, DAC 044 (Stryker Neurovascular, Fremont, CA, USA), was placed through the guiding catheter and a microcatheter (Prowler 21, Codman & Sheurtleff, Inc. USA) through the smaller DAC (Fig. 30.2a). Loop of microguidewire was formed to push against the edge of the stent; the same maneuver was done with tip of microcatheter as well as the DAC (Fig. 30.2b, c). Final angiogram revealed almost complete opening of the flow diverter (Fig. 30.2d). Follow-up DSA revealed complete occlusion of the aneurysm with completely patent stent. Patient was discharged with no new focal neurological deficits.

Tips and Tricks

1. Partially open flow diverter can result in thromboembolism or occlusion of the stent. Careful evaluation of images is mandatory to detect this potential complication.

V. Gupta
Neurointerventional Surgery, Stroke unit, Artemis Agrim Institute of Neuroscience, Gurgaon, India
e-mail: vipul.gupta@artemishospitals.com

V. Gupta et al. (eds.), *100 Interesting Case Studies in Neurointervention: Tips and Tricks*,
https://doi.org/10.1007/978-981-13-1346-2_30

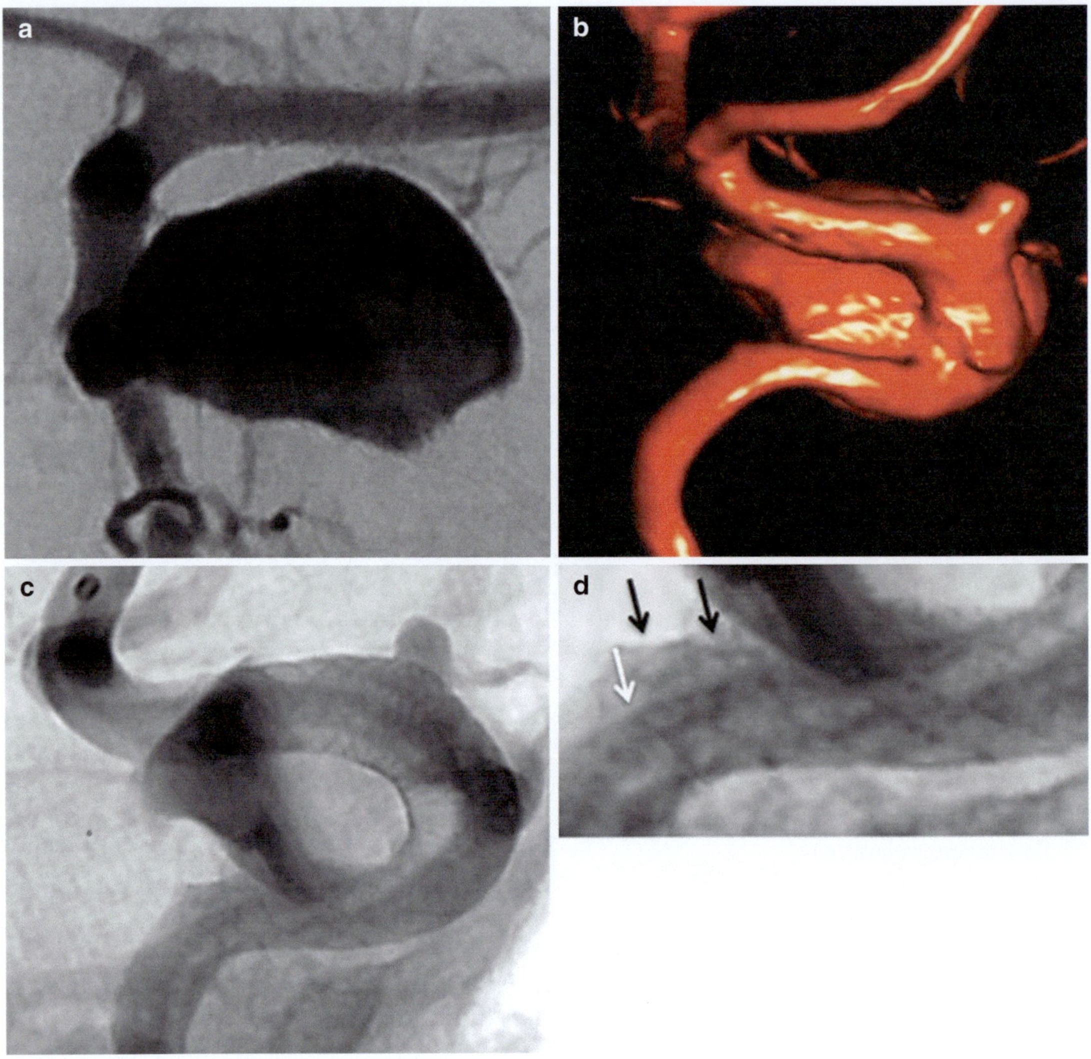

Fig. 30.1 (**a**, **b**) DSA and 3D angiography images show a giant partially thrombosed left ICA aneurysm along with a small paraclinoidal ophthalmic aneurysm. (**c**) Flow diverter placement shows partial opening of proximal end of the device. (**d**) Magnified view of **c** showing partial opening of the FD (*white arrow*). Black arrow denotes the ICA margins

2. It is not uncommon to have incomplete opening of proximal end of the device. Key feature for complete opening is to foreshorten the device for complete expansion.
3. Navigation of flow diverter delivery microcatheter may help in opening up of the device. As shown in the case, pushing against the edge of the FD with a loop of wire, microcatheter or a distal access catheter helps in foreshortening and opening up of the device.

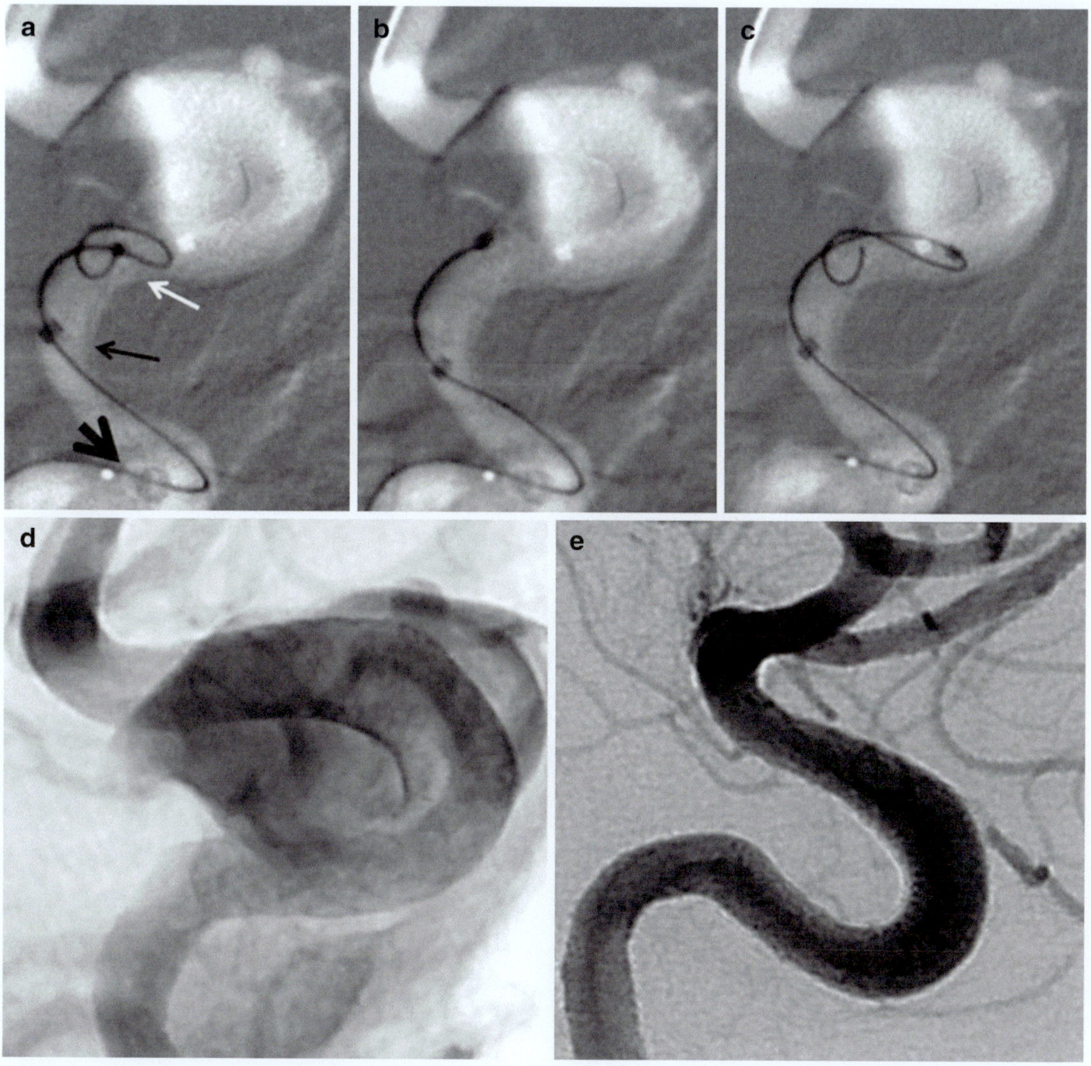

Fig. 30.2 (**a**) Catheter manipulation to open the device. DAC 044 (*thin black arrow*) was placed through the 6 F DAC (*thick black arrow*) and a microcatheter (*white arrow*) through the smaller DAC. A loop of microguidewire was formed to engage the proximal end of flow diverter. (**b**) Microcatheter edge against the edge of device so as to foreshorten the stent. (**c**) Microcatheter inside the device and over it the smaller DAC was navigated to push against the end of FD. (**d**) Final angiogram showing well open FD. (**e**) Follow-up DSA image with complete occlusion and patent artery

"Catheter Pull" Technique to Open Flow Diverter

31

Vipul Gupta

Case

A 62-year-old lady presented with subarachnoid haemorrhage (Fig. 31.1a), Hunt and Hess Grade II. DSA revealed broad neck small para-clinoidal aneurysm (Fig. 31.1b). Case was planned for flow diverter placement.

Issue

Lack of opening flow diverter during the procedure.

Management

Procedure was performed under general anaesthesia. A 6 F long sheath (Cook Corp) was placed in the left common carotid artery and thereafter a 6 F guiding catheter (DAC 6F, Stryker) in the left ICA. A Pipeline embolization device (5 × 30, Medtronic) was placed across the aneurysms. Incomplete opening of the proximal end of the device was seen over the bend between laceral and cavernous ICA (Fig. 31.2a, b). Stent delivery microcatheter (Marksman, Medtronic) was taken across the stent; however it didn't result in any significant opening of the stent (Fig. 31.2c). Thereafter a sharp tug was given to the microcatheter along with the delivery wire so as to create a downward force on the stent (as shown by the arrows, Fig. 31.2c). The manoeuver resulted in remarkable opening of the device (Fig. 31.2d). Thereafter, angioplasty was performed with hypercomplaint balloon (Scepter XC, Microvention) to further expand the stent (Fig. 31.2e). Final angiogram revealed almost complete opening of the flow diverter. Patient was extubated intact neurological condition.

Tips and Tricks

1. It is critical to open the flow diverter device to prevent stent thrombosis or embolic phenomenon.
2. In selected cases a sharp tug on the microcatheter along with the delivery wire can lead to outward force on the unopened stent with expansion of the device. The to and fro movement of microcatheter helps, as in our case. The initial forward movement displaced the stent upwards and further sudden withdrawal helped to open the stent.
3. Angioplasty can also help to open the stent. We prefer to navigate the stent delivery microcatheter beyond the incompletely opened stent and then exchange with a hypercomplaint balloon. This manoeuver prevents loss of access across the stenosed stent.

V. Gupta
Neurointerventional Surgery, Stroke unit, Artemis Agrim Institute of Neuroscience, Gurgaon, India
e-mail: vipul.gupta@artemishospitals.com

V. Gupta et al. (eds.), *100 Interesting Case Studies in Neurointervention: Tips and Tricks*,
https://doi.org/10.1007/978-981-13-1346-2_31

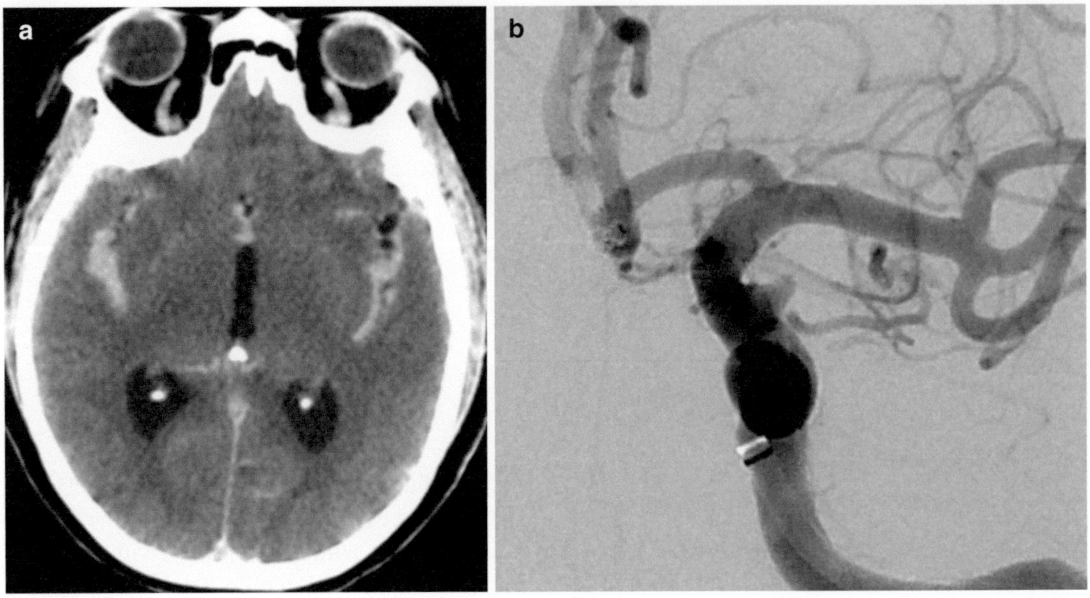

Fig. 31.1 (**a**) Non-contrast CT showing diffuse subarachnoid haemorrhage. (**b**) DSA image showing a broad neck para-clinoidal aneurysm

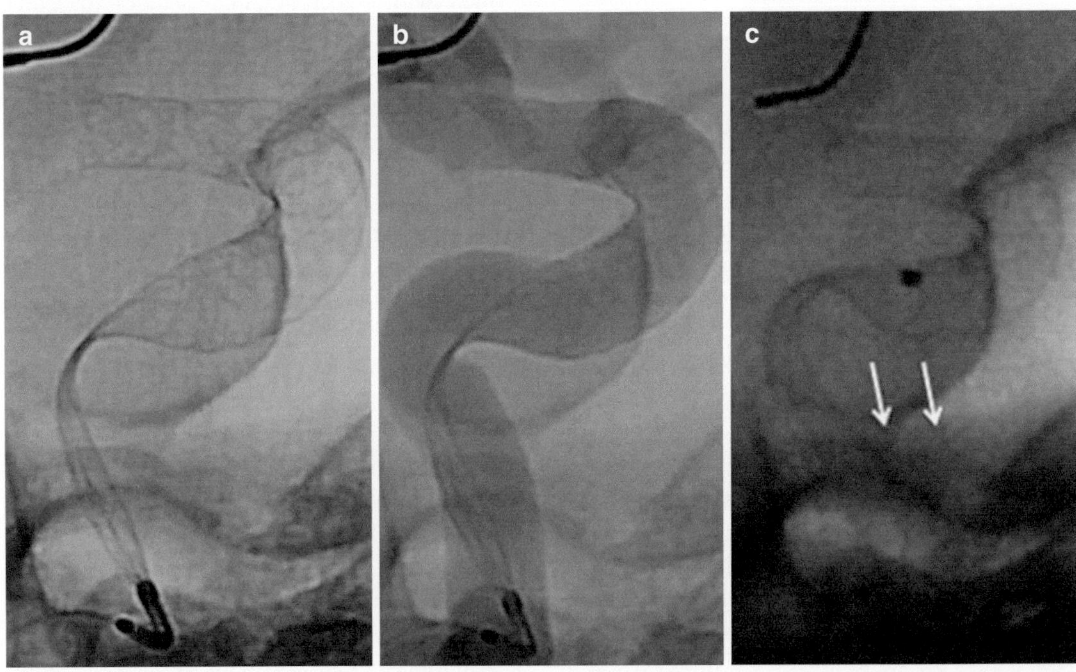

Fig. 31.2 (**a**, **b**) Native and angiographic images showing incomplete opening of the flow diverter. (**c**) Microcatheter navigation across the device didn't result in any significant change. However, the stent has been pushed to the outer wall of ICA. Thereafter, the microcatheter along with delivery wire was pulled backwards with a jerk resulting in a downward tug on the device, as shown by the direction of the arrows. (**d**) Native images show significant opening of the stent. (**e**) Further angioplasty was performed with a Scepter XC balloon. (**f**) Final angiogram showing almost complete opening of the stent and patent ICA

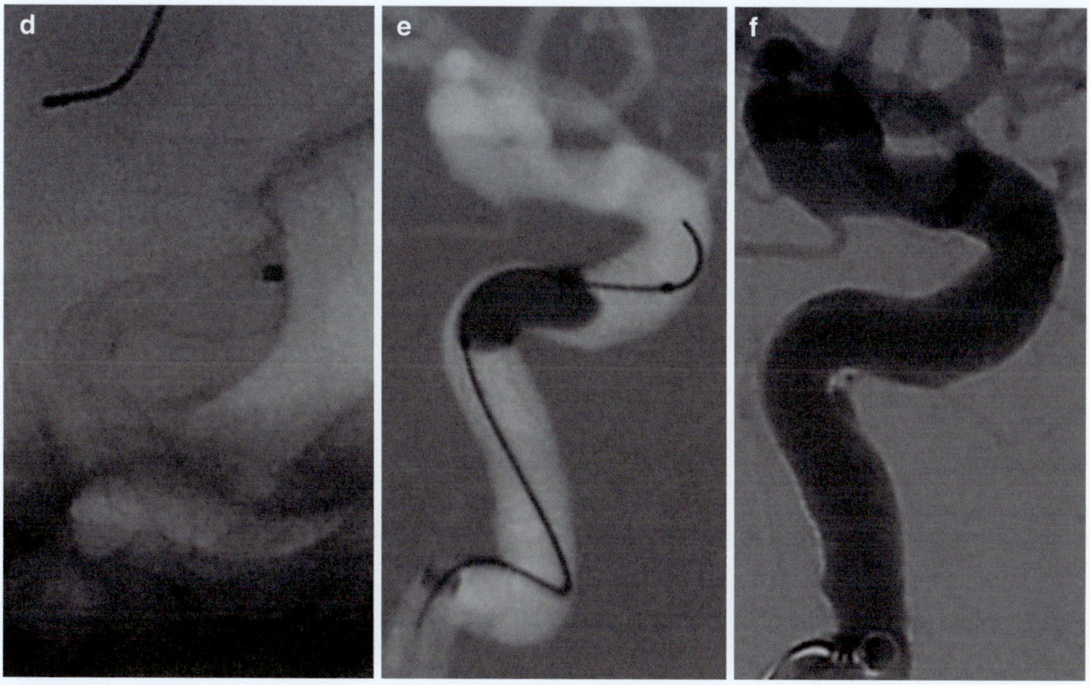

Fig. 31.2 (continued)

"Balloon-Push" Technique to Open Flow Diverter

32

Vipul Gupta

Case

A 64-year-old lady presented with headaches and diminution of vision for 1 year. MRI (not shown) revealed a giant internal carotid artery (ICA) aneurysm of the left ICA with compression of optic apparatus. DSA revealed giant paraclinoidal aneurysm (Fig. 32.1a). The case was planned for flow diverter placement.

Issues

Incomplete opening of flow diverter device during the procedure.

Management

The procedure was performed under general anesthesia. A flow diverter (Pipleline, Medtronic) was placed across the aneurysm. However, incomplete opening of the proximal part of the device was seen (Fig. 32.1a, b). Maneuvering the stent delivery microcatheter (Marksman, Medtronic Corp) through the device didn't make any significant difference. Balloon catheter (Scepter C 4 × 20, Microvention) was taken across the stent. However, balloon inflation didn't result in any significant opening of stent. Thereafter, partially inflated balloon was pushed to and fro, so as to push and foreshorten the stent (Fig. 32.1d). The maneuver resulted in almost complete opening of the device (Fig. 32.1e). Final angiogram revealed well-patent stent, and the patient was extubated in intact clinical condition.

Tips and Tricks

1. Partially open flow diverter can result in thromboembolism or occlusion of the stent. Careful evaluation of images is mandatory to detect this potential complication.
2. Balloon inflation can help in opening the device; however, one should understand that flow diverters open by foreshortening of the stent. As in our case, using the balloon catheter to push the device forward in an attempt to shorten the stent is more likely to result in opening of the proximal free edge.

Similar maneuver in a companion case (Fig. 32.2)

V. Gupta
Neurointerventional Surgery, Stroke unit, Artemis Agrim Institute of Neuroscience, Gurgaon, India
e-mail: vipul.gupta@artemishospitals.com

V. Gupta et al. (eds.), *100 Interesting Case Studies in Neurointervention: Tips and Tricks*,
https://doi.org/10.1007/978-981-13-1346-2_32

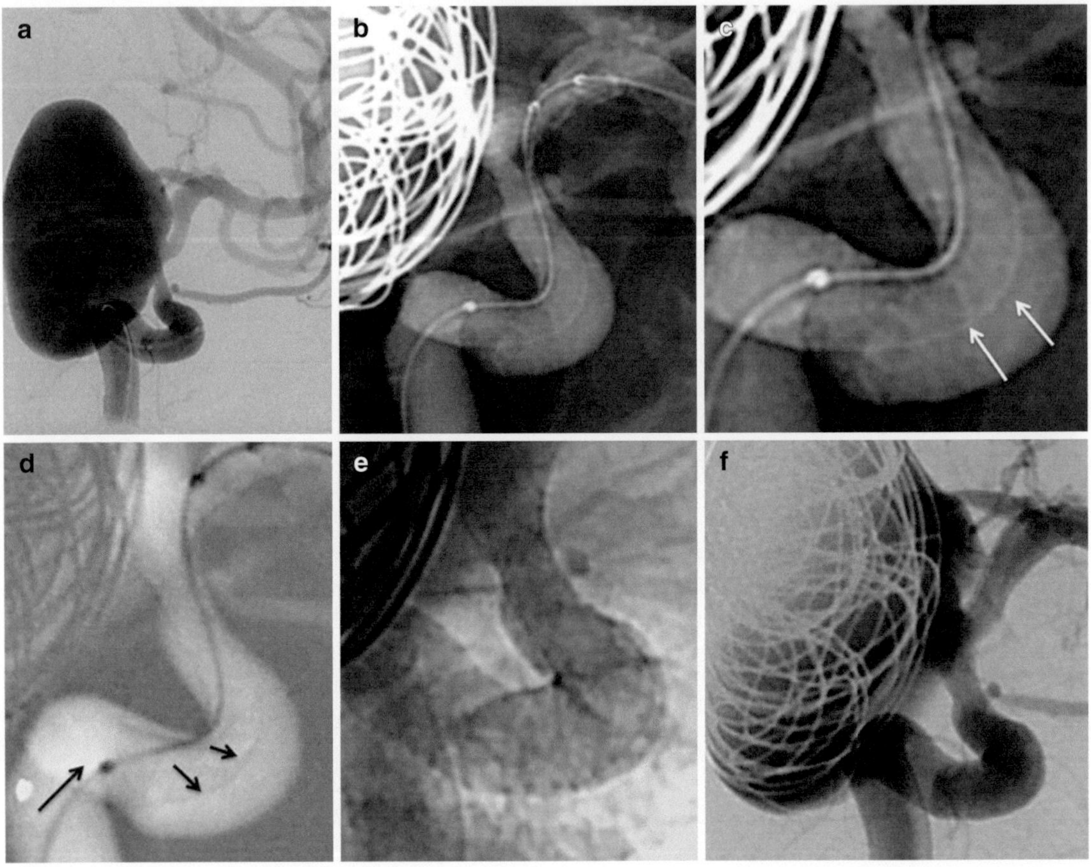

Fig. 32.1 (**a**) DSA image showing a giant para-clinoidal aneurysm. (**b**, **c**) Native DSA image showing partially open flow diverter, well seen (*arrows*) in magnified image (*arrows*, **c**). Balloon catheter was taken across the device. Balloon inflation didn't make any significant difference. (**d**) Thereafter the inflated balloon catheter was moved to and fro so as to push the stent against the wall of ICA in an attempt to foreshorten the stent. (**e**) Image showing almost completely open stent. Notice the shortening of the device as compared to previous image. (**f**) DSA showing well-patent stent

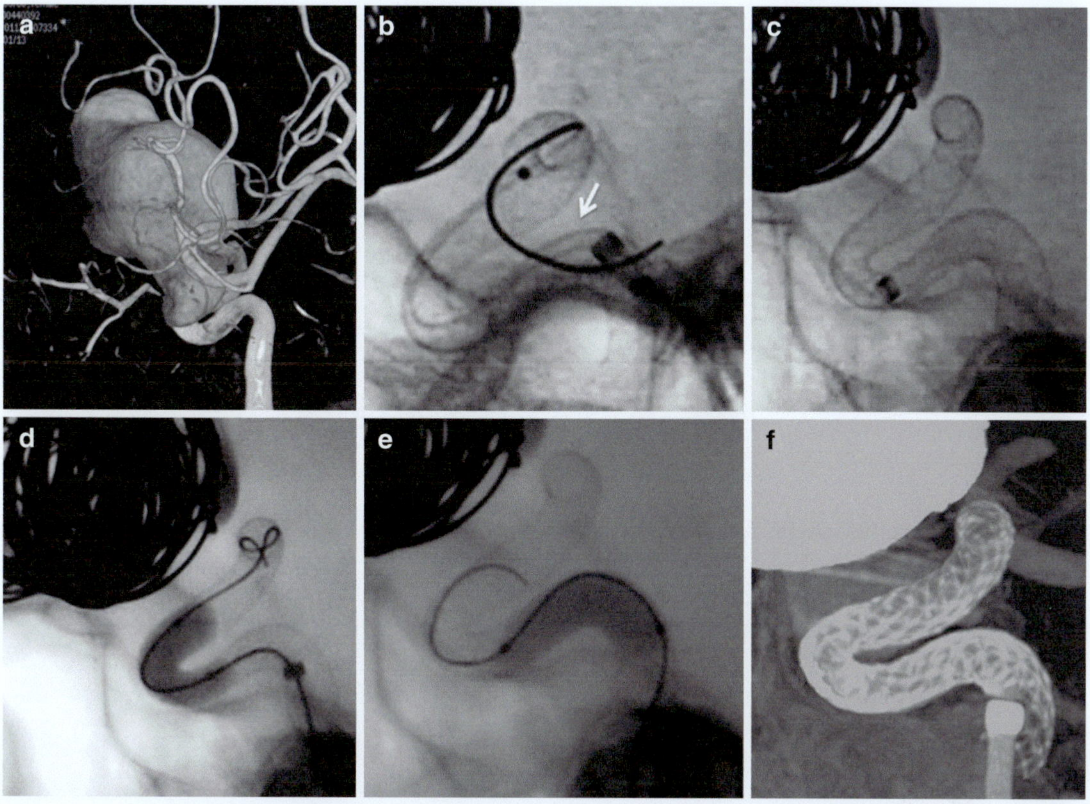

Fig. 32.2 (**a**) 3D angiogram showing giant ICA aneurysm. (**b**, **c**) Flow diverter placement with incomplete opening in the cavernous segment. The guiding catheter (AXS Catalyst 5, Stryker) was navigated into the device over the stent delivery microcatheter (**b**) and taken across the narrowed segment (**c**) in an attempt to completely expand the device. (**d**, **e**) Balloon angioplasty was tried (**d**) followed by balloon inflation proximal to the under-expanded stent, and the whole system (balloon as well as guidewire) was advanced together in effort to foreshorten the stent. (**f**) Post-embolization Vaso CT shows well-expanded flow diverter

Endovascular Techniques for Achievement of Better Flow Diverter Wall Apposition: Telescopic Device Placement

33

Ajit S. Puri and Rajsrinivas Parthasarathy

Case

Two patients in whom a wall apposition was achieved by deploying a second device in a telescopic manner.

Issue

- Device malapposition leads to persistent endoleak and aneurysm filling.

Management

Flow diverter deployment tips and tricks:

- Size: The diameter of the device according to the diameter of the artery at the proximal landing zone
- Length: Allow for the foreshortening that can occur particularly at the aneurysmal segment and take measurements from a straight proximal to the distal landing segment.
- Device expands by foreshortening; therefore, one should attempt device expansion by foreshortening during deployment rather than mechanical dilatation after deployment.
- If the proximal end of the device ends at a bend, this can prevent the device from expanding as it tends to *ovalize at a bend*. This in turn *causes malapposition of the proximal end* of the device resulting in endoleak. Crossing the device without dislodging or damaging the stent can be technically challenging.
- Deployment technique: *Pushing* the device results in unsheathing; this should be followed with *fluffing* wherein you push the device along with the microcatheter to open the stent. To avoid kinking of the device at the bend, a *push and pull* technique is followed. Aim to bring the delivery microcatheter to the center of the artery by pulling back on the microcatheter after every push and fluff maneuver.

Malapposition correction:

Maneuver 1: Overlapping PEDs. If there is a significant discrepancy in the diameter of the artery in the proximal and the distal landing zone, one may have to deploy a larger diameter second device in a telescopic fashion to enable adequate proximal wall apposition (Figs. 33.1 and 33.2).

Maneuver 2: Proximal open cell design stent placement in a telescopic fashion. This can be attempted when the proximal end of the stent

A. S. Puri (✉)
Radiology, and Neurosurgery,
Division of Neurointerventional Surgery,
Neurointerventional Fellowship Program,
University of Massachusetts Medical Center,
Worcester, MA, USA
e-mail: ajit.puri@umassmemorial.org

R. Parthasarathy
Vascular Neurology and Neurointerventional Surgery,
Artemis Agrim Institute of Neuroscience,
Gurgaon, India

V. Gupta et al. (eds.), *100 Interesting Case Studies in Neurointervention: Tips and Tricks*,
https://doi.org/10.1007/978-981-13-1346-2_33

lands at bend such that a wall of the stent is projecting into the lumen. Deploy a second open cell design stent in a telescopic fashion; there should be adequate overlap of the second over the first stent in a straight segment. The proximal landing zone for the second stent should also be at a straight segment (Fig. 33.3).

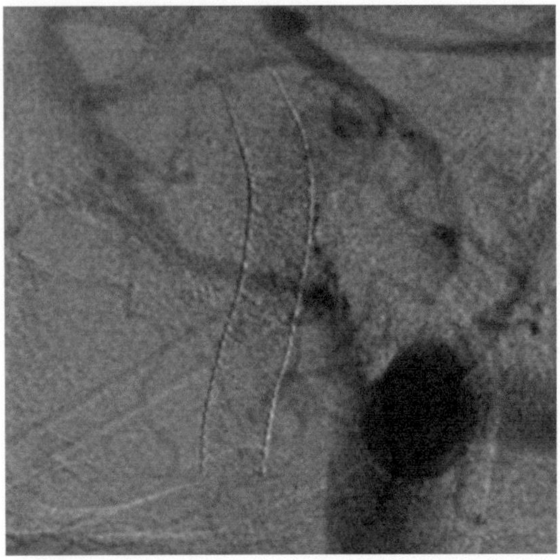

Fig. 33.1 Placement of another flow diverter within the previously placed FD to better oppose the ends. The second PED will be placed in telescopic fashion

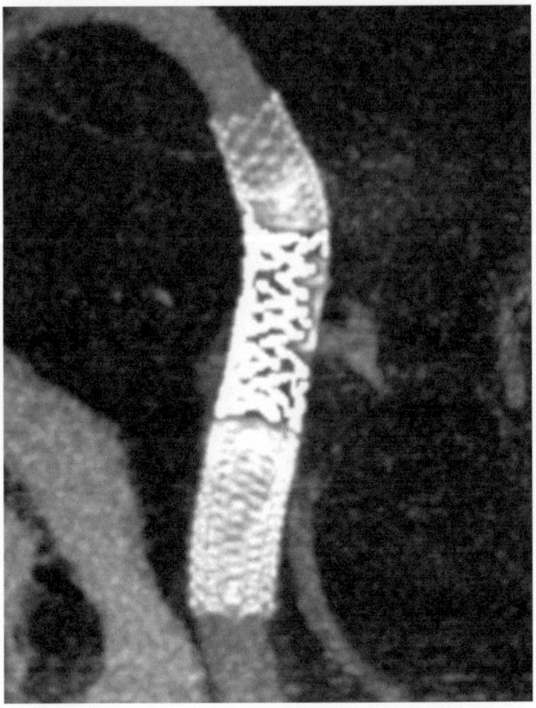

Fig. 33.2 Cone-beam CT confirms proper vessel wall apposition of the devices

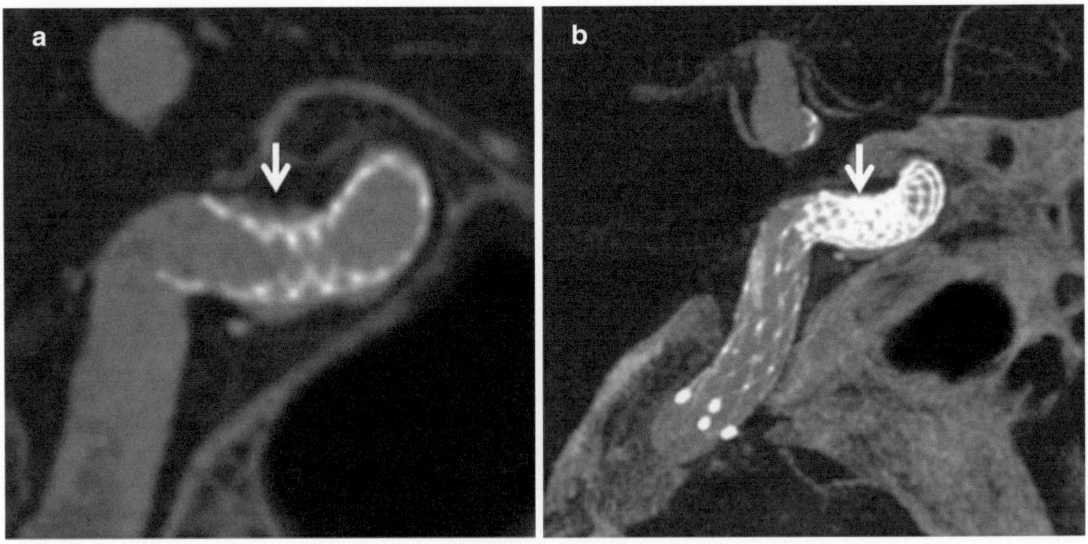

Fig. 33.3 Placement of an open-cell stent in telescopic fashion across the mal-apposed proximal part of the FD; (**a**) Malapposition of the PED detected on cone-beam CT image post device placement (*arrow*). (**b** – **d**) Confirmed overlap of the proximal to mid portion of the open-cell stent with the proximal aspect of the PED on multiplanar 3D reconstruction images acquired after stent placement (*arrows*)

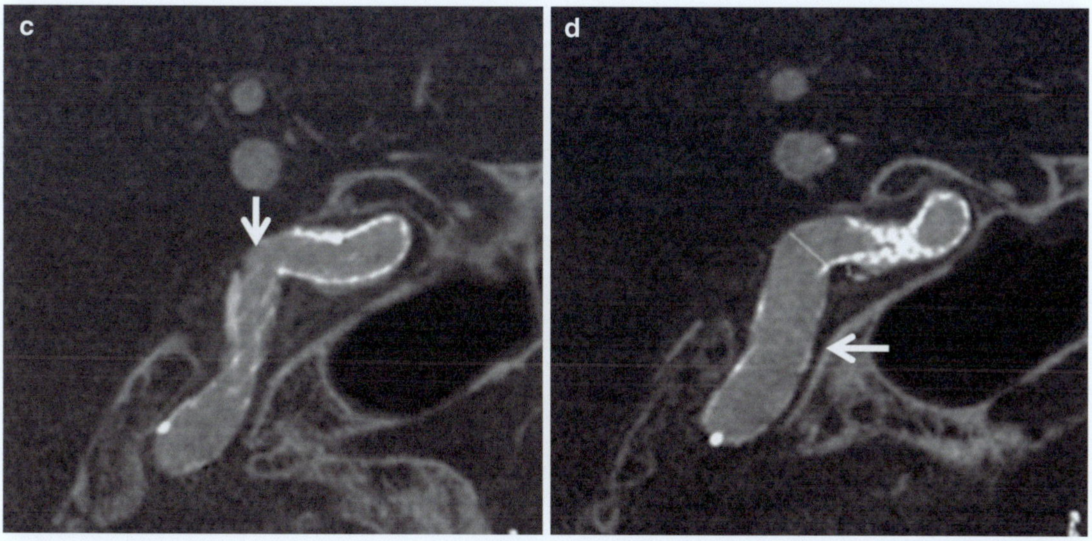

Fig. 33.3 (continued)

Suggested Reading

Kühn AL, et al. Use of self-expanding stents for better intracranial flow diverter wall apposition. Interv Neuroradiol. 2016;23(2):129–36.

34 pCONus Reconstruction for Basilar Top Aneurysm

Hans Henkes and Marta Aguilar Pérez

Case

This 46-year-old male presented with confusion and massive headache due to a spontaneous SAH. His clinical condition was equivalent to Hunt and Hess III; the Fisher grade was IV (Fig. 34.1). DSA showed a wide-necked aneurysm of the bifurcation of the basilar artery with a fundus diameter of 10 mm and a neck diameter of 8 mm (Fig. 34.2a, b).

Issue

The ruptured aneurysm of the basilar bifurcation was not considered an ideal target for microsurgical clipping or conventional coiling. WEB would have been an option but was not available. Crossing stents would have been our choice prior to the availability of pCONus but has several disadvantages: the need to get access to the efferent vessels, placing more metal into the vessel bifurcation, and sometimes less efficacious coil retention.

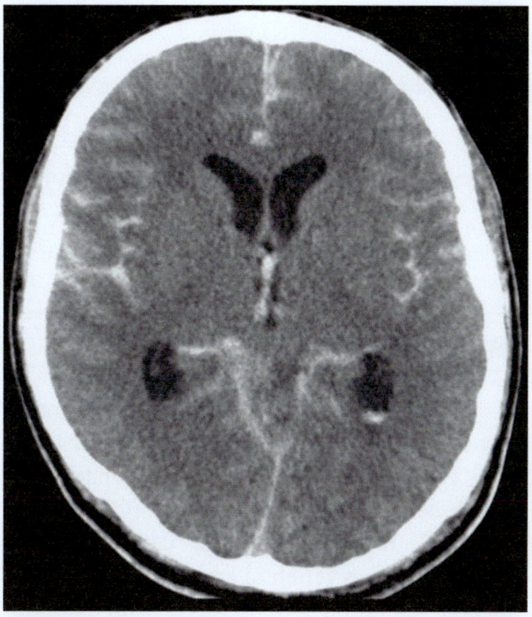

Fig. 34.1 Cranial CT showing a spontaneous SAH with blood in the hemispheric sulci and in the third ventricle (Fisher grade IV)

H. Henkes (✉) · M. A. Pérez
Neuroradiological Clinic, Klinikum Stuttgart,
Stuttgart, Germany

V. Gupta et al. (eds.), *100 Interesting Case Studies in Neurointervention: Tips and Tricks*,
https://doi.org/10.1007/978-981-13-1346-2_34

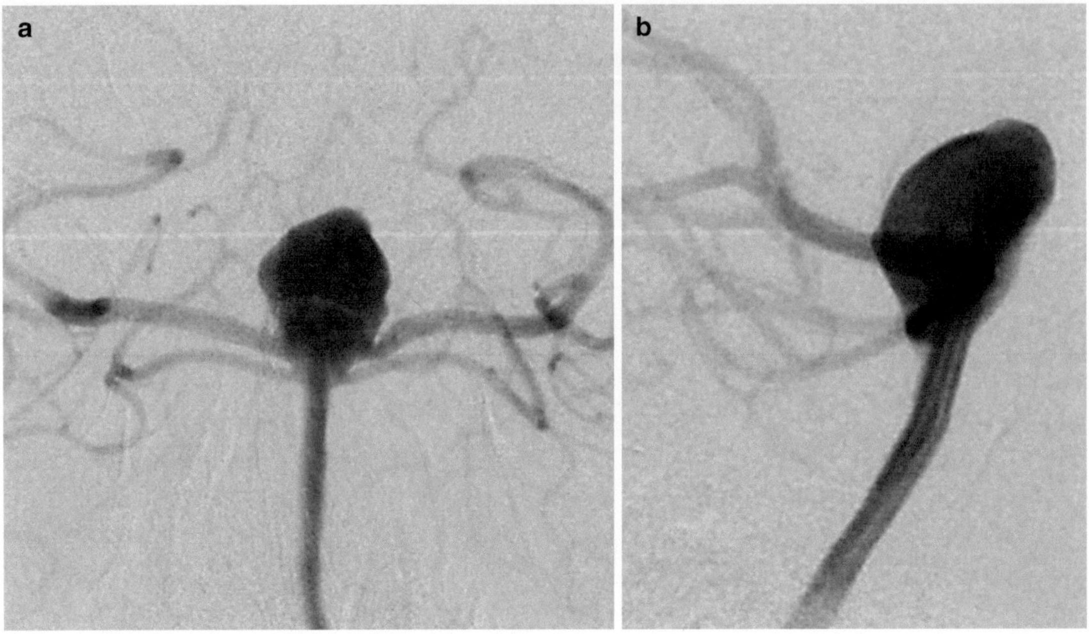

Fig. 34.2 DSA of a ruptured wide-necked aneurysm of the bifurcation of the basilar artery, with a fundus diameter of 10 mm and a neck diameter of 8 mm (**a**) AP view and (**b**) lateral view

Management

An external ventricular drainage was performed prior to the angiography and endovascular treatment. Under general anesthesia via bilateral 6F femoral sheaths, 6F Envoy MPC (Codman & Sheurtleff, Inc. USA) guide catheters were inserted into both vertebral arteries. Dual platelet function inhibition was induced with 500 mg ASA IV and 600 mg clopidogrel PO via a gastric tube. For the pCONus a Prowler select plus 45° microcatheter was inserted via the left vertebral artery. A pCONus1 4-25-10 was deployed at the neck level of the aneurysm (Fig. 34.3). Through the pCONus (Phenox GmbH, Lise-Meitner-Allee 31, D-44801 Bochum, Germany), an Echelon10 45° microcatheter was inserted into the aneurysm (Fig. 34.4). A Morpheus 3D coil 9/28 (ev3 Inc., Irvine, California, USA) was too large, not well retained by the pCONus and therefore removed (Fig. 34.5). Complete occlusion of the aneurysm was achieved by using nine coils [Deltamaxx (Codman & Sheurtleff, Inc. USA): 2× 8/35, 3× 6/25, 1× 4/15, MicroPlex10: 1× 4/8, 2× 5/8] (Fig. 34.6). The patient recovered without a permanent neurological deficit. Follow-up DSA examinations, the last performed 30 months after the treatment, confirmed the persistent complete occlusion of the aneurysm (Fig. 34.7).

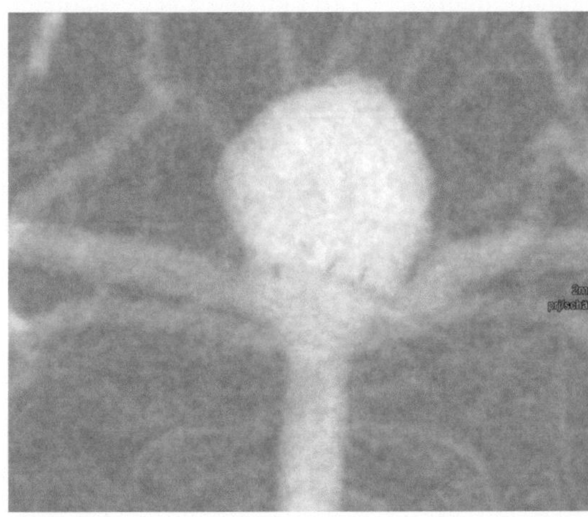

Fig. 34.3 A pCONus1 4-25-10 is deployed inside the aneurysm

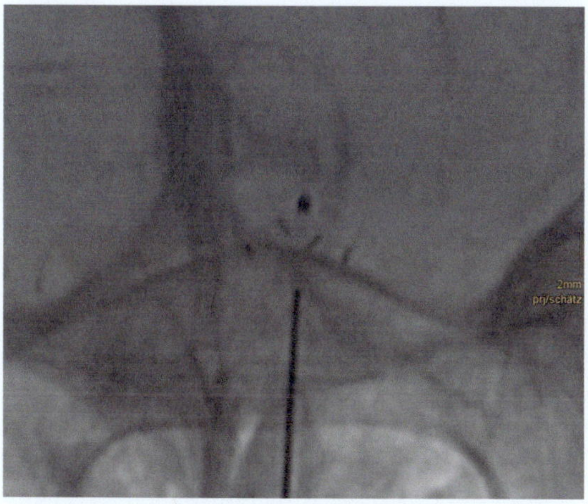

Fig. 34.4 An Echelon10 microcatheter is inserted through the pCONus into the aneurysm

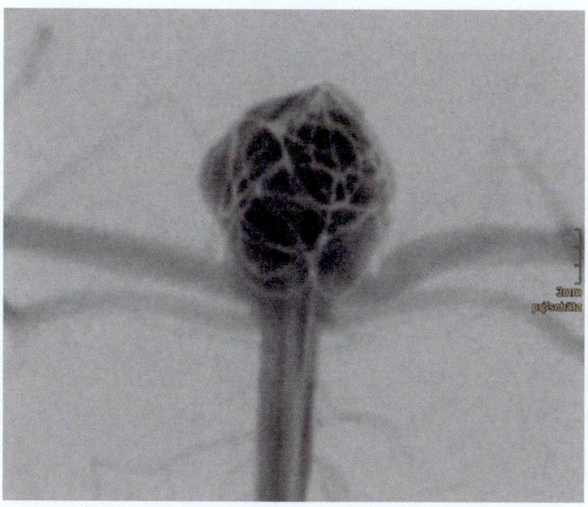

Fig. 34.5 A Morpheus 3D coil 9/28 was not properly retained in the aneurysm by the pCONus1 and therefore removed. The level of occlusion shown by this image goes too far proximal

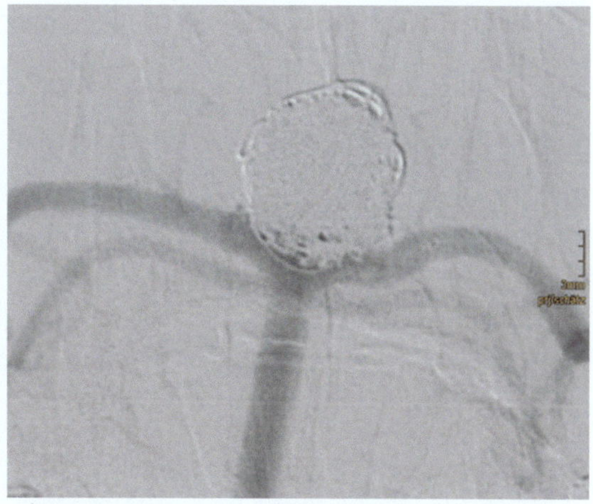

Fig. 34.6 Final DSA run after complete occlusion of the aneurysm by nine coils. Both origin of the PCAs are not compromised. No thrombus formation inside the stent shaft

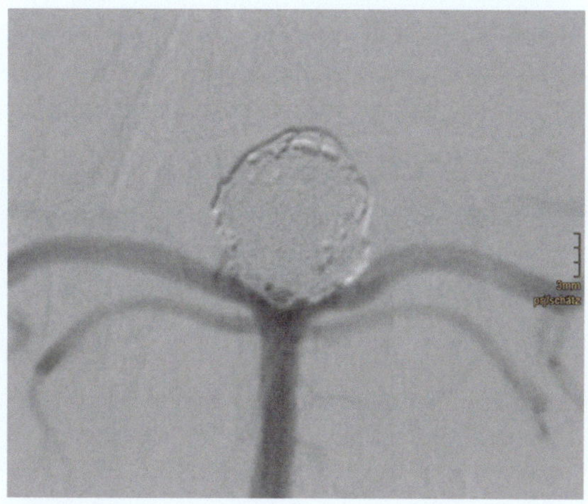

Fig. 34.7 Follow-up DSA 30 months after the treatment, confirming the persistent complete occlusion of the aneurysm

Tips and Tricks

1. *Premedication, postmedication:* In patients with a severe SAH, we usually perform an external ventricular drainage prior to any anti-aggregation. Once the decision is made to use a pCONus, 500 mg ASA IV and 180 mg ticagrelor PO or 600 mg clopidogrel PO are given. The platelet function inhibition effect of ticagrelor starts more rapid and is more reliable. As soon as the pCONus is deployed, a body weight-adapted bolus of eptifibatide IV is added. Our postmedication comprises currently 1× 100 mg ASA PO daily forever and 2× 90 mg ticagrelor PO daily for 3 months.
2. *Selection of the microcatheter for pCONus:* Microcatheters with either 0.021″ or 0.027″ inner diameter are suitable; with the 0.027″ microcatheter, the deployment and positioning of the pCONus are usually more accurate.

3. *Sizing*: The pCONus comes with three numbers (e.g., 4-25-10); the first number indicates the shaft diameter (4 mm), the second number indicates the shaft length (25 mm), and the third number indicates the wingspan of the petals (10 mm); this is the critical number; the nominal diameter or wingspan of the petals of the pCONus should be one size larger than the largest diameter of the aneurysm neck.
4. *Positioning of the pCONus*: The microcatheter is inserted into the middle of the aneurysm. The pCONus is advanced to this position. The pCONus will be held in place, while the microcatheter is slowly pulled back. The pCONus must not move more distally during this process. Once the petals of the pCONus are fully open, the microcatheter will be pulled back together with the half-deployed pCONus. The final position of the petals of the pCONus is just at the neck of the aneurysm. Once this position is reached, the pCONus is held in place, and the microcatheter is slowly withdrawn, deploying the shaft of the pCONus.
5. *Time of detachment*: We prefer to keep the pCONus undetached until the aneurysm is completely obliterated with coils.
6. *Microcatheter* for coils, jailing, or insertion through the pCONus: Jailing the microcatheter for coiling is possible but not necessary. In general the catheterization of the deployed pCONus is straightforward. The non-jailed microcatheter allows reaching the entire space of the aneurysm sac.
7. *Which coil*: Sizing of the coils follows the accepted rules for plain coil occlusion. Oversizing should be avoided. We prefer to start with a 3D coil with a diameter slightly smaller than the diameter of the aneurysm fundus. Dense packing is required. Adjacent to the aneurysm neck and the pCONus petals, short coils with a small diameter (e.g., 2 mm/2 cm) should not be used since they may not be retained by the petals.
8. Follow-up: DSA follow-up 6 and 24 months after the treatment is recommended. pCONus has no hemodynamic effect and does not direct the blood flow toward the aneurysm. However, these are usually wide-necked aneurysms with a certain risk of reperfusion. In the case of coil compaction or aneurysm growth, recoiling can and should be done. The pCONus will retain the coil loops in the same way as it was the case during the first treatment.

Suggested Reading

Pérez MA, Bhogal P, Moreno RM, Wendl C, Bäzner H, Ganslandt O, Henkes H. Useof the pCONus as an adjunct to coil embolization of acutely ruptured aneurysms. J Neurointerv Surg. 2017;9(1):39–44. https://doi.org/10.1136/neurintsurg-2016-012508.

35 Recurrent Wide-Necked Bifurcation Aneurysm: Treatment Using PulseRider® as an Adjunctive Device

Helen Cliffe and Tufail Patankar

Case

A 53-year-old female had an anterior communicating artery (ACOM) aneurysm (Fig. 35.1a) treated electively with balloon-assisted coiling (Fig. 35.1b, c). Six months later, a repeat catheter angiogram showed significant recurrence of the aneurysm (Fig. 35.1d). Treatment options were assessed and the pros and cons discussed in a neurovascular multidisciplinary team meeting. The patient was offered either surgery or endovascular treatment and she opted for the former. However, after failed attempt at surgical management, the endovascular options were re-evaluated, and a PulseRider® (Pulsar Vascular, San Jose, CA, USA) assisted coiling was considered (Fig. 35.2).

Issues

- Wide-necked aneurysm recurrence makes coiling (± balloon assistance) undesirable due to risk of further recurrence.
- Y and T stenting is a highly complex procedure, particularly in cases where the access is challenging, such as ACOM aneurysms.
- Surgical clipping is difficult and had failed in this case due to the absence of a true neck and subsequent inability to place a clip safely.

H. Cliffe · T. Patankar (✉)
Leeds Teaching Hospitals NHS Trust, Leeds, UK

Procedure

The patient was treated with dual platelet therapy (aspirin and clopidogrel) prior to the procedure. Right common femoral artery access was obtained. An 8F Neuron Max (Penumbra Inc., Alameda, CA, USA) was placed distally in the right common carotid artery, and a 6F Navien (Covidien Vascular Therapies, Mansfield, MA, USA) was advanced into the right internal carotid artery. 3D rotational angiogram was performed, demonstrating the ACOM aneurysm recurrence with a 5 mm neck, a working projection was obtained, and a 2.75 × 8.6 mm PulseRider device was selected (Fig. 35.3a).

A Synchro (Stryker, Freemont, CA, USA) 0.014 microwire was placed at the aneurysm neck and Prowler Plus Select (Codman Neurovascular, Miami Lakes, FL, USA) microcatheter navigated over it. The PulseRider device was sited across the aneurysm neck with the device limbs within the A2 vessels bilaterally and the body extending along the right A1 (Fig. 35.3b–d). The aneurysm was catheterised using a Synchro 0.014 microwire and an Excelsior SL10 (Stryker Neurovascular, Fremont CA, USA) microcatheter, and five coils were placed within the aneurysm. Complete occlusion was achieved. The PulseRider device was detached (Fig. 35.3e–f). The patient was neurologically intact on waking. Follow-up DSA at 6 months and MRA at 18 months demonstrate complete aneurysm occlusion.

V. Gupta et al. (eds.), *100 Interesting Case Studies in Neurointervention: Tips and Tricks*,
https://doi.org/10.1007/978-981-13-1346-2_35

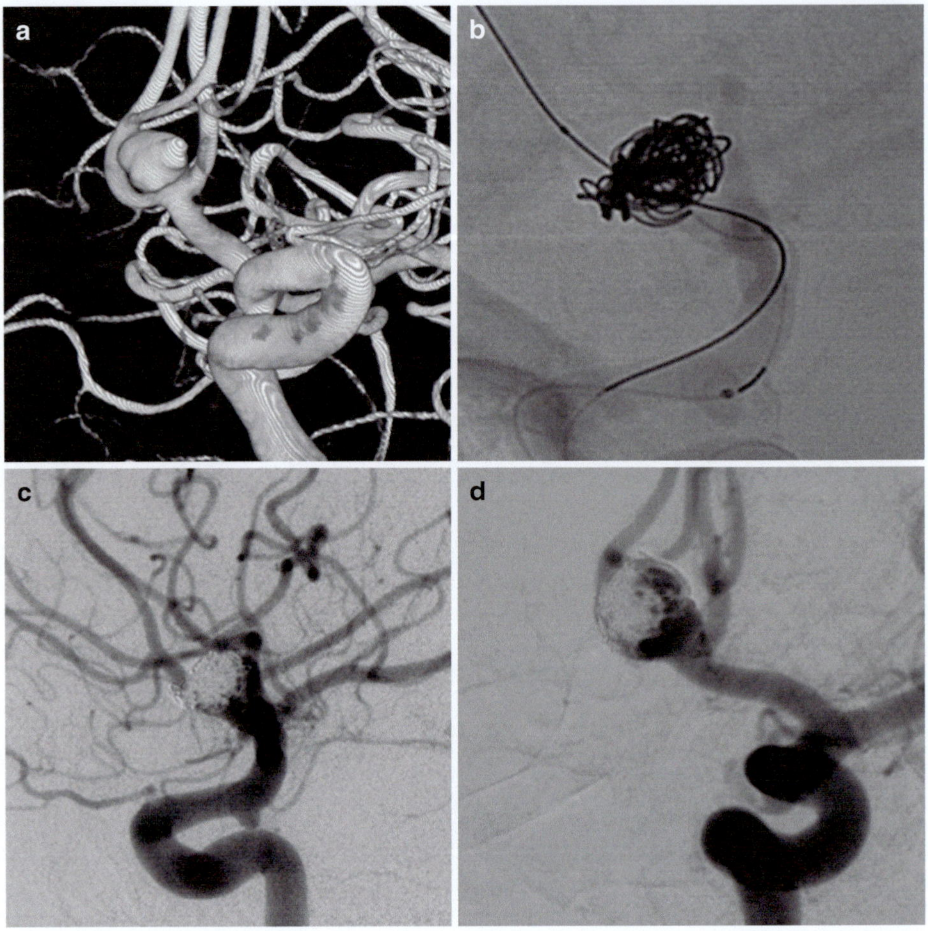

Fig. 35.1 (**a**) Three-dimensional rotational cerebral angiogram demonstrates a wide-necked ACOM bifurcation aneurysm. (**b**) Left ICA catheter angiogram illustrates (CodmanNeurovascular, MiamiLakes, FL, USA) a balloon across the ACOM neck and Headway 17 (Microvention-Terumo, Tustin, CA, USA) microcatheter being employed to insert coils into the aneurysm. (**c**) At the end of the procedure, the aneurysm is occluded. (**d**) Six months later, repeat left ICA catheter angiography illustrates recurrence at the base of the aneurysm

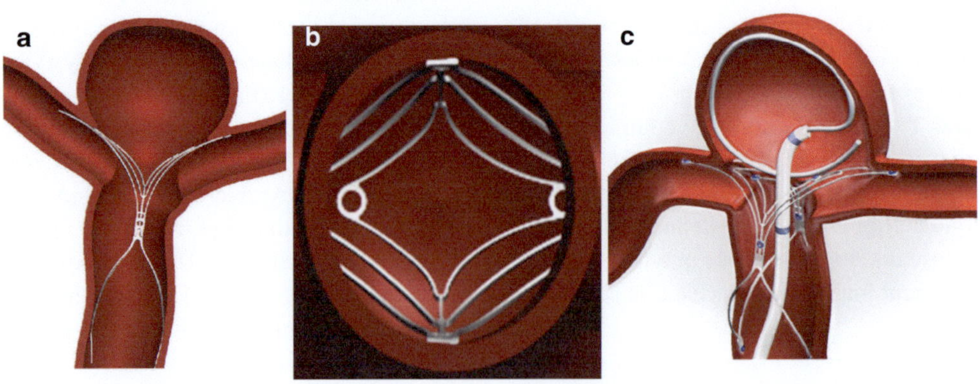

Fig. 35.2 (**a**) Coronal schematic illustrates the position of the PulseRider device relative to the aneurysm neck, with the device body across the neck and the limbs extending along the bifurcation vessels. (**b**) Axial schematic demonstrates a reduced metalwork burden at the aneurysm base compared to stenting. (**c**) Oblique coronal schematic illustrates the position of the microcatheter and microwire, beyond the device within the aneurysm, to allow for deployment of coils. Images used with permission from Pulsar Vascular (San Jose, CA, USA)

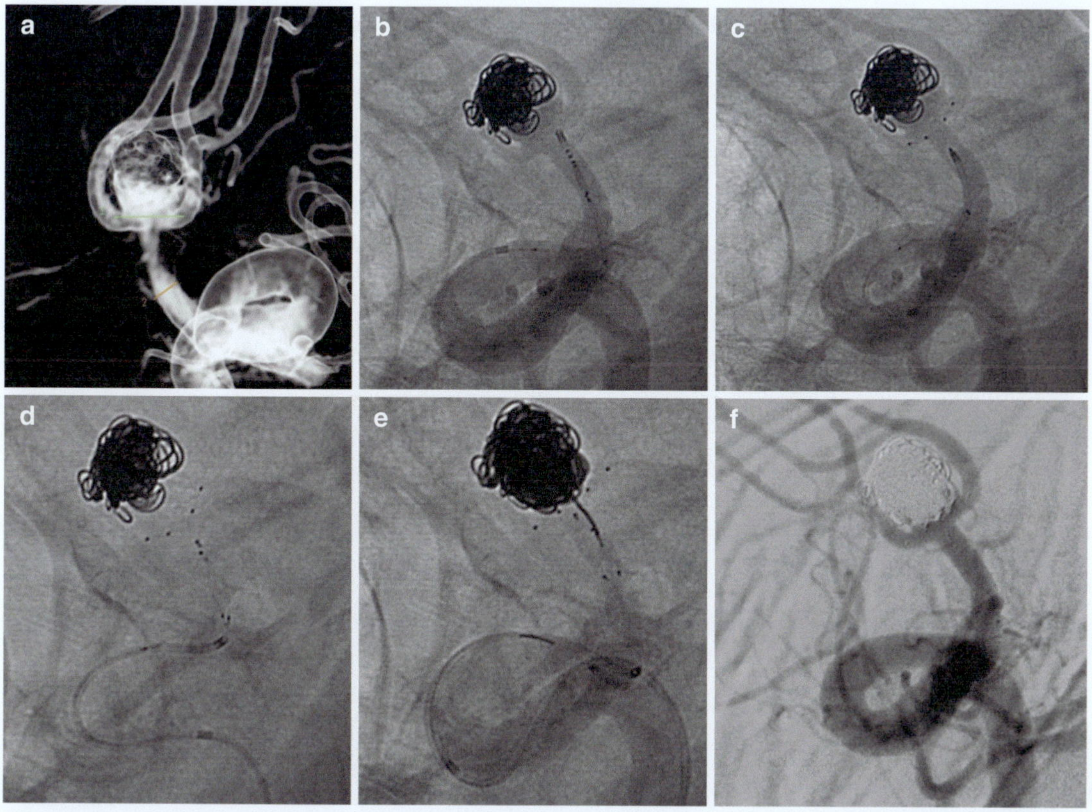

Fig. 35.3 (**a**) Three-dimensional rotational cerebral angiogram demonstrates a recurrent wide-necked ACOM bifurcation aneurysm, with measurements of the neck and right A1 access dimensions. Selected DSA images (**b–d**): (**b**) Manipulation of the Prowler Plus Microcatheter to the aneurysm base. (**c**) Deployment of the limbs of the PulseRider into the A2 vessels bilaterally. (**d**) Deployment of the body of the device into the right A1. (**e**) Placement of coils into the aneurysm via a distally sited Excelsior SL10 microcatheter. (**f**) End of procedure with complete occlusion of the aneurysm

Tips and Tricks

1. The PulseRider device is a self-expanding Nitinol implant, which is designed to better maintain intraluminal patency, compared to other T or Y stenting techniques.
2. May be considered less complex than T or Y stenting and can be placed without the catheterisation of branch vessels.
3. Pre-procedure dual antiplatelet therapy is required.
4. To position the PulseRider device, use a 6F guide catheter and then use a microcatheter navigated over a microwire, positioned at aneurysm neck.
5. The PulseRider device can be deployed in a 'T' or a 'Y' configuration.
6. Sometimes it is better to catheterise the side branch and unsheath the device. If this is not possible, the device can be safely pushed forward across the neck of the aneurysm.
7. A push and pull technique is often required if deploying against the neck of the aneurysm.
8. A microcatheter can then be navigated over a microwire through the PulseRider device into the aneurysm.
9. Avoid jailing of microcatheter, as Echelon and Excelsior SL10 can be easily navigated through the device.
10. After deployment of the PulseRider, use an assistant to hold the microcatheter to stabilise the device in position whilst you coil the

aneurysm—this will prevent the PulseRider from getting displaced by the coils.

11. Detach the device once the aneurysm is coiled completely.
12. In de novo aneurysms, the PulseRider leaflets can be also placed within the aneurysm to cover the neck for coiling; alternatively, one leaflet can be placed in aneurysm and another in the artery if needed. This is a distinct advantage of the device compared to alternatives like pCONus (Phenox, Bochum, Germany).
13. Continue dual antiplatelet therapy post-procedure for 6 weeks and aspirin for life.

Suggested Reading

Gory B, Spiotta AM, Mangiafico S, Consoli A, Biondi A, Pomero E, Killer-Oberpfalzer M, Weber W, Riva R, Labeyrie PE, Turjman F. PulseRider stent-assisted coiling of wide-neck bifurcation aneurysms: periprocedural results in an international series. Am J Neuroradiol. 2016;37(1):130–5.

Mukherjee S, Chandran A, Gopinathan A, Putharan M, Goddard T, Eldridge PR, Patankar T, Nahser HC. PulseRider-assisted treatment of wide-necked intracranial bifurcation aneurysms: safety and feasibility study. J Neurosurg. 2017;127:61–8.

Starke RM, Turk A, Ding D, Crowley RW, Liu KC, Chalouhi N, Hasan DM, Dumont AS, Jabbour P, Durst CR, Turner RD. Technology developments in endovascular treatment of intracranial aneurysms. J Neurointerv Surg. 2016;8:135–44.

Wide-Necked Bifurcation Aneurysm: Treatment with Woven EndoBridge (WEB) Device

36

Helen Cliffe and Tufail Patankar

Case

A 62-year-old female was diagnosed with an incidental wide-necked anterior communicating artery (ACOM) aneurysm with partial involvement at the neck of the right A2 vessel (Fig. 36.1a) on CTA. Sequential CT scans demonstrated interval growth and the patient requested treatment. Endovascular management options include balloon-assisted coiling, stent-assisted coiling, and treatment with WEB (Sequent Medical Palo Alto, CA, USA). The alternatives were evaluated in the neurovascular multidisciplinary team meeting, and WEB was decided upon. Two attempts at elective WEB embolization were unsuccessful due to difficult access with tortuous internal carotids (Fig. 36.1b) and an angulated ICA/A1 junction bilaterally (Fig. 36.1c). A third attempt was planned (Figs. 36.2 and 36.3).

Issues

- Difficult access with sharp angulation at the ICA/A1 junction bilaterally.
- A wide aneurysm neck makes coiling alone undesirable.
- Thromboembolic risks of balloon-assisted coiling in the ACOM territory are significant.
- The need to occlude aneurysm whilst preserving the involved right A2 makes stent-assisted embolization less preferable.
- There is a desire to avoid stenting and subsequent long-term dual platelet therapy in a relatively young patient where possible.

Procedure

The patient was treated with dual platelet therapy prior to the procedure. Right common femoral artery access was obtained using an 8F sheath. A 6F Neuron Max (Penumbra Inc., Alameda, CA, USA) was placed in the left common carotid artery and advanced into the left internal carotid artery for proximal support (Fig. 36.3a). 3D angiographic images were obtained; a satisfactory working projection for WEB placement was achieved, and the aneurysm was measured in two planes AP (width and height) and lateral (width and height). The neck width was also assessed. Due to the challenging access, an Echelon 10 microcatheter (eV3 Neurovascular, Inc., Irvine, CA, USA) was advanced into the right internal carotid, and a 6F Navien was tracked over it as the distal support catheter. The Echelon 10 was then replaced by a VIA 27 microcatheter over a 0.014 Synchro exchange guidewire. A WEB SL

H. Cliffe · T. Patankar (✉)
Leeds Teaching Hospitals NHS Trust, Leeds, UK

V. Gupta et al. (eds.), *100 Interesting Case Studies in Neurointervention: Tips and Tricks*,
https://doi.org/10.1007/978-981-13-1346-2_36

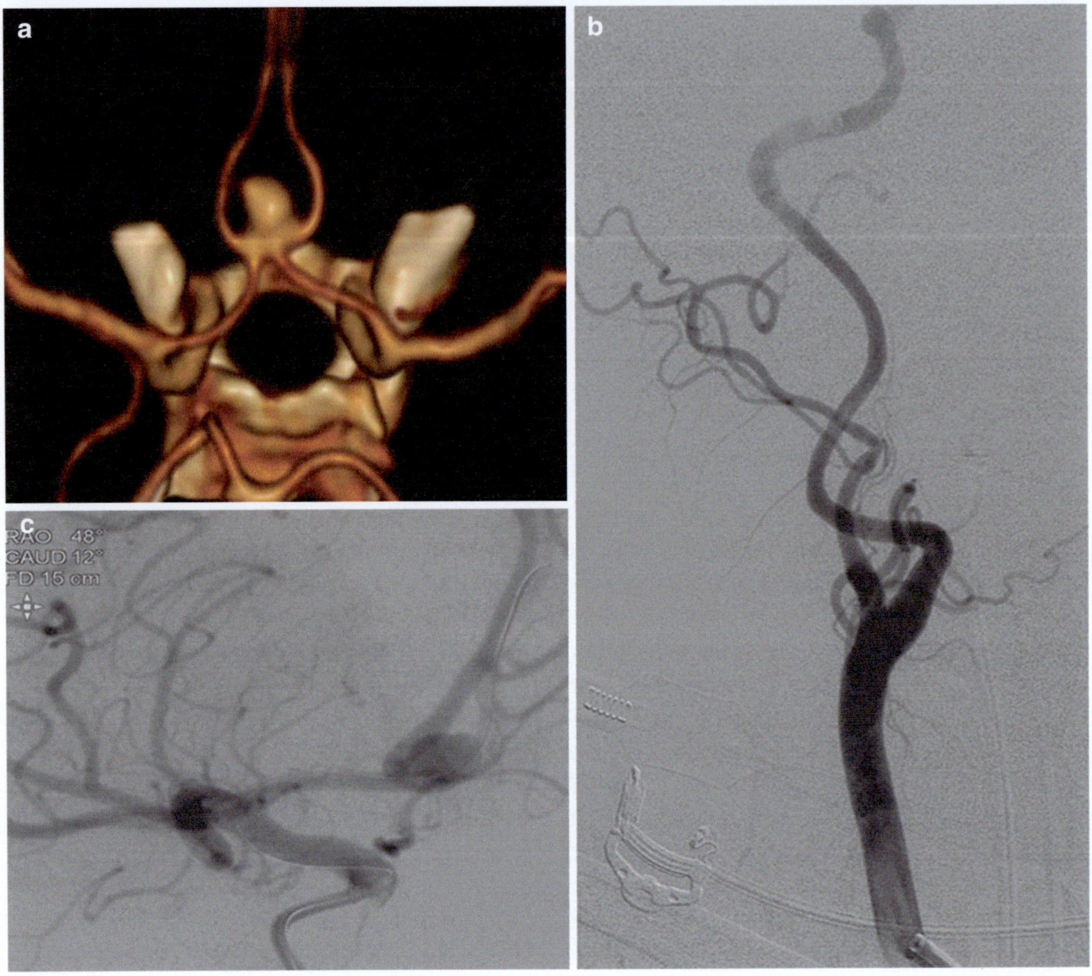

Fig. 36.1 (**a**) Three-dimensional reformat of a CT angiogram demonstrates the wide-necked right ACOM bifurcation aneurysm. (**b**) Digital subtraction angiography (DSA) image of the right carotid bifurcation illustrates a gracile and tortuous internal carotid artery. (**c**) DSA image of the right ICA bifurcation demonstrates a 5F Navien (Covidien Vascular Therapies, Mansfield, MA, USA) in the distal right ICA and a Synchro (Stryker, Freemont, CA, USA) microwire crossing the aneurysm neck; however, the VIA 27 (Sequent Medical/MicroVention Terumo, Tustin, CA, USA) could not be manipulated into the aneurysm

7x3 mm was selected. The VIA 27 microcatheter was negotiated into the ACOM aneurysm and the WEB device deployed (Fig. 36.3b–e). Immediate stasis was obtained in the aneurysm. The aneurysm remained occluded at 2-year follow-up.

Tips and Tricks

1. WEB is a good option for wide-necked bifurcation aneurysms.
2. Peri-procedural dual antiplatelet therapy is not essential but should be considered. In the absence of contraindications, the authors recommend 500 mg of intravenous aspirin immediately after deployment and 75 mg aspirin after the procedure for 6 weeks to avoid thromboembolic complications.
3. If access is tricky, consider an alternative vascular approach, using smaller catheters, or an additional distal support catheter.
4. Always use good proximal support and distal access catheters for WEB.
5. Use appropriate size of VIA catheter depending on WEB sizes. Beware: the VIA 32 catheter is short in length.

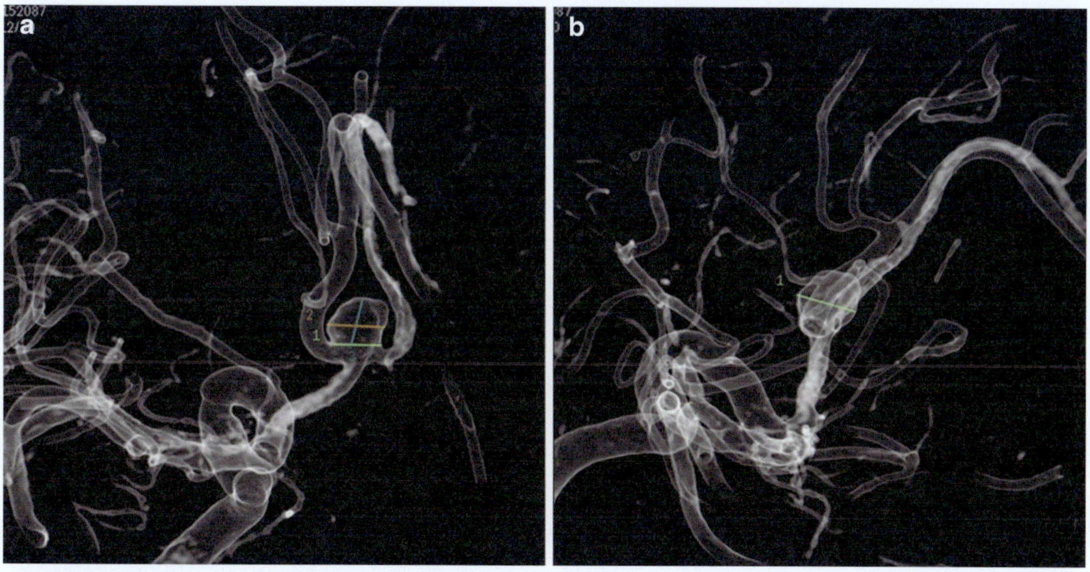

Fig. 36.2 Images from a three-dimensional rotational angiogram in AP (**a**) and lateral (**b**) projections illustrate the ACOM aneurysm with maximal height, width, and neck measurements. Ideally, height and width measurements in both planes are required for WEB sizing

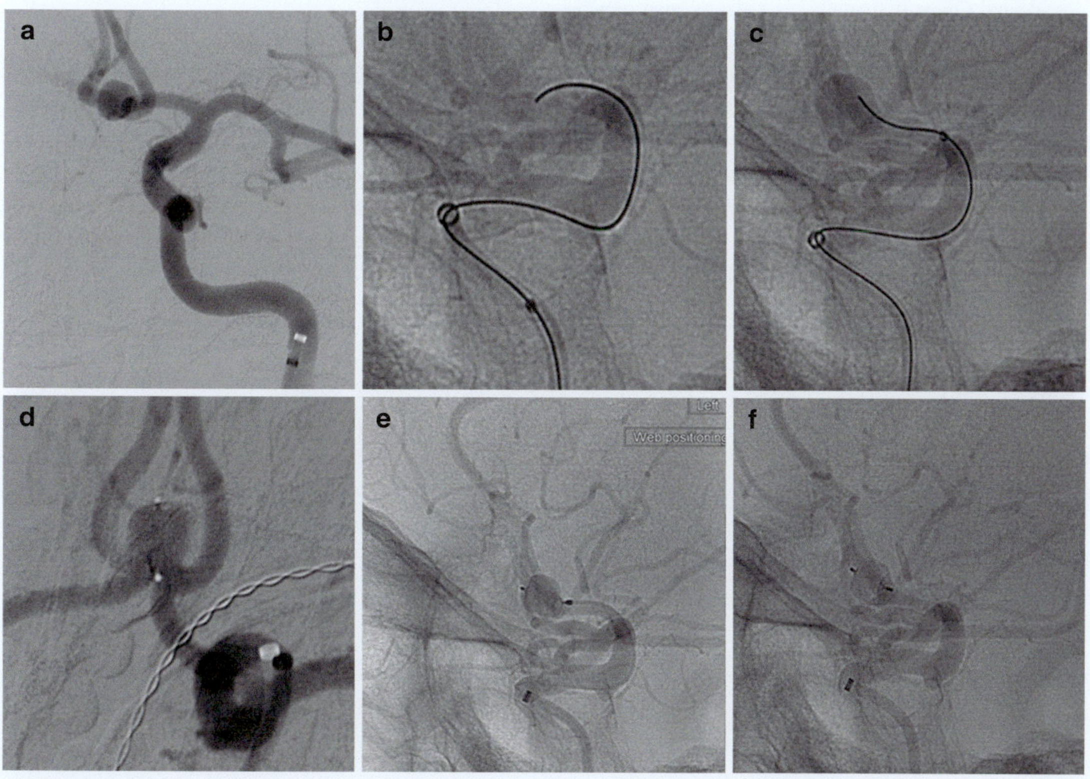

Fig. 36.3 Selected DSA images. (**a**, **b**, **c**) Navien guiding catheter within the distal ICA. A VIA 27 microcatheter is advanced over a Synchro microwire sited within the distal A1. (**d**, **e**) Placement and deployment of the WEB device into the aneurysm, the markers are sited at the apex and base of the aneurysm indicating appropriate sizing. (**f**) Post deployment of the WEB with occlusion of the aneurysm

6. Be careful with WEB sizing; the operator should take time to make the decision. Undersizing results in recanalization; oversizing compromises adjacent vessels and risks thrombus formation and the need for permanent antiplatelet therapy.
7. If unsure of the best size, go up 1 mm in width if needed, provided it does not compromise the parent vessel. Always remember to think of the simultaneous increase in height of the device if the WEB width is oversized.
8. Always use a biplane angiographic view to assess the position of the VIA catheter before deployment.
9. The mode of deployment depends on position of catheter; one can push the device or unsheath the device depending on the position of the microcatheter.
10. Until the WEB device flowers it is stiff, so don't push it against the wall of the aneurysm. Once it flowers, it softens and can be deployed safely.
11. Before detachment of the WEB, make sure all tension has been released from the system.
12. Know when not to WEB—some aneurysms are very challenging for WEB and alternative techniques should be considered. Such cases include carotico-ophthalmic aneurysms, sidewall distal MCA aneurysms, and partially thrombosed aneurysms.
13. WEB 17 appears promising in acutely ruptured aneurysms.

Suggested Reading

Anil G, Goddard AJ, Ross SM, Deniz K, Patankar T. WEB in partially thrombosed intracranial aneurysms: a word of caution. Am J Neuroradiol. 2016;37(5):892–6.

Lawson A, Goddard T, Ross S, Tyagi A, Deniz K, Patankar T. Endovascular treatment of cerebral aneurysms using the Woven EndoBridge technique in a single center: preliminary results. J Neurosurg. 2017;126(1):17–28.

Lawson A, Molyneux A, Sellar R, Lamin S, Thomas A, Gholkar A, Patankar T. Safety results from the treatment of 109 cerebral aneurysms using the Woven EndoBridge technique: preliminary results in the United Kingdom. J Neurosurg. 2018;128:144–53.

Lubicz B, Klisch J, Gauvrit JY, Szikora I, Leonardi M, Liebig T, Nuzzi NP, Boccardi E, Paola FD, Holtmannspötter M, Weber W. WEB-DL endovascular treatment of wide-neck bifurcation aneurysms: short-and midterm results in a European study. Am J Neuroradiol. 2014;35(3):432–8.

Lubicz B, Mine B, Collignon L, Brisbois D, Duckwiler G, Strother C. WEB device for endovascular treatment of wide-neck bifurcation aneurysms. Am J Neuroradiol. 2013;34(6):1209–14.

Pierot L, Liebig T, Sychra V, Kadziolka K, Dorn F, Strasilla C, Kabbasch C, Klisch J. Intrasaccular flow-disruption treatment of intracranial aneurysms: preliminary results of a multicenter clinical study. Am J Neuroradiol. 2012;33(7):1232–8.

37 Glue Occlusion of Dissecting Aneurysm After Induced Cardiac Asystole

Hans Henkes

Case

A 27-year-old man sustained a severe facial and cranial trauma. The initial CT examination showed several fractures of the facial and skull base bones, a frontal epidural hematoma, and a traumatic SAH. CTA at this time did not reveal an aneurysm of the anterior communicating artery ACom A (Fig. 37.1). Recurrent right frontal intraparenchymal and intraventricular hemorrhages (Fig. 37.2) requiring decompressive craniectomy and an external ventricular drainage was noted on the 9th and 10th day following trauma. Repeat cerebral angiography now revealed a dissecting aneurysm of the AcomA (Fig. 37.3). nBCA glue occlusion of the sac under adenosine-induced asystole was undertaken.

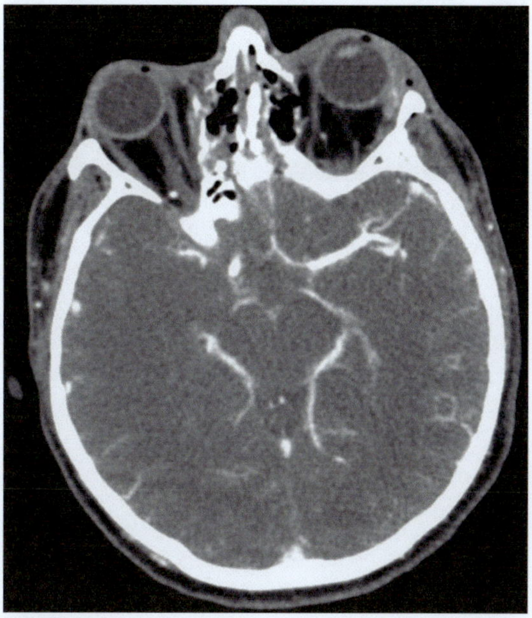

Fig. 37.1 CTA following a severe trauma to the face and skull with fractures of the facial bones but no aneurysm of the AcomA

Issues

Dissecting intracranial aneurysms are not rare but easily missed. The majority of dissecting intradural aneurysms occurs spontaneously, but a preceding trauma may well result in arterial dissection and aneurysm formation. Dissecting aneurysms of intracranial arteries carry a high risk of rupture. The treatment of these lesions can be difficult since they are actually pseudoaneurysms, covered only by the adventitia of the concerning vessel. Any impact on the wall of the dissecting aneurysm can result in an instantaneous (re-)rupture. This may happen during

H. Henkes
Neuroradiological Clinic, Klinikum Stuttgart,
Stuttgart, Germany

V. Gupta et al. (eds.), *100 Interesting Case Studies in Neurointervention: Tips and Tricks*,
https://doi.org/10.1007/978-981-13-1346-2_37

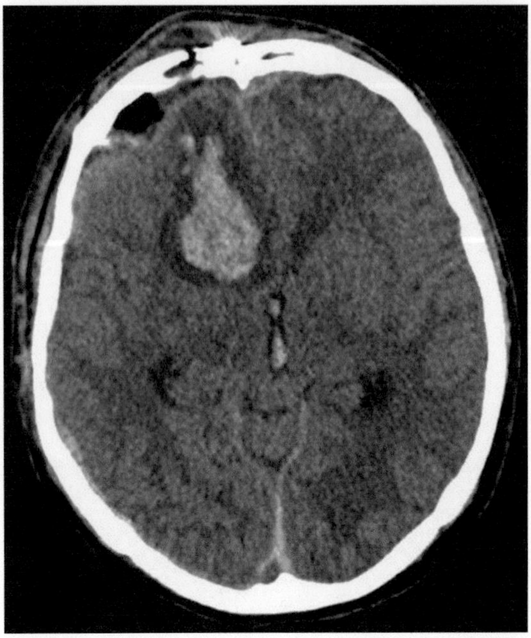

Fig. 37.2 Right frontal intraparenchymal hemorrhage 9 days after the trauma

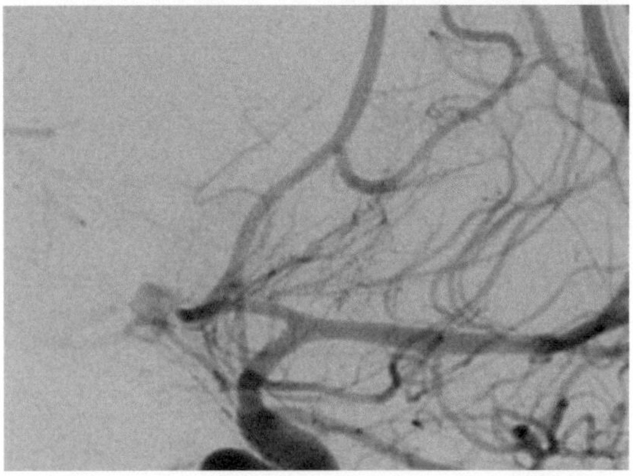

Fig. 37.3 Presumably dissecting AcomA aneurysm as the most likely source of the frontal lobe hematoma

attempted clipping or coil occlusion. Therefore alternatives such as parent vessel occlusion, flow diversion, or the usage of liquid embolic agents should be considered.

nBCA glue has the advantage of very rapid polymerization within seconds, good visibility under fluoroscopy, and strong adhesion to the vessel wall. Injection of a liquid polymer into an aneurysm carries the risk of an uncontrolled escape of this liquid into the parent or efferent artery.

The distribution of other liquid embolic agents (e.g., ethylene vinyl alcohol copolymer; Onyx) can be controlled by a temporary vessel occlusion with a balloon catheter. This is not the case with nBCA (e.g., Glubran, Histoacryl) since the available balloon catheters are disintegrated by contact with this embolic agent.

Cardiac arrest for several seconds allows a better control of the distribution of a polymerizing liquid embolic agent. Asystole can be induced by a temporary pacemaker, which is set on 400 beats per minute (rapid overpacing). The usage of an IV adenosine bolus injection is less cumbersome, and the effect is more reliable.

Management

An external ventricular drainage and a decompressive craniectomy were performed prior to the angiography and endovascular treatment. Under general anesthesia via a right femoral arterial access, a 6F femoral sheath and a 6F Guider were inserted. Also from the right groin, a 4F sheath and a Tempo4 diagnostic catheter were introduced in the femoral vein, and the tip of the catheter was placed at the level of the right atrium. The left ICA was catheterized. Gentle injection of the left ICA confirmed the dissecting AcomA aneurysm with a fundus diameter of about 5 mm (Fig. 37.4). An Echelon10_45° microcatheter using a Traxcess14 microguidewire was inserted into the aneurysm avoiding any contact to the presumably very fragile aneurysm wall (Fig. 37.5). Injection of the left ICA with the microcatheter tip inside the aneurysm did not show any opacification of the aneurysm (Fig. 37.6). This confirmed that the aneurysm was hemodynamically isolated from the parent vessel due to the inserted microcatheter. The liquid embolic agent Glubran2 was mixed with an equal amount of lipiodol. The microcatheter was gently and very slowly flushed with a 40% glucose solution. The dead space of the microcatheter was filled with the Glubran2/lipiodol mixture. Through the venous 4F catheter, a bolus of 36 mg adenosine (Adrekar) was injected and asystole induced for about 15 s. Under DSA with six frames per second, a small amount of the liquid embolic agent was injected

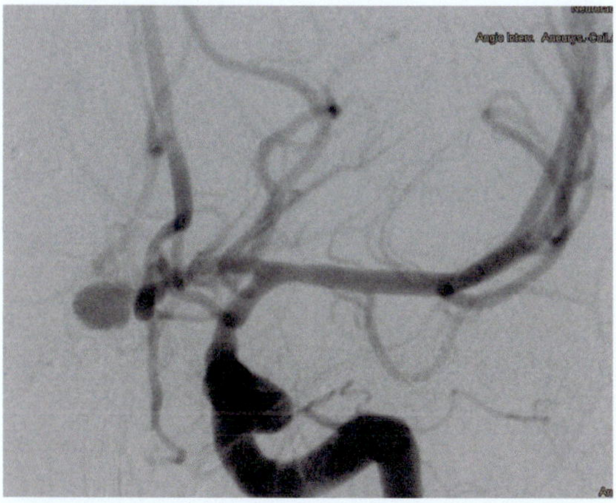

Fig. 37.4 The dissecting AcomA aneurysm on the following day prior treatment

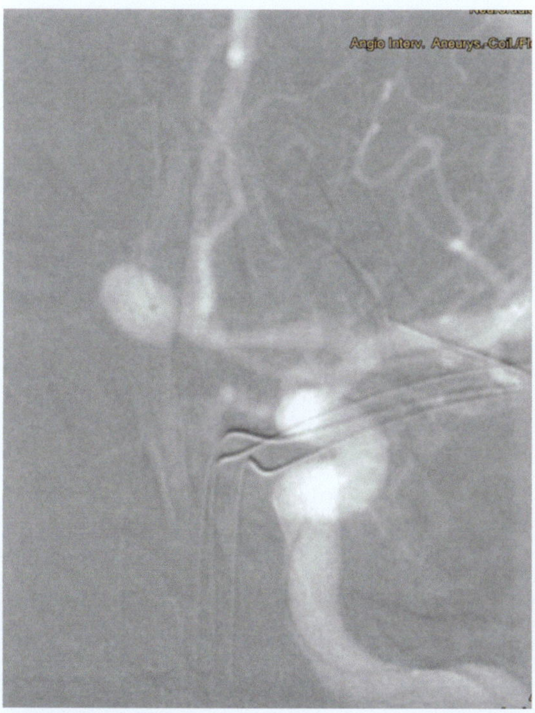

Fig. 37.5 Road map was used to insert an Echelon10 microcatheter

(Fig. 37.7). The polymerizing liquid remained inside the aneurysm. The injection was stopped for 5 s to allow for complete solidification of the polymer, and the microcatheter was rapidly withdrawn. Subsequent injection of the left ICA confirmed the complete occlusion of the dissecting aneurysm without injury to the afferent or emboli

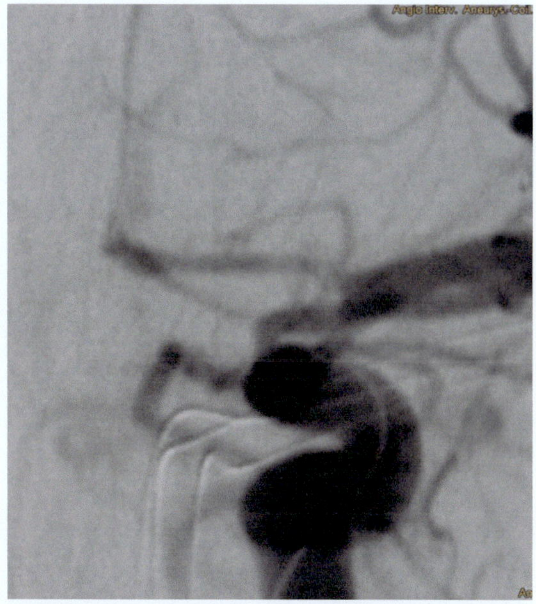

Fig. 37.6 The neck of the dissecting aneurysm was so narrow that the catheterization of the aneurysm already interrupted the blood circulation in the aneurysm sac

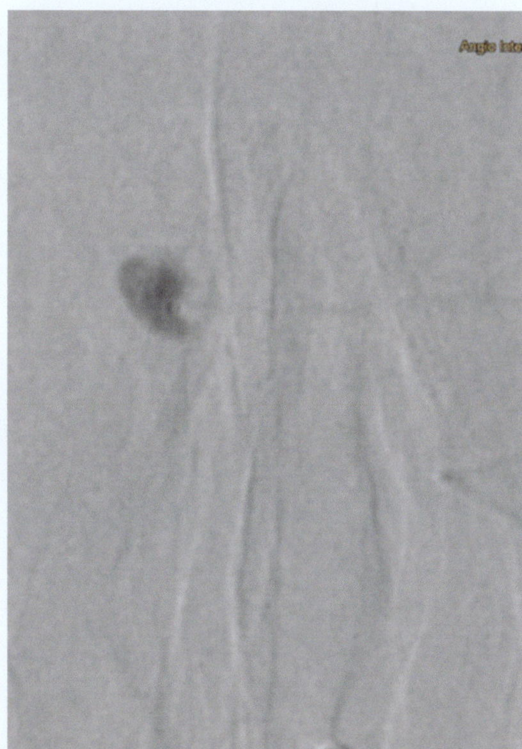

Fig. 37.7 Under adenosine-induced asystole and using DSA with a six per second frame rate, a small amount of Glubran2/lipiodol was very slowly injected. The polymerizing liquid remained entirely within the aneurysm

into the efferent vessels (Fig. 37.8). DSA 1 week later showed posthemorrhagic vasospasm but no aneurysm perfusion (Fig. 37.9). On follow-up DSA examinations 15 months (Fig. 37.10) and

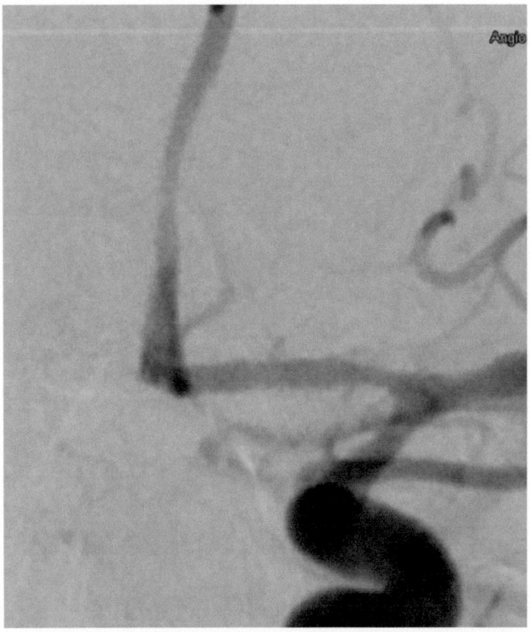

Fig. 37.8 DSA with injection of the left ICA confirmed the complete occlusion of the aneurysm

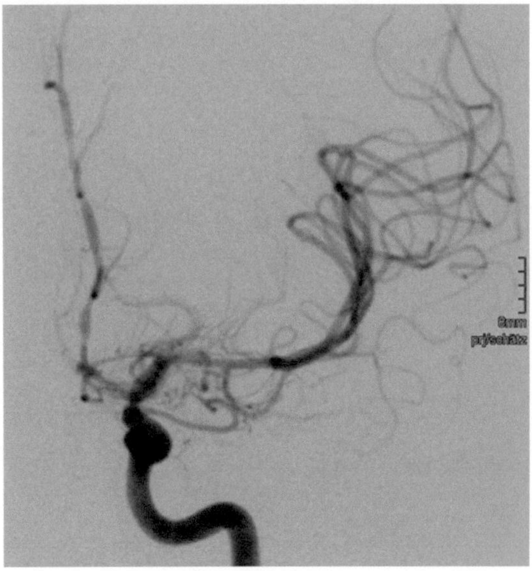

Fig. 37.9 One week later, massive posthemorrhagic vasospasm but no aneurysm perfusion was found

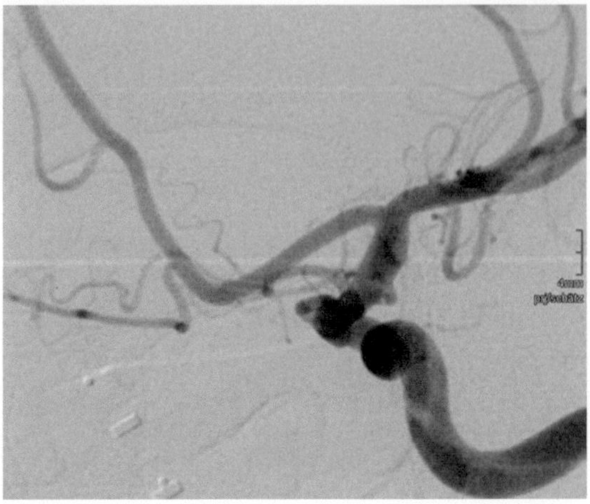

Fig. 37.10 Follow-up DSA 15 months later. The vasospasm is completely resolved, and the aneurysm remains occluded

40 months after the treatment, neither the previous aneurysm nor chronic vasospasm was found.

Tips and Tricks

1. A typical feature of dissecting aneurysms is their rapid formation, a change in size and shape within days, and the propensity for (recurrent) rupture. In the acute phase after a first rupture, we sometimes wait three to four ways until we treat these aneurysms. This strategy exposes the patient to the risk of another hemorrhage but helps to avoid intervening in the initial phase after a rupture when the aneurysm wall is very vulnerable.
2. The typical usage of Glubran2 or Histoacryl mixed with lipiodol is in the embolization of brain AVMs. This application is certainly more forgiving than the treatment of aneurysms with glue. Using glue for aneurysm occlusion should be done only by experienced operators.
3. The bolus injection of adenosine to induce asystole is reliable and in our experience safe. A standard dosage of 36 mg per bolus is recommended. The preferred way of application is via a venous catheter adjacent to the right atrium. The average duration of the induced asystole is about 15 s. In patients with massive

arteriovenous shunts, significantly increased dosages are sometimes required. As a safety measure, patients undergoing induced asystole as an elective treatment should have had a comprehensive cardiac examination. We always have a defibrillator ready but fortunately never had to use it. Induced asystole is an off-label use of adenosine.

Suggested Reading

Henkes H, Reinartz J, Preiss H, Miloslavski E, Kirsch M, Kühne D. Endovascular treatment of small intracranial aneurysms: three alternatives to coil occlusion. Minim Invasive Neurosurg. 2006;49(2):65–9.

Lee SH, Kwun BD, Kim JU, Choi JH, Ahn JS, Park W, Yun JH. Adenosine-induced transient asystole during intracranial aneurysm surgery: indications, dosing, efficacy, and risks. Acta Neurochir (Wien). 2015;157(11):1879–86; discussion 1886. Epub 2015 Sep 18. https://doi.org/10.1007/s00701-015-2581-7.

Powers CJ, Wright DR, McDonagh DL, Borel CO, Zomorodi AR, Britz GW. Transient adenosine-induced asystole during the surgical treatment of anterior circulation cerebral aneurysms: technical note. Neurosurgery. 2010;67(2 Suppl Operative):461–70. https://doi.org/10.1227/NEU.0b013e3181f7ef46.

Selcuk H, Soylu N, Albayram S, Selcuk D, Ozer H, Kocer N, Islak C. Endovascular treatment of persistent epistaxis due to pseudoaneurysm formation of the ophthalmic artery secondary to nasogastric tube. Cardiovasc Intervent Radiol. 2005;28(2):242–5.

Teng MM, Chen CC, Lirng JF, Chen SS, Lee LS, Chang T. N-butyl-2-cyanoacrylate for embolisation of carotid aneurysm. Neuroradiology. 1994;36(2):144–7.

Wright JM, Huang CL, Sharma R, Manjila S, Xu F, Dabb B, Bambakidis NC. Cardiac standstill and circulatory flow arrest in surgical treatment of intracranial aneurysms: a historical review. Neurosurg Focus. 2014;36(4):E10. https://doi.org/10.3171/2014.2.

Anterior Communicating (ACOM) Artery Aneurysm; Acute Angle Between A1 and A2: Microwire Shaping

38

Rajsrinivas Parthasarathy and Vipul Gupta

Case

A 40-year-old male was shifted from another hospital with a diagnosis of subarachnoid haemorrhage. His clinical condition was good with a Hunt and Hess grade 2. CT scan showed Fisher grade 2 haemorrhage. DSA (Fig. 38.1) revealed a broad-based lobulated ACOM aneurysm. Balloon-assisted coiling was planned.

Issues

1. Large broad neck aneurysm
2. Navigating the microwire across the aneurysm sac

Management

Procedure was performed under general anaesthesia. A 6F guiding catheter was placed in the right ICA. The A2 ACA was arising at an acute angle from the A1 ACA (Fig. 38.1). A

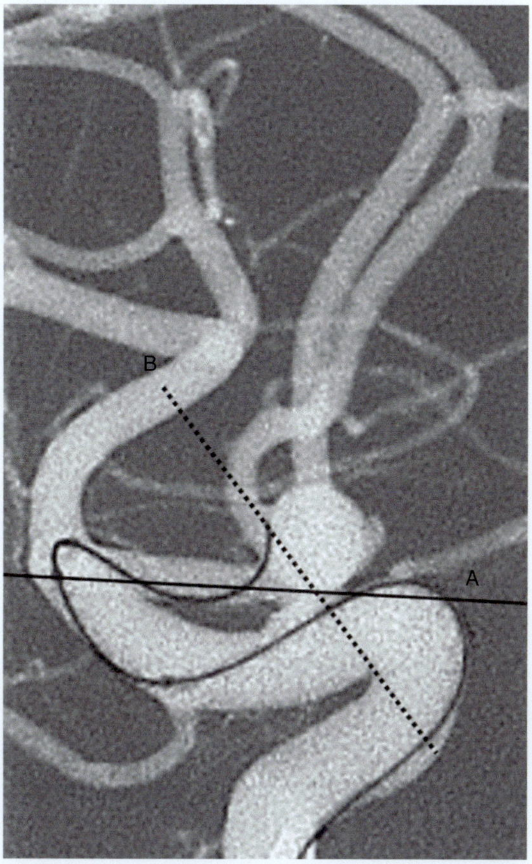

Fig. 38.1 Axis A is along the A1 ACA; axis B is along the A2 ACA origin. Note the acute angle between the A1 and A2 ACA

R. Parthasarathy (✉)
Vascular Neurology and Neurointerventional Surgery, Artemis Agrim Institute of Neuroscience, Gurgaon, India

V. Gupta
Neurointerventional Surgery, Stroke Unit, Artemis Agrim Institute of Neuroscience, Gurgaon, India
e-mail: vipul.gupta@artemishospitals.com

V. Gupta et al. (eds.), *100 Interesting Case Studies in Neurointervention: Tips and Tricks*, https://doi.org/10.1007/978-981-13-1346-2_38

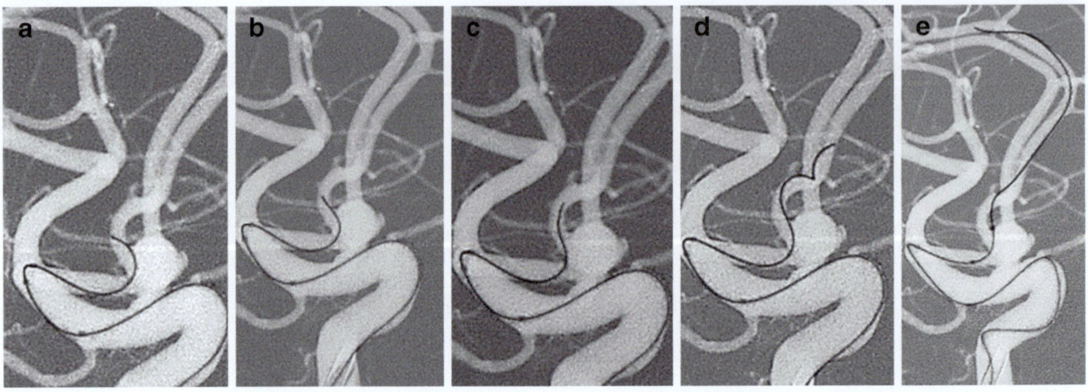

Fig. 38.2 (**a**–**e**) Note wire access of the left A2 ACA

balloon catheter (Scepter XC, Microvention, Tustin, California, USA) was navigated across the aneurysm neck using a 0.014 guidewire (Synchro, Stryker Neurovascular, CA, USA) that was appropriately shaped (Fig. 38.2, 38.3), and the coiling microcatheter was placed into the aneurysm sac. Thereafter, coiling was performed using balloon remodelling. The balloon was allowed to bulge into the neck of the aneurysm in order to spare the pathway for the A2 ACA that was arising at a relatively acute angle to the A1 ACA. Some coils were seen to project into the neck after coil embolization. The balloon was inflated, and a new blank roadmap (without dye injection) was acquired. Balloon deflation did not reveal displacement of coil loops. This indicated that the coils were in aneurysm sac either anterior or posterior to the neck. Final angiogram revealed complete occlusion of the aneurysm with preservation of all arteries (Fig. 38.4). Patient made a slow but progressive recovery and was independent on interval follow-up. Interval cerebral angiography showed stable result with no recanalization.

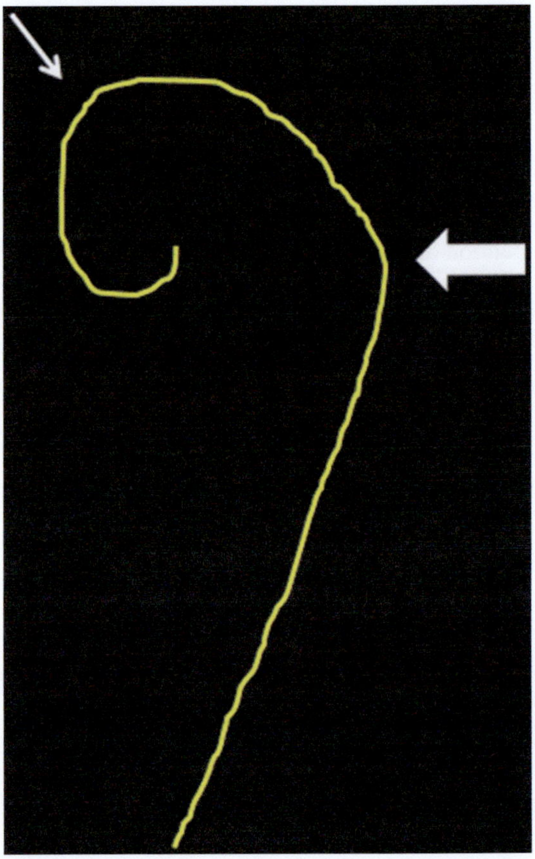

Fig. 38.3 Distal tight curve (*white arrow*); proximal 90° curve (*bold white arrow*)

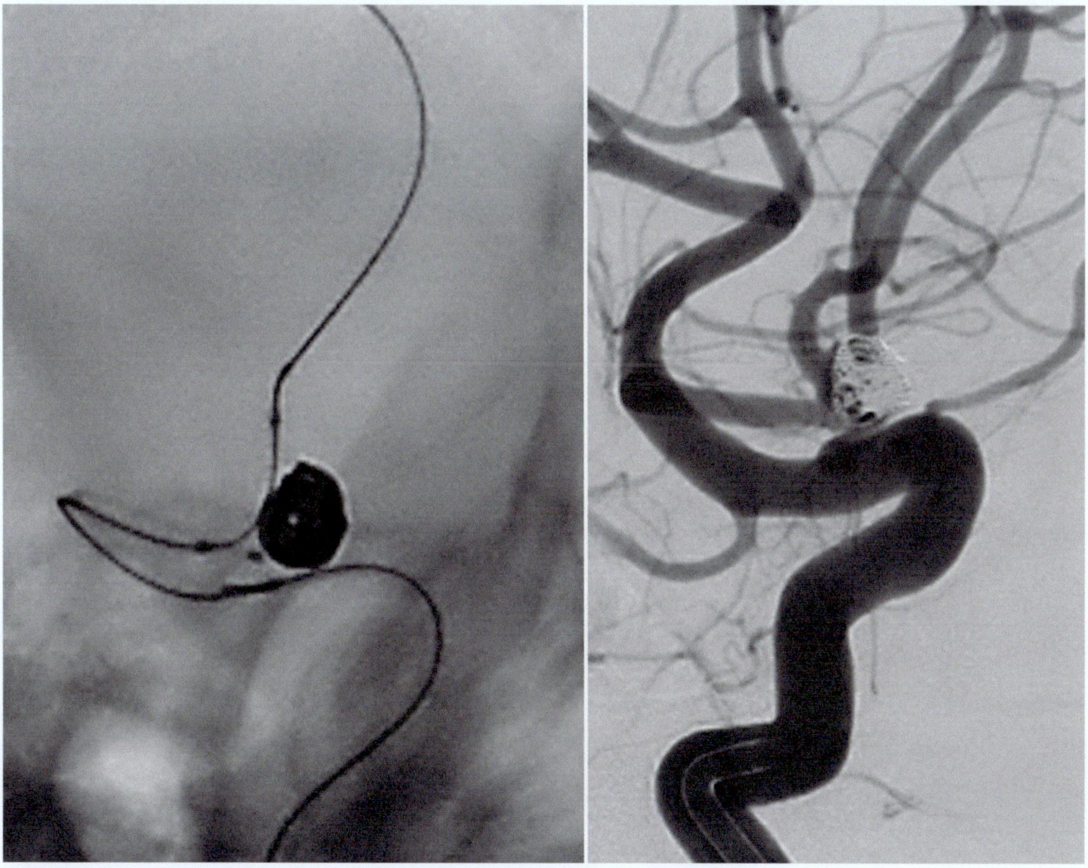

Fig. 38.4 Native and DSA image showing aneurysm occlusion post procedure

Tips and Tricks

1. Understanding the neck anatomy is crucial to achieving satisfactory coil occlusion of the aneurysm sac while preserving the patency of the artery harbouring the aneurysm.
2. In circumstances where the A2 ACA makes an acute angle with the A1 ACA, balloon placement can be challenging.
   (a) Use a double-lumen balloon in difficult anatomy. There is a portion of the catheter beyond the balloon; this catheter segment allows for easier navigation across the bends.
   (b) A dual-lumen balloon allows for changing the wire shape with ease.
   (c) A Synchro 0.014′ wire offers better torqueability and navigation across acute bends and therefore in authors' experience is the wire of choice in difficult anatomy.
   (d) Wire shape is the key to navigate across the acute bends. A distal pigtail-like curve and a proximal 90° curve allow for navigating across the bend without entering the sac (Fig. 38.4).

Suggested Reading

Fiorella D, Woo HH. How I treat: balloon assisted treatment of intracranial aneurysms: the conglomerate coil mass technique. J Neurointerv Surg. 2009;1(2):121–31.

Broad Neck Dysplastic Anterior Communicating Artery Aneurysm: Compartmental Packing

39

Vipul Gupta

Case

A 66-year-old female presented with subarachnoid hemorrhage (Hunt and Hess IV). The angiogram revealed an anterior communicating artery aneurysm (Fig. 39.1). The aneurysm had a broad neck involving origin of both the anterior cerebral arteries. The A1 segment of left ACA was absent. Two lobules were seen near the neck of aneurysm (Fig. 39.1c). Balloon-assisted coiling was planned.

Issues

1. In view of broad neck, the coil stability was an issue in spite of the balloon. Since the width of the aneurysm was much more than the length, the coils were likely to bulge into the parent vessel.
2. The angle showing the neck of the aneurysm (Fig. 39.1b) could not be achieved by the C-arm.
3. The lobules near the neck indicate potential friability and it was critical to occlude this part of aneurysm.

Management

Balloon-assisted coiling was undertaken. Since the angle profiling the neck could not be achieved, an end-on view profiling both the ACAs was used as working angle. In the other angle, the near the neck lobules were profiled. The width of the aneurysm sac (10 mm) was greater than the length/depth (from neck to fundus 6.4 mm). A coil that is bigger than the depth of the sac could prolapse into the parent artery. Therefore, the first coil that was used was a 6 mm coil (Fig. 39.2b, c). After checking for the stability of the first coil, multiple coils were placed in a single inflation, achieving adequate occlusion of upper part of aneurysm. Thereafter, the coiling microcatheter was reshaped and navigated to lower residual part of aneurysm, and further coil placement was performed leading to complete occlusion. In the later stages, the coils could be placed in the lobules near the neck (Fig. 39.2e). This was done carefully under clear visualisation and complete occlusion was achieved with preservation of the parent arteries (Fig. 39.3). Patient achieved complete recovery.

V. Gupta
Neurointerventional Surgery, Stroke Unit,
Artemis Agrim Institute of Neuroscience,
Gurgaon, India
e-mail: vipul.gupta@artemishospitals.com

V. Gupta et al. (eds.), *100 Interesting Case Studies in Neurointervention: Tips and Tricks*,
https://doi.org/10.1007/978-981-13-1346-2_39

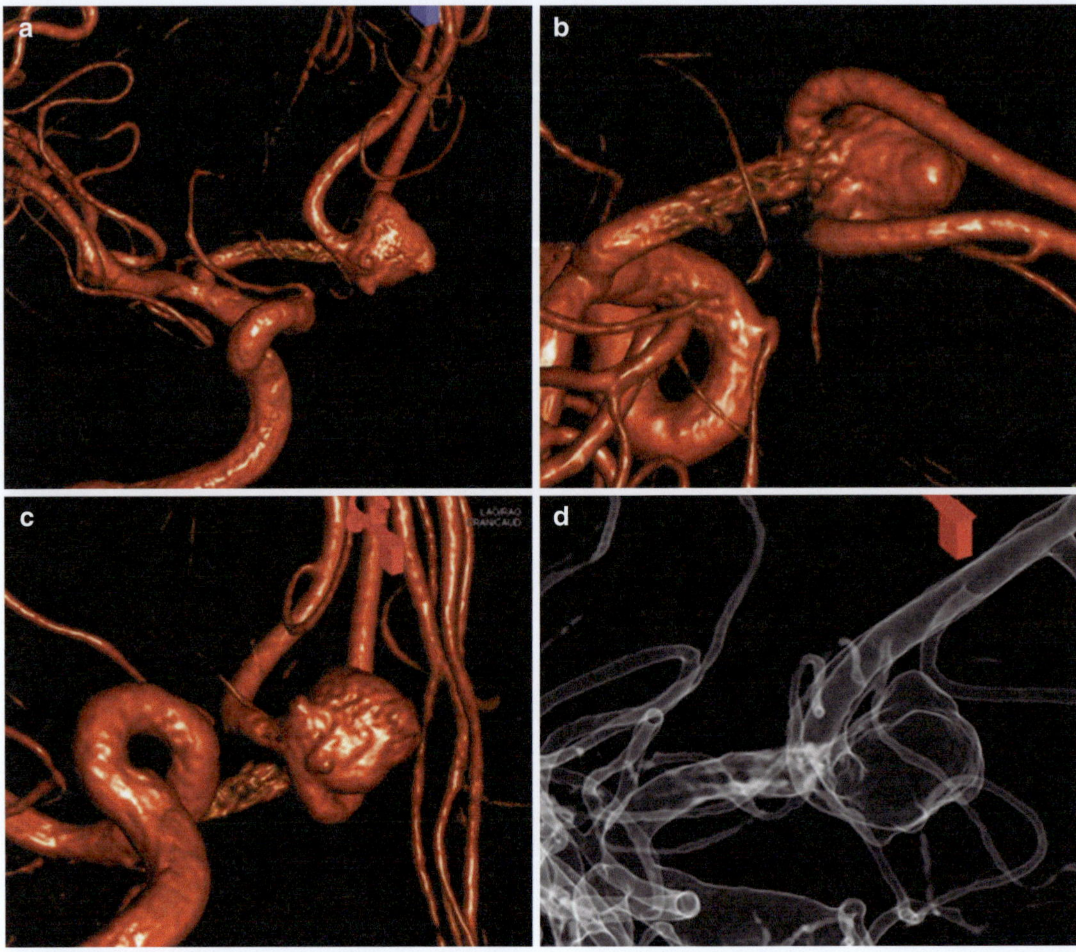

Fig. 39.1 (**a**) 3D reconstruction images show a large broad neck aneurysm in anterior communicating artery. (**b**) Image showing the neck; however this angle was impossible to achieve with the C-arm. The aneurysm is involving origin of both anterior cerebral arteries. (**c**) Two lobulations seen near the neck region, indicating probable weak spots. (**d**) See-through reconstruction image showing origin of both ACAs in end-on manner. This angle was used as working angle during the procedure

Tips and Tricks

1. Broad neck aneurysms with width more than the length, one may have to do compartmental packing. After packing one part of the aneurysm, the catheter can be repositioned (if need be after reshaping) to treat residual aneurysm.
2. In the event the neck cannot be profiled due to extreme angulation, an option is to work in an end-on view after placing the balloon. As shown above, this technique enabled us to profile origin of the both the ACAs. The "see-through/translucent" reconstruction after rotational angiography is extremely useful to get this view.
3. In cases with near the neck lobules, it is critical to secure these potential weak spots. It is prudent to profile these weak spots in one of the views, as coiling of these should be performed with clear visualization.

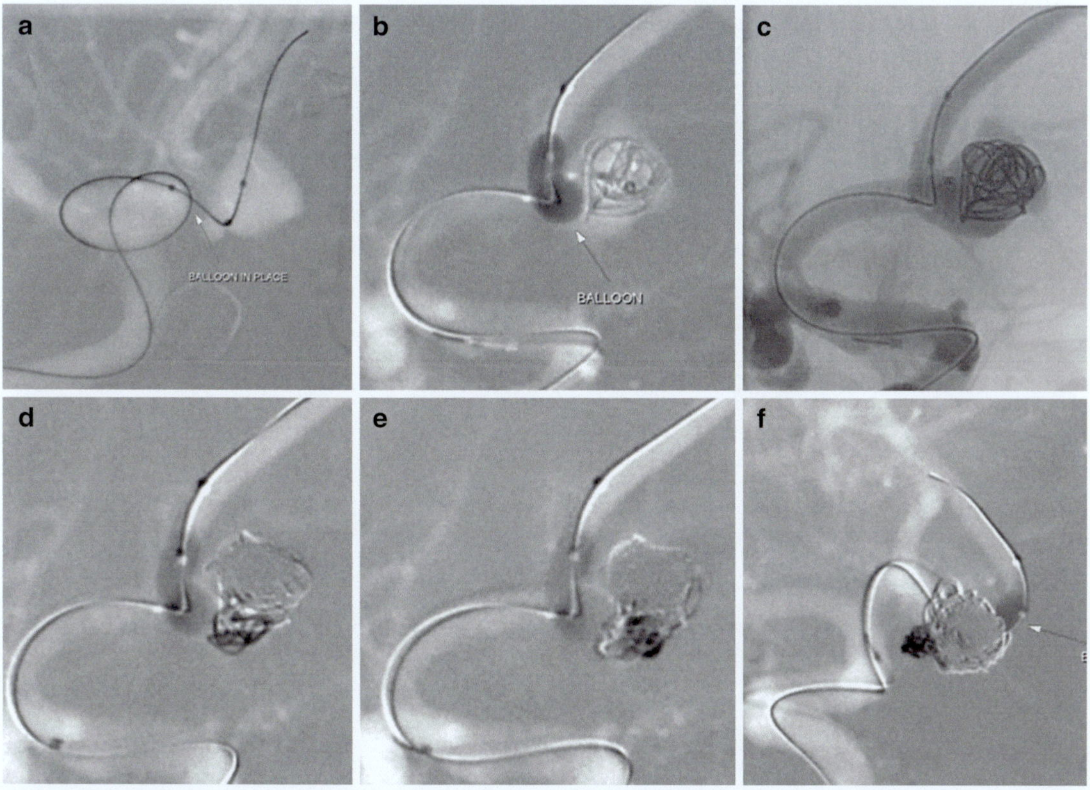

Fig. 39.2 (**a**) Road map image with balloon placement in left ACA. After placing the balloon microcatheter, working angles used were as shown in Fig. 39.1d. (**b**, **c**) Placement of first coil. The coil was not well anchored onto the walls. (**d**, **e**) After packing upper part of aneurysm, the catheter was navigated into lower lobule and was coiled. (**f**) Shows coil placement in lobules near the neck (refer to Fig. 39.1c)

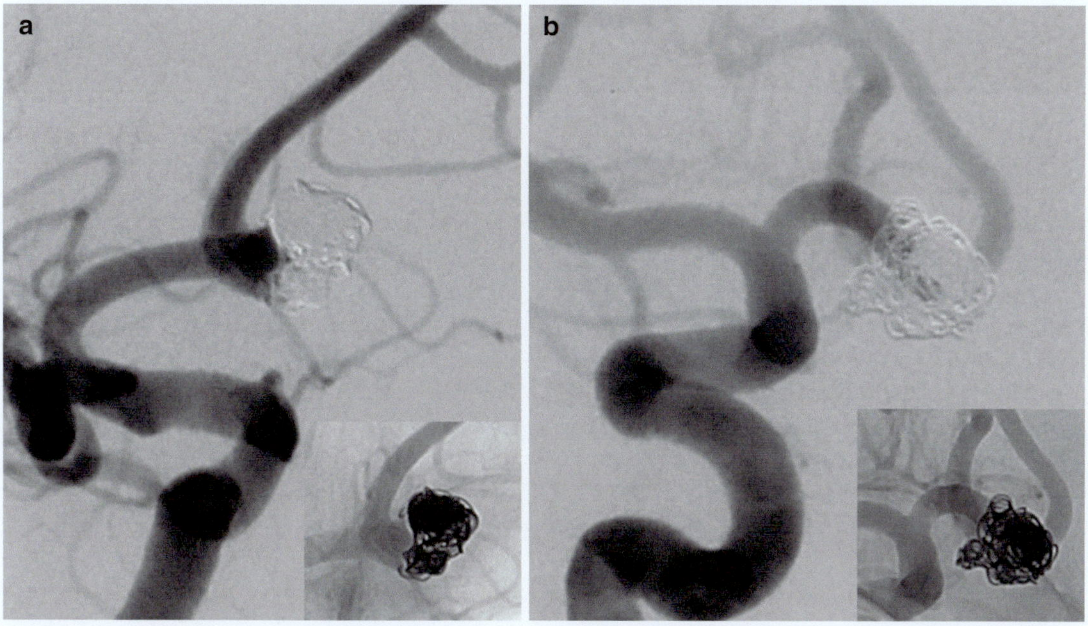

Fig. 39.3 (**a**, **b**) Post-embolization angiograms showing complete occlusion of the aneurysm. The inset in image **b** clearly shows sparing of origins of ACAs

4. Single inflation technique is useful if the first coil that has been used is less likely to oppose all the walls of the sac as it usually is the case when the width is greater than the length/depth of the aneurysm sac. This allows for coil stability.
5. During coiling of broad neck aneurysms, adequate care should be taken regarding heparinization, particularly in the later stages of procedure.

Suggested Reading

Gonzalez N, Sedrak M, Martin N, Vinuela F. Impact of anatomic features in the endovascular embolization of 181 anterior communicating artery aneurysms. Stroke. 2008;39:2776–82.

Tsutsumi M, Aikawa H, Onizuka M, Kodama T, Nii K, Matsubara S, et al. Endovascular treatment of tiny ruptured anterior communicating artery aneurysms. Neuroradiology. 2008;50:509–15.

Broad Neck Basilar Top Aneurysm: Understanding the Neck

40

Vipul Gupta

Case

A 64-year-old male presented with subarachnoid hemorrhage (Fischer grade III). He was well preserved (Hunt and Hess II). DSA revealed a broad neck basilar top aneurysm pointing superiorly (Fig. 40.1a). An anteriorly projecting lobule seen in the lateral view was the probable site of rupture (Fig. 40.1b).

Issue

- Coiling of broad neck aneurysm with preservation of both posterior cerebral arteries
- Complete occlusion of the anteriorly projecting lobule

Management

Careful consideration was given to the evaluation of the anatomy of the neck of the aneurysm. In selected cases of bifurcation aneurysm, a slight bulge of the coil at the neck is likely to recreate the true bifurcation geometry and is considered desirable (Fig. 40.1c). Procedure was performed under general anesthesia and a 6 F guiding catheter was placed in left vertebral artery. First coil was deployed with care (Fig. 40.1d) so as to form a cage that opposed the walls of the aneurysm sac. In doing so, a slight bulge of the coil loop was noted at the neck of the aneurysm. However, the coil loop was not repositioned as it was mimicking the true anatomy of the bifurcation as described above. The path for both posterior cerebral arteries was clear. Thereafter, multiple soft coils were placed achieving complete occlusion in all the views including of the anteriorly projecting lobule. Patient had uneventful recovery. Angiography follow-up at 6 months showed stable occlusion of aneurysm (Fig. 40.2).

Tips and Tricks

1. Due consideration should be given to the anatomy of the neck.
2. In selected cases, a slight bulge of the coils recreates the true bifurcation and should be considered as the neck of the aneurysm.

V. Gupta
Neurointerventional Surgery, Stroke unit, Artemis Agrim Institute of Neuroscience, Gurgaon, India
e-mail: vipul.gupta@artemishospitals.com

V. Gupta et al. (eds.), *100 Interesting Case Studies in Neurointervention: Tips and Tricks*, https://doi.org/10.1007/978-981-13-1346-2_40

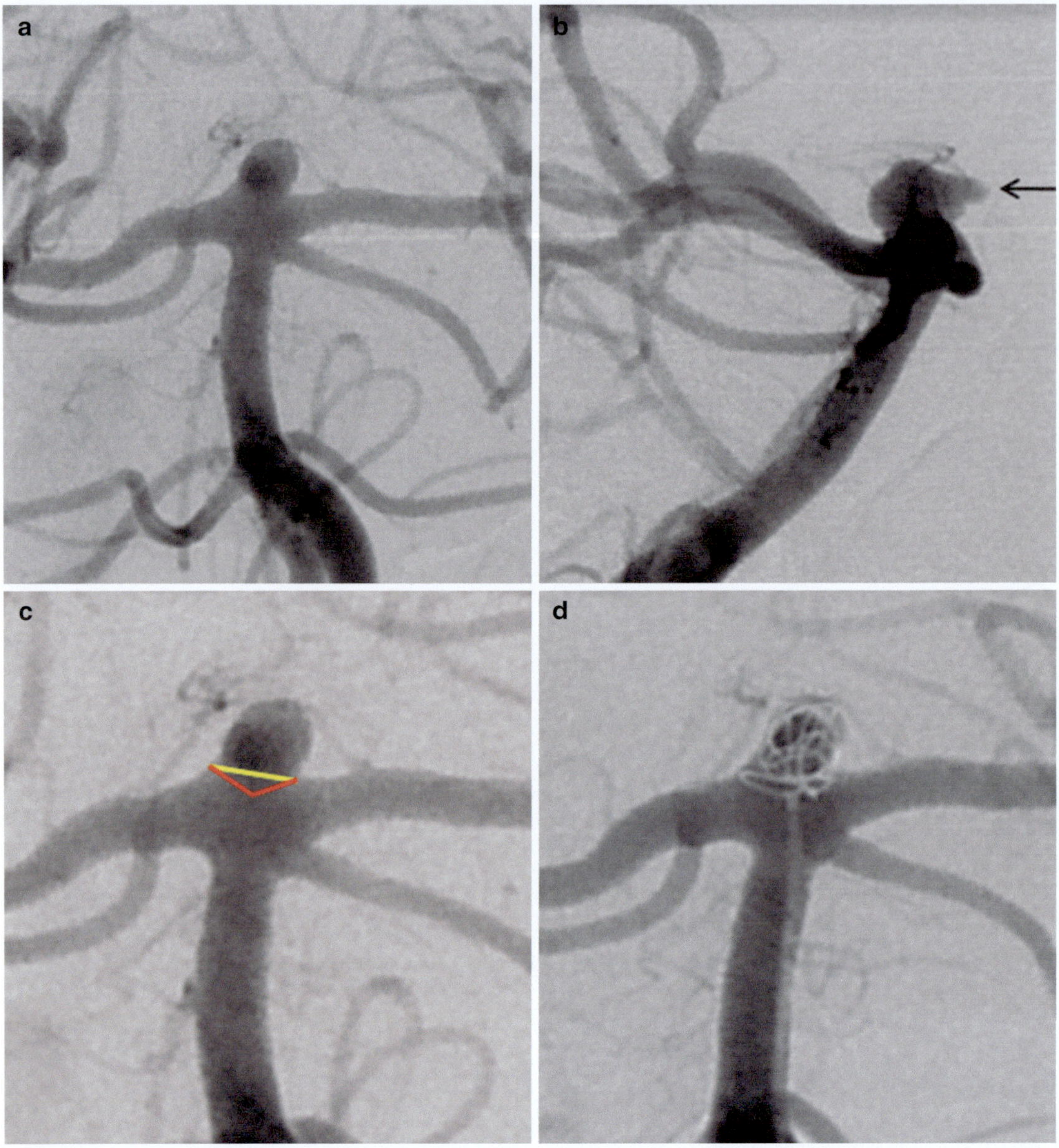

Fig. 40.1 (**a**) DSA image showed a broad neck basilar top aneurysm. (**b**) Lateral view showing an anterior pointing lobule (*black arrow*), the probable rupture point. (**c**) DSA demonstrating neck. Yellow line marks the conventional view of the neck, while the red denoted the true neck which will reform the bifurcation. (**d**) DSA after first coil placement showed the coil bulging into the bifurcation, forming the true neck according to the red line in the image **c**

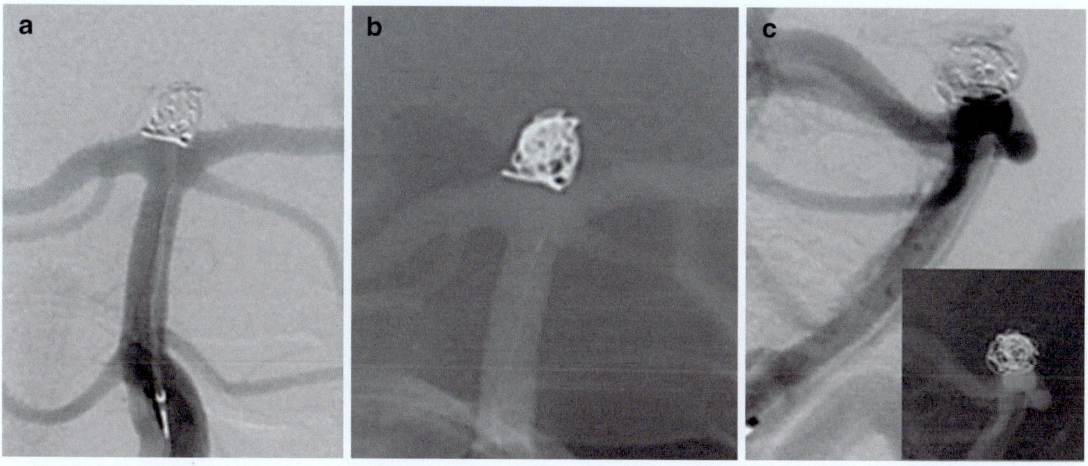

Fig. 40.2 (**a**) Post-embolization, check DSA image showing complete occlusion of the aneurysm. (**b**) Depicting the coil mass. (**c**) Lateral view showing complete occlusion of the aneurysm including anteriorly projecting lobule

Suggested Reading

Fernandez Zubillaga A, Guglielmi G, Vinuela F, Duckwiler GR. Endovascular occlusion of intracranial aneurysms with electrically detachable coils: correlation of aneurysm neck size and treatment results. Am J Neuroradiol. 1994;15:815–20.

Vallee JN, Pierot L, Bonafe A, Turjman F, Flandroy P, Berge J, et al. Endovascular treatment of intracranial wide-necked aneurysms using three-dimensional coils: predictors of immediate anatomic and clinical results. Am J Neuroradiol. 2004;25:298–306.

Aneurysm Rupture During Coiling: Key Actions

41

Vipul Gupta

Case

A 43-year-old female presented with subarachnoid hemorrhage (Hunt and Hess grade II). DSA (Fig. 41.1a–c) revealed left middle cerebral artery aneurysm. Patient was planned for coiling.

Issue

There was tortuosity of cervical ICA with a tight bend in the mid cervical segment (Fig. 41.1c). Placement of the guiding catheter proximal to the tight bend would result in less control over the microcatheter.

Management

Procedure was performed under general anesthesia. The guiding catheter tip was placed below the tight bending the cervical ICA. The aneurysm sac was catheterized and coiling was undertaken (Fig. 41.2a). During manipulation to place the third coil, the microcatheter suddenly moved forward and perforated through the fundus (Fig. 41.2b). DSA revealed contrast medium extravasation into subarachnoid space. No attempt was made to withdraw the microcatheter, and very soft small coils were used. After a few coils loops were deployed in the potential subarachnoid space outside the aneurysm margin, the catheter was slowly withdrawn and the rest of the coils deposited within the sac. Protamine was administered to reverse the effect of heparin and level of anesthesia was deepened with thiopentone. Mannitol was given to reduce the ICP. The rupture was controlled within few minutes, and repeat DSA revealed completely occluded aneurysm with no leakage of contrast and patent arteries (Fig. 41.2c). Immediate angioCT revealed subarachnoid dye and bleed in left sylvian fissure (Fig. 41.2d). On CT head there was no evidence of ventricular dilatation, large hematoma or midline shift. Patient was extubated the next day in intact neurological condition.

Tips and Tricks

1. In patients with tortuous anatomy, considerable tension can build up in the microcatheter. This may get released during the procedure resulting in sudden forward migration of the catheter tip. This may be avoided by releasing the tension in catheter soon after placement in the aneurysm by withdrawing to straighten the proximal loops. This maneuver should be done under fluoroscopy to avoid movement of the tip.

V. Gupta
Neurointerventional Surgery, Stroke unit, Artemis Agrim Institute of Neuroscience, Gurgaon, India
e-mail: vipul.gupta@artemishospitals.com

V. Gupta et al. (eds.), *100 Interesting Case Studies in Neurointervention: Tips and Tricks*,
https://doi.org/10.1007/978-981-13-1346-2_41

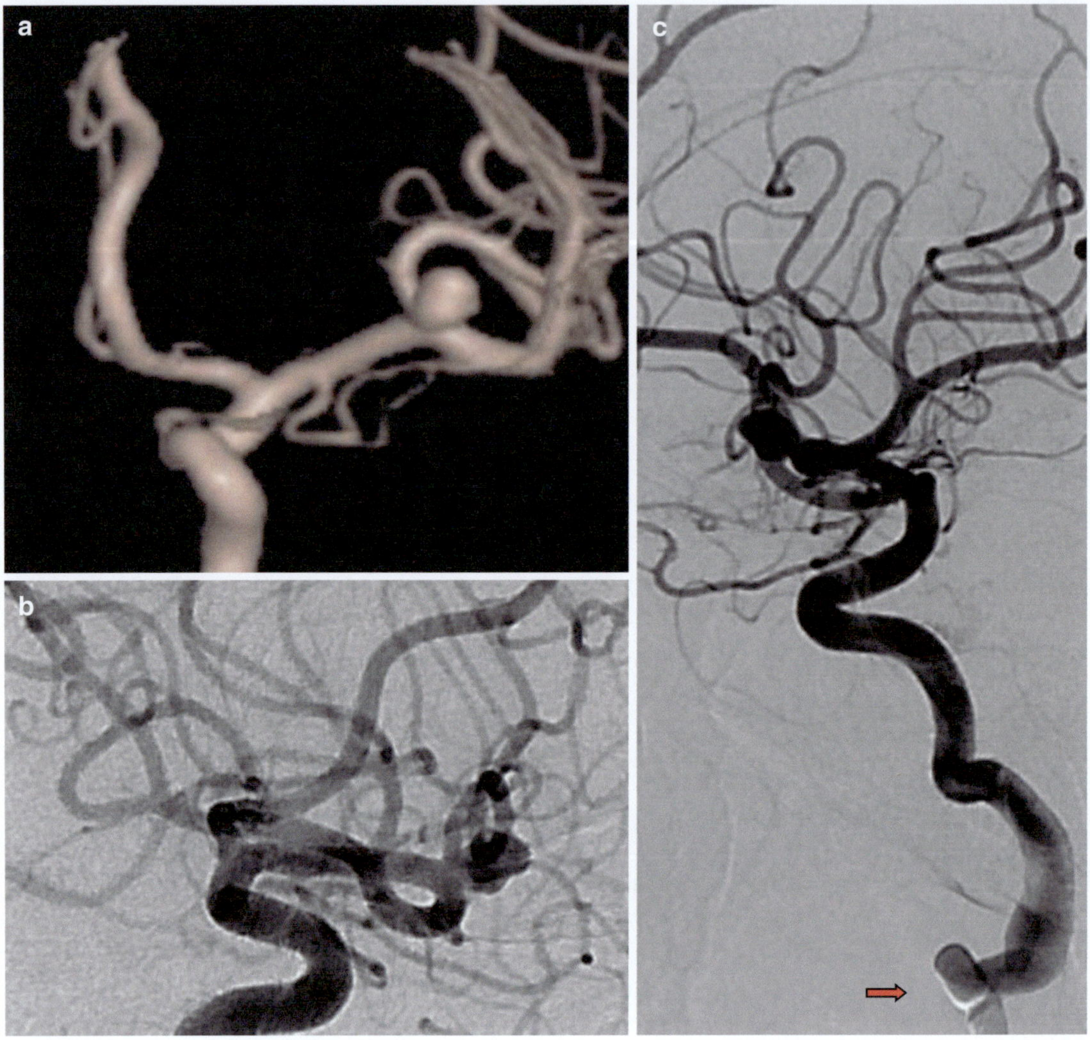

Fig. 41.1 (**a**) 3D DSA showing left middle cerebral artery aneurysm. (**b**) DSA profiling the aneurysm. (**c**) Tortuous ipsilateral cervical ICA with a kink (*red arrow*)

2. In small aneurysms, it is crucial to be aware of the location of tip of microcatheter. This can be difficult to judge particularly after few coils have been deployed. The position of the proximal marker on the microcatheter acts as a surrogate marker for the microcatheter tip location and is very useful to gauge if the microcatheter tip has migrated forward within the sac.
3. A new or a blank road map taken during coil placement can indicate position of catheter tip.
4. In general coils should not be pushed against resistance. In case of doubt, the microcatheter should be withdrawn partially to ensure that the catheter is not under tension. This allows for catheter tip to back out in case of resistance during coil placement.

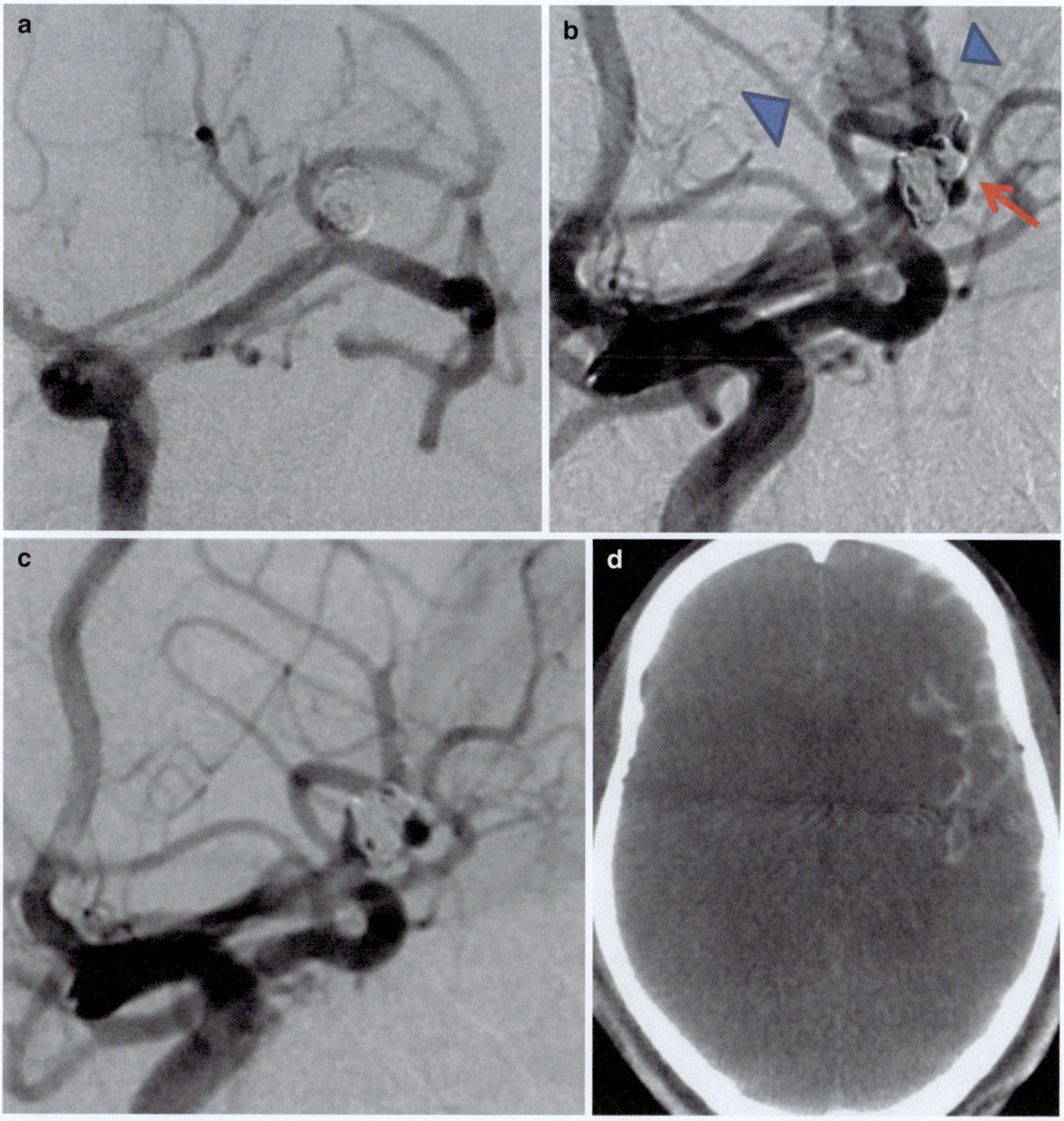

Fig. 41.2 (**a**) DSA shows after placement of three coils showing almost complete occlusion of the aneurysm. (**b**) Another coil placement was attempted, sudden catheter movement was seen along with coil protrusion from the fundus (*arrows*) along with leakage of contrast (*arrowheads*). (**c**) Further coil placement was done with occlusion of the leak. (**d**) Immediate angioCT shows fresh bleed and dye in left sylvian fissure

5. In case of rupture during coiling, one should not withdraw the microcatheter; rather, continue with coil placement even if few coil loops are outside the aneurysm margin. Multiple small soft coils should be placed as quickly as possible. At the same time, microcatheter itself can contribute to hemostasis. Data shows that rupture after a few coils have been placed can

be controlled by further coiling with good outcomes in most of the patients.

6. In case of rupture, the anesthetist should be warned immediately, and heparin should be reversed by protamine. Intracranial pressure should be lowered by anesthetists by using drugs such as mannitol. If external ventricular drain is in place, it should be opened completely to drain CSF and reduce the ICP.
7. As soon as possible, angioCT or regular CT should be done to assess for amount of bleed, ventricular dilatation, or sizable hematoma. Neurosurgery should be given a call to prepare for EVD insertion or to drain a big hematoma.

Suggested Reading

Doerfler A, Wanke I, Egelhof T, et al. Aneurysmal rupture during embolization with Guglielmi detachable coils: causes, management, and outcome. Am J Neuroradiol. 2001;22(10):1825–32.

Ross IB, Dhillon GS. Complications of endovascular treatment of cerebral aneurysms. Surg Neurol. 2005;64(1):12–8. discussion 8–9

43 Coil Rupture During Balloon-Assisted Coiling

Vipul Gupta

Case

A 54-year-old male presented with sudden severe headache. CT scan revealed Fisher grade III SAH. He was clinically well preserved (Hunt and Hess grade II). DSA with 3D imaging revealed a large broad neck aneurysm with both anterior cerebral arteries from the base of the aneurysm (Fig. 43.1a, b). The plan was to do a balloon-assisted coiling.

Issues

1. Preservation of both ACAs while achieving complete occlusion of the aneurysm sac

Management

The procedure was performed under general anaesthesia. A guiding catheter (Envoy, Boston Scientific Corp, Fremont CA) was placed in the left internal carotid artery. Thereafter, a balloon catheter (Eclipse, Balt Extrusion, Montmorency, France) was placed in right ACA (Fig. 43.1a, b). A microcatheter (Excelsior SL10, Stryker Neurovascular, CA, USA) was placed over a microguidewire (Transend, Stryker Neurovascular, CA, USA). During placement of the coil with inflated balloon, the tip of the coil was seen to protrude beyond the aneurysm margin into the subarachnoid space (Fig. 43.1d). As aneurysm rupture was suspected, coiling was continued, and in the same inflation three coils were further placed in quick succession. Meanwhile, the anaesthetist administered protamine to reverse the effect of heparin. The angiogram performed after deflating the balloon (Fig. 43.1d) showed no evidence of contrast extravasation. Coiling was continued with complete aneurysm occlusion (Fig. 43.1e, f). Post-embolization CT did not reveal any fresh haemorrhage. Patient was extubated in intact clinical condition.

Tips and Tricks

1. In case of suspected aneurysm rupture during coiling due to protrusion of the coil tip/loop beyond the aneurysm margin, do not deflate the balloon; rather, place a few more coils in an attempt to seal the suspected rupture site.
2. The authors prefer to keep the balloon inflated for 8–10 min, and deflate only after adequate coil occlusion of the sac has been achieved and heparin effect has been reversed.

V. Gupta
Neurointerventional Surgery, Stroke unit,
Artemis Agrim Institute of Neuroscience,
Gurgaon, India
e-mail: vipul.gupta@artemishospitals.com

V. Gupta et al. (eds.), *100 Interesting Case Studies in Neurointervention: Tips and Tricks*,
https://doi.org/10.1007/978-981-13-1346-2_43

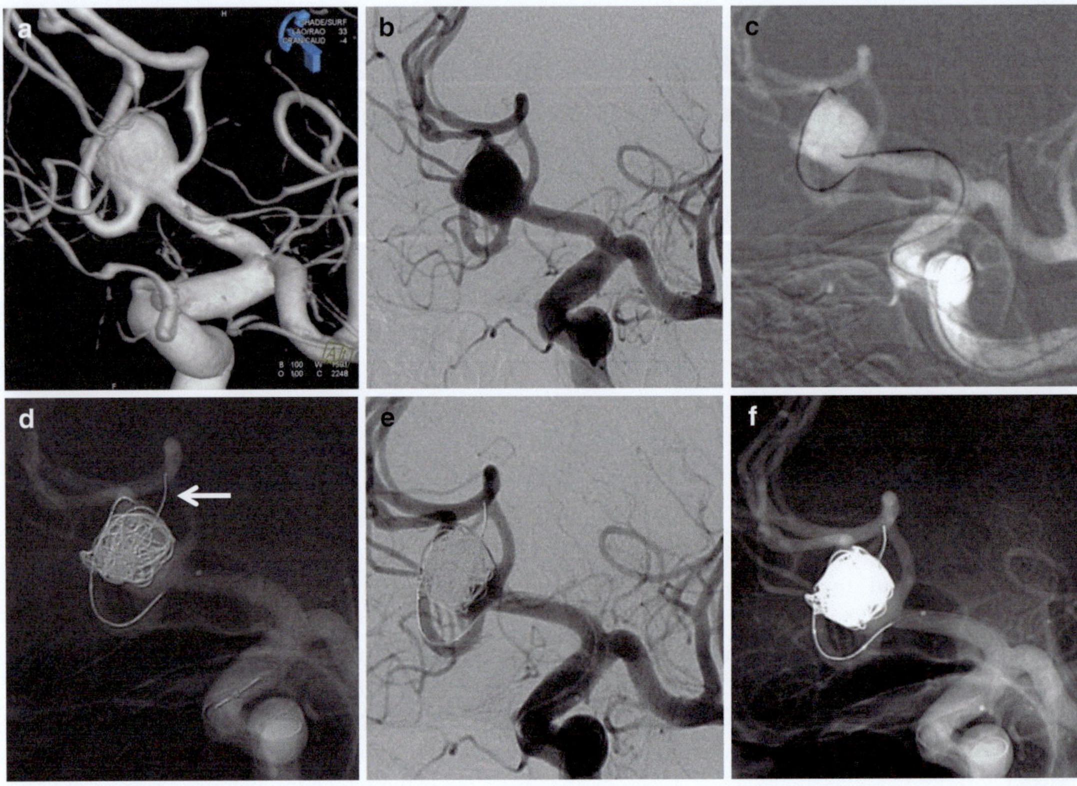

Fig. 43.1 (**a**, **b**) 3D reconstruction (**a**) and DSA image (**b**) shows a broad neck anterior communicating artery aneurysm. (**c**) Road map image showing balloon catheter in right ACA and coiling microcatheter at the neck of the aneurysm. (**d**) Image showing tip of coil (*arrow*) outside the confines of the aneurysm. (**e**, **f**) Final DSA (**e**) and native (**f**) images showing completely occluded aneurysm with adequate packing

Suggested Reading

Levy E, Koebbe CJ, Horowitz MB, et al. Rupture of intracranial aneurysms during endovascular coiling: management and outcomes. Neurosurgery. 2001;49:807–11.

Ross IB, Dhillon GS. Complications of endovascular treatment of cerebral aneurysms. Surg Neurol. 2005;64(1):12–8.

Zheng Y, Liu Y, Leng B, Xu F, Tian Y. Periprocedural complications associated with endovascular treatment of intracranial aneurysms in 1764 cases. J Neurointerv Surg. 2016;8:152–7.

44 Aneurysm Rupture After Flow Diversion with a Braided Stent

Vipul Gupta

Case

A 52-year-old lady presented with headaches and feeling of weakness of all four limbs. On examination patient had a power of 3+/5 in the upper and lower limbs and gait ataxia. MRI revealed giant aneurysm compressing upon the brain stem (Fig. 44.1a). DSA showed a giant fusiform aneurysm involving mid and lower third of the basilar artery trunk (Fig. 44.1b). Case was planned for overlapping Leo stent placement to create flow diversion.

Issues

1. Long segment of the aneurysm necessitating use of multiple overlapping stents or a single long stent
2. Crossing the aneurysmal segment
3. Rupture after flow diversion

Management

The procedure was planned under general anesthesia. A 6 F long sheath (Flexor Check-Flo Introducer, Raabe Modification, Cook) was placed in right subclavian artery, and a 5 F distal access catheter (DAC, Stryker) was navigated to V 4 segment of the right vertebral artery. Thereafter a microcatheter (Echelon 10, Medtronic) was used to cross the aneurysm after forming a loop (not shown) and then exchanged with a balloon catheter (Scepter XC, Microvention) (Fig. 44.1c). The balloon was inflated and pulled back to straighten the loop and exchanged with stent delivery microcatheter (Vasco, Balt). Leo 4.5 x 75 was delivered (Fig. 44.1d) extending from right posterior cerebral artery to right vertebral artery (Fig. 44.1e). Post-stenting angiogram revealed remarkable change in flow dynamics with partial filling of aneurysm along with stasis of contrast in the sac. Although the original plan was to place overlapping stents, in view of change in hemodynamics, the procedure was stopped. Postoperative angio-CT was unremarkable, and patient was discharged in 2 days with no change in her neurological condition. A week later, she presented with complaints of headache and dizziness. There were no neurological signs. MRI (Fig. 44.2a, b) and MR angiography revealed almost complete thrombosis of the aneurysm with small residual filling in the posterior component. There were no new parenchymal changes. Patient was treated with injectable steroids; however, after 2 days patient had massive subarachnoid hemorrhage (Fig. 44.2c, d) and expired.

V. Gupta
Neurointerventional Surgery, Stroke Unit, Artemis Agrim Institute of Neuroscience, Gurgaon, India
e-mail: vipul.gupta@artemishospitals.com

V. Gupta et al. (eds.), *100 Interesting Case Studies in Neurointervention: Tips and Tricks*,
https://doi.org/10.1007/978-981-13-1346-2_44

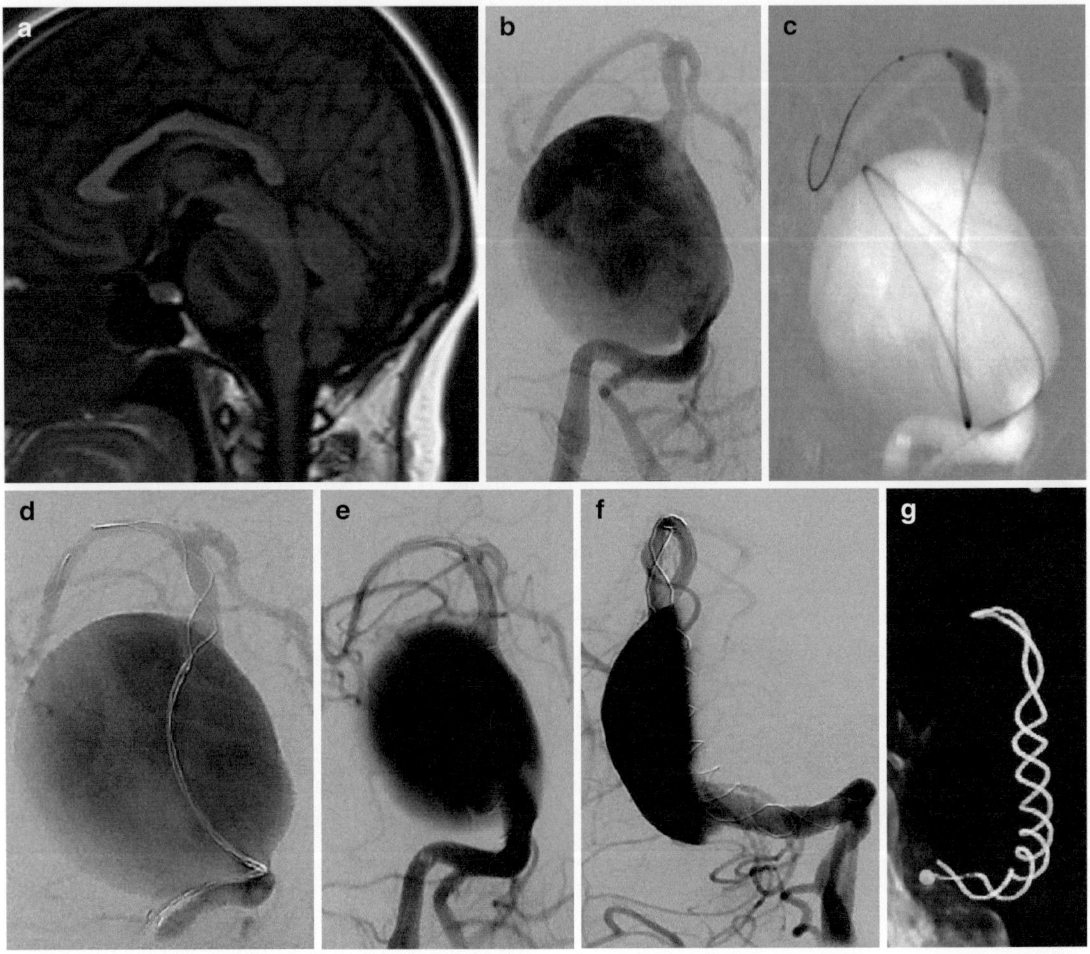

Fig. 44.1 (**a**) T1-weighted sagittal image showing basilar aneurysm with compression of brain stem. (**b**) DSA image reveals giant fusiform aneurysm of basilar trunk. (**c**) Roadmap image showing balloon loop technique to cross the aneurysm. Thereafter, the catheter was straightened with inflated balloon and exchanged with stent delivery catheter. (**d**) Stent delivery. (**e, f**) Post-stenting image revealing considerable flow modification with stagnation of contrast in the aneurysm. (**g**) Angio-CT image of the stent

Tips and Tricks

1. Giant posterior circulation aneurysms have poor prognosis. One of the options is to perform flow diversion treatment. Flow diverter stents can be used, or like in our case, single/overlapping braided stent like Leo can be used for this purpose. It was our strategy to avoid excessive flow diversion and rapid aneurysm thrombosis, and therefore a single device that could cover the entire length of the aneurysm was used.
2. As seen in our case, these aneurysms are not easy to cross; balloon loop technique can be used. In our case, we had to use the microcatheter to cross the aneurysm and then exchange with balloon catheter. Thereafter balloon was inflated so as to fix the catheter, and the loops in the aneurysm were straightened. Exchange was performed to place the stent delivery microcatheter to finally deliver the stent.
3. Aneurysmal rupture following flow diversion is a known phenomenon. One of the theories is that intra-aneurysmal thrombus formation activates

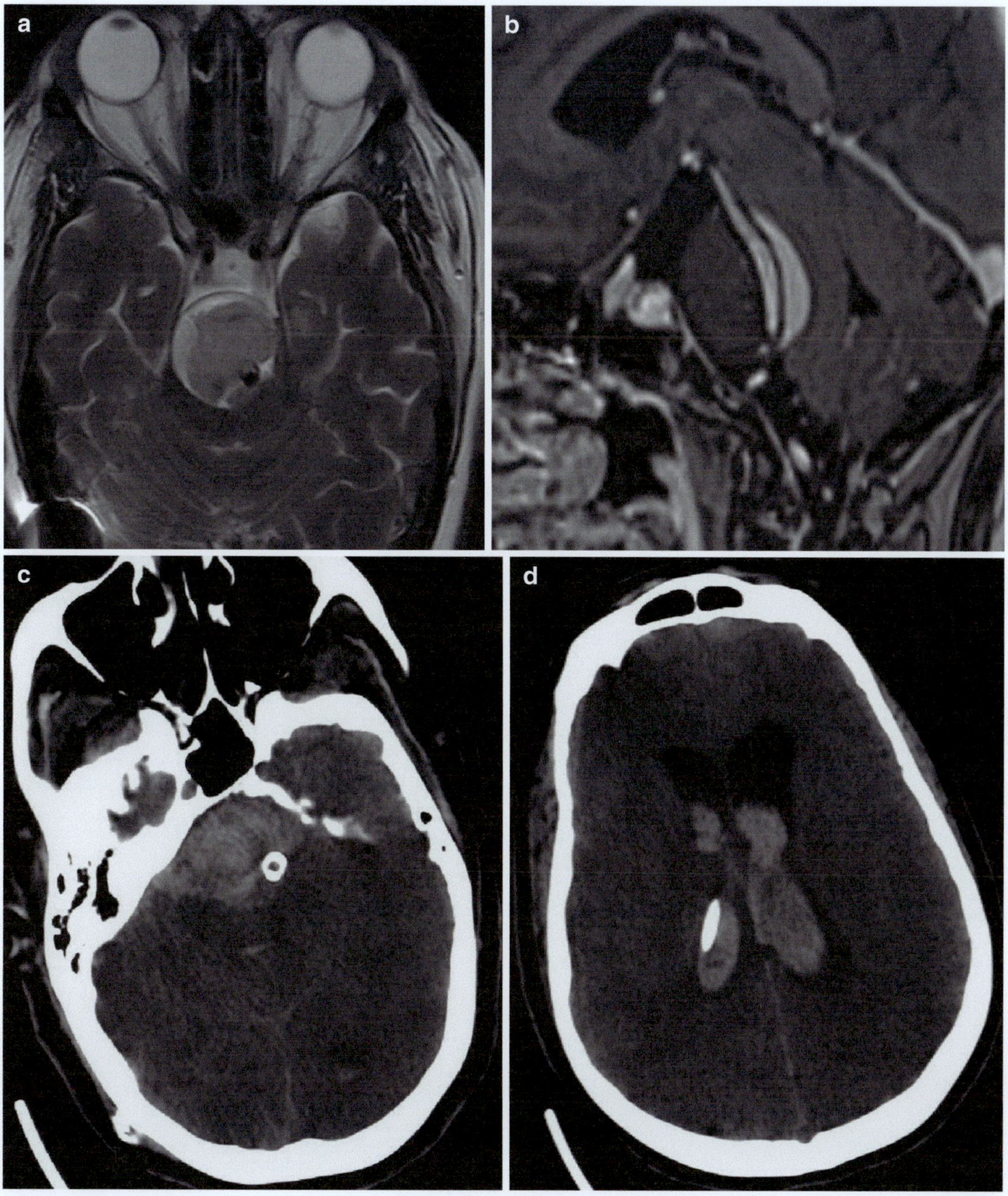

Fig. 44.2 (**a**) MRI 8-days after the procedure showing thrombosis within the aneurysm. (**b**) Contrast-enhanced MR confirms thrombosis of most of the aneurysm. (**c**, **d**) Non-contrast CT 3 days after the MRI shows subarachnoid and intraventricular hemorrhage

an inflammatory cascade and increased level of proteases, which leads to aneurysmal wall degradation with rupture. In our case, we observed a remarkable drop in aneurysm flow after placing single stent. Despite a single stent deployment we saw rapid aneurysm thrombosis and rupture. One of the options is to heparinize the patient for few weeks so as to prevent early massive thrombosis. Another is to perform partial coiling of the aneurysm to reduce the thrombus load. Intravenous followed by oral steroids are also used in these cases. It is author's practice to perform partial coiling before flow diverter placement in large anterior circulation aneurysms; however, in posterior circulation that may result in persistent/increase in mass effect, and heparinization may be preferable.

Suggested Reading

Fox B, Humphries WE, Doss VT, et al. Rupture of giant vertebrobasilar aneurysm following flow diversion: mechanical stretch as a potential mechanism for early aneurysm rupture. J Neurointerv Surg. 2015;7(11):e37.

Kulcsár Z, Houdart E, Bonafé A, et al. Intra-aneurysmal thrombosis as a possible cause of delayed aneurysm rupture after flow-diversion treatment. Am J Neuroradiol. 2011;32:20.

Prolapse of Coil Loop: Balloon-Repositioning Technique

45

Vipul Gupta

Case

A 42-year-old female presented with subarachnoid hemorrhage (Fisher Grade III). Patient was well preserved (Hunt and Hess II). DSA revealed a superiorly pointing ACOM aneurysm. The aneurysm had a broad neck with the left ACA arising from the base of the aneurysm (Fig. 45.1a, b).

Issues

Occlusion of the aneurysm while preserving both the ACAs.

Management

Balloon-assisted coiling was considered the most appropriate strategy to treat this broad necked aneurysm. Procedure was done under general anesthesia. A guiding catheter (0.070″ DAC, Concentric Medical, Inc. Mountain View, CA) was placed in the petrous ICA. Under road map guidance, a balloon (Sceptre XC, Microvention, Inc.) was placed over a micro-guidewire (Synchro®-14, BOSTON SCIENTIFIC CORP, Fremont CA) into the left ACA (Fig. 45.1c). Thereafter, coiling was performed uneventfully (Fig. 45.2a). After detachment of the last coil, the last loop prolapsed into the parent vessel (Fig. 45.2b, c, f). This loop could result in thromboembolism in spite of preserved patency of the parent artery. Therefore, a bolus dose of unfractionated heparin (1500 IU) was administered intravenously and was followed with interval doses of heparin every 30 min to maintain an activated coagulation time (ACT) of more than 300 s. The balloon was inflated slightly more than what was done during the procedure to reposition the coil loop. The inflation was maintained for few minutes. On deflation it was noted that the coil loop (Fig. 45.2d, e, g) remained within the aneurysm sac without any recurrent prolapse. Final DSA showed patent vessels with no coil prolapse.

Tips and Tricks

1. Coil loops can prolapse after detachment particularly if the last loop is not entangled in the coil mass and is partly anchored within the microcatheter by the pusher wire.

V. Gupta
Neurointerventional Surgery, Stroke unit,
Artemis Agrim Institute of Neuroscience,
Gurgaon, India
e-mail: vipul.gupta@artemishospitals.com

V. Gupta et al. (eds.), *100 Interesting Case Studies in Neurointervention: Tips and Tricks*,
https://doi.org/10.1007/978-981-13-1346-2_45

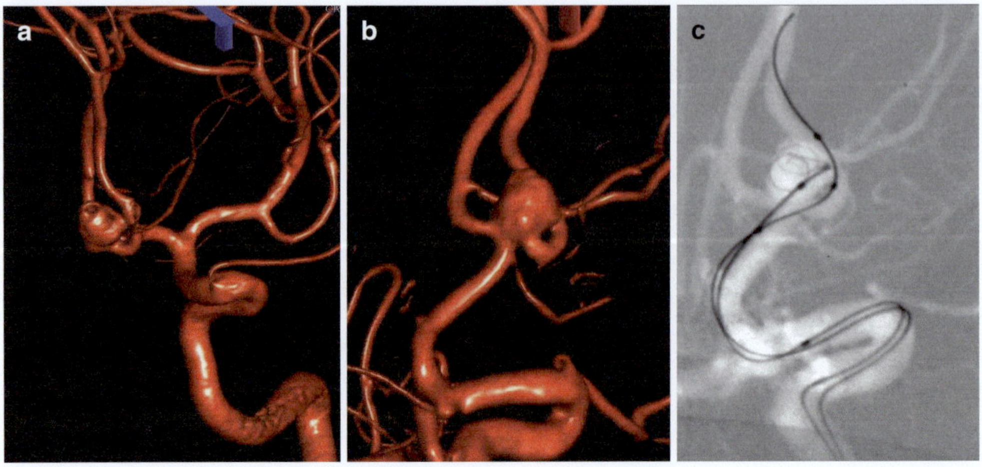

Fig. 45.1 (**a**, **b**) DSA with three-dimensional reconstruction shows a broad neck ACOM aneurysm. (**c**) Road map image in working projection (same as image **b**) with balloon in left ACA and coiling microcatheter in the aneurysm

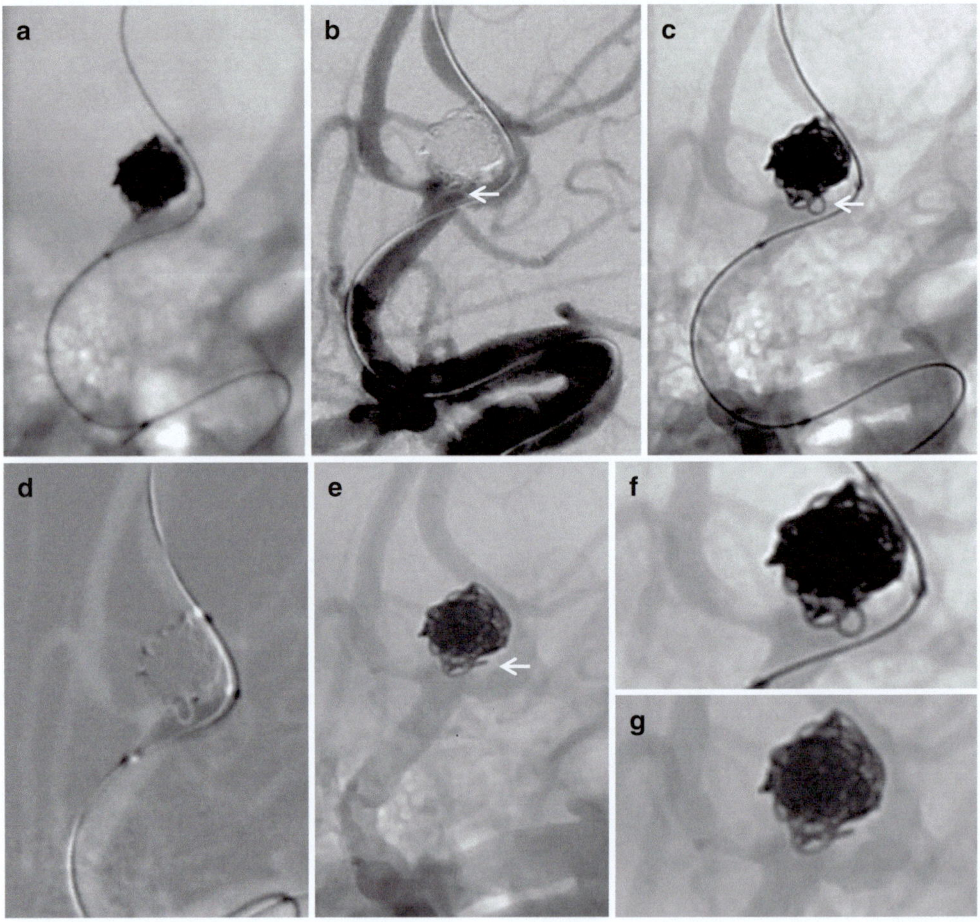

Fig. 45.2 (**a**) Placement of coils with balloon assistance. (**b**) DSA after deflation reveals prolapse of a coil loop in to the left ACA (*arrow*). (**c**, **f**) Native images showing the prolapsed loop (*arrow*). (**d**) A fresh road map was taken and balloon was inflated, resulting in repositioning of the loop into the aneurysm. (**e**, **g**) DSA after balloon deflation shows that the loop is now well anchored in the aneurysm and is no longer prolapsing into the parent vessel

2. If a coil loop prolapses, we prefer to administer intravenous heparin with an aim to maintain ACT at 300–350 s. Repeat interval runs should be undertaken and carefully examined for a thromboembolism.
3. If a balloon is in place, an attempt is made to reposition the coil loop by balloon inflation. We opt to slightly overinflate the balloon in an attempt to entangle the loop in the coil mass.
4. If the loop cannot be repositioned, we are inclined to commence antiplatelet therapy preferably on the operating table through a Ryles tube.
5. Final option is to place a stent if the coil cannot be repositioned by the above maneuver.

Suggested Reading

Ding D, Liu KC. Management strategies for intraprocedural coil migration during endovascular treatment of intracranial aneurysms. J Neurointerv Surg. 2014;6(6):428–31.

Fiorella D, Woo HH. How I treat: balloon assisted treatment of intracranial aneurysms: the conglomerate coil mass technique. J Neurointerv Surg. 2009;1(2):121–31.

Ladner TR, He L, Davis BJ, Froehler MT, Mocco J. Simultaneous stent expansion/balloon deflation technique to salvage failed balloon remodeling. J Neurointerv Surg. 2016;8:e15.

Suju K, Martin JB, Jean B, et al. Rescue balloon procedure for an emergency situation during coil embolization for cerebral aneurysms: technical note. J Neurosurg. 2002;96:373–6.

Yoo E, Kim DJ, Kim DI, Lee JW, Suh SH. Bailout stent deployment during coil embolization of intracranial aneurysms. Am J Neuroradiol. 2009;30(5):1028–34.

Coil Prolapse: Balloon-Repositioning and Coil Fixation Technique

46

Vipul Gupta

Case

A 34-year-old male presented with subarachnoid hemorrhage (Hunt and Hess grade II, Fisher grade III) due to a broad neck basilar top aneurysm (Fig. 46.1a, b). Although both the PCAs were involved, the aneurysm was predominantly committed to the right side and the plan was to do balloon-assisted coiling with remodeling balloon in the right PCA.

Issues

- Complete coil occlusion of the large broad neck aneurysm
- Preservation of both PCAs

Management

The procedure was performed under general anesthesia. A 6F guiding catheter (Chaperon, Microvention, Tustin, California, USA) was placed in left vertebral artery. As is authors practice, a bolus of unfractionated heparin (3000 IU) was given intravenously at start of the procedure and was followed with 2000 IU every hour to keep activated coagulation time (ACT) at twice the baseline. Under road map guidance, a remodeling balloon catheter (Scepter Balloon, Microvention, Tustin, California, USA) was placed in right PCA over a microguidewire (Traxcess, Microvention, Tustin, California, USA). Thereafter a microcatheter (Echelon-10, ev3 Inc., Irvine, California, USA) was placed in the aneurysm sac (Fig. 46.1c). Coiling was then performed with a slightly overinflated balloon in an attempt to provide coverage of as much of the aneurysm neck as possible. After placement of third coil, the DSA revealed prolapse of few loops into the origin of left PCA (Fig. 46.1d). Patient was given another bolus of heparin to prevent clot formation. It was decided to withdraw the balloon from right PCA and place it into the left one to reposition the loops. This was done under a new road map in order to monitor for coil loop displacement during navigation of wire and the balloon into the left PCA (Fig. 46.2a). Balloon inflation resulted in coil loops being pushed back into the aneurysm, and this was seen as "white" cast on the road map image as a new map was obtained after the prolapse occurred (Fig. 46.2b, c). The balloon was kept inflated and further coils were deployed to "fix" the prolapsed loops and prevent repeat prolapse after the deflation of the

V. Gupta
Neurointerventional Surgery, Stroke unit,
Artemis Agrim Institute of Neuroscience,
Gurgaon, India
e-mail: vipul.gupta@artemishospitals.com

V. Gupta et al. (eds.), *100 Interesting Case Studies in Neurointervention: Tips and Tricks*,
https://doi.org/10.1007/978-981-13-1346-2_46

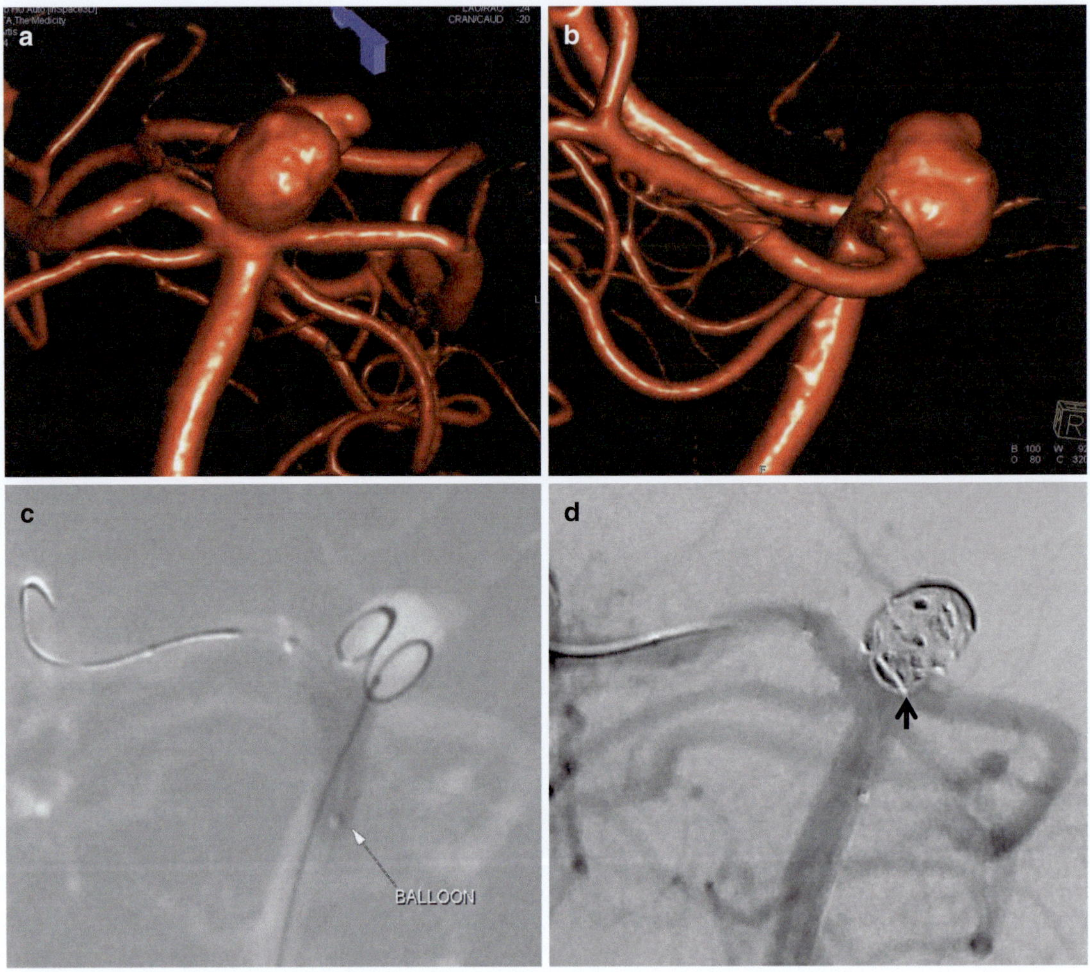

Fig. 46.1 (**a**, **b**) 3D reconstructed images show a broad neck basilar tip aneurysm with involvement of origin of PCAs, probably more on right side. (**c**) Road map image showing balloon-assisted coiling with slightly overinflated balloon in right PA in an attempt to protect the neck of aneurysm. (**d**) DSA after placement of third coil showing prolapse of coil loops into left PCA

balloon. The technique proved to be successful, and final angiogram revealed well-occluded aneurysm with preservation of both the PCAs.

Tips and Tricks

1. Prolapsed coil loop can be repositioned into the aneurysm by balloon inflation.
2. In cases of bifurcation aneurysms, the balloon can be repositioned into the branch in which the coil has prolapsed. This should be done carefully to prevent further prolapse and migration due to manipulation of microguidewire and balloon catheter in the artery. *We feel a new road map is useful under these circumstances so that any movement in the prolapsed loops will be readily observed.*
3. Even if coil has been pushed back into the aneurysm, they can prolapse back into the parent vessel after balloon deflation. An attempt can be made to "fix" the loops in the coil mass by placing more coils under balloon inflation. This can result in entanglement of the unstable coil loops into the freshly placed one and may prevent recurrent prolapse.
4. It is advisable to administer further heparin to maintain activated coagulation time high as

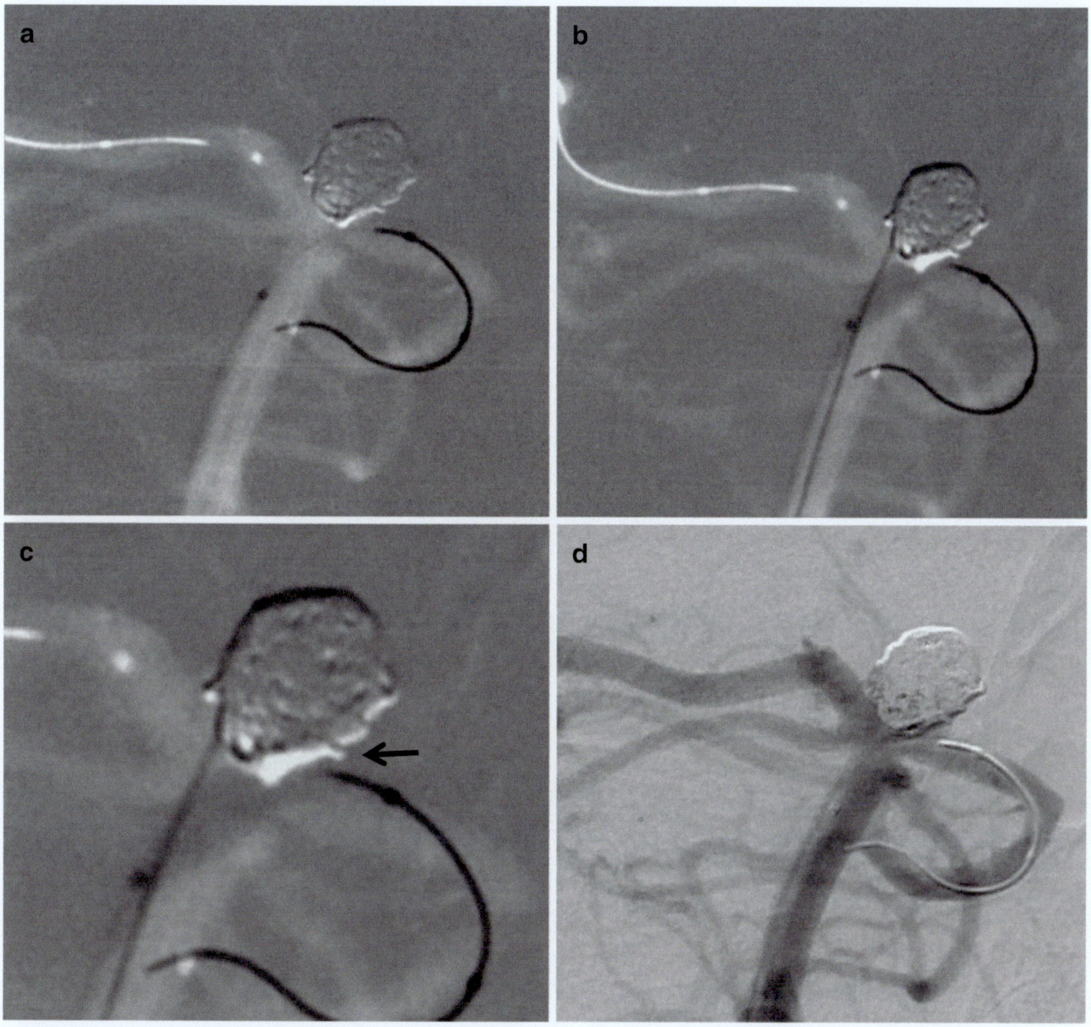

Fig. 46.2 (**a**) Road map image was taken after the prolapse and the balloon has been placed into the left PCA. (**b**, **c**) Balloon inflation has resulted in coils being pushed back into the aneurysm seen as "white" cast on the road map image since a new map was acquired after the prolapse. (**d**) Final DSA image showing well-occluded aneurysm with preserved PCAs

soon as such a complication happens in an attempt to prevent thromboembolism.

5. Another option is to place a second balloon in the left PCA—a "double balloon technique" to coil the aneurysm.

Suggested Reading

Ding D, Liu KC. Management strategies for intraprocedural coil migration during endovascular treatment of intracranial aneurysms. J Neurointerv Surg. 2014;6(6):428–31.

Eddleman CS, Welch BG, Vance AZ, et al. Endovascular coils: properties, technical complications and salvage techniques. J Neurointerv Surg. 2013;5(2):104–9.

Fiorella D, Woo HH. How I treat: balloon assisted treatment of intracranial aneurysms: the conglomerate coil mass technique. J Neurointerv Surg. 2009;1(2):121–31.

Zheng Y, Liu Y, Leng B, Xu F, Tian Y. Periprocedural complications associated with endovascular treatment of intracranial aneurysms in 1764 cases. J Neurointerv Surg. 2016;8:152–7.

Coil Prolapse: Emergency Stent Placement

47

Vipul Gupta

Case

A 58-year-old lady presented with subarachnoid hemorrhage (Hunt and Hess grade II, Fisher grade III). Cerebral angiography revealed an ACOM aneurysm filling from left ICA injection (Fig. 47.1a). Endovascular coiling was undertaken.

Issues

1. Achieve adequate coil occlusion of small aneurysm sac.
2. Coil prolapse during coiling: Evaluation of management strategies and implementation.

Management

Balloon- or stent-assisted coiling was proposed as the apt endovascular management strategy. Procedure was performed under general anesthesia, and a guiding catheter (Neuron, 6F, Penumbra, Inc. CA) was placed in left ICA. Under road map guidance, a microcatheter (Echelon 10, ev3 Inc., Irvine, California, USA) was placed in the base of the aneurysm over a micro-guidewire (Traxcess, Microvention, Tustin, California, USA). A coil (2 mm × 2 cm, Cosmos) was placed in the aneurysm (Fig. 47.1b) and detached uneventfully. During subsequent injection, sudden coil movement and prolapse of loops into the left ACA (A2 segment) was observed (Fig. 47.1c). The part of the coil loops within the parent vessel was moving freely raising concern over further prolapse. Therefore, the decision to deploy a retrievable stent, Solitaire (4 × 20 mm), with a view to stabilize the prolapsed coil loop was made. The stent delivery microcatheter (Prowler Select Plus, Codman & Sheurtleff, Inc., Raynham, Massachusetts) was taken across the prolapsed loops (Fig. 47.2a, b). Care was taken during guidewire manipulation (Fig. 47.2a) to minimize the risk of further coil herniation. Despite this, progressive herniation of coil was seen and can be attributed to blood flow (Fig. 47.2a–d). The stent was partially delivered to stabilize the coil loops (Fig. 47.2c), and a bolus dose of unfractionated heparin was administered to raise the ACT to 300 s. The coil delivery microcatheter was navigated to the neck of the aneurysm and another coil (2 mm × 2 cm) was placed in the aneurysm. As soon as the coil was placed, antiplatelet agents (Tab Ecosprin 150 mg and Tab Ticagrelor 180 mg) were given through Ryles tube.

V. Gupta
Neurointerventional Surgery, Stroke unit,
Artemis Agrim Institute of Neuroscience,
Gurgaon, India
e-mail: vipul.gupta@artemishospitals.com

V. Gupta et al. (eds.), *100 Interesting Case Studies in Neurointervention: Tips and Tricks*,
https://doi.org/10.1007/978-981-13-1346-2_47

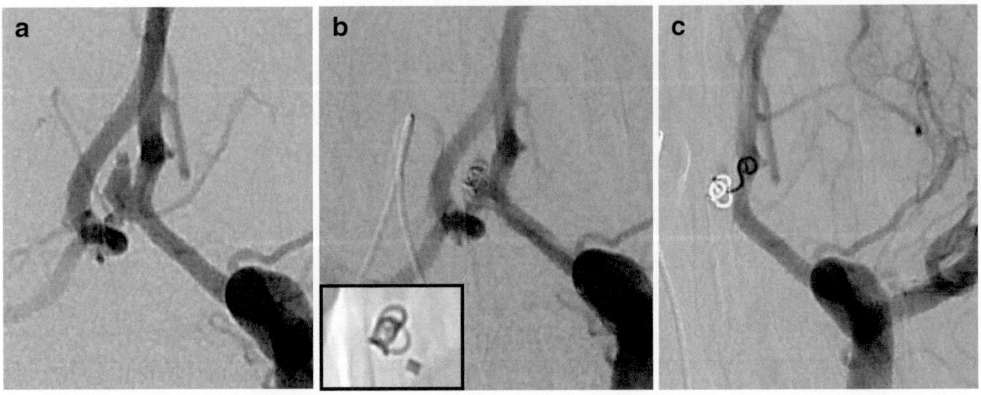

Fig. 47.1 (**a**) DSA image showing ACOM aneurysm filling from left ICA injection. (**b**) SA after placement of first coil (coil mass shown in the inset). (**c**) DSA after the coil detachment showing coil prolapse during the injection

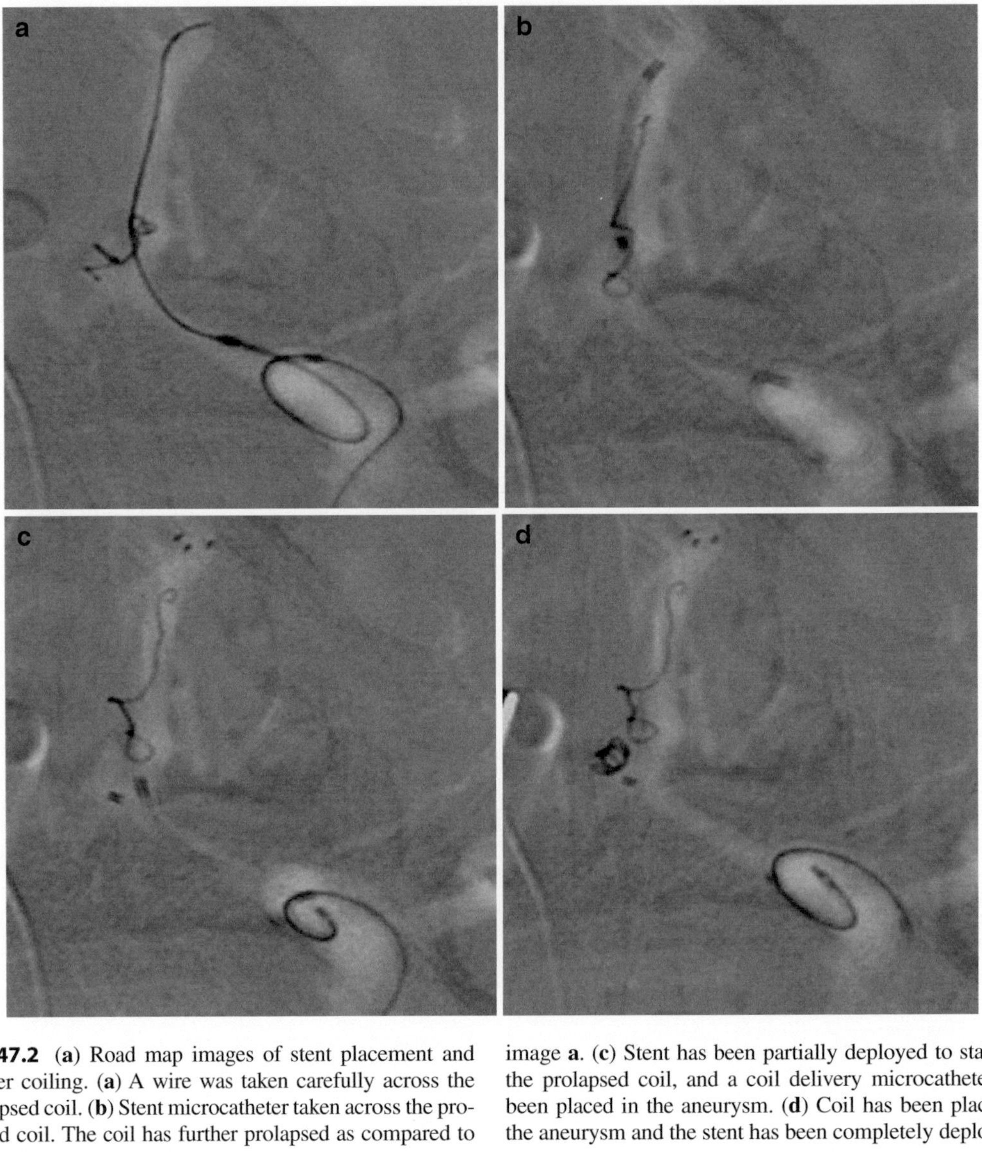

Fig. 47.2 (**a**) Road map images of stent placement and further coiling. (**a**) A wire was taken carefully across the prolapsed coil. (**b**) Stent microcatheter taken across the prolapsed coil. The coil has further prolapsed as compared to image **a**. (**c**) Stent has been partially deployed to stabilize the prolapsed coil, and a coil delivery microcatheter has been placed in the aneurysm. (**d**) Coil has been placed in the aneurysm and the stent has been completely deployed

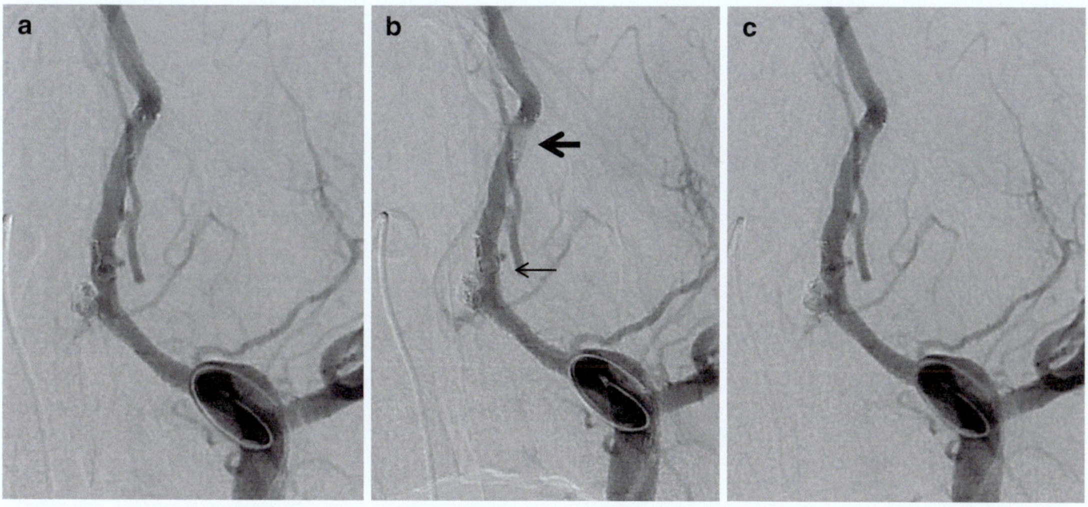

Fig. 47.3 (**a**) DSA after placement of second coil shows almost complete occlusion of the aneurysm. (**b**) Thrombus formation seen at distal end of stent (*bold arrow*) and prolapsed coil loops (*thin arrow*). (**c**) DSA after abciximab infusion shows almost complete resolution of the clot (I/A ReoPro given 10 mg)

Another small coil (Ultrasoft 1 mm × 2 cm) was placed in the aneurysm to achieve near complete occlusion (Fig. 47.3a). The stent was completely delivered and the coiling microcatheter was withdrawn. Interval angiogram revealed thrombus formation in the parent vessel (Fig. 47.3b). Intra-arterial abciximab was given (10 mg over 10 min) with near complete resolution of the clot (Fig. 47.3c). Final angiogram revealed patent arteries with occluded aneurysm. AngioCT did not reveal any fresh bleed and patient made an uneventful recovery.

Tips and Tricks

Coil prolapse after detachment can be handled by many strategies.

1. Minor prolapse can be managed by anticoagulant and antiplatelet drugs. However, major prolapse, as in our case, is dealt with by retrieving the coil or by stabilizing the coil by way of jailing (plastering the coil against) on to the arterial wall by means of a stent.
2. Initially, we deployed the stent partially to enable navigation of coil delivery catheter. The stent was completely deployed and detached after embolizing the aneurysm. Antiplatelet drugs were administered as soon as the aneurysm was coiled (Tab Ticagrelor was given as it has faster onset of effect as compared to clopidogrel).
3. Another option in this case could have been to retrieve the coil using the Solitaire. However in trying to do so, there was the danger of distal migration of the coil. Therefore it was considered safer to jail the coil against the arterial wall with a stent.
4. Patient was carefully watched for 30 min after delivery of stent for any thromboembolism. Intra-arterial gpIIb/IIIa inhibiting agents such as abciximab can be used to lyse the thrombus.

Suggested Reading

Linfante I, Etezadi V, Andreone V, et al. Intra-arterial abciximab for the treatment of thrombus formation during coil embolization of intracranial aneurysms. J Neurointerv Surg. 2010;2(2):135–8.

Yoo E, Kim DJ, Kim DI, Lee JW, Suh SH. Bailout stent deployment during coil embolization of intracranial aneurysms. Am J Neuroradiol. 2009;30(5):1028–34.

Coil Migration During Coiling: Retrieval by Snare

48

Vipul Gupta

Case

A 48-year-old female presented with a history of subarachnoid haemorrhage along with haematoma in the right medial temporal lobe 1 year ago. No investigations were performed then. She now had a re-bleed due to a right posterior communicating artery aneurysm (Fig. 48.1). The aneurysm sac was bilobed and coiling was planned.

Issue

1. Aneurysm was bilobed which may necessitate separate catheterization of the lobules.
2. Coil migration during the procedure—how to manage?

Procedure

Procedure was performed under general anaesthesia. No balloon or stent assistance was used. The bigger lobule was embolized uneventfully. Thereafter, the microcatheter was reshaped and the small lobule was catheterized. A small (2 mm × 2 cm Orbit, Codman neurovascular) coil was placed in the aneurysm sac (Fig. 48.1). However, as soon as the coil was detached, it unravelled and migrated out of the aneurysm to the middle cerebral artery (MCA) bifurcation (Fig. 48.1c). A bolus of heparin was given to raise the ACT to more than 300 s. It was decided to retrieve the coil using a 2 mm snare (ev3 Inc., Irvine, California, USA). Therefore a stent delivery microcatheter (Prowler 21, Codman Neurovascular) was carefully navigated across the coil. However, this resulted in further migration of coil into the M2 segment (Fig. 48.1d). Henceforth, the catheter was navigated with great caution, and once taken across the coil (Fig. 48.1e), the retriever was deployed and the coil was snared and taken out. Final angiogram revealed patent arteries (Fig. 48.1f) and stent-assisted coiling was planned for at a later date.

Tips and Tricks

1. Coil migration is a recognized complication and a retriever should be available at all times in the interventional laboratory.
2. Progressive migration of coil loops to smaller distal vessels is common, and one should be

V. Gupta
Neurointerventional Surgery, Stroke unit,
Artemis Agrim Institute of Neuroscience,
Gurgaon, India
e-mail: vipul.gupta@artemishospitals.com

V. Gupta et al. (eds.), *100 Interesting Case Studies in Neurointervention: Tips and Tricks*,
https://doi.org/10.1007/978-981-13-1346-2_48

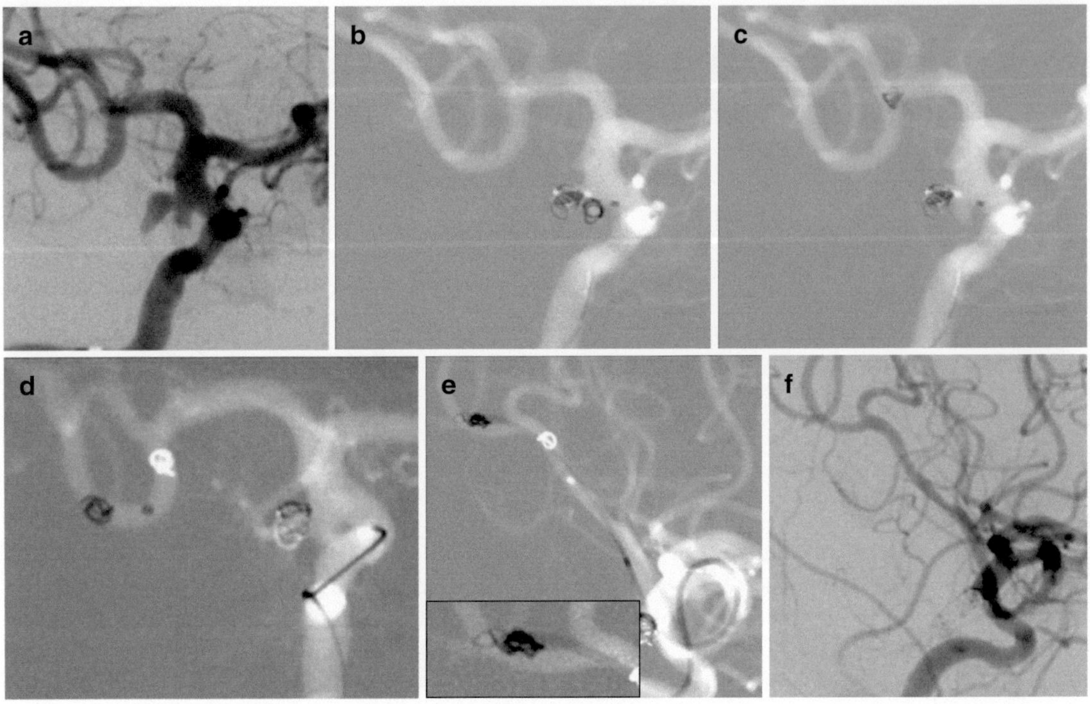

Fig. 48.1 (**a**) DSA image showing bilobed right posterior communicating aneurysm. (**b**) The upper larger lobe was coiled successfully. Thereafter a coil was placed in the smaller lobule. (**c**) Soon after detachment, the coil migrated to middle cerebral artery. (**d**) During the attempt to navigate the microcatheter across the coil, further migration was seen. (**e**) Finally a snare could be deployed across the coil. (**f**) Final angiogram showing patent arteries

careful while navigating the wire or catheter across the prolapsed loops.

3. Multiple attempts may be required to retrieve the coil. An important trick can be to take the catheter across the coil, deliver the retriever, and then *withdraw the system to engage the coil*. Once the coil is engaged, the loop of the retriever is closed to grasp the coil loop.
4. Heparin bolus should be given immediately to prevent clot formation. If clot formation is seen, one may have to use agents such as Gp IIb/IIIa inhibitors.
5. In retrospect, balloon- or stent-assisted coiling could have avoided the complication.

Suggested Reading

Ding D, Liu KC. Management strategies for intraprocedural coil migration during endovascular treatment of intracranial aneurysms. J Neurointerv Surg. 2014;6(6):428–31.

Eddleman CS, Welch BG, Vance AZ, et al. Endovascular coils: properties, technical complications and salvage techniques. J Neurointerv Surg. 2013;5(2):104–9.

49 Thrombus Formation During Coiling: Heparinization Protocol

Vipul Gupta

Case

A 54-year-old male presented with subarachnoid hemorrhage (Hunt and Hess II, Fisher grade 4). DSA with 3D angiography showed aneurysm at vertebrobasilar junction associated with a fenestration (Fig. 49.1a, b). Patient was planned for coiling under GA.

Issue

During coiling such cases, one has to be careful to keep both the limbs of fenestration patent. Placement of balloon or stent in one of the limbs may not give complete coverage at the neck. Small arteries such as these are more likely to develop clot formation at the coil-artery interface as compared to a bigger vessel.

Management

Under general anesthesia coiling was performed in biplane laboratory. The working angle during coiling was chosen in a manner to visualize both limbs of fenestration (Fig. 49.1). Baseline ACT was 136 s. At the start of procedure, 3000 U of heparin was given followed by 2000 U every hour. The heparinized saline (1000 U in 1 L of saline) infusion was given through the guiding catheter. During the procedure small hazy filling defect was seen in one of the limbs of the fenestration suggestive of clot formation (Fig. 49.1c). Immediately, 1500 U of heparin was given as bolus. Repeat ACT was 290 s and additional 1000 U of heparin was given. During this period coiling was continued. Repeat angiograms revealed slow resolution of the thrombus (Fig. 49.1d); both the limbs of the fenestration were patent with no evidence of coil prolapse or clot (Fig. 49.1e, f). Patient awoke uneventfully and was given low molecular weight heparin (Inj. Clexane 0.4 mL twice a day) for 2 days.

Tips and Tricks

1. Various heparinization protocols are used in different institutions. We give 3000 IU heparin at start of procedure followed by bolus of 2000–2500 U every hour.
2. Early detection of filling defect or haziness allows for use of aggressive measures to prevent

V. Gupta
Neurointerventional Surgery, Stroke unit,
Artemis Agrim Institute of Neuroscience,
Gurgaon, India
e-mail: vipul.gupta@artemishospitals.com

V. Gupta et al. (eds.), *100 Interesting Case Studies in Neurointervention: Tips and Tricks*,
https://doi.org/10.1007/978-981-13-1346-2_49

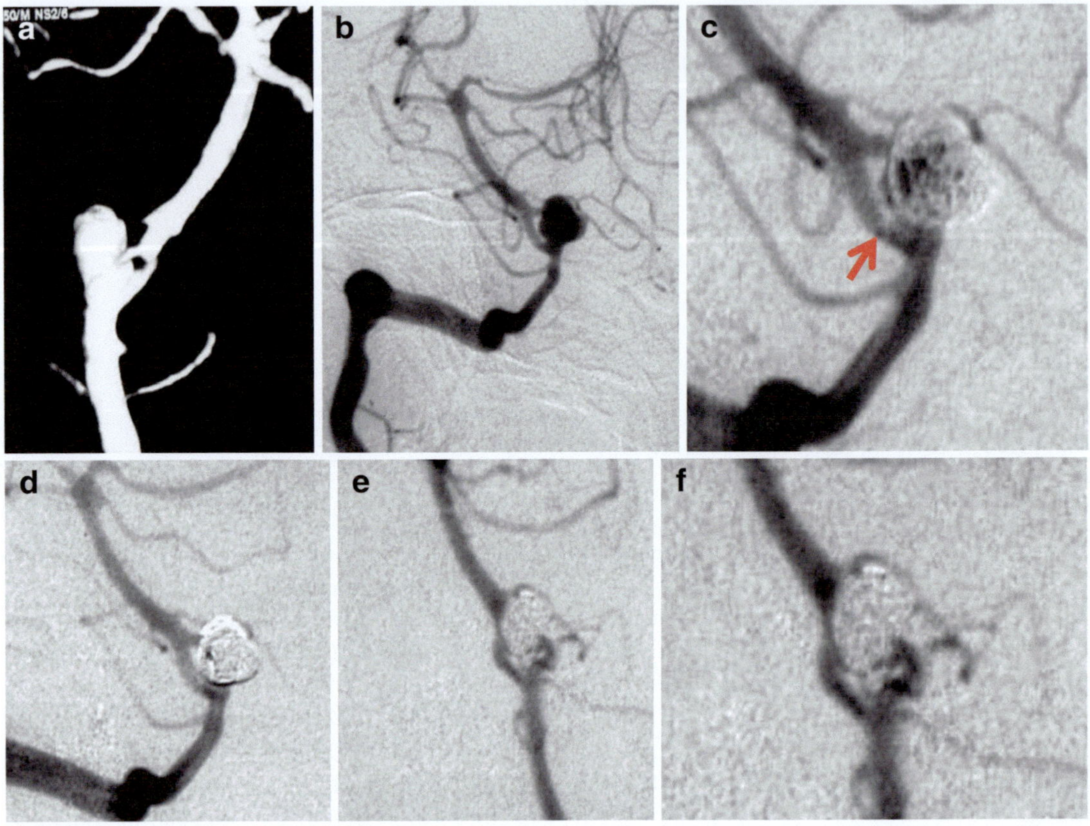

Fig. 49.1 (**a**) 3-DRA image showing a vertebrobasilar aneurysm associated with fenestration. (**b**) DSA image showing of the same. (**c**) DSA after placement of few coils show irregular, hazy filling defect in one of the limbs of fenestration, indicating thrombus formation (*arrow*). (**d**) After giving additional heparin, partial resolution of thrombus seen. (**e**, **f**) Final angiogram reveals complete occlusion of aneurysm, with preservation of both limbs of fenestration. Thrombus has completely resolved

further progression and preventing a clinical complication.

3. In cases with clot formation during coiling, additional heparin should be given immediately to raise the ACT 2–2.5 times of base value. If baseline ACT has not been done, heparin is given to raise it to 300–350 s.
4. If treated early, in most cases clot progression is halted, and in many clot resolution occurs. If it doesn't resolve, additional agents such as GpIIb–IIIa inhibitors can be given.

Suggested Reading

Debrun GM, Viñuela FV, Fox AJ. Aspirin and systemic heparinization in diagnostic and interventional neuroradiology. Am J Roentgenol. 1982;139:139–42.

Derdeyn CP, Cross DT 3rd, Moran CJ, Brown GW, Pilgram TK, Diringer MN, et al. Postprocedure ischemic events after treatment of intracranial aneurysms with Guglielmi detachable coils. J Neurosurg. 2002;96:837–43.

Park HK, Horowitz M, Jungreis C, et al. Periprocedural morbidity and mortality associated with endovascular treatment of intracranial aneurysms. Am J Neuroradiol. 2005;26(3):506–14.

50 Delayed Thromboembolism After Balloon-Assisted Coiling

Vipul Gupta

Case

A 44-year-old lady presented with subarachnoid haemorrhage (Hunt and Hess grade II, Fischer-I). MRA (not shown) followed by DSA (Fig. 50.1a) revealed two aneurysms in the left ICA in the ophthalmic segment. The ophthalmic artery was arising from the base of the proximal one. Balloon-assisted coiling was considered to be the most appropriate management strategy.

Issue

- In view of the uncertainty over which aneurysm bled, there is the need to treat both the aneurysms in the same session.
- Preservation of the ophthalmic artery origin while treating the proximal aneurysm.

Management

Procedure was performed under general anaesthesia. Heparin (intra-arterial, 3000 IU) was given as a bolus at the start of the procedure. This was followed with interval intravenous blouses of heparin (1000–2000 units) every hour so as to maintain the activated clotting time at 2–2.5 times the baseline. After placing the guiding catheter, a balloon catheter (Eclipse, Balt Extrusion, Montmorency, France) was placed across the neck of the aneurysms. Distal aneurysm was coiled first followed by the proximal one. Coiling of both the aneurysms was uneventful (Fig. 50.1b–d). During coiling of the proximal aneurysm, the balloon was overinflated so as to bulge it into the base of the aneurysm sac (Fig. 50.1c). This enabled the sparing of the base of aneurysm sac from which the ophthalmic artery was arising. No evidence of any thrombus formation or coil protrusion was observed. In accordance to our practice, a repeat interval angiogram was performed after 10 min. It revealed barely discernable filling defects along the distal aneurysm base (Fig. 50.2a, b). Thrombus formation was suspected and additional bolus of heparin was given to raise the ACT above 300 s. However, progressive increase in clot burden was observed (Fig. 50.2c). Therefore, intra-arterial abciximab (10 mg) was given through the guiding catheter over 8 min. Marked resolution of the clot was noted with only minimal residual thrombus along the vessel (Fig. 50.2d). Patient

V. Gupta
Neurointerventional Surgery, Stroke unit,
Artemis Agrim Institute of Neuroscience,
Gurgaon, India
e-mail: vipul.gupta@artemishospitals.com

V. Gupta et al. (eds.), *100 Interesting Case Studies in Neurointervention: Tips and Tricks*,
https://doi.org/10.1007/978-981-13-1346-2_50

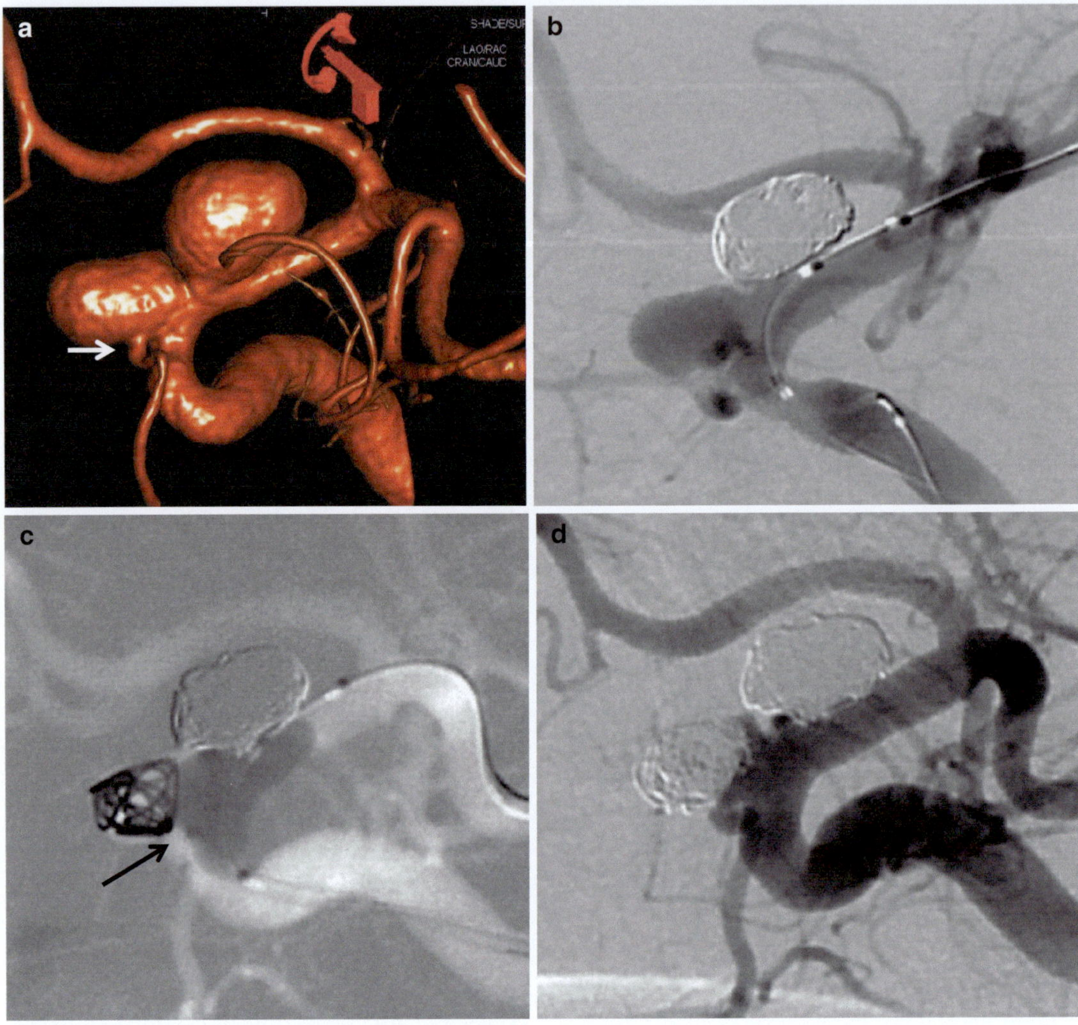

Fig. 50.1 (**a**) Three-dimensional reconstructed image shows two aneurysms in the paraclinoidal region of left ICA. The ophthalmic artery was arising from the base of the proximal aneurysm (*arrow*). (**b**) Balloon-assisted coiling of distal aneurysm. (**c**) Road map image during coiling of the proximal aneurysm showing the overinflated balloon protruding in to the base of aneurysm so as to spare the ophthalmic artery (*arrow*). (**d**) Post-embolization angiogram showing almost complete occlusion of the proximal aneurysm with sparing of the neck to preserve the ophthalmic artery

was extubated in intact clinical condition. She was given LMWH (Inj. Clexane 0.4 cc twice a day) for the next 48 h followed by Ecosprin 150 mg for the next 6 weeks.

Tips and Tricks

1. Delayed thrombus formation is not uncommon and can occur after uneventful coiling. Therefore, the author prefers to do an interval angiogram at 10–15 min after completion of the procedure.
2. One should carefully study the angiogram for small filling defects or irregularity of vascular margins as this may indicate early clot formation.
3. It is our practice to give additional bolus of heparin for small thrombus and raise the ACT to up to 300–350 s.

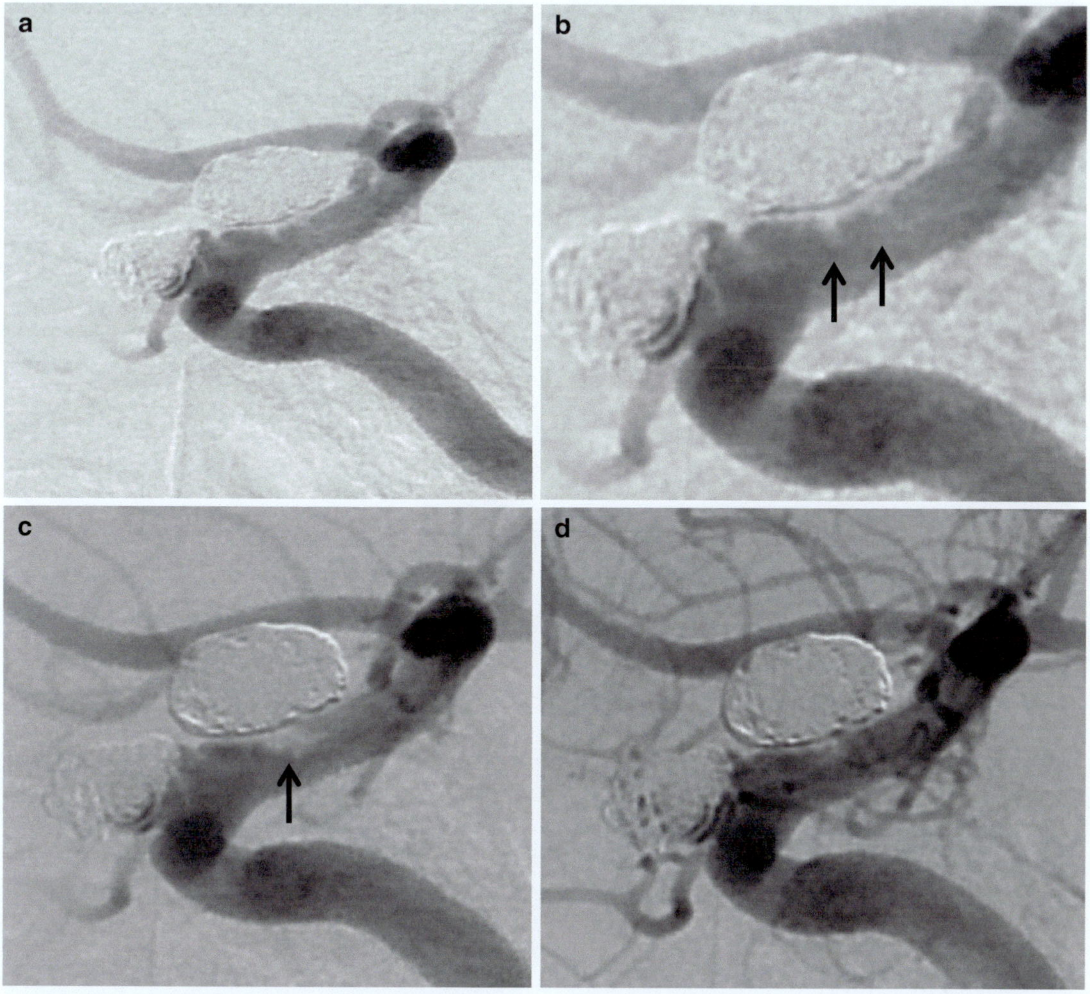

Fig. 50.2 (**a**) Repeat angiogram done 10 min after the completion of procedure shows ill-defined filling defects along the coil mass. (**b**) Magnified image showing the filling defect suggestive of clot formation (*arrows*). (**c**) Repeat angiogram 5 min after giving additional heparin. Marked increase in clot mass is seen. (**d**) Angiogram after intra-arterial abciximab infusion seen marked resolution of thrombus

4. If progressive increase in thrombus size is noted, a Gp IIb/IIIa inhibitor is administered. We prefer intra-arterial injection over 8–10 min.
5. As described above, overinflation of balloon can be done to preserve the normal branches arising from the base of aneurysm. *We prefer an extra-compliant over the usual compliant balloon used in ICA to achieve reasonable protrusion of the balloon into the base of the aneurysm sac.*

Suggested Reading

Brinjikji W, McDonald JS, Kallmes DF, Cloft HJ. Rescue treatment of thromboembolic complications during endovascular treatment of cerebral aneurysms. Stroke. 2013;44(5):1343–7.

Layton KF, Cloft HJ, Gray LA, Lewis DA, Kallmes DF. Balloon-assisted coiling of intracranial aneurysms: evaluation of local thrombus formation and symptomatic thromboembolic complications. Am J Neuroradiol. 2007;28(6):1172–5.

Linfante I, Etezadi V, Andreone V, et al. Intra-arterial abciximab for the treatment of thrombus formation during coil embolization of intracranial aneurysms. J Neurointerv Surg. 2010;2(2):135–8.

Air Embolism During Coiling Procedure

51

Vipul Gupta

Case

A 48-year-old male presented with subarachnoid hemorrhage (Fig. 51.1a). He was clinically well preserved. DSA and 3D angiography revealed a dissecting aneurysm of right vertebral artery (Fig. 51.1b, c). Left vertebral artery was also dissected with almost complete occlusion (not shown). The case was planned for stent-assisted coiling.

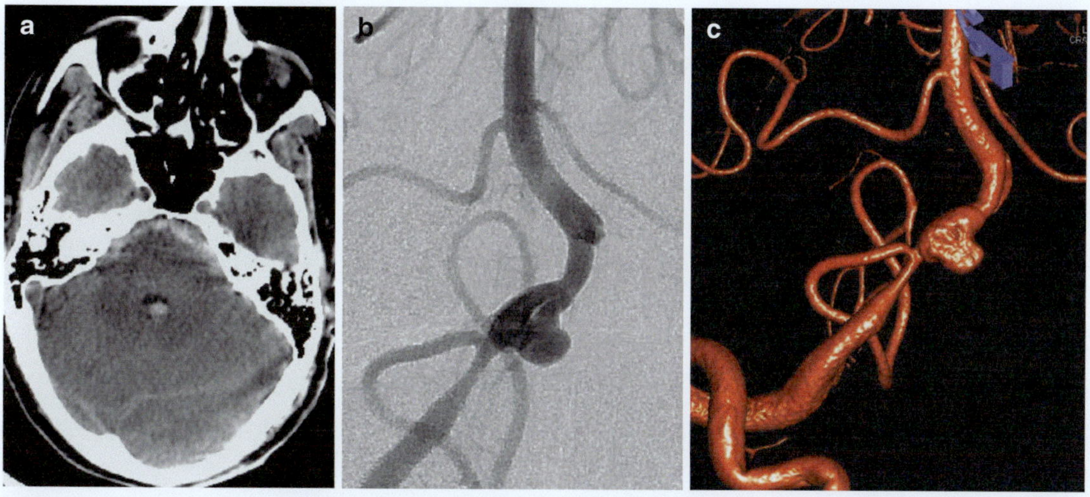

Fig. 51.1 (**a**) Non-contrast CT shows subarachnoid hemorrhage along with blood in the fourth ventricle. (**b**, **c**) DSA and 3D angiography images reveal fusi-saccular aneurysm of V4 segment of right vertebral artery, likely to be dissecting. One can also observe a linear filling defect, likely to be a dissection flap

V. Gupta
Neurointerventional Surgery, Stroke Unit, Artemis Agrim Institute of Neuroscience, Gurgaon, India
e-mail: vipul.gupta@artemishospitals.com

V. Gupta et al. (eds.), *100 Interesting Case Studies in Neurointervention: Tips and Tricks*, https://doi.org/10.1007/978-981-13-1346-2_51

Issues

1. Air embolism during the procedure

Management

After general anesthesia, guiding catheter (Envoy 6F, Codman Neurovascular) was placed in right vertebral artery. Angiogram revealed a new round filling defect in the aneurysm (Fig. 51.2a), which was swirling around in the sac, suggestive of air embolism. Patient was given pure oxygen through the endotracheal tube; the FiO2 was increased to 100%, and the repeat angiograms revealed progressive decrease in size of bubble, and finally complete disappearance of the filling defect was seen (Fig. 51.2b, c, e-g). Careful observation of the drip line tubing did not reveal any air, and it was assumed that it was injected through the syringe during dye injection. DSA revealed patency of all the vessels. Stent-assisted coiling was performed uneventfully, and patient was extubated in intact clinical condition (Fig. 51.2d).

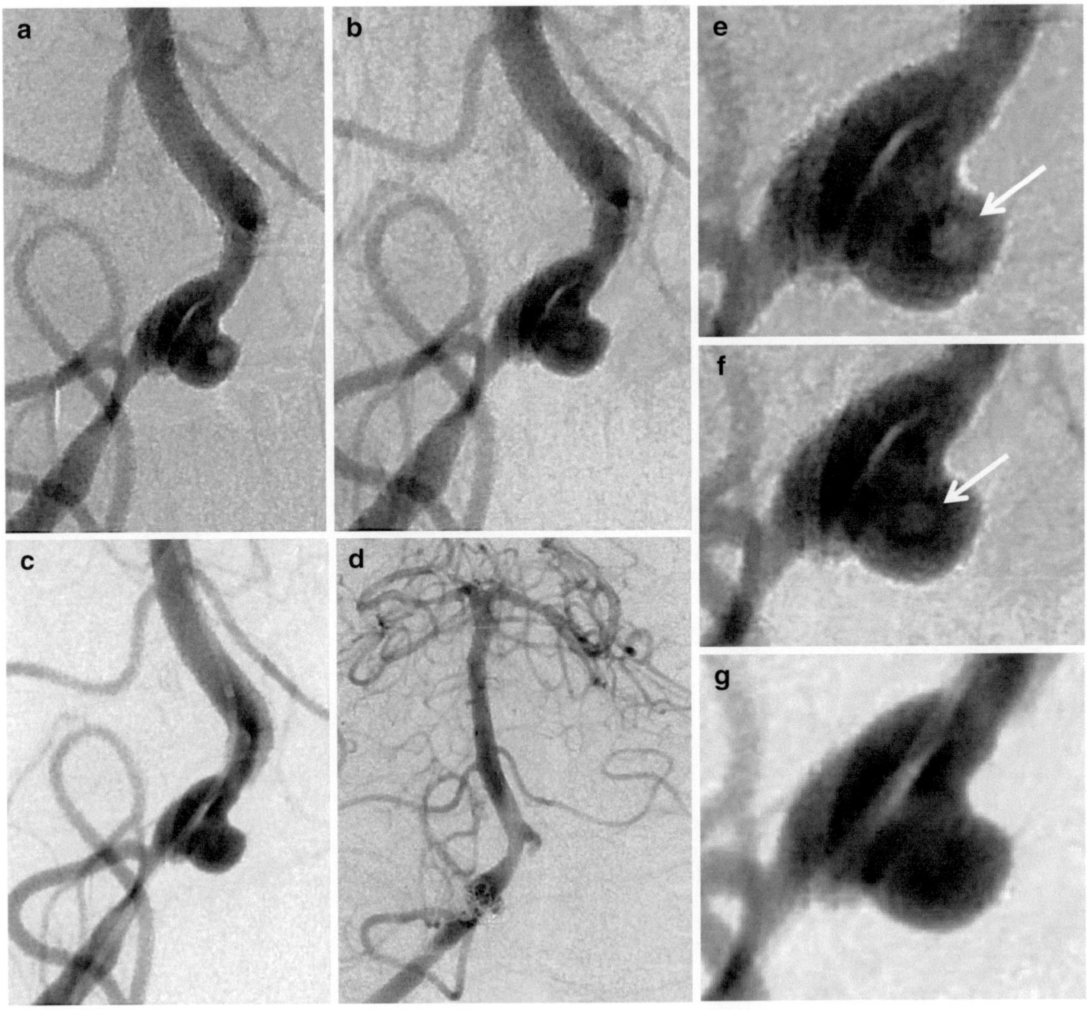

Fig. 51.2 (**a**) Patient was planned for stent-assisted coiling. DSA at start of the procedure showed a round filling defect in the aneurysm; this was observed to swirl around in the aneurysm, suggesting an air embolus. (**b**) Pure oxygen was given and the repeat angiogram shows decrease in size of bubble (note the different location as compared to previous image). (**c**) Complete resolution of the air bubble was seen (microcatheter in situ for stent placement). (**d**) Post-embolization angiogram shows occlusion of aneurysm and patent intracranial vessels. Image (**e**), (**f**), and (**g**) magnified view of image (**a**), (**b**), and (**c**), respectively

Tips and Ticks

1. One should take all the precautions to prevent air embolism, including using luerlock syringes, keeping the syringes erect during injection, careful clearing of drip line tubing set of air, and degassing of pressure bag.
2. However, air embolism can happen and very small air bubbles may not result in major complications in most cases.
3. In case of small non-occlusive air embolism (like ours), one can give pure (100%) oxygen to dilute the nitrogen in air emboli and facilitate absorption of air. It usually results in dissolution of the bubble.
4. In case of major occlusive air embolism, one should perform immediate suction, raise the blood pressure, increase heparinization level, and give antiepileptics.
5. In selected case of occlusion of major vessels, distal aspiration technique can be used.

Suggested Reading

Belton PJ, Nanda A, Alqadri SL, Khakh GS, Chandrasekaran PN, Newey C, Humphries WE. Paradoxical cerebral air embolism causing large vessel occlusion treated with endovascular aspiration. J Neurointerv Surg. 2017;9(4):e10.

Tan LA, Keigher KM, Lopes DK. Symptomatic cerebral air embolism during stent-assisted coiling of an unruptured middle cerebral artery aneurysm: intraoperative diagnosis and management of a rare complication. J Cerebrovasc Endovasc Neurosurg. 2014;16:93.

52 Coil Retrieval: Stent-Assisted Retrieval Techniques

Rajsrinivas Parthasarathy and Vipul Gupta

Case 1

Balloon-assisted coiling was undertaken for a right MCA bifurcation aneurysm in a 45-year-old male patient. After detachment of the third coil, the fourth coil was introduced (Fig. 52.1a–c). However, there was resistance while trying to deliver the fourth coil, and the coil would neither come out of the tip of the microcatheter nor could be with drawn into the microcatheter. Therefore, the microcatheter had to be pulled back. During the process, the previous coil tip was noted to be stuck to the tip of the microcatheter. Therefore, the microcatheter along with the previous coil attached to the tip of the microcatheter was gradually withdrawn into the distal end of the guiding catheter.

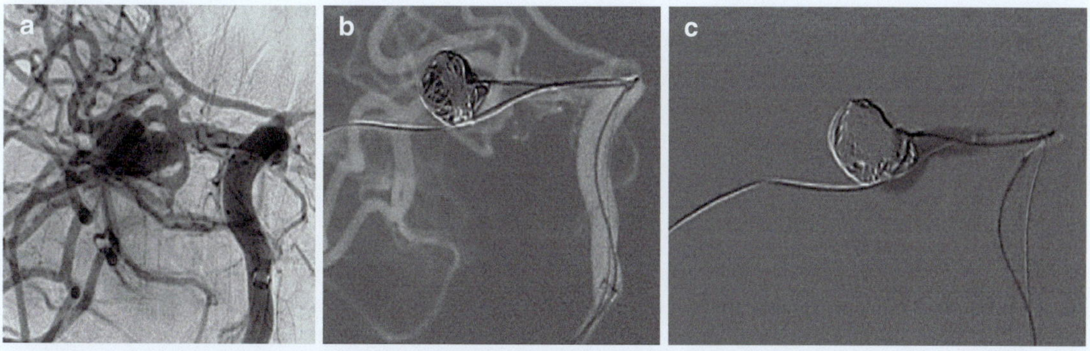

Fig. 52.1 (**a**) R MCA bifurcations aneurysm; (**b**) balloon placed across the neck of the aneurysm with the coiling microcatheter in the aneurysm sac; (**c**) resistance with backing of microcatheter while deploying the fourth coil

R. Parthasarathy (✉)
Vascular Neurology and Neurointerventional Surgery, Artemis Agrim Institute of Neuroscience, Gurgaon, India

V. Gupta
Neurointerventional Surgery, Stroke Unit, Artemis Agrim Institute of Neuroscience, Gurgaon, India
e-mail: vipul.gupta@artemishospitals.com

V. Gupta et al. (eds.), *100 Interesting Case Studies in Neurointervention: Tips and Tricks*, https://doi.org/10.1007/978-981-13-1346-2_52

Issues

1. Risk of losing the coil in the parent artery while withdrawing the microcatheter
2. Coil retrieval in the event of coil deposition in the parent artery

Management

Balloon jailing technique (Fig. 52.2): Initially balloon jailing technique was undertaken. The microcatheter with the proximal tip of the coil was pulled back into the distal end of the guiding catheter. Thereafter, the balloon (Transform balloon; 4 × 10, Stryker Neurovascular, USA) was pulled back such that part of the balloon is within the guiding catheter and was inflated to gain hold onto the coil (Fig. 52.2a). Then the guiding catheter along with the inflated balloon and the tip of the coil was pulled back (Fig. 52.2b). However, the hold on the coil was not adequate, and the coil migrated into the parent lumen (Fig. 52.2c).

Stent-assisted retrieval (Figs. 52.3, 52.4, 52.5, and 52.6)**: The "open and grab" technique**: The coil migrated progressively from the ICA to the MCA bifurcation when angiographic run was taken and while attempting to navigate

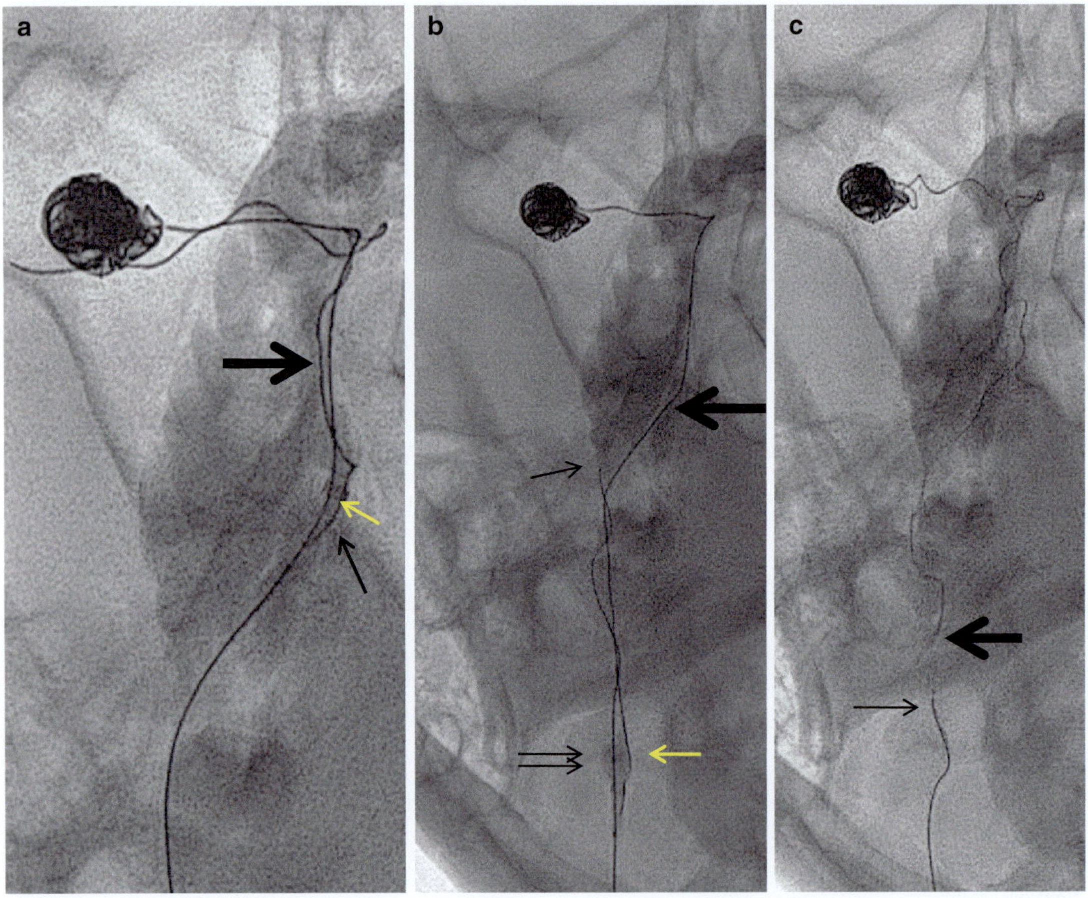

Fig. 52.2 (**a**) Prolapsed coil in the parent lumen (bold arrow); tip of the coil at the tip of the guiding catheter (*thin black arrow*); tip of the guiding catheter (*thin yellow*). (**b**) Coil in the parent artery (*bold arrow*); tip of the balloon wire (*thin black arrow*); balloon inflated at the tip of the guiding catheter jailing the coil between the balloon and the guiding (*double black arrow*); tip of the guiding catheter (yellow arrow). (**c**) The lost grip on the coil; proximal end of the coil (*bold arrow*); distal wire tip of the balloon (*thin black arrow*)

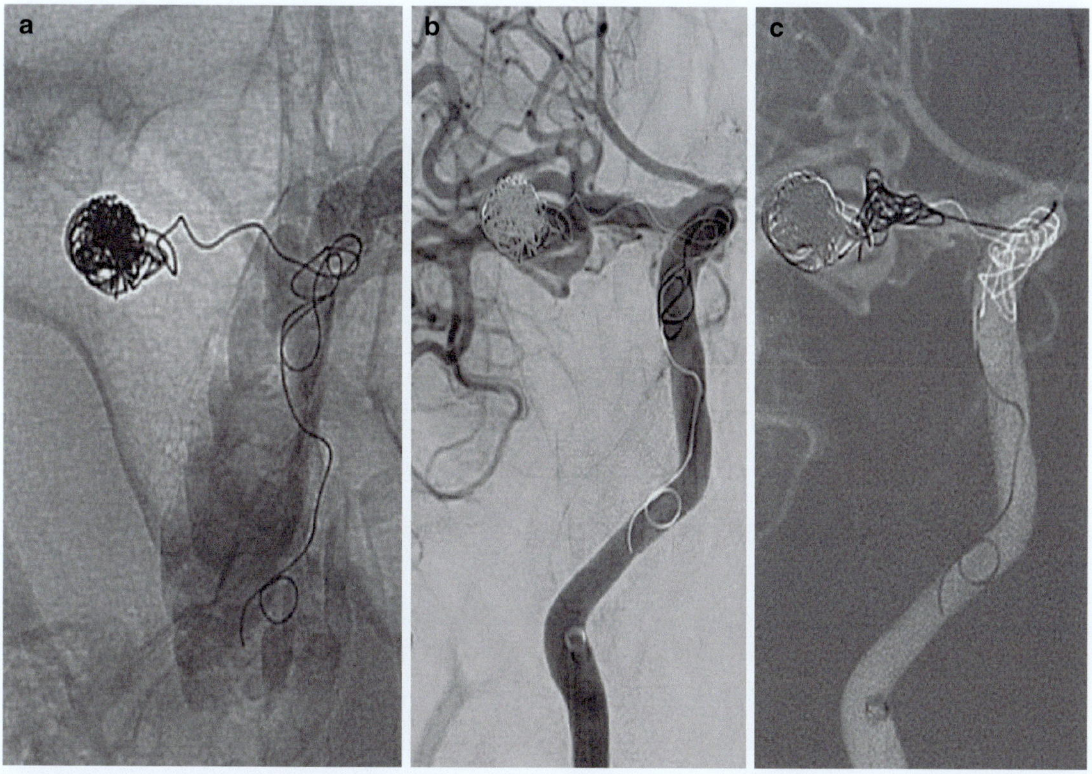

Fig. 52.3 (**a–c**) Progressive migration of coil to the bifurcation following a DSA injection

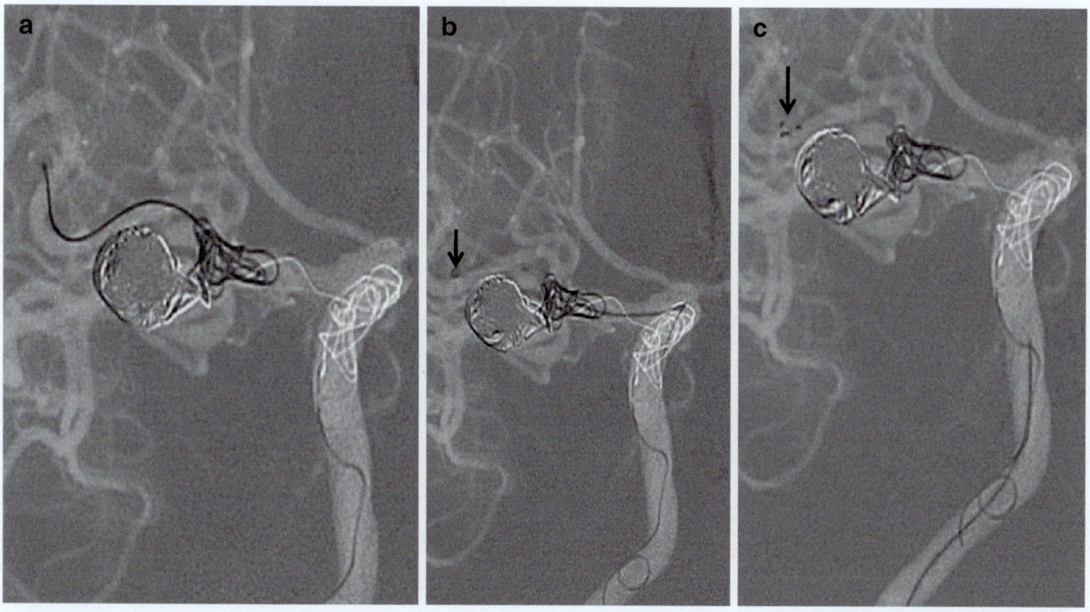

Fig. 52.4 (**a**) Coils noted against the bifurcation, the microwire navigated through the coils and across the neck of the aneurysm into the superior division; (**b**) Rebar 21 microcatheter navigated over the wire into the superior division; (**c**) solitaire 6 × 30 deployed across the neck and then re-sheathed in an attempt to capture the coil

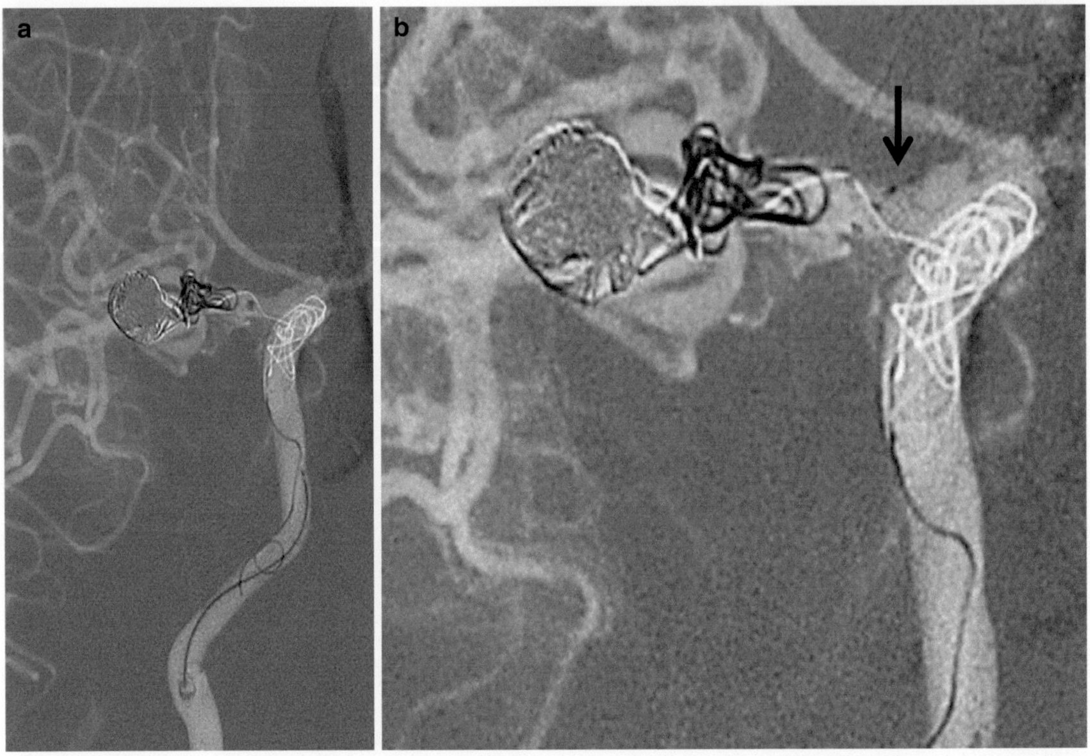

Fig. 52.5 (**a**) Rebar 27 microcatheter proximal to the coil mass; (**b**) solitaire 6 × 30 deployed proximal to the coil mass and then advanced in an attempt to engage the coil loops

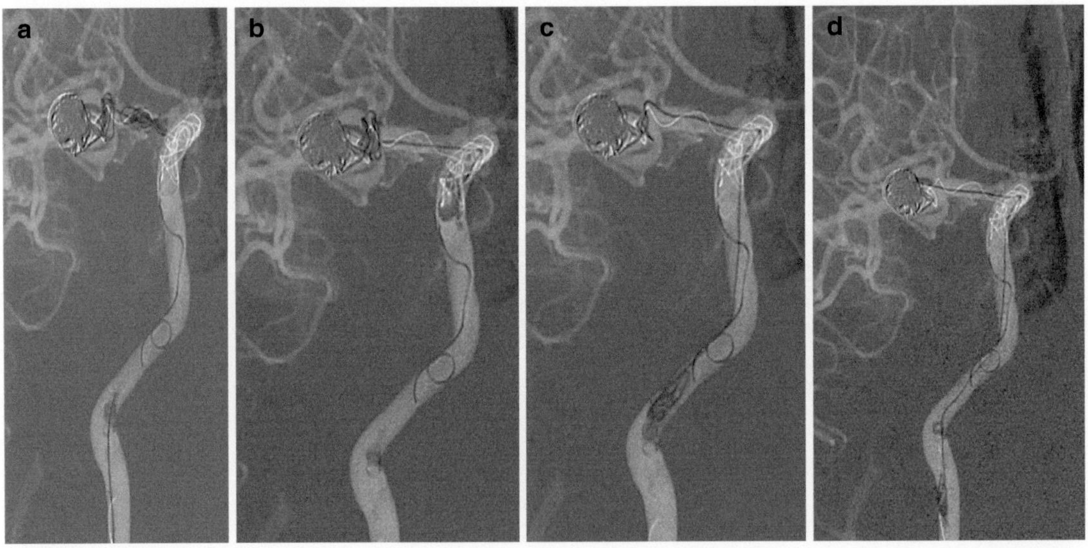

Fig. 52.6 (**a–d**) The stent is re-sheathed into the microcatheter, and during this process, the coils are captured, and the whole setup is pulled out together

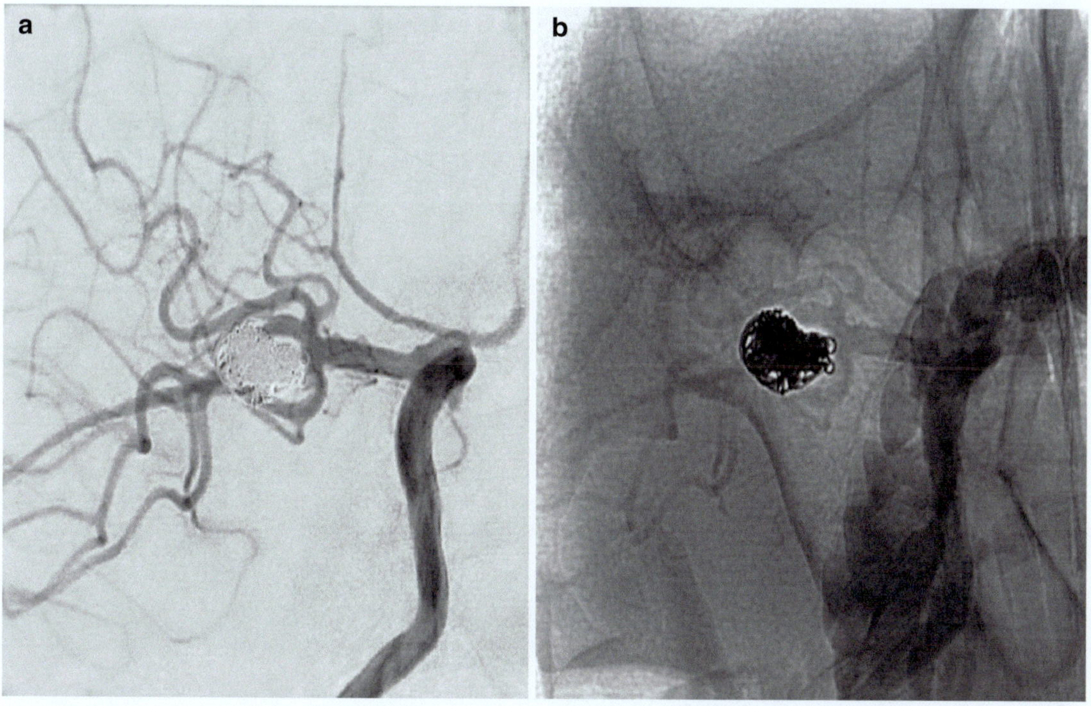

Fig. 52.7 Post-procedure angiography showed complete aneurysm occlusion (**a**) subtracted and (**b**) native images

the Rebar 0.027 (Fig. 52.3) microcatheter beyond the coil loops (Fig. 52.3a–c). The Rebar 0.027 (Medtronic, CA) microcatheter was first navigated beyond the aneurysm neck and into the superior division (Fig. 52.4a, b). A solitaire 6 × 30 mm (Medtronic, CA) stent was then deployed across the coil loop in the parent artery with the distal end of the stent beyond the coil loops (Fig. 52.4c). The stent was re-sheathed until resistance was encountered and then pulled back; however, this did not engage the loops in the parent artery. Therefore, an "open and grab technique" was employed. The solitaire was partly deployed proximal to the loops in the parent artery (Fig. 52.5a, b). Then the stent along with the microcatheter was advanced forward in an attempt to engage the prolapsed loops. Once the stent has been advance through the loops, it is re-sheathed till resistance is encountered to provide an adequate hold on to the coil. Following this, the stent microcatheter is withdrawn along with the coil loops (Fig. 52.6a–d). The rest of the coiling was continued. The post procedure angiography showed complete occlusion (Fig. 52.7a, b).

Case 2

A 65-year-old female presented with a rebleed. During diagnostic angiography, active extravasation was noted from a left MCA bifurcation aneurysm. In view of this, immediate coiling was undertaken. The blood pressure was lowered, heparin effect was reversed, and the DAC 0.07 (Stryker Neurovascular) was parked in the distal left ICA. The first coil was delivered. The

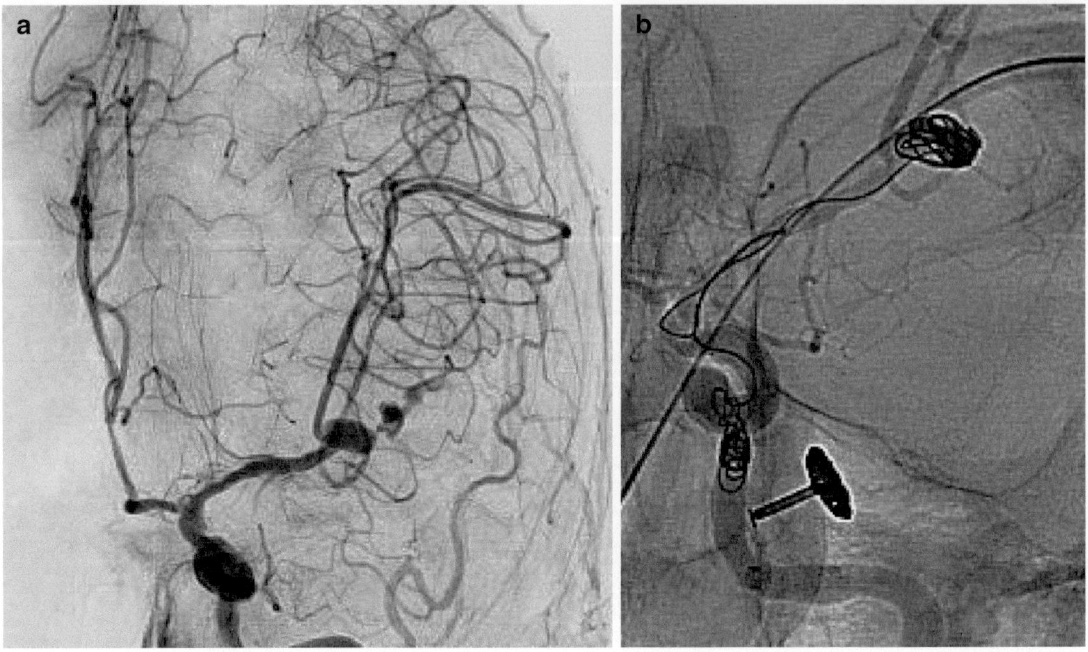

Fig. 52.8 (**a**) acute rupture during angiography; (**b**) coil prolapse in parent artery after attempted removal of the second coil failed, and the microcatheter had to be pulled back

second coil was partly delivered; following this, there was resistance and any attempt at deploying or retrieving the coil failed. While attempting to withdraw the microcatheter into the guiding catheter, the coil detached and prolapsed into the parent artery (Fig. 52.8).

Issues

1. Coil retrieval in the event of coil deposition in the parent artery

Management

The Rebar 0.027 (Medtronic, CA) microcatheter was navigated beyond the coil loops in the parent artery. A solitaire 6 × 30 mm stent was deployed across the loops and then re-sheathed. The stent held on to the loop of the coil, and the stent microcatheter was pulled back into the guiding catheter (Fig. 52.9).

Tips and Tricks

1. During angiographic run, coils can migrate distally into smaller caliber artery. Avoid taking a run unless required.
2. Careful navigation of the microcatheter beyond the prolapsed loops should be undertaken to avoid distal migration of the loops.
3. When the loops are compacted at the bifurcation, an "open and grab" technique can be a useful method to retrieve the coils. Going beyond and deploying across might not be as helpful a technique as it would be in a straight arterial segment.

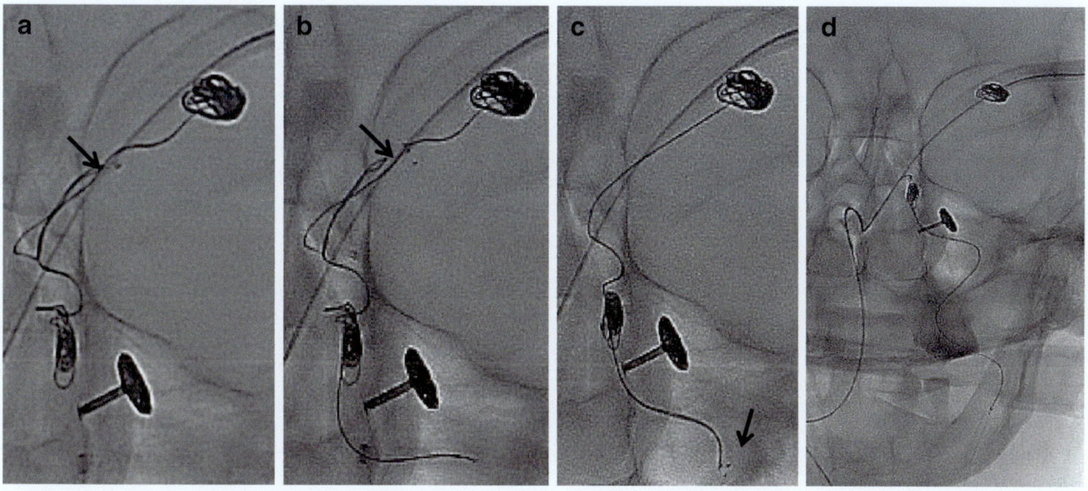

Fig. 52.9 (**a**) The Rebar 27 microcatheter was taken beyond the prolapsed coil; (**b**) the 6 × 30 solitaire was deployed across the coil loops, and then the stent resheathed until resistance is encountered to engage the coil loops; (**c**, **d**) the stent microcatheter along with the captured coil is pulled back

4. A 6 × 30 mm stent as opposed to a 4 × 40 mm solitaire stent would be ideal in a large artery to engage the coils. This would necessitate taking a larger bore microcatheter that can potentially cause distal migration. However, we had not faced major issues with navigating a larger bore catheter in the ICA and proximal MCA.

Suggested Reading

Chen XP, Wang ZF, Guang Z, Liu XZ. Retrievable stent for migrated coil removal: literature review. Neurol India. 2015;63:992–5.

Nikoubashman O, et al. Retrieval of migrated coils with stent retrievers: an animal study. Am J Neuroradiol. 2015;36(6):1162–6.

53 Wire Retrieval Method: Stent- and Snare-Based Retrieval Technique

Vipul Gupta

Case 1

A 48-year-old male presented with brainstem stroke due to a giant fusiform basilar aneurysm. During the planned stent placement, the tip of the Traxcess 14 guidewire (Micorvention, CA, USA) detached in the vertebral artery (Fig. 53.1a).

Case 2

A 72-year-old male presented with subarachnoid hemorrhage due to ruptured blister aneurysm in left ICA. During flow diverter placement procedure, the distal wire of pipeline embolization device (ev3-covidien, Irvine, CA, USA) detached in the left middle cerebral artery (MCA) (Fig. 53.2a).

Issues

1. Detached wire in cerebral artery can lead to thrombo-embolism and injury to vessel wall.

V. Gupta
Neurointerventional Surgery, Stroke Unit, Artemis Agrim Institute of Neuroscience, Gurgaon, India
e-mail: vipul.gupta@artemishospitals.com

Management

Case 1

The DAC038 catheter (Concentric Medical, CA, USA) was taken over the wire. During the process, further displacement of wire was observed (Fig. 53.1b). A solitaire stent (Medtronic, US) was deployed across the wire (Fig. 53.1c). With the stent in stable position, the catheter was threaded over the stent till resistance was felt, indicating entrapment of the wire in the stent mesh (Fig. 53.1d). Thereafter, the catheter along with the stent and the detached wire was withdrawn (Fig. 53.1e). Angiogram didn't reveal any evidence of vessel injury, and stent procedure was performed uneventfully.

Case 2

The microcatheter, Prowler Select Plus (Codman Neurovascular, US) was taken across the detached wire over a Traxcess 14 guidewire (Micorvention, CA, USA) (Fig. 53.2b, c). Care was taken to not to displace the detached wire during the maneuver. A 2-mm microsnare (Amplatz Goose neck Microsnare, ev3, MN, USA) was opened distal to the tip of detached wire (Fig. 53.2d) and carefully withdrawn such that the ring of the snare loops around the detached wire (Fig. 53.2e). Following this, the loop was closed by threading the

V. Gupta et al. (eds.), *100 Interesting Case Studies in Neurointervention: Tips and Tricks*,
https://doi.org/10.1007/978-981-13-1346-2_53

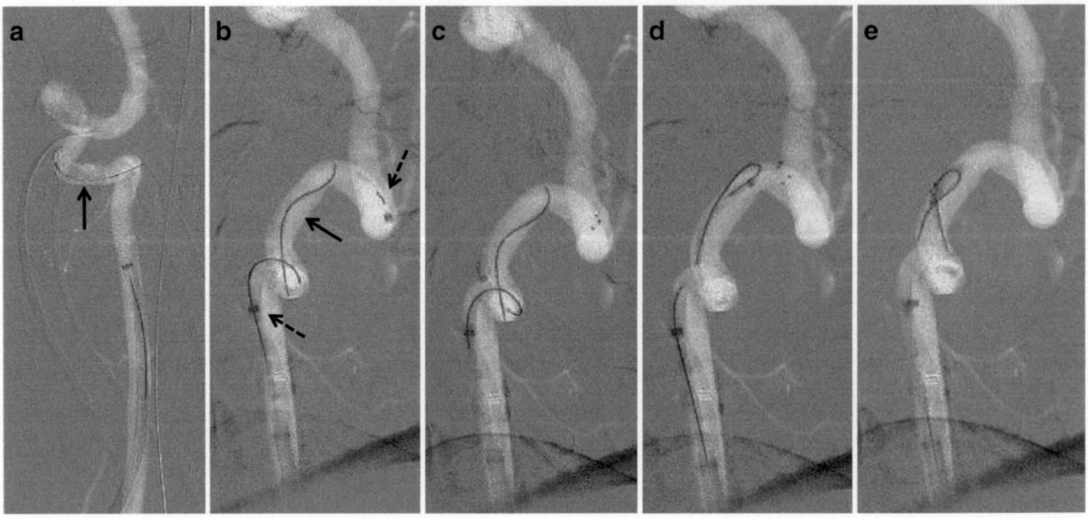

Fig. 53.1 (**a**) Roadmap image in AP view shows the detached wire (*arrow*) in vertebral artery. (**b**) Roadmap image in lateral view—catheter was taken across the wire. During the manipulation the detached wire was displaced distally (*arrow*). Solitaire stent can be seen in the catheter (*broken arrows*). (**c**) Stent released across the wire. (**d**) The catheter was threaded over the stent till resistance was felt, indicating entrapment of the wire in the stent. (**e**) The stent along with the wire were withdrawn

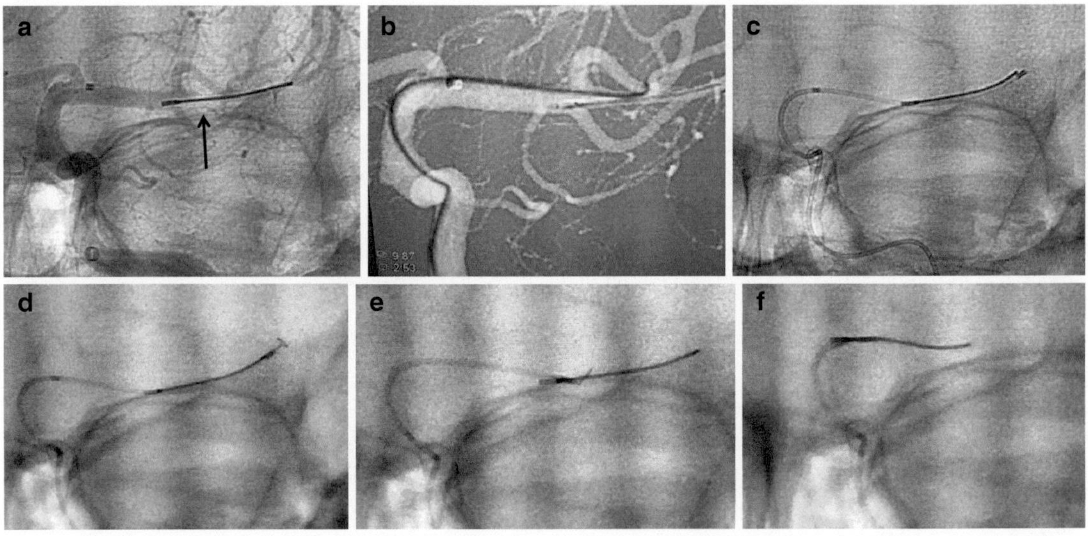

Fig. 53.2 (**a**) DSA AP view shows the detached distal wire (*arrow*) of pipeline device in the left middle cerebral artery (MCA). (**b**, **c**) Microwire (**b**) and microcatheter (**c**) were taken across the detached wire; care was being taken to not to displace it further into the MCA. (**d–f**) Microsnare opened distal to the wire tip (**d**), slid around the wire, (**e**) and tightened across the wire by sliding the microcatheter forward

microcatheter over the ring of the snare (Fig. 53.2f). The catheter, snare, and detached wire were withdrawn across the deployed flow diverter.

Tips and Tricks

1. Though rare, wire tips can get detached. In both the cases, patients were on antiplatelet regimen; otherwise, we give bolus of heparin in these cases so as prevent any thrombus formation.
2. Detached wire can be retrieved using snare or stent retriever.
3. Care has to be taken in navigating catheter across the wire as it can be further displaced. Migration into smaller vessel may make it difficult to retrieve and increases chances of any complication.
4. After engaging the wire in the snare or stent retriever, it is critical to fix the wire to the retrieval device by taking the catheter forward over the snare or stent retriever.
5. At times it is difficult to engage the wire; however, change of position of wire may make it amenable to be retrieved.

Suggested Reading

Gunnarsson T, Da Costa L, Souza MPS, et al. Guidewire tip detachment during Stent-Assisted coiling of an intracranial aneurysm. Interv Neuroradiol. 2009;15:93.

54 Very Small (Less Than 2 mm) Aneurysm with Severe Vasospasm: Pretreatment Dilatation

Vipul Gupta

Case

A 56-year-old female presented with left lower limb weakness following a 1-week history of sudden severe headache. CT scan revealed subarachnoid haemorrhage and small areas of infarction in the right anterior cerebral artery (ACA) territory. Digital subtraction angiography (DSA) revealed a very small (≤1.5 mm) anterior communicating artery aneurysm (Fig. 54.1) with severe vasospasm of anterior and middle cerebral arteries and distal internal carotid artery (Fig. 54.1a, b).

Issue

- Vasospasm management prior to coil embolization of the aneurysm sac—how safe is it?
- Evaluation of geometry of aneurysm on 3D rotational angiography to allow for safe sac catheterization.

Management

The procedure was performed under general anaesthesia. A 6F guiding catheter was placed in the right ICA and intra-arterial vasodilatation was performed with 3-mg of intra-arterial nimodipine given over 40-min. Repeat angiogram showed adequate resolution of vasospasm and a very small ACOM artery aneurysm (≤1.5 mm) (Fig. 54.1c, d) which was evaluated by rotational angiogram and 3D reconstruction. Angio-CT (DynaCT, Siemens, Erlangen, Germany) did not reveal any fresh bleed or change in mass effect due to the infarcts. A pre-shaped microcatheter was used as it was likely to point into the aneurysm sac. It was carefully navigated over a microguidewire under road map guidance up to the neck of the aneurysm. No attempt was made to enter the aneurysm as the catheter was pointing towards the aneurysm in both the planes (Fig. 54.2a, b). A very small soft coil (Micrus 1.5 mm × 1 cm) was placed in the aneurysm slowly, and with increase in resistance, the catheter was allowed to back off so as to avoid any increase in intra-aneurysmal pressure (Fig. 54.2c). The coil was detached, and the final angiogram revealed complete thrombosis of the aneurysm (Fig. 54.2d, e) with good flow in the intracranial arteries (Fig. 54.2f). Patient made complete recovery.

Tips and Tricks

1. Intra-arterial vasodilatation can be performed safely before treating the aneurysm. We prefer to perform partial dilatation under general anaesthesia followed by coiling.

V. Gupta
Neurointerventional Surgery, Stroke Unit, Artemis Agrim Institute of Neuroscience, Gurgaon, India
e-mail: vipul.gupta@artemishospitals.com

V. Gupta et al. (eds.), *100 Interesting Case Studies in Neurointervention: Tips and Tricks*,
https://doi.org/10.1007/978-981-13-1346-2_54

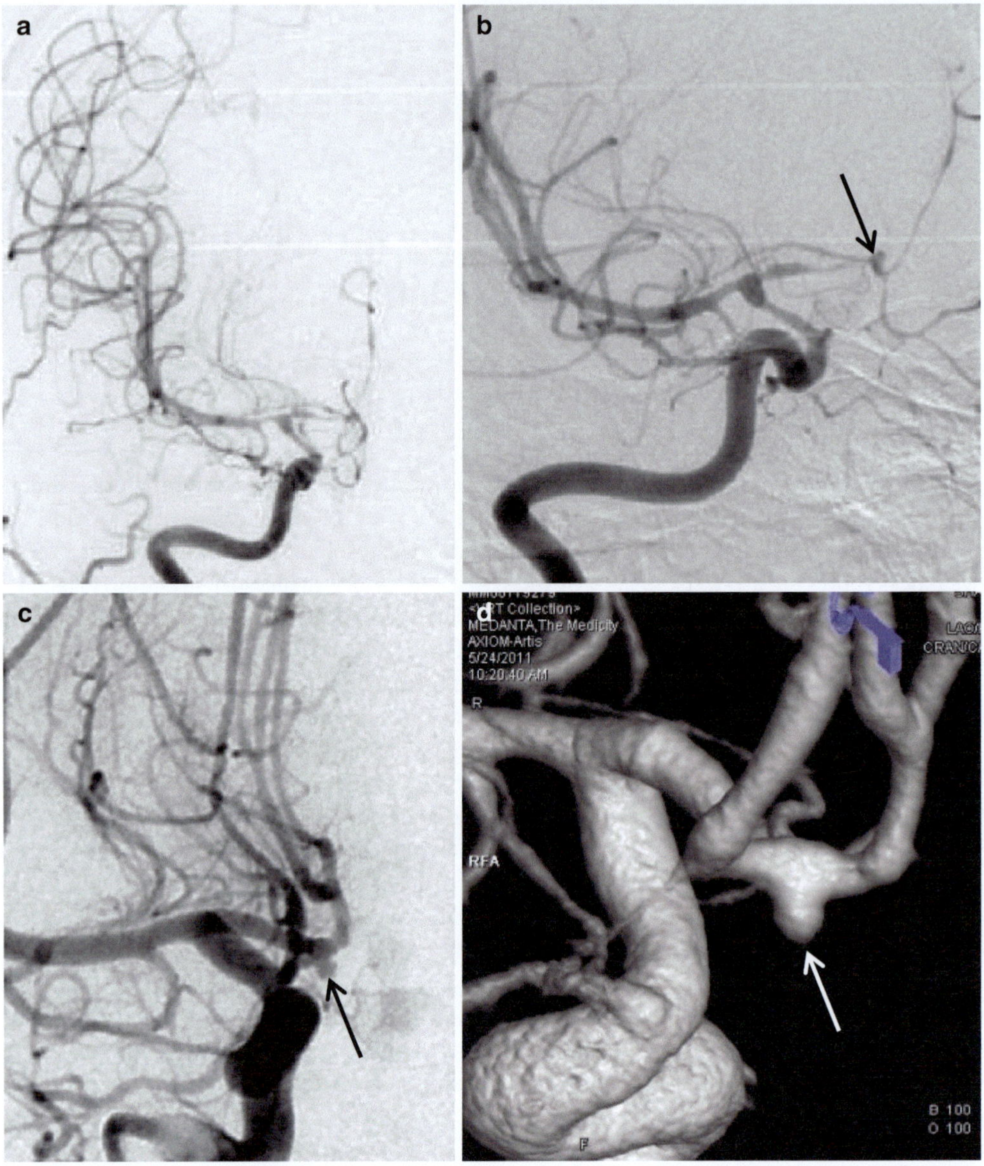

Fig. 54.1 (**a**) Right ICA DSA (AP view) showing severe vasospasm of ACAs, MCAs and distal internal carotid arteries. (**b**) Oblique shows a probable very small aneurysm in relationship to the ACA (*arrow*). (**c**, **d**) DSA and 3D images obtained after intra-arterial vasodilatation clearly showed a very small aneurysm in anterior communication region (*arrow*)

2. In our experience, intra-arterial dilatation with nimodipine is more effective if given over relatively longer period (40–45 min) as compared to the same amount given over short period (2-min or so).
3. Very small aneurysm can be difficult to visualize; rotational angiography with 3D reconstruction is crucial in identification and evaluation of these aneurysms.
4. Coiling of very small aneurysm can be difficult and can result in intra-operative rupture if adequate precautions are not taken. We prefer to place the catheter tip near the neck rather than at the dome of small and friable aneurysms.

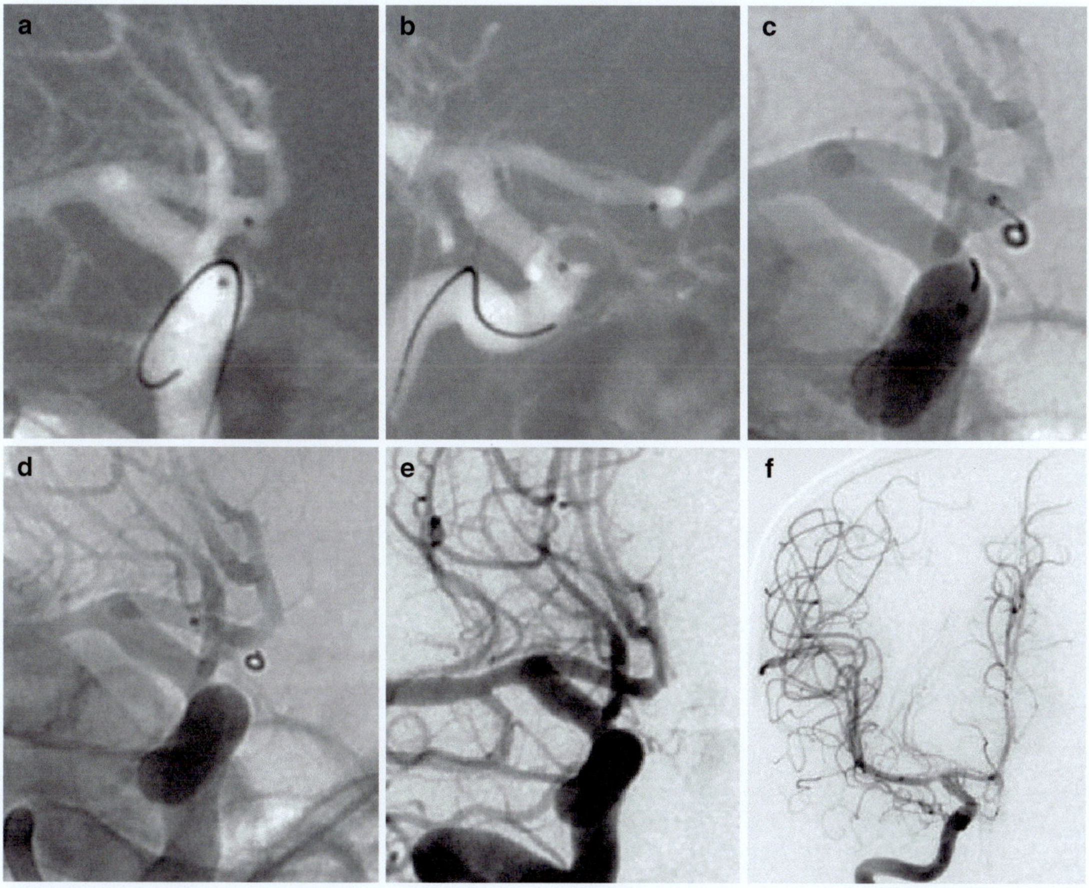

Fig. 54.2 (**a**, **b**) Road map images showing the microcatheter position at the neck of the aneurysm. (**c**) Coil placement done with microcatheter tip outside the aneurysm. (**d**) Microcatheter withdrawn after detachment. (**e**, **f**) Post-embolization check angiogram showing complete occlusion of aneurysm (**e**) and good opacification of intracranial arteries

This avoids the possibility of rupture due to wire or microcatheter manipulation. Coil size should be chosen carefully, and in most instances a single coil is adequate to achieve sac occlusion by promoting thrombosis in very small aneurysms. If during coiling, resistance is felt, it is better to release the tension from the microcatheter by withdrawing it slightly, rather than risk a rupture.

Suggested Reading

1. Moret J, Pierot L, Boulin A, Castaings L, Rey A. Endovascular treatment of anterior communicating artery aneurysms using Guglielmi detachable coils. Neuroradiology. 1996;38:800–5.
2. Suzuki S, Kurata A, Ohmomo T, et al. Endovascular surgery for very small ruptured intracranial aneurysms. Technical note. J Neurosurg. 2006;105:777–80.

55 Severe Diffuse Vasospasm: B/L Intraarterial Vasodilatation Followed by Coiling

Rajsrinivas Parthasarathy and Vipul Gupta

Case

A 35-year-old female had sudden severe headache without associated neurological deficits. Although CT scan revealed diffuse SAH, she was treated conservatively. Ten days after the ictus she became drowsy and was shifted to our hospital. At the time of admission, she had right hemiparesis with a score of E3M5V1 on the Glasgow coma scale. Repeat CT scan revealed residual SAH (Fig. 55.1a) and left frontal infarct (Fig. 55.1b). DSA revealed severe vasospasm of B/L ACAs in the A1 and A2 segments (Fig. 55.2c–f) and the left MCA. A very small aneurysm was discernible in the ACOM region.

Issues

The management of vasospasm prior to coil embolization of the aneurysm sac

R. Parthasarathy (✉)
Vascular Neurology and Neurointerventional Surgery, Artemis Agrim Institute of Neuroscience, Gurgaon, India

V. Gupta
Neurointerventional Surgery, Stroke Unit, Artemis Agrim Institute of Neuroscience, Gurgaon, India
e-mail: vipul.gupta@artemishospitals.com

Management

Intraarterial vasodilatation followed by aneurysm coiling in the same session was considered to be the most appropriate management strategy. The procedure was performed under general anaesthesia. Through transfemoral route, guiding catheters (Envoy 5F, Codman & Sheurtleff, Inc. USA) were placed in both cervical ICAs. Initially, nimodipine (3 mg) was infused in both internal carotid artery territories over 30 min. However, in view of inadequate reopening, a further 2 mg was given in both the territories over 30 min. Volume expanders and vasopressors were administered to maintain blood pressure to preoperative levels. Post-dilatation angiogram revealed marked decrease in vasospasm along with good antegrade flow in both ACAs and MCAs (Fig. 55.2a). The aneurysm sac was better appreciated and looked bigger than in the initial angiogram. An AngioCT (DynaCT, Siemens, Erlangen) performed post-procedure did not reveal fresh haemorrhage. Thereafter, the aneurysm was coiled, and complete occlusion was achieved (Fig. 55.2b). Patient showed remarkable improvement in consciousness and could be extubated the next day. She recovered with mild residual paresis in the right ankle. Follow-up angiogram after 6 months revealed satisfactory coil occlusion of the aneurysm sac (Fig. 55.2c).

V. Gupta et al. (eds.), *100 Interesting Case Studies in Neurointervention: Tips and Tricks*,
https://doi.org/10.1007/978-981-13-1346-2_55

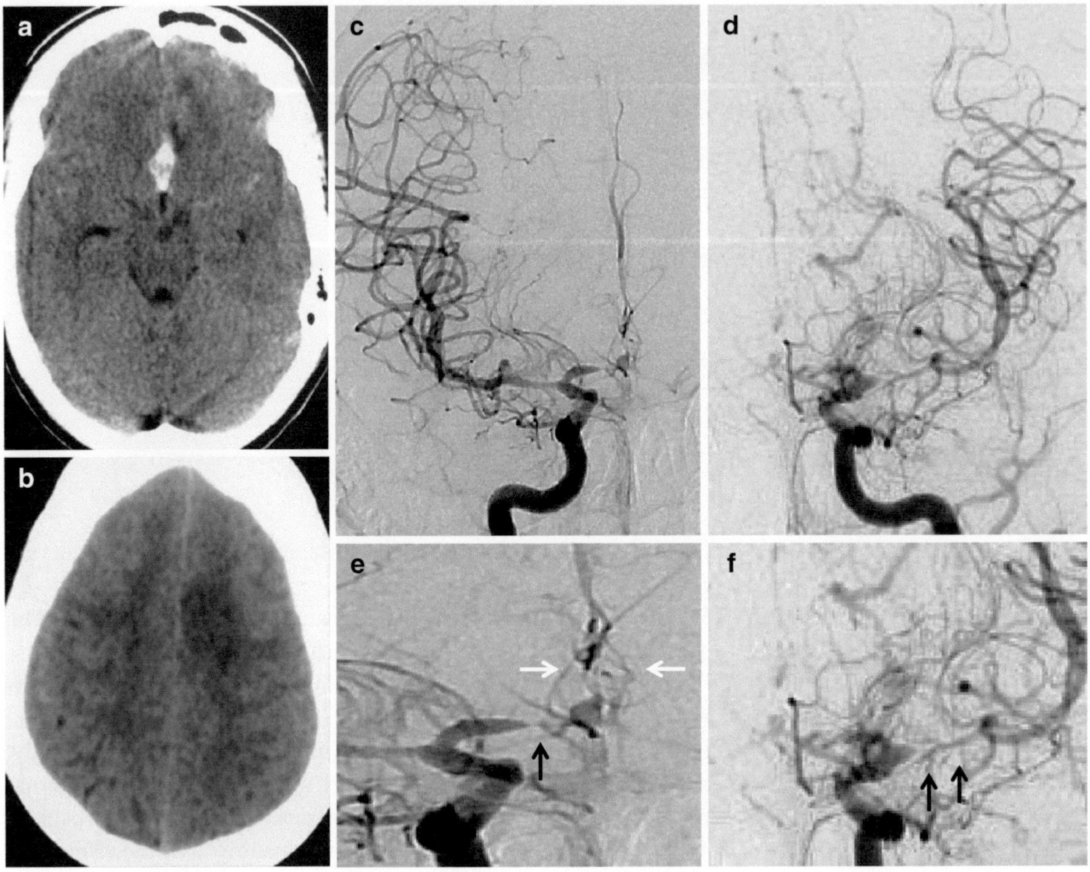

Fig. 55.1 (**a**, **b**) CT scan images showing SAH (**a**) and left frontal infarction (**b**). (**c**, **e**) Right ICA angiogram showing severe vasospasm in A1 (*black arrow*, **e**) segment of right ACA and B/L A2 (*white arrows*, **e**) segments. Leptomeningeal collaterals are seen from right MCA. Small aneurysm is seen in ACOM region. (**d**, **f**) Left ICA injection showing severe vasospasm of left ACA and M1 segment (*arrows*, **f**) of left MCA

Tips and Tricks

1. Severe vasospasm can potentially respond to intraarterial vasodilatation. It is authors' view that a slow and prolonged infusion of nimodipine is required to achieve the desired result.
2. Spasm involving the ACA does respond to an infusion from the catheter placed in the cervical ICA.
3. Small aneurysms can be better visualized after vasodilatation.
4. AngioCT can be performed to evaluate for fresh haemorrhage if this is suspected post vasodilatation.
5. Vasodilatation can be safely performed when small infarcts are present. Caution should be exercised when large infarcts are noted as reperfusion haemorrhage and oedema can occur.
6. Interval repeat doses of heparin are administered during the period of vasodilatation to prevent thromboembolism. In our experience, vasodilatation has not resulted in repeat haemorrhage.

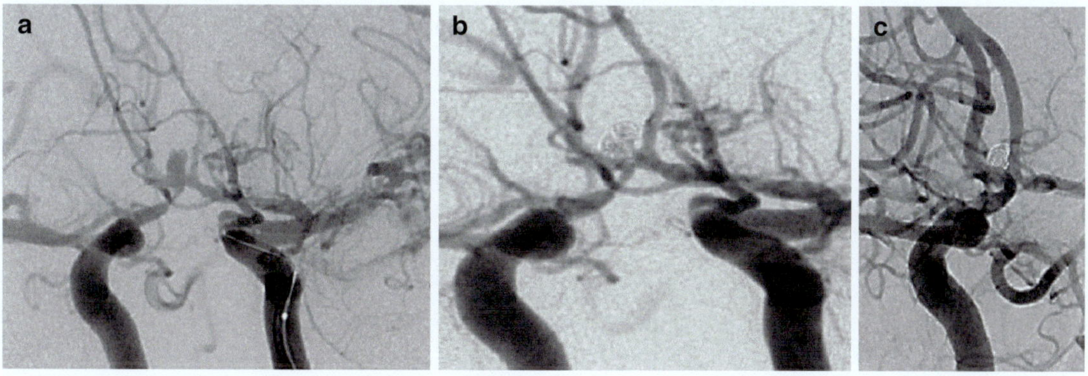

Fig. 55.2 (**a**) DSA after vasodilatation showing reopening of the previously spastic vessels. The aneurysm in ACOM region is seen better. (**b**) AngioCT after the dilatation—no fresh haemorrhage could be seen. (**c**) Post-coiling angiogram showing complete occlusion. (**d**) Follow-up DSA showing stable result

Suggested Reading

Anand S, Goel G, Gupta V. Continuous intra-arterial dilatation with nimodipine and milrinone for refractory cerebral vasospasm. J Neurosurg Anesthesiol. 2014;26(1):92–3.

Oran I, Cinar C. Continuous intra-arterial infusion of nimodipine during embolization of cerebral aneurysms associated with vasospasm. AJNR. 2008;29(2):291–5.

Velat GJ, Kimball MM, Mocco JD, Hoh BL. Vasospasm after aneurysmal subarachnoid hemorrhage: review of randomized controlled trials and meta-analyses in the literature. World Neurosurg. 2011;76(5):446–54.

Intraarterial Dilatation in Subarachnoid Haemorrhage-Induced Vasospasm

56

Rajsrinivas Parthasarathy and Vipul Gupta

Case

A 40-year-old lady with history of sudden onset headache was diagnosed with subarachnoid haemorrhage. Digital subtraction angiography revealed a left MCA bifurcation aneurysm, which was subsequently coiled successfully (Fig. 56.1).

On the seventh day since the ictus, she developed weakness of right arm and leg and expressive aphasia. She underwent an urgent cerebral angiography to assess for vasospasm (Fig. 56.2a).

Issues

1. Severe spasm of intracranial vessels can result in large brain infarctions.

Management

A 4F small sheath (Cordis) was used to access the right femoral artery. Following this a 5F diagnostic catheter (Cook) was positioned in the left internal carotid artery. Initially, 1 mg of nimodipine is administered as bolus over 3–5 min, followed by slow infusion of 2 mg over 20 min (total of 3 mg) (Fig. 56.2b, e). Following this, 6–8 mg of milrinone is infused over 30 min. The intraarterial dilatation is more pronounced due to the synergistic action of nimodipine and milrinone (Fig. 56.2c, f).

Patient had improvement in the neurological status with no deficits clinically or radiologically (Fig. 56.2g).

Tips and Tricks

1. The occurrence of vasospasm in SAH can be detrimental. It is imperative to diagnose and treat vasospasm early to avoid cerebral infarction.
2. Serial TCD monitoring allows for early detection and appropriate management of vasospasm; the operator experience determines the reliability with which the insonation velocities can be interpreted with confidence.
3. CT perfusion imaging is an alternate excellent tool to look at decrease in cerebral perfusion and can be a very useful tool to diagnose cerebral vasospasm.
4. Traditionally, intraarterial dilatation with calcium channel blockers, like nimodipine or verapamil, was the norm.

R. Parthasarathy (✉)
Vascular Neurology and Neurointerventional Surgery, Artemis Agrim Institute of Neuroscience, Gurgaon, India

V. Gupta
Neurointerventional Surgery, Stroke Unit, Artemis Agrim Institute of Neuroscience, Gurgaon, India
e-mail: vipul.gupta@artemishospitals.com

V. Gupta et al. (eds.), *100 Interesting Case Studies in Neurointervention: Tips and Tricks*,
https://doi.org/10.1007/978-981-13-1346-2_56

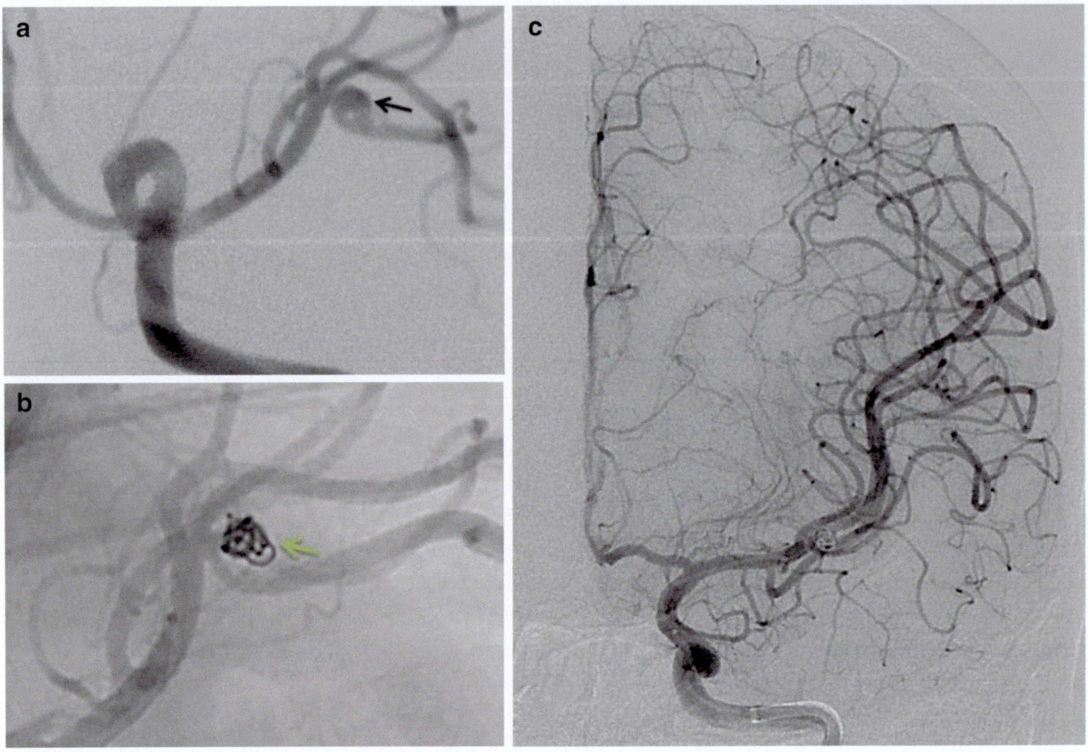

Fig. 56.1 (**a**) DSA image showing small let MCA bifurcation aneurysm (*arrow*). (**b**) Coiling of the aneurysm (*green arrow*). (**c**) Post-coiling DSA left ICA AP view showing normal flowing arteries

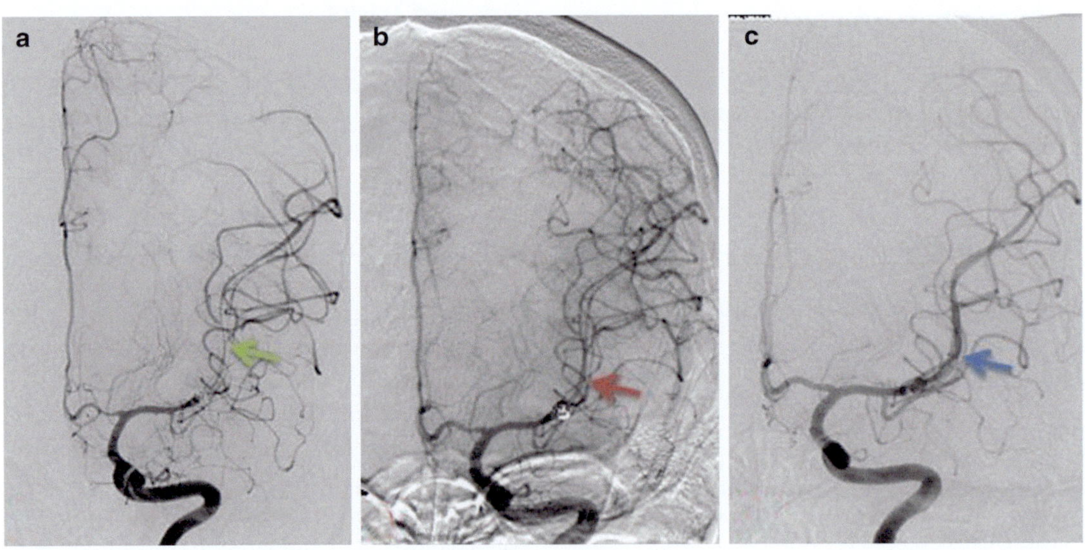

Fig. 56.2 (**a**) DSA showing severe spasm of intracranial arteries particularly in M2 segment (*arrow*) of MCA with secondary hypoperfusion. (**b**) DSA after nimodipine infusion reveal partial improvement. (**c**) Milrinone infusion resulted in further significant improvement in calibre of arteries particularly in M2 segment (**d–f**). Magnified view of MCA M2 segment from images (**a–c**). (**g**) CT scan showing normal parenchyma

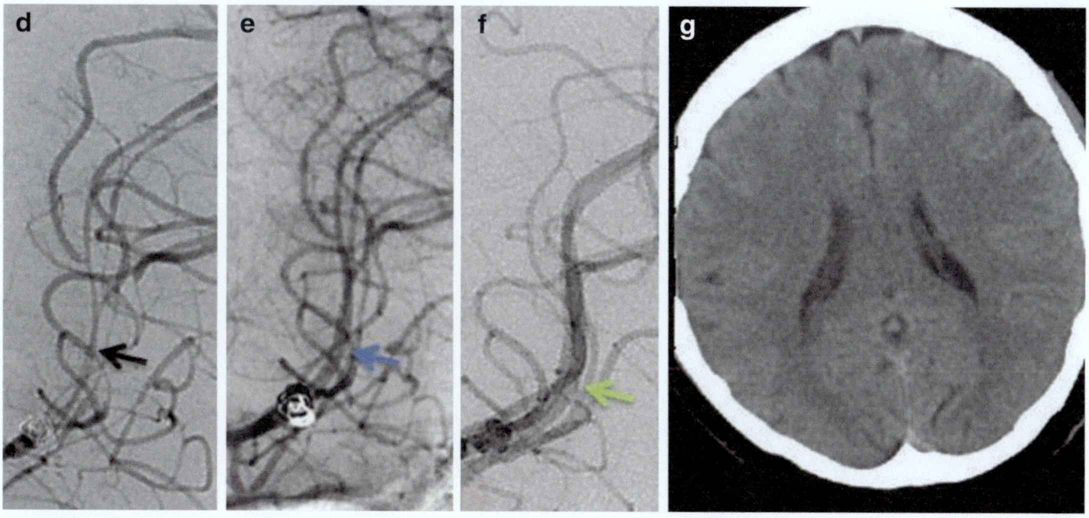

Fig. 56.2 (continued)

5. In our experience milrinone, a phosphodiesterase-3 inhibitor augments the vasodilatory effect achieved with nimodipine. Milrinone increases intracellular cyclic AMP. An increase in cAMP inhibits myosin light chain kinase and consequent phosphorylation of myosin light chain resulting in vasodilatation.
6. The effect of nimodipine and milrinone is synergistic and therefore results in better dilatation of the involved vessel.
7. Nimodipine (dose, 3 mg over 20 min) is followed with milrinone (dose, 8 mg over 30–40 min).
8. The factors that limit the dose and rate of milrinone infusion are hypotension and tachycardia. It is imperative to maintain the mean arterial pressure over 90–100 to maintain the cerebral perfusion. This can be achieved by titrating up the rate of infusion of noradrenaline. Tachycardia can precipitate myocardial infarction and therefore reduce the rate of infusion in the event the heart rate exceeds >130 bpm.
9. Acute subarachnoid haemorrhage can result in procoagulant state. Therefore, adequate heparinization should be maintained during the procedure to avoid thromboembolism.
10. Balloon angioplasty also requires GA, is expensive and can cause rupture of the spastic arteries, and henceforth not recommended by the authors as first line measure by us.

Suggested Reading

Anand S, Goel G, Gupta V. Continuous intra-arterial dilatation with nimodipine and milrinone for refractory cerebral vasospasm. J Neurosurg Anesthesiol. 2014;26(1):92–3.

Oran I, Cinar C. Continuous intra-arterial infusion of nimodipine during embolization of cerebral aneurysms associated with vasospasm. AJNR. 2008;29(2):291–5.

Velat GJ, Kimball MM, Mocco JD, Hoh BL. Vasospasm after aneurysmal subarachnoid hemorrhage: review of randomized controlled trials and meta-analyses in the literature. World Neurosurg. 2011;76(5):446–54.

Continuous Intra-arterial Dilatation in Refractory/Malignant Vasospasm

57

Rajsrinivas Parthasarathy and Vipul Gupta

Case 1

A 52-year-old lady with history of sudden onset headache was diagnosed with subarachnoid hemorrhage. Digital subtraction angiography revealed a ACOM aneurysm, which was subsequently coiled successfully (Fig. 57.1).

On the fifth day since the ictus, she became drowsy. She underwent an urgent cerebral angiography to assess for vasospasm (Fig. 57.2a).

She improved post dilatation with nimodipine (Fig. 57.2b) and milrinone (Fig. 57.2c). However, she needed dilatations on a daily basis and was diagnosed with malignant spasm, and therefore was planned for continuous intra-arterial dilatation after the third session.

Issues

1. Malignant spasm of intracranial vessels

Management

A 5F diagnostic catheter (Cook) was positioned in the left internal carotid artery. Initially, 1 mg of nimodipine is administered as bolus over 3–5 min, followed by slow infusion of 2 mg over 20 min (total of 3 mg). Following this, 6–8 mg of milrinone is infused over 30 min. The intra-arterial dilatation was more pronounced due to the synergistic action of nimodipine and milrinone. Following that, a 0.021' microcatheter was positioned in the distal cervical ICA, and the diagnostic catheter was withdrawn into the arch of the aorta (Fig. 57.3). The microcatheter was connected to a continuous infusion of nimodipine (40 mg) and milrinone (20 mg) mixed in 1 L of normal saline. The diagnostic catheter is connected to a continuous flush line. Heparin 2000 U is added to both the bags. The microcatheter was left in place for 3 days. Patient had improved and made complete recovery.

Case 2

A 65-year-old male was diagnosed with subarachnoid hemorrhage. He was diagnosed with right PCOM aneurysm, and endovascular coiling was undertaken. He developed left arm and face weakness on the sixth day after ictus.

He needed three sessions of intra-arterial dilatations (Fig. 57.4a, b). He had refractory and malignant vasospasm and therefore continuous intra-arterial dilatation (Figs. 57.5 and 57.6).

R. Parthasarathy (✉)
Vascular Neurology and Neurointerventional Surgery, Artemis Agrim Institute of Neuroscience, Gurgaon, India

V. Gupta
Neurointerventional Surgery, Stroke Unit,Artemis Agrim Institute of Neuroscience, Gurgaon, India
e-mail: vipul.gupta@artemishospitals.com

V. Gupta et al. (eds.), *100 Interesting Case Studies in Neurointervention: Tips and Tricks*, https://doi.org/10.1007/978-981-13-1346-2_57

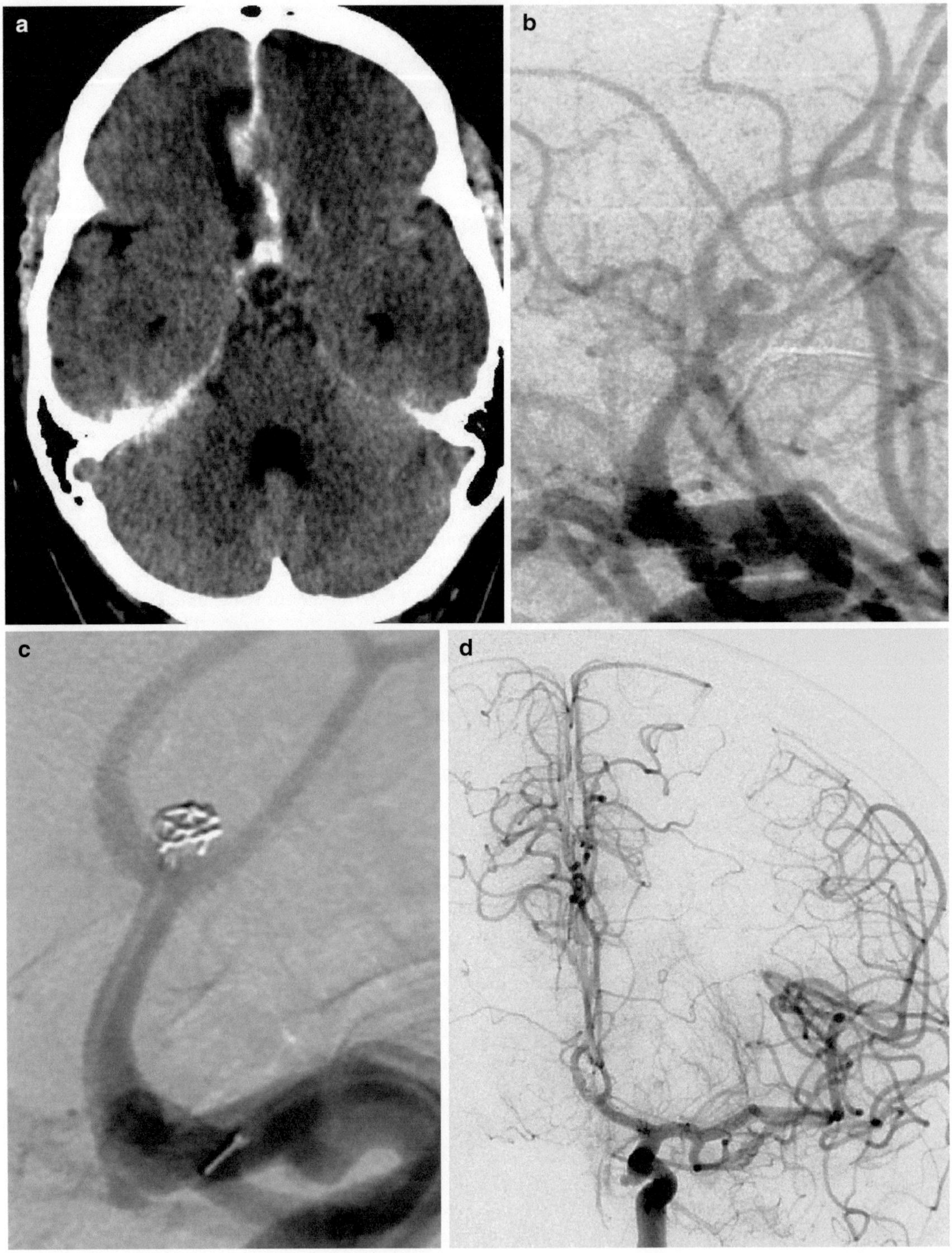

Fig. 57.1 (**a**) CT head showing diffuse SAH; (**b**) DSA image showing ACOM aneurysm; (**c**) coiling of the aneurysm undertaken successfully; (**d**) post-coiling DSA left ICA AP view showing normal flowing arteries

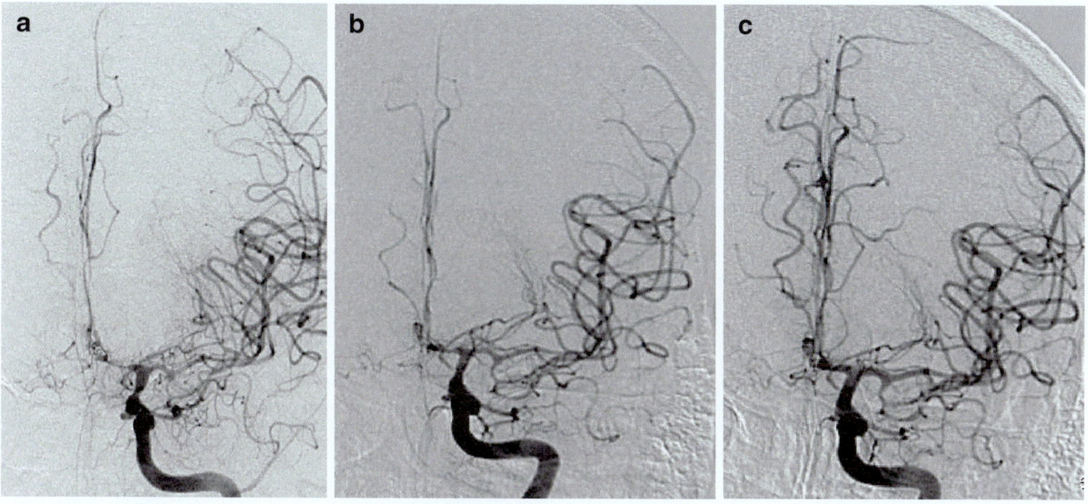

Fig. 57.2 (**a**) DSA showing severe spasm, of intracranial arteries particularly in M1 and A1 ACA. (**b**) DSA after nimodipine infusion reveals partial improvement. (**c**) Milrinone infusion resulted in further significant improvement in caliber of arteries

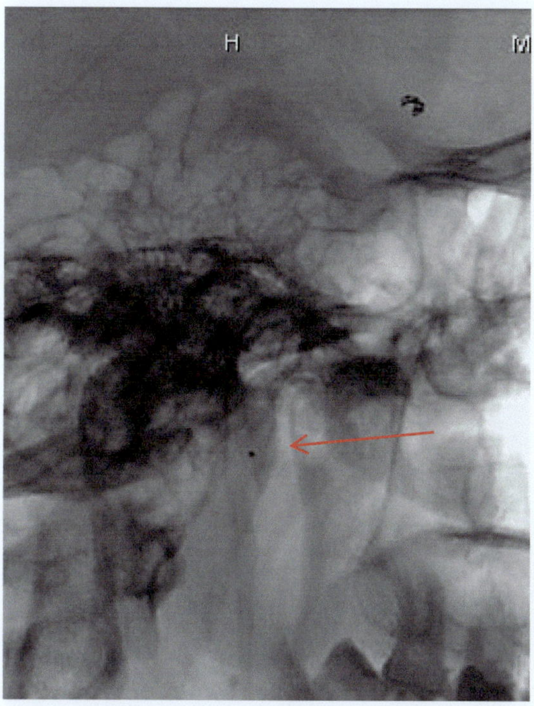

Fig. 57.3 Microcatheter tip noted in the distal cervical ICA

Tips and Tricks

1. Continuous intra-arterial dilatation is performed when three or more intra-arterial dilatations have been performed and/or if the effect of the dilatation lasts less than 24 h.
2. Systemic hypotension due to large doses of intravenous milrinone is not uncommon and may require two or more inotropes to maintain the mean arterial pressure above 90–100.
3. Continuous delivery of drug in the ipsilateral ICA allows for reduction in the total dose of milrinone delivered over 24 h and therefore allows for the reduction in the dose of vasopressors required.
4. The microcatheter tip is positioned in the distal cervical ICA. Avoid parking at bends or loops to prevent clot formation around the catheter.
5. The microcatheter infusion mixture contains nimodipine (40 mg) + milrinone (20 mg) + heparin (2000 IU). Single-strength mixture is started at 16 drops per minute and titrated according to the clinical response and the need for vasopressors. Volume overload can be frequently encountered, and in those instances a double strength preparation can be used [nimodipine (80 mg) + milrinone (40 mg) in 1 L NS].
6. The microcatheter is left in place, while the diagnostic catheter is pulled back into the arch of aorta to minimize the risk of cerebral thromboembolism. The diagnostic catheter is connected to a heparinized flush line.

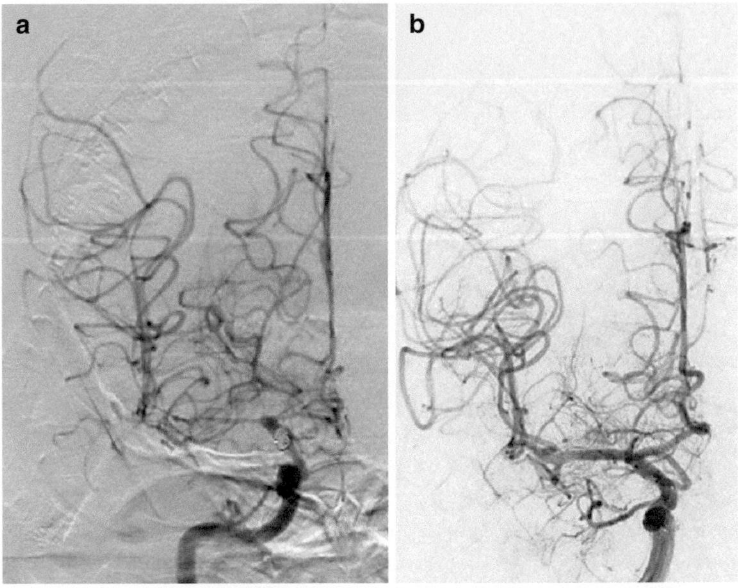

Fig. 57.4 (**a**) Severe spasm involving both M1 MCA and A1 ACA. (**b**) Post dilatation with nimodipine and milrinone

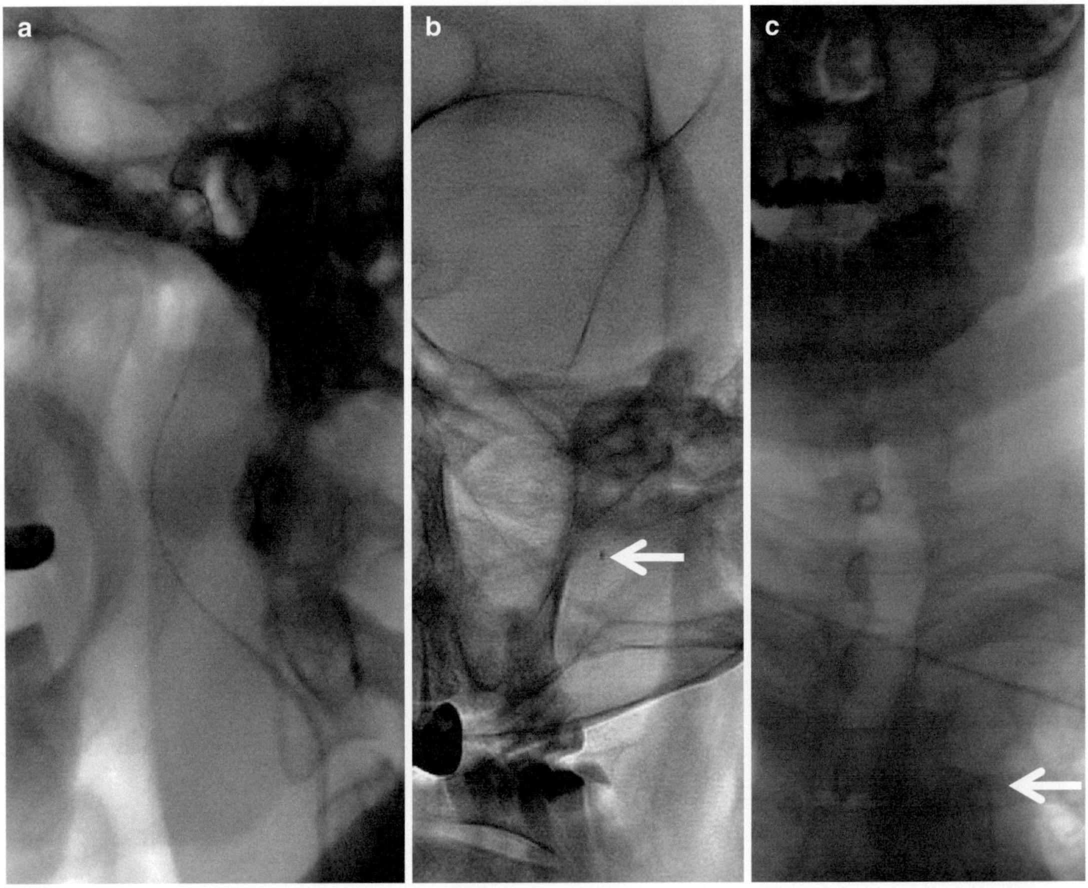

Fig. 57.5 (**a**) Diagnostic catheter was placed in the cervical ICA with microcatheter in the distal cervical ICA. (**b**) Microcatheter in the distal cervical ICA in a straight segment. (**c**) Diagnostic catheter withdrawn into the arch

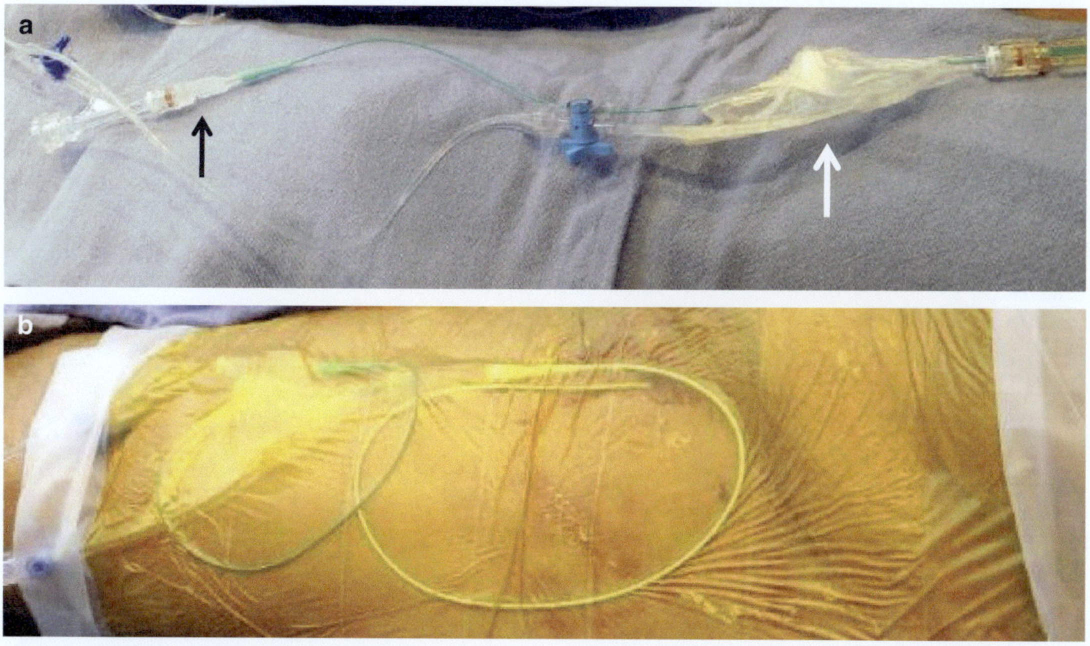

Fig. 57.6 (**a**) Microcatheter is taped on to the rotating hemostatic valve (RHV) of the diagnostic catheter using a Tegaderm (*white arrow*); microcatheter connected to a RHV and flush line containing a mixture of nimodipine, milrinone, and heparin (*black arrow*). (**b**) Fixation of the diagnostic catheter—microcatheter system on to the thigh using a Ioban

7. A Tegaderm is used to tape the microcatheter on to the RHV of the diagnostic catheter. Following this, the microcatheter (MC) and the diagnostic catheter are taped on to the thigh using an Ioban.
8. Clexane 0.4 cc is administered subcutaneously twice daily to prevent clot formation around the microcatheter.
9. The MC can be left in place for 72 h. During this period intravenous antibiotics are administered to avoid systemic sepsis.

Suggested Reading

Anand S, Goel G, Gupta V. Continuous intra-arterial dilatation with nimodipine and milrinone for refractory cerebral vasospasm. J Neurosurg Anesthesiol. 2014;26(1):92–3.

Oran I, Cinar C. Continuous intra-arterial infusion of nimodipine during embolization of cerebral aneurysms associated with vasospasm. AJNR. 2008;29(2):291–5.

Velat GJ, Kimball MM, Mocco JD, Hoh BL. Vasospasm after aneurysmal subarachnoid hemorrhage: review of randomized controlled trials and meta-analyses in the literature. World Neurosurg. 2011;76(5):446–54.

58 CT Perfusion Imaging to Diagnose Vasospasm After Subarachnoid Hemorrhage

Rajsrinivas Parthasarathy and Vipul Gupta

Case 1: History

A 28-year-old lady with a history of sudden-onset headache was diagnosed with subarachnoid hemorrhage on CT scan. Cerebral angiography revealed a left anterior choroidal artery aneurysm which was subsequently coiled successfully (Fig. 58.1).

On day 6 she became confused, with weakness on right side. Her NCCT brain showed no acute infarct (Fig. 58.2a). She was evaluated with a CT angio and CT perfusion to rule out vasospasm (Fig. 58.2). Cerebral perfusion imaging revealed reduced cerebral blood flow (CBF) (Fig. 58.2b), prolonged mean transit

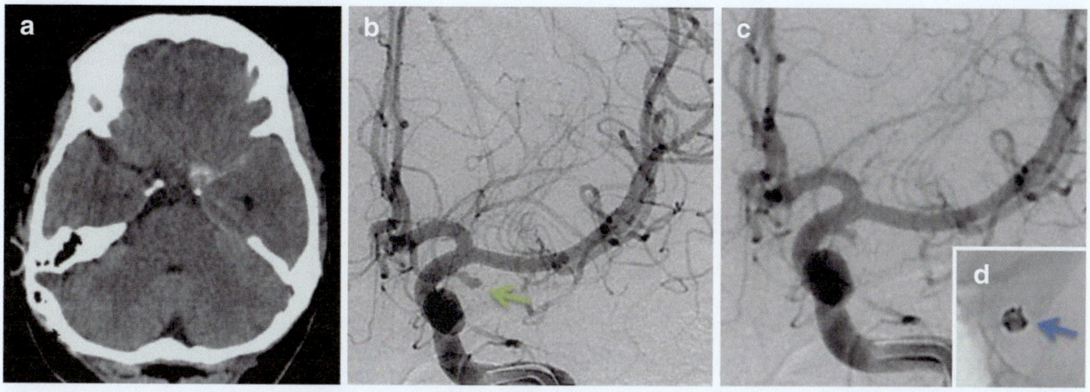

Fig. 58.1 (**a**) CT scan showing diffuse SAH. (**b**) Left ICA AP view demonstrating left anterior choroidal artery aneurysm. (**c**) Post coiling of the aneurysm with coil mass in inset (**d**)

R. Parthasarathy (✉)
Vascular Neurology and Neurointerventional Surgery,
Artemis Agrim Institute of Neuroscience,
Gurgaon, India

V. Gupta
Neurointerventional Surgery, Stroke Unit,
Artemis Agrim Institute of Neuroscience,
Gurgaon, India
e-mail: vipul.gupta@artemishospitals.com

V. Gupta et al. (eds.), *100 Interesting Case Studies in Neurointervention: Tips and Tricks*,
https://doi.org/10.1007/978-981-13-1346-2_58

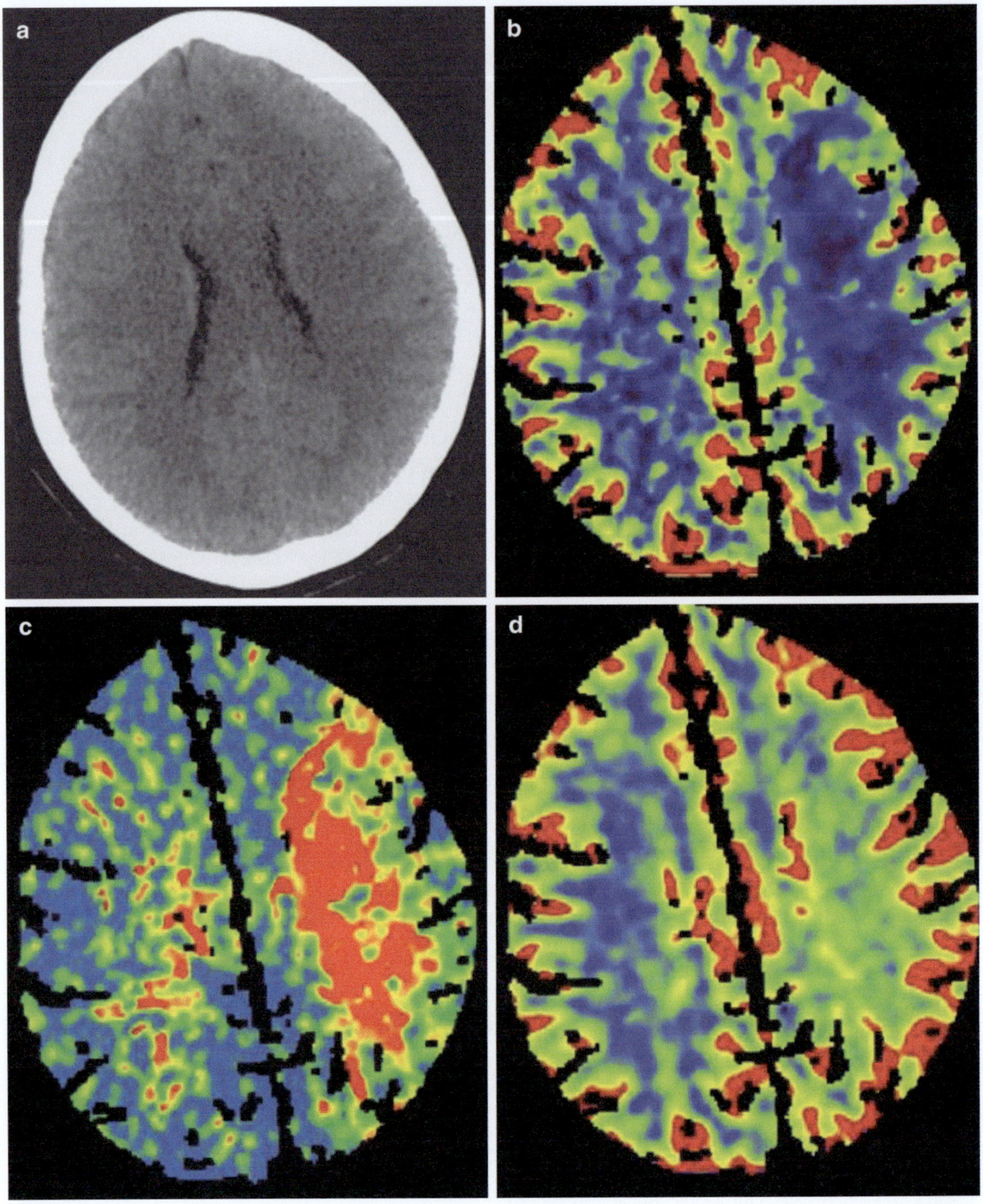

Fig. 58.2 (**a**) CT scan showing no infarct. (**b–d**) There is a large mismatch between CBF (**b**), MTT (**c**), and CBV (**d**) maps in the left MCA territory suggestive of penumbra

time (MTT) (Fig. 58.2c) and preserved cerebral blood volume (CBV) (Fig. 58.3d) suggestive of impaired perfusion (penumbra) without infarct.

Issues

1. Severe spasm of the intracranial vessels can cause large brain infarctions.

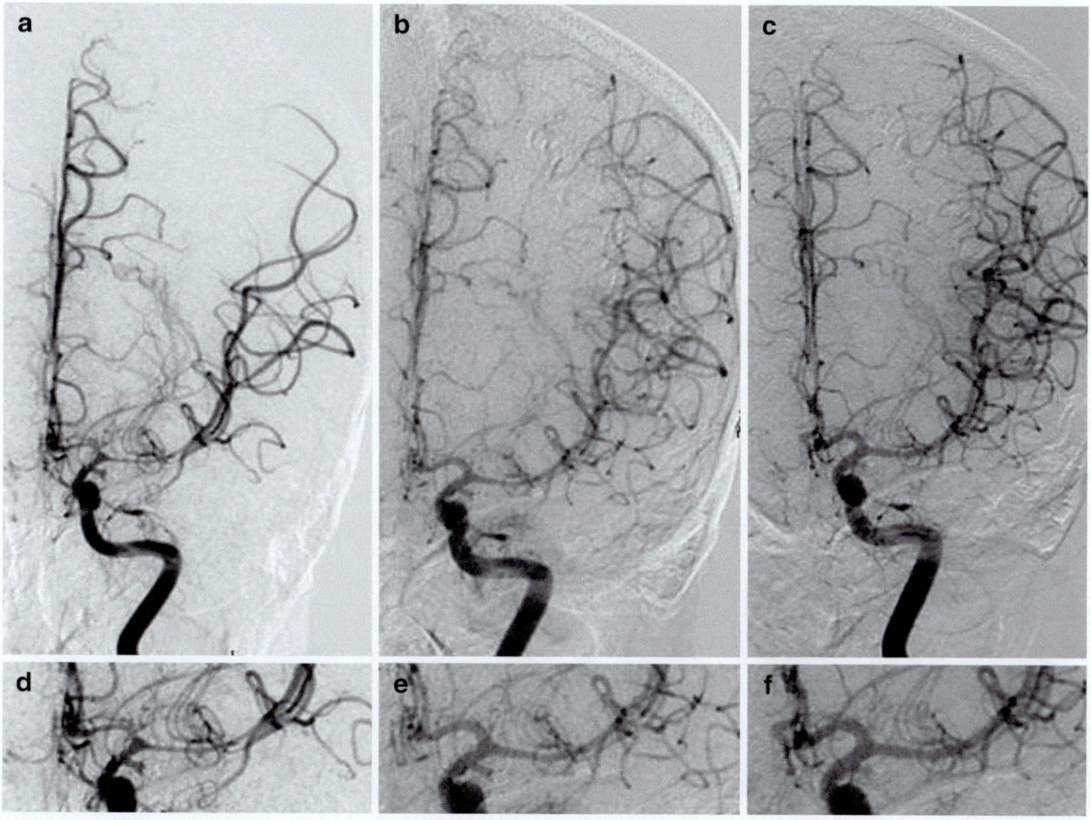

Fig. 58.3 (**a**) DSA showing severe spasm of the intracranial arteries particularly in M1 segment of MCA with secondary hypoperfusion. (**b**) DSA after nimodipine infusion reveals partial improvement. (**c**) Milrinone infusion resulted in further significant improvement in the caliber of arteries particularly in M1 segment. (**d–f**) Magnified view of MCA M2 segment from images (**a–c**)

Procedure

A small 11-cm-long, 5F sheath (Cordis) was used to access the right femoral artery. Following this a 5F diagnostic catheter (Cook) was positioned in the left internal carotid artery. Cerebral run revealed severe spasm involving the left M1 MCA (Fig. 58.3a). Initially, 1 mg of nimodipine is administered as bolus over 3–5 min, followed by slow infusion of 2 mg over 20 min (total of 3 mg). Therefore, 6–8 mg of Milrinone was, infused over 25–30 min. The intra-arterial dilatation was more pronounced due to the synergistic action of nimodipine and milrinone (Fig. 58.3c). Patient had improvement in her neurological status with no deficits clinically or radiologically.

Companion Case 2

A 50-year-old male presented with diffuse SAH. Cerebral angiography revealed right PCOM aneurysm. Endovascular coiling was undertaken (Fig. 58.4a–c).

On day 12, patient developed weakness of the left arm and leg. CTA and CTP were undertaken (Fig. 58.5). Large area of penumbra was noted in the right MCA territory.

Cerebral angiography revealed severe spasm affecting the right M1 and M2 MCA and probably the right A1 ACA. Intra-arterial dilatation was performed (Fig. 58.6).

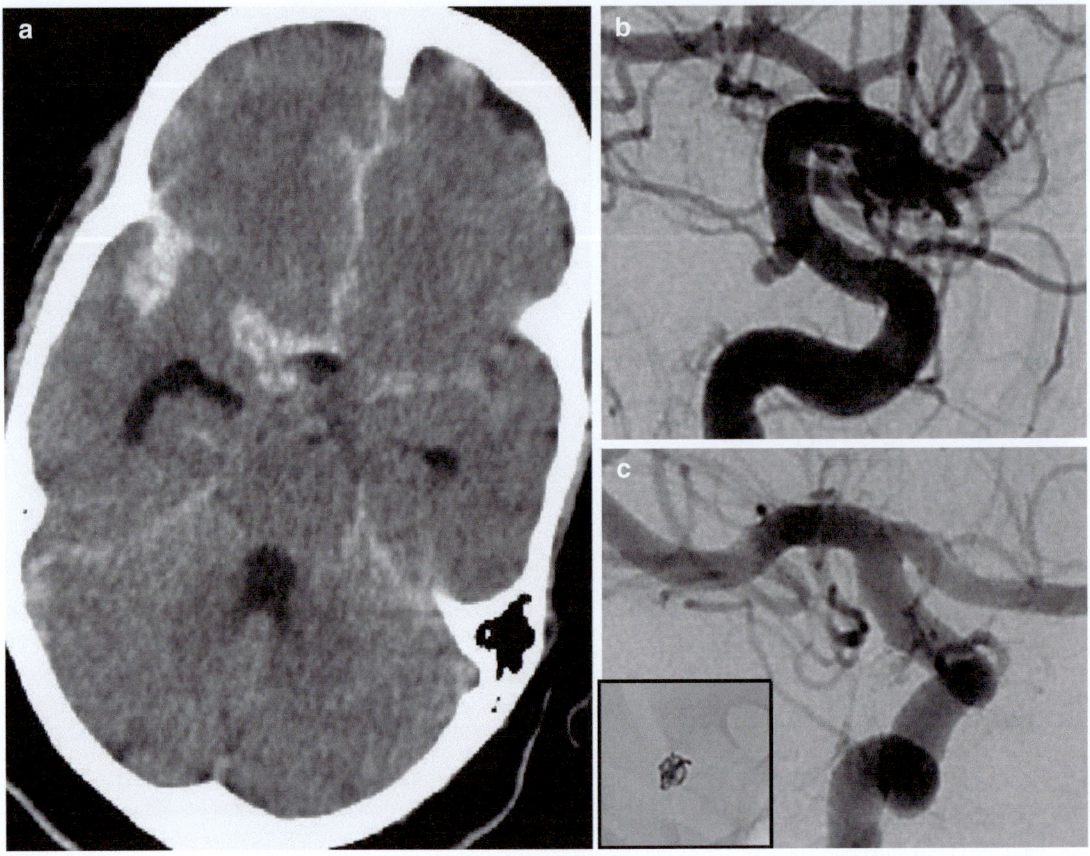

Fig. 58.4 (**a**) Diffuse SAH on NCCT brain, (**b**) right PCOM aneurysm, (**c**) post-procedure notice coils within the aneurysm sac

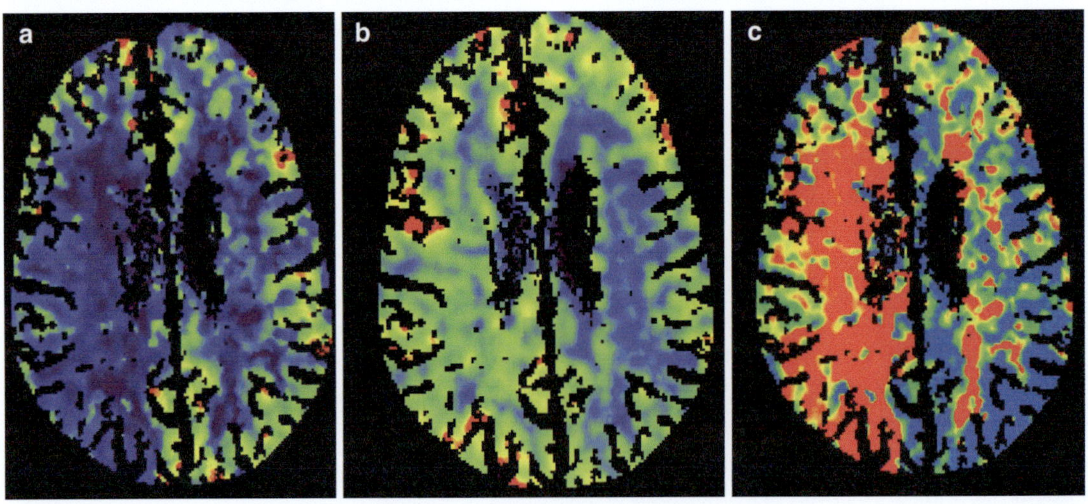

Fig. 58.5 (**a**) CBF map showing reduced flow, (**b**) CBV map showing preserved volume, (**c**) MTT map showing prolonged transit time, (**d** and **e**) right MCA narrow caliber suggestive of spasm

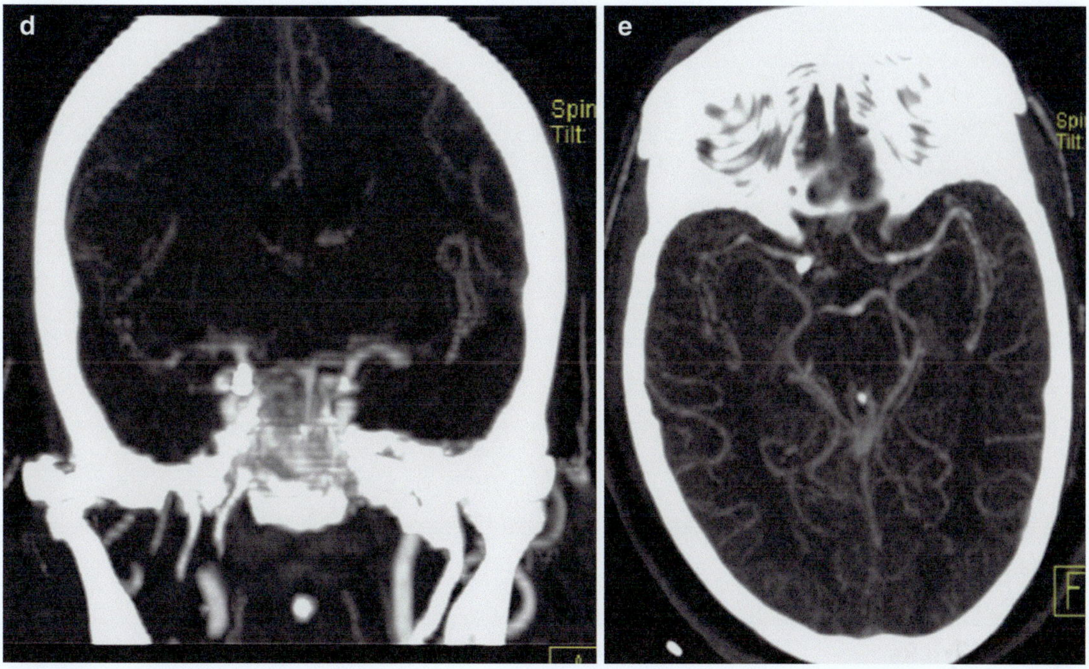

Fig. 58.5 (continued)

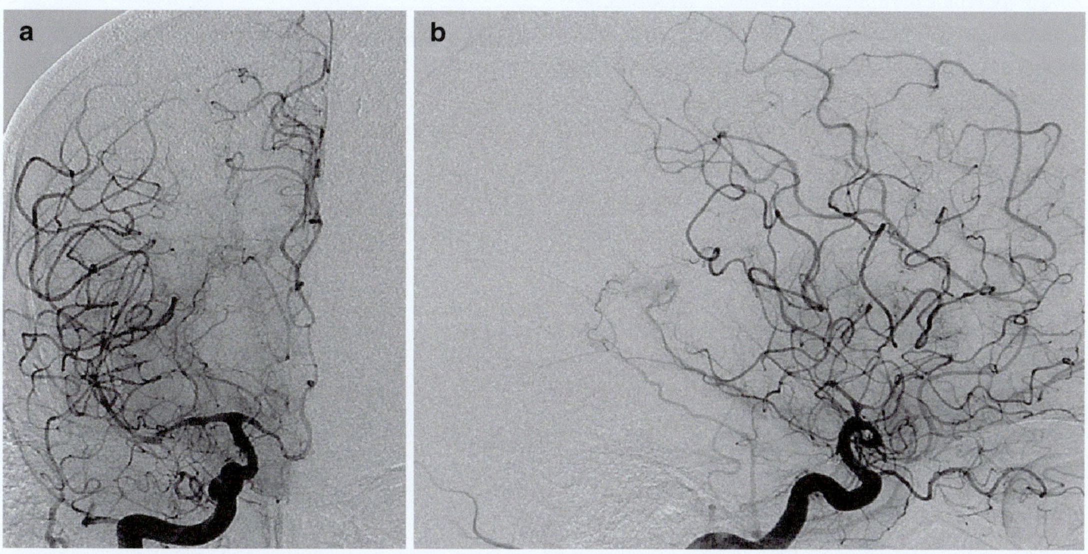

Fig. 58.6 (**a**, **b**) DSA showing severe spasm involving both MCA and ACA in AP and lateral projection; (**c**, **d**) post-dilatation showing normal caliber arteries in AP and lateral projection

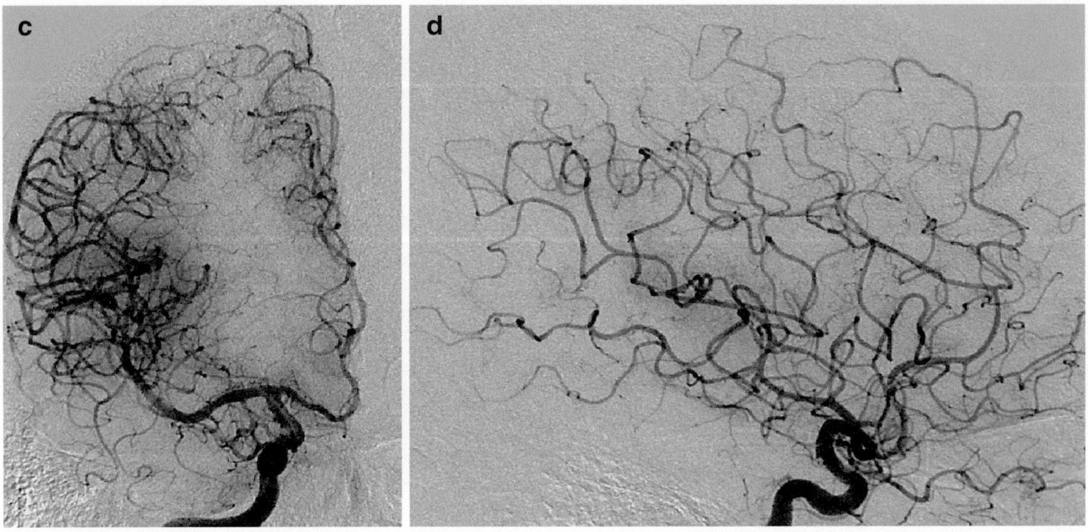

Fig. 58.6 (continued)

Tips and Tricks

1. The vasospasm in SAH can be detrimental. It is imperative to diagnose the vasospasm.
2. CT perfusion imaging provides an objective measure of cerebral perfusion. Infarct core and the penumbra can be identified reliably. CBV maps give the core volume, whereas CBF and MTT maps quantify the infarct core and the tissue at risk.
3. Perfusion imaging is more accurate than transcranial Doppler in diagnosing cerebral vasospasm.
4. The aim is quick diagnosis and early dilatation of the involved vessels.
5. Use of both nimodipine and milrinone is synergistic and achieves better dilatation of the involved vessel.

Suggested Reading

Binaghi S, Colleoni ML, Maeder P, et al. CT angiography and perfusion CT in cerebral vasospasm after subarachnoid hemorrhage. Am J Neuroradiol. 2007;28(4):750–8.

Greenberg ED, Gobin YP, Riina H, et al. Role of CT perfusion imaging in the diagnosis and treatment of vasospasm. Imaging Med. 2011;3(3):287–97.

Part II

Arteriovenous Malformation

Cavernous Sinus Dural Arteriovenous Fistula (AVF): Trans-venous Approach Through Inferior Petrosal Sinus

59

Vipul Gupta

Case

A 48-year-old lady presented with proptosis and congestion of the right eye. MRI revealed enlarged right cavernous sinus along with dilated right ophthalmic vein. DSA showed a right cavernous sinus dural arteriovenous fistula draining through right ophthalmic vein. Feeders were from bilateral external and left internal carotid arteries (Fig. 59.1). Stenosis was seen in ophthalmic vein at its exit from orbit and was draining into multiple small venous channels. Right inferior petrosal sinus was not visualized. Case was planned for trans-venous coil embolization.

Issues

- To access the cavernous sinus through the thrombosed inferior petrosal sinus
- Complete occlusion of fistula

Management

Procedure was performed under general anaesthesia. Diagnostic catheters were placed in right external carotid and left common carotid arteries. A 6F long sheath (Cook Medical, Bloomington, USA) was placed in the right internal jugular vein through trans-femoral route. A soft tip 4F diagnostic catheter (MPA, Cook Medical, Bloomington, USA) was placed in the distal end of the inferior petrosal sinus (Fig. 59.2a). Thereafter, a road map was taken from arterial catheters, and Echelon-10 microcatheter (ev3 Neurovascular, USA) was navigated through the soft tip diagnostic catheter over a Transend 014 microguidewire (Stryker Neurovascular, CA, USA) (Fig. 59.2a). Care was taken that in both anteroposterior and lateral planes, it travelled along the usual course of inferior petrosal sinus. Once the catheter entered the cavernous sinus, it was taken to the origin of ophthalmic vein (Fig. 59.2b). After confirming the position, coil embolization was done with care being taken to embolize the origin of ophthalmic vein (Fig. 59.2c). Whole of cavernous sinus segment was occluded by coils, and final angiograms revealed complete occlusion of the fistula (Fig. 59.2d, e).

Tips and Tricks

1. Cavernous sinus dural AVF usually needs trans-venous approach. Unlike dural AVFs at other sites, trans-arterial embolization using liquid agent such as onyx is dangerous because of possibility of reflux in to internal carotid arteries and possibility of cranial nerve injury.

V. Gupta
Neurointerventional Surgery, Stroke Unit, Artemis Agrim Institute of Neuroscience, Gurgaon, India
e-mail: vipul.gupta@artemishospitals.com

V. Gupta et al. (eds.), *100 Interesting Case Studies in Neurointervention: Tips and Tricks*,
https://doi.org/10.1007/978-981-13-1346-2_59

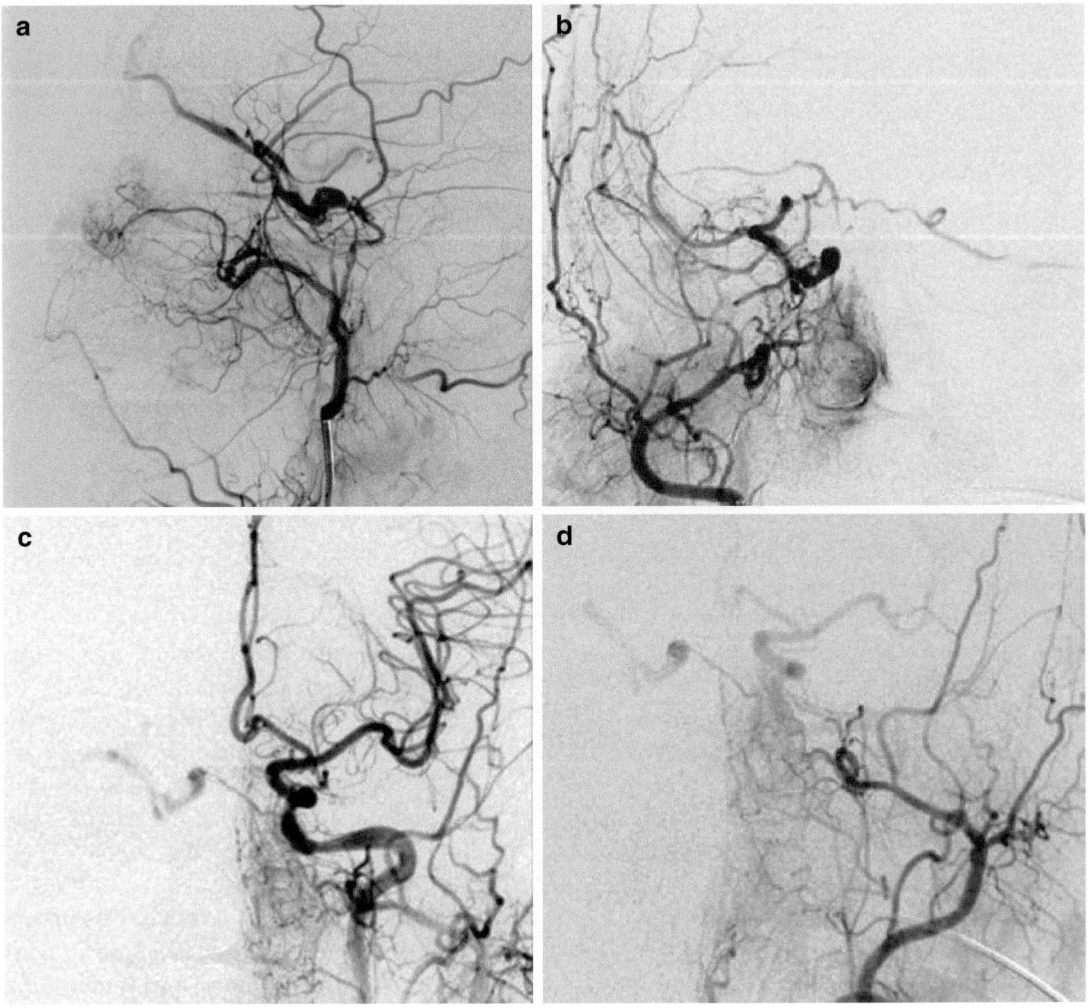

Fig. 59.1 (**a**, **b**) Right external carotid artery angiogram lateral (**a**) and anteroposterior (**b**) projections reveals a dural AVF of right cavernous sinus draining through ophthalmic vein. Right inferior petrosal sinus is occluded. (**c**) Left ICA injection reveals a small feeder to the AVF. (**d**) Left ECA injection also reveals small feeder to the fistula

2. Ophthalmic vein or inferior petrosal sinus approach are the favoured routes.
3. Even if the inferior petrosal sinus is thrombosed, navigation is mostly possible by probing along its path. Place the diagnostic catheter at the distal end of the sinus to provide the necessary support to microcatheter system. Navigate carefully confirming the course along the usual direction of the sinus under biplane fluoroscopy.
4. It is advisable to coil the origin of ophthalmic vein and whole of patent segment of cavernous sinus so as to prevent recurrences.
5. In few recent reports, onyx has also been used for trans-venous embolization, particularly after incomplete occlusion with coils. However, one should exercise caution to ensure that there is no reflux into the carotid particularly if there are internal carotid artery feeders.

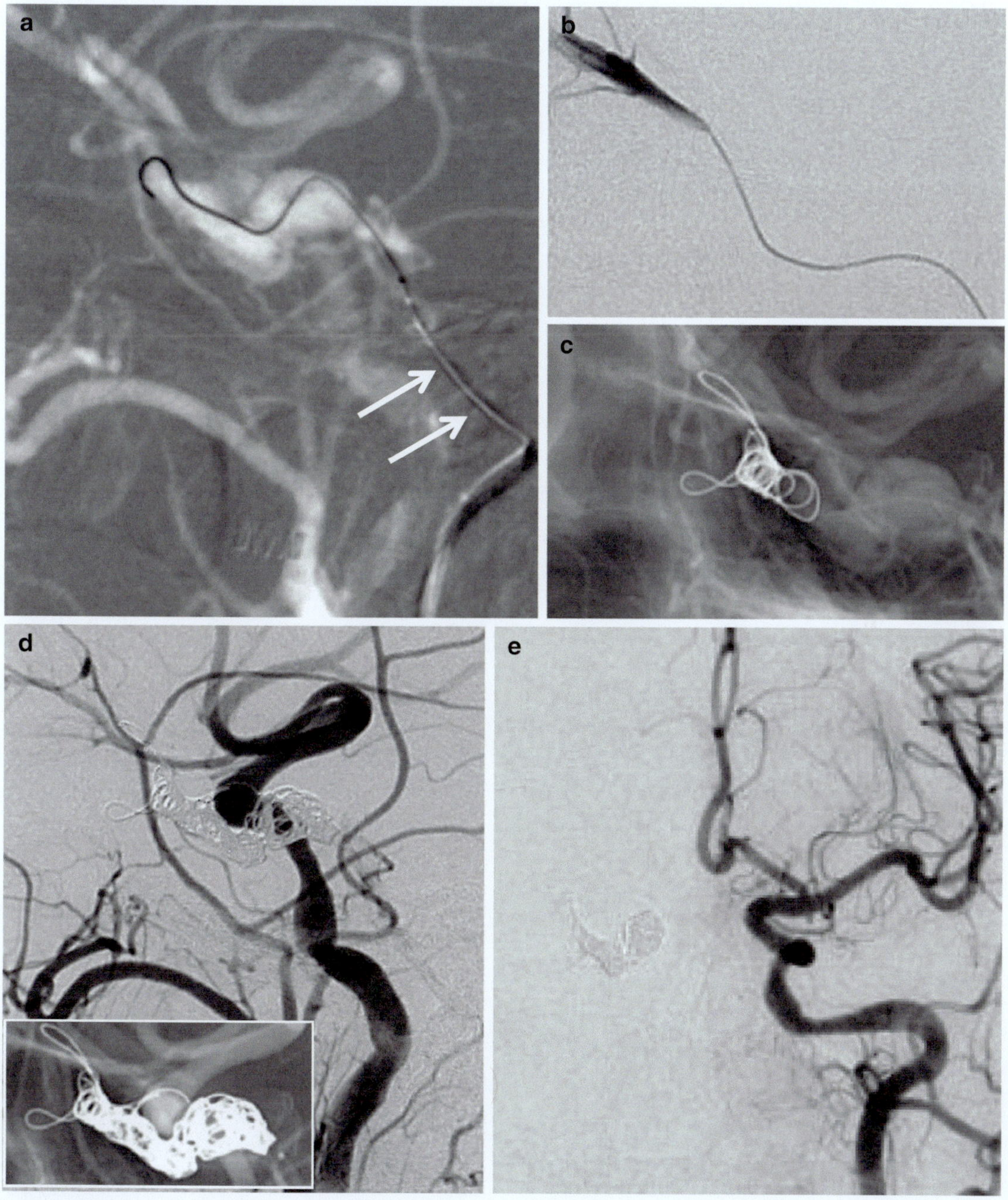

Fig. 59.2 (**a**) Road map image showing catheterization of the cavernous sinus via the inferior petrosal sinus. Arrows point to the diagnostic catheter placed in the inferior segment of sinus through which microcatheter was placed. (**b**) Microcatheter injection in ophthalmic vein. (**c**) First coil placement with coil loops in both divisions of the vein. (**d**, **e**) Post-embolization right (**d**) and left (**e**) common carotid angiograms showing complete occlusion of the AVF

Suggested Reading

Gemmete J, Ansari SA, Gandhi D. Endovascular treatment of carotid cavernous fistulas. Neuroimaging Clin N Am. 2009;19(2):241–55.

Lekkhong E, Pongpech S, ter Brugge K, Geibprasert S, Krings T. Transvenous embolization of intracranial dural arteriovenous shunts through occluded venous segments: experience in 51 patients. AJNR Am J Neuroradiol. 2011;32(9):1738–44.

Cavernous Dural Arteriovenous Fistula (AVF): Angio-CT-Guided Fistula Site Localization

60

Vipul Gupta

Case

A 34-year-old male presented with left eye conjunctival congestion and proptosis. MRI (not shown) revealed dilated left superior ophthalmic vein as well as prominence of left cavernous sinus. Cerebral DSA was performed which showed left cavernous sinus dural AVF with feeders from left internal and external carotid arteries (Fig. 60.1a–c). The AVF was draining via left ophthalmic vein into the left facial vein (Fig. 60.1c). No obvious drainage into the petrosal system was observed. Transvenous embolization with detachable coils was planned.

Issue

1. Transvenous access for embolization of the AVF. Access through the inferior petrosal sinus is less challenging; however, it was completely occluded.
2. Accurate localization of site of fistula and occlusion of the fistulous communication is crucial to prevent residual/delayed recurrence.

V. Gupta
Neurointerventional Surgery, Stroke Unit, Artemis Agrim Institute of Neuroscience, Gurgaon, India
e-mail: vipul.gupta@artemishospitals.com

Management

Embolization was undertaken under general anaesthesia. To accurately localize the fistula site, a diagnostic catheter was placed in the left common carotid artery, and angio-CT (DynaCT, Siemens, Erlangen, Germany) was performed with intraarterial injection of contrast. The DynaCT angiogram (Fig. 60.1d) revealed a small venous sac (arrows, Fig. 60.1e) draining into the dilated ophthalmic vein. Once the localization was done with the help of DynaCT angiogram, the fistula site was better appreciated on 2D DSA image (Fig. 60.1f). It was crucial to access this sac and occlude it completely. Occlusion of posterior end of ophthalmic vein without occlusion of the venous end of the fistula can result in persistence/delayed recurrence with change in direction of venous drainage. For the venous access, a 6F long sheath (Raphe, Cook) was placed in the left internal jugular vein. Thereafter, a 4F diagnostic catheter with a soft tip was placed in the left facial vein (arrow, Fig. 60.2a), and a microcatheter (Echelon 10, Micro Therapeutics, Inc. d/b/a ev3 Neurovascular, Irvine, California) was navigated under road map guidance into the left ophthalmic vein (Fig. 60.2a, b). The venous sac was carefully accessed with a microguidewire (Fig. 60.2c). Following that, the microcatheter was navigated into venous aspect of the fistula, and the sac was embolized with detachable coils with few coil loops at the origin of ophthalmic vein (Fig. 60.2d).

V. Gupta et al. (eds.), *100 Interesting Case Studies in Neurointervention: Tips and Tricks*,
https://doi.org/10.1007/978-981-13-1346-2_60

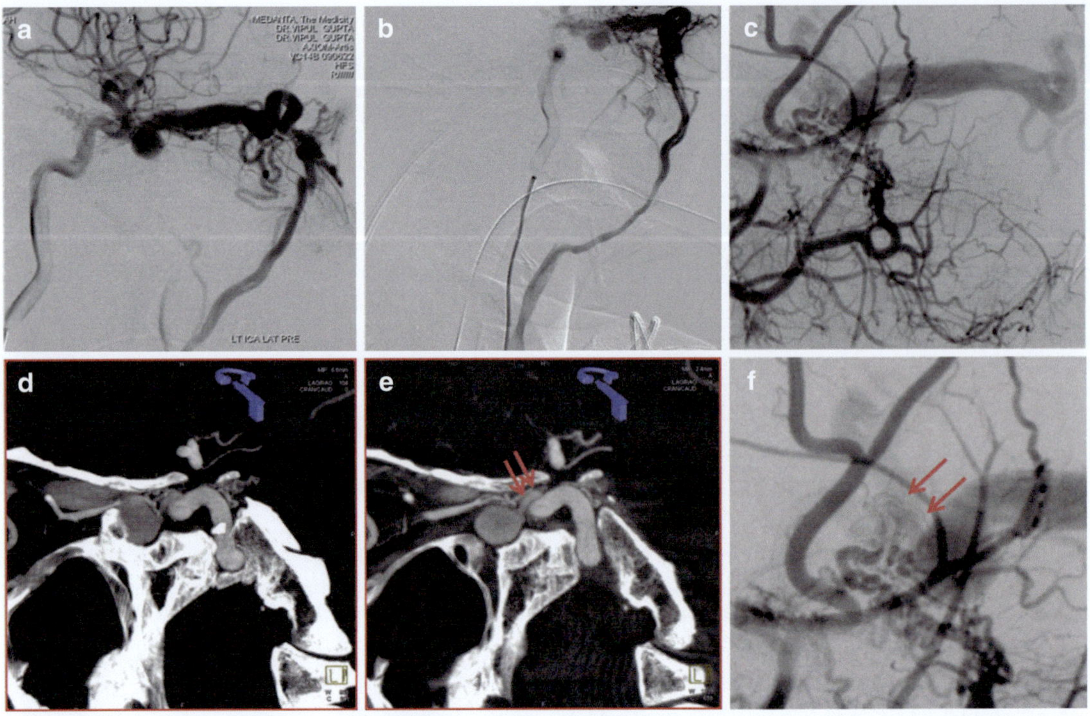

Fig. 60.1 Left ICA injection (**a**, **b**) and left ECA (**c**) reveal dural AVF of left cavernous sinus draining via the facial vein (**b**). Angio-CT with intraarterial injections (**d**, **e**) shows a small sac (*arrows*, **e**) which is draining in to the ophthalmic vein. This is the true site of the AVF. Enlarged image of ECA injection (**f**) with arrows pointing at the site of dural AVF as was seen in the angio-CT images

Final angiogram revealed complete occlusion of the dural AVF. Over next few days, patient's symptoms improved almost completely.

Tip and Trick

1. It is important to localize the exact site of dural AVF in order to achieve complete and lasting occlusion. Occlusion at a location distal to the site of the fistula may result in residual or a recurrent AVF with drainage into different set of veins.
2. DynaCT (angio-CT) with intraarterial injection can be useful in difficult cases to delineate the anatomy of the AVF.
3. Coaxial placement of a low-profile diagnostic/guide catheter in the facial vein is useful in catheterization of ophthalmic vein and cavernous sinus in these cases.

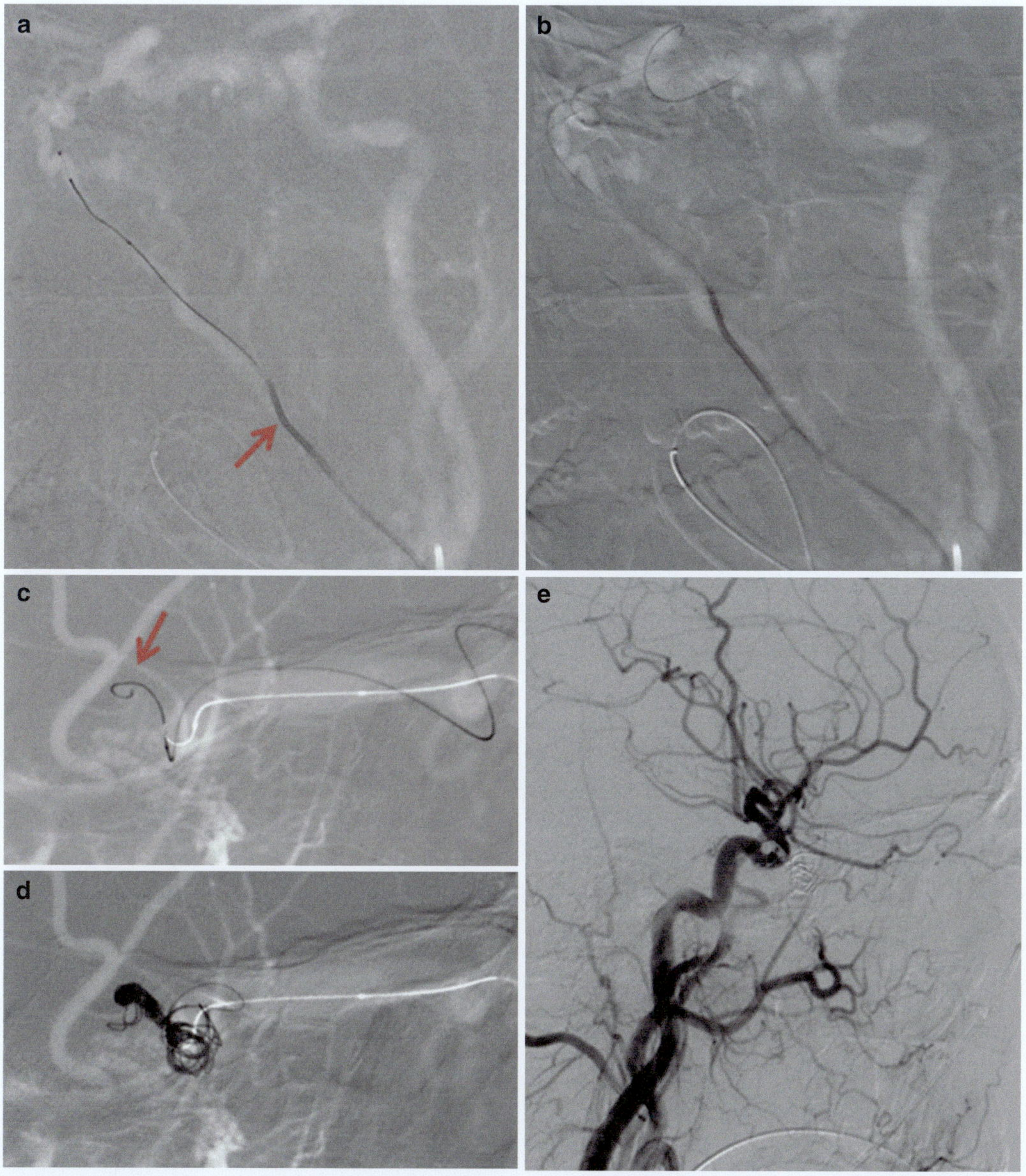

Fig. 60.2 Embolization of cavernous sinus dural AVF. (**a**) A 4F diagnostic catheter (*arrow*, **a**) was placed in the left facial vein under road map guidance. A microcatheter was navigated through it into the ophthalmic vein (**b**). Under road map guidance, the cavernous venous sac which was the site of AVF was catheterized (**c**) and was embolized with detachable coils (**d**). Final angiogram revealed complete occlusion of the dural AVF

Suggested Reading

Bink A, Berkefeld J, Lüchtenberg M, et al. Coil embolization of cavernous sinus in patients with direct and dural arteriovenous fistula. Eur Radiol. 2009;19:1443.

Bink A, Goller K, Lüchtenberg M, et al. Long-term outcome after coil embolization of cavernous sinus arteriovenous fistulas. AJNR Am J Neuroradiol. 2010;3:1216.

Kiyosue H, Hori Y, Okahara M, et al. Treatment of intracranial dural arteriovenous fistulas: current strategies based on location and hemodynamics, and alternative techniques of transcatheter embolization. Radiographics. 2004;24:1637.

Coil Embolization of Direct Carotid Cavernous Fistula (CCF)

61

Vipul Gupta

Case

A 34-year-old female presented with history of right eye proptosis and conjunctival congestion for 2 weeks. She had history of road traffic accident 5 weeks back. MRI brain revealed dilated right ophthalmic vein and prominent right cavernous sinus. DSA (Fig. 61.1a, b) revealed high flow direct CCF filling from the right internal carotid artery (ICA). ICA distal to fistula was not opacified. Venous drainage was through the cavernous sinus into ipsilateral ophthalmic vein and posteriorly into petrosal vein and thereafter into the cerebellar veins. Cortical reflux into the Sylvian veins was also seen.

Issue

- Localization of exact site of the fistula
- Embolization of the fistula while preserving the internal carotid artery

Management

Embolization was performed under general anesthesia. To locate the exact site of fistula, vertebral artery injection was performed (Fig. 61.2a) with occlusion of ICA using a balloon (Hyperglide 4 × 20 mm). Retrograde filling of the right ICA was seen through the posterior communicating artery with filling of the fistula at junction of lacerum and cavernous segments of ICA. This technique depicted the site of the fistula. Coil occlusion of the fistula was planned with use of balloon assistance. Bilateral femoral accesses were used. A 6F guiding catheter was placed in the ICA, and a diagnostic catheter was placed in the vertebral artery. Thereafter, the balloon wire was taken across the fistula into the distal ICA. VA injection was done with balloon inflated to allow for retrograde filling of the ICA distal to the fistula (Fig. 61.2b). This helped to document that the balloon wire was in the ICA and not in one of the veins. Thereafter, the balloon was navigated across the fistula. A microcatheter was then navigated into the venous sac. Embolization was done using detachable coils with balloon assistance to preserve the parent artery (Fig. 61.2c). Using this technique one could be sure of preserving the ICA even when coils in the venous sac overlapped the artery. During the later stage of procedure, new road map was taken without dye injection (Fig. 61.2d). This helped in clear visualization of the coil being placed and its relationship with the parent artery. Complete occlusion of the fistula was achieved (Fig. 61.3). Although there was superimposition of coils on the ICA in both the planes, one can be certain that the parent artery was preserved due to balloon

V. Gupta
Neurointerventional Surgery, Stroke Unit, Artemis Agrim Institute of Neuroscience, Gurgaon, India
e-mail: vipul.gupta@artemishospitals.com

V. Gupta et al. (eds.), *100 Interesting Case Studies in Neurointervention: Tips and Tricks*,
https://doi.org/10.1007/978-981-13-1346-2_61

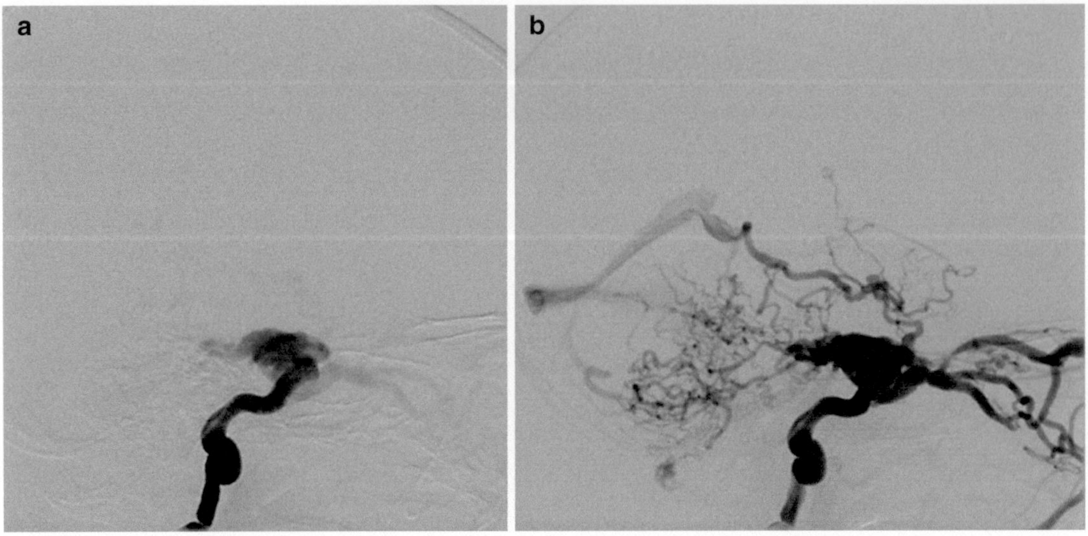

Fig. 61.1 DSA (lateral view) showing direct CCF with drainage into the ophthalmic and pial veins

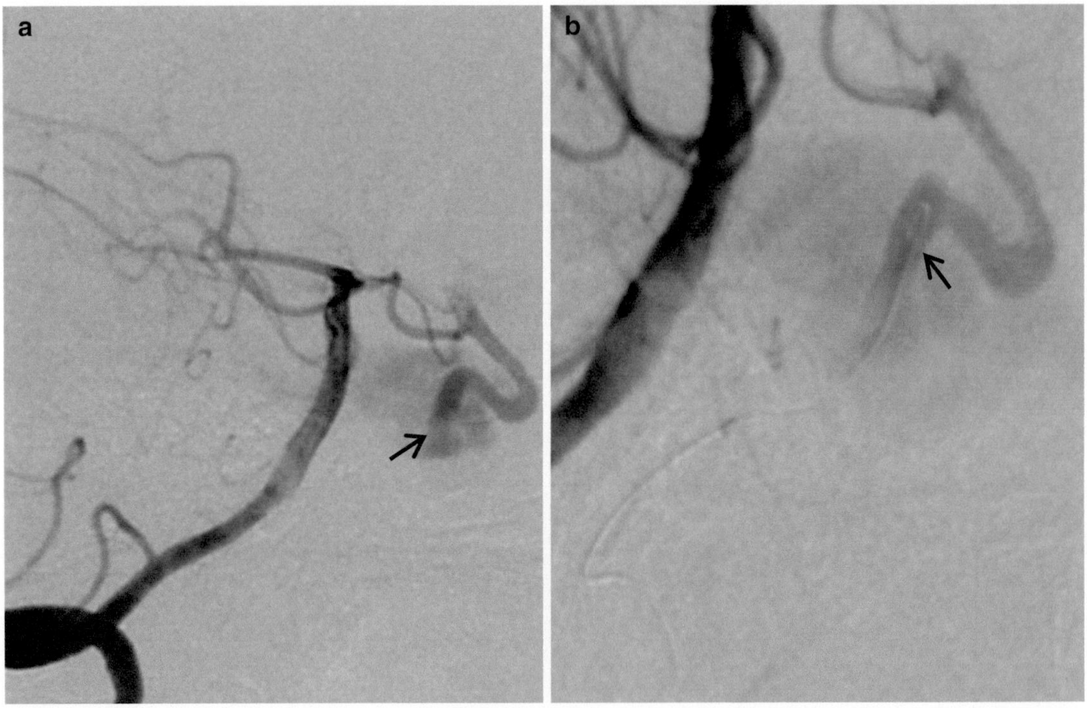

Fig. 61.2 Vertebral artery injection with balloon occlusion (**a**) shows retrograde filling of ICA with clear visualization of the site of fistula. Similar injection performed to opacify the distal ICA during placement of balloon wire (*arrow*, **b**) into ICA distal to the fistula. Coil embolization was done with balloon assistance (**c**). During embolization, road map was taken without dye injection for clear visualization of the coil being placed

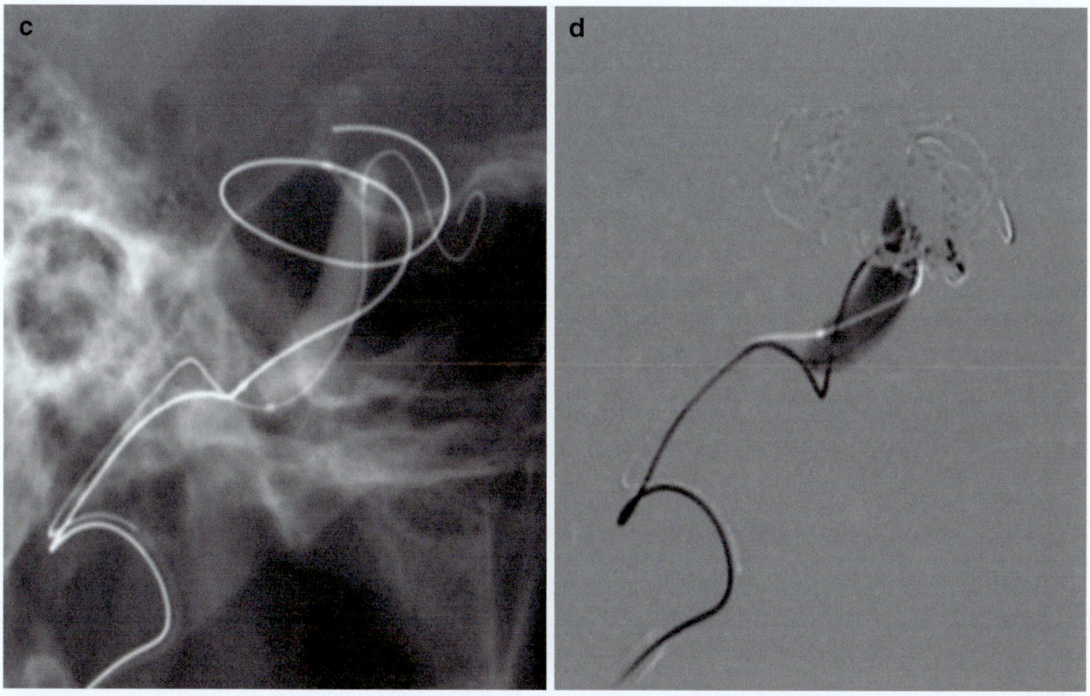

Fig. 61.2 (continued)

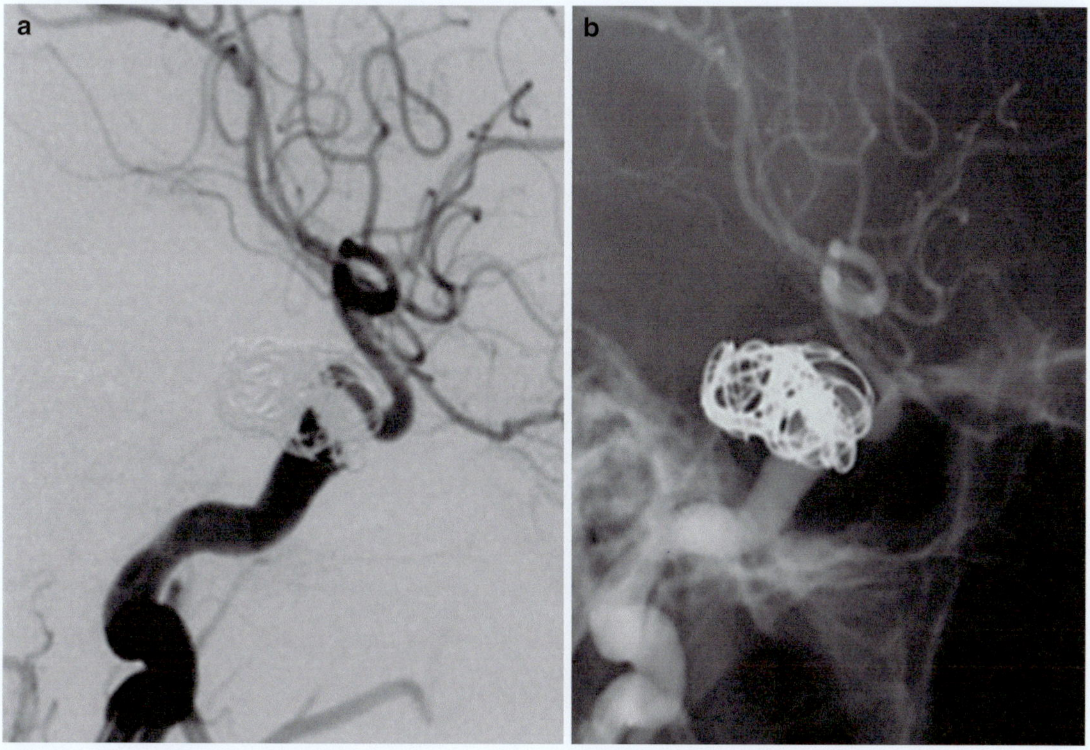

Fig. 61.3 Post-embolization angiogram (**a**) shows complete occlusion of CCF with antegrade flow in ICA. Although coils were overlapping the ICA in both lateral (**b**) and anteroposterior (**c**) views, ICA was well preserved because of use of balloon remodeling. Repeat DSA after 6 months shows stable result (**d**)

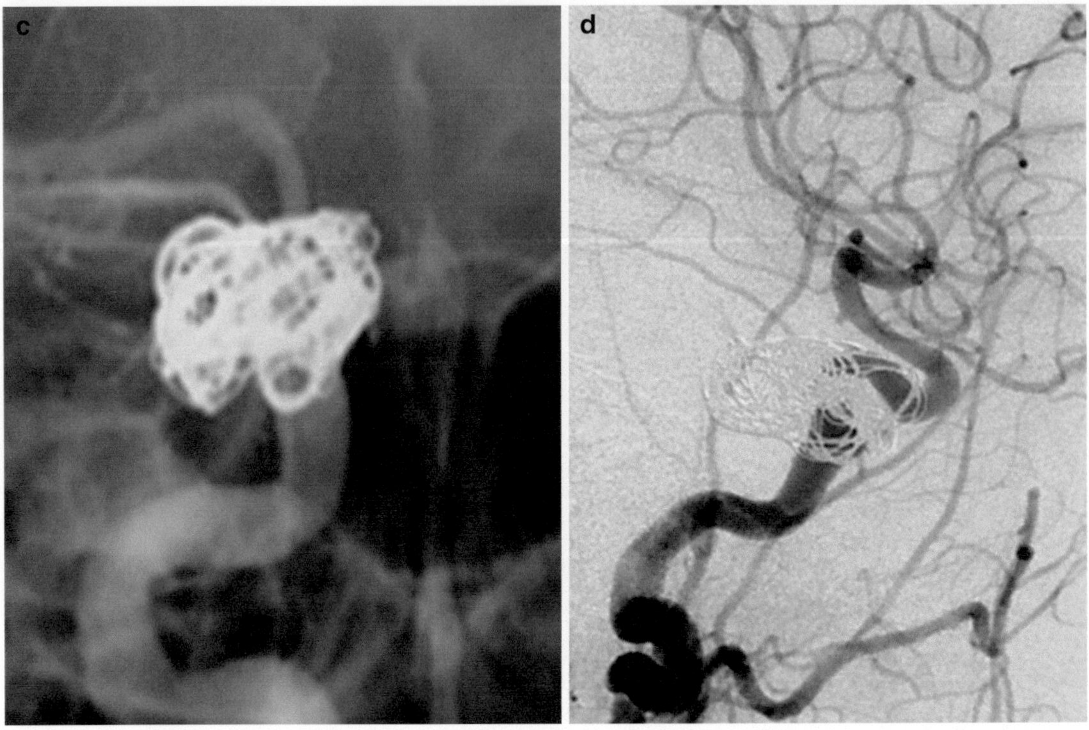

Fig. 61.3 (continued)

inflation during coil deployment. Six months follow-up revealed persistent occlusion of the fistula with remodeling of the ICA.

Tips and Tricks

1. Embolization using detachable coils has emerged as a good alternative for use of detachable balloons for the treatment of direct CCF. Since the venous sac frequently overlaps the parent vessel (ICA), it can be difficult to exclude coil protrusion into the parent artery. Using balloon assistance, the parent artery can be preserved, and complete occlusion can be achieved while preserving the ICA.
2. Balloon also helps in stabilizing the microcatheter and achieving complete occlusion of the fistula.
3. One can change to a new road map without contrast to visualize coil placement.
4. To exactly visualize the site of fistula, vertebral artery/contralateral ICA injections while occluding the ICA proximal to site of fistula helps in visualizing the exact site of rent in the ICA.

Suggested Reading

Bink A, Goller K, Lüchtenberg M, Neumann-Haefelin T, Dützmann S, Zanella F, Berkefeld J, du Mesnil de Rochemont R. Long-term outcome after coil embolization of cavernous sinus arteriovenous fistulas. AJNR Am J Neuroradiol. 2010;31:1216–21.

Ducruet AF, Albuquerque FC, Crowley RW, McDougall CG. The evolution of endovascular treatment of carotid cavernous fistulas: a single-center experience. World Neurosurg. 2013;80(5):538–48.

Tsai YH, Wong HF, Weng HH, Chen YL. Comparison of the risk of oculomotor nerve deficits between detachable balloons and coils in the treatment of direct carotid cavernous fistulas. AJNR Am J Neuroradiol. 2010;31:1123–6.

Combined Trans-arterial and Balloon-Assisted Transvenous Onyx Embolization of Dural AVF

62

Vipul Gupta

Case

A 30-year-old man presented with history of blurring of vision of both eyes since one and half years. Ophthalmological evaluation had revealed bilateral papilloedema. MRI had showed cerebral sino-venous thrombosis (CVT) involving the right transverse sinus and superior sagittal sinus, and he was treated with anticoagulants. Subsequently he developed tinnitus in the right ear. Repeat MRI and MRA revealed dural AV fistula of the right transverse sinus. Cerebral angiography (Fig. 62.1a–e) showed high flow dural AV fistula of the right transverse sinus supplied by multiple transosseous hypertrophied branches of bilateral occipital arteries, parietal branch of right MMA, and small contribution from meningo-hypophyseal trunk from the right ICA and dural branch of the right AICA. Occlusion of the right transverse sinus at the junction with sigmoid sinus with contrast reflux into the torcula, straight sinus, superior sagittal sinus, and left transverse-sigmoid sinus was noted. No obvious cortical venous reflux was seen. The right cerebral hemisphere was seen to have venous drainage into the left transverse sinus except the vein of Labbe which was draining into the right transverse sinus.

V. Gupta
Neurointerventional Surgery, Stroke Unit, Artemis Agrim Institute of Neuroscience, Gurgaon, India
e-mail: vipul.gupta@artemishospitals.com

Issues

- Vein of Labbe which was draining into the right transverse sinus has to be preserved to avoid venous infarct in the temporal lobe.
- Complete occlusion of dural AV fistula is challenging in view of left ECA feeders which were seen to enter near the torcula.

Management

The procedure was performed via bilateral transfemoral arterial access under general anesthesia. A 6F long sheath (Cook Medical, Bloomington, USA) was placed in the right common carotid artery. A 5F short sheath was placed in the left common femoral artery so that simultaneous bilateral angiograms can be done. Careful review of pre-procedure right CCA (Fig. 62.2a–e) revealed another separate venous channel superior and parallel to the right transverse sinus. Using permanent pen marker, we marked both the venous compartments and confirmed that the vein of Labbe was entering the superior channel (Fig. 62.2f, g). In order to preserve the vein of Labbe, the decision to place a compliant dual-lumen onyx-compatible balloon across the upper channel was taken.

A 6F long sheath (Cook Medical, Bloomington, USA) was placed via the right common femoral vein and positioned in the left internal jugular

V. Gupta et al. (eds.), *100 Interesting Case Studies in Neurointervention: Tips and Tricks*,
https://doi.org/10.1007/978-981-13-1346-2_62

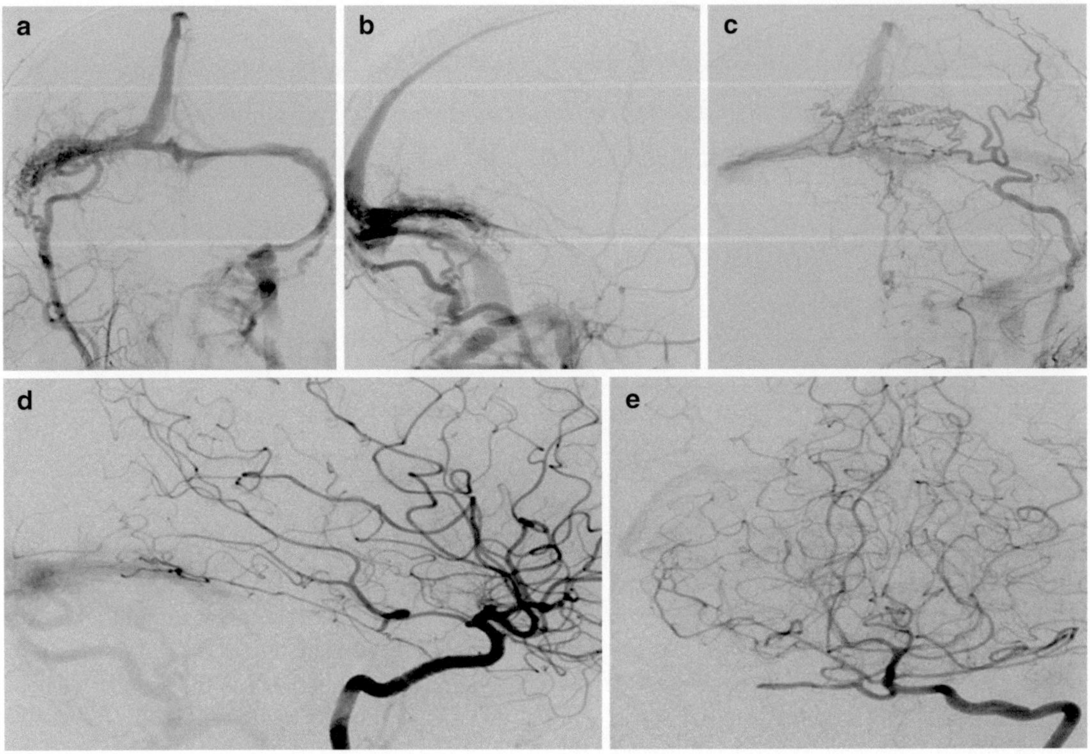

Fig. 62.1 (**a**–**c**) Right ECA angiogram AP (**a**) and lateral views (**b**) and left ECA angiogram AP view (**c**) show dural AV fistula of the right transverse sinus supplied by multiple transosseous hypertrophied branches of bilateral occipital arteries and parietal branch of right MMA. Occlusion of the right transverse sinus at the junction with sigmoid sinus with contrast reflux was noted into the torcula, straight sinus, superior sagittal sinus, and left transverse-sigmoid sinus. No obvious cortical venous reflux seen. (**d**) Right ICA angiogram lateral view shows meningo-hypophyseal trunk, and (**e**) left vertebral angiogram AP view shows dural branch of right AICA supplying the fistula

vein. Thereafter, a DAC 070 (Concentric Medical, CA, USA) was placed in the left transverse sinus through which 4 × 20 mm Scepter C balloon (MicroVention, Tustin, CA, USA) was advanced into the venous compartment superior and parallel to the right transverse sinus where the vein of Labbe was seen to enter (Fig. 62.3a).

A 6F Chaperon guide catheter (MicroVention, Tustin, CA, USA) was placed in the right distal ECA through which Marathon microcatheter (ev3 Inc., Irvine, CA, USA) over Mirage microwire (ev3 Inc., Irvine, CA, USA) was positioned in the right middle meningeal artery proximal to the fistula (Fig. 62.3b). Once in the optimal position, 0.23 mL DMSO followed by 5 mL of Onyx was injected in the AVF under biplane fluoroscopic guidance with inflation of the balloon to avoid occlusion of superior venous compartment (Fig. 62.3c–e). To occlude fistula at the medial aspect supplied by left ECA feeders, balloon was navigated more medially but still covering the vein of Labbe and further onyx embolization carried out (Fig. 62.3g). There was still a small residual component of dural AV fistula at the lateral aspect of superior venous channel (Fig. 62.4a). Balloon catheter was then advanced into more lateral position (Fig. 62.4c). Thereafter with balloon inflated, DMSO followed by Onyx was injected through the lumen of the balloon catheter (Fig. 62.4d). Post-procedure, right CCA and left ECA angiograms showed complete obliteration of the dural AV fistula with preservation of the vein of Labbe (Fig. 62.5a–c).

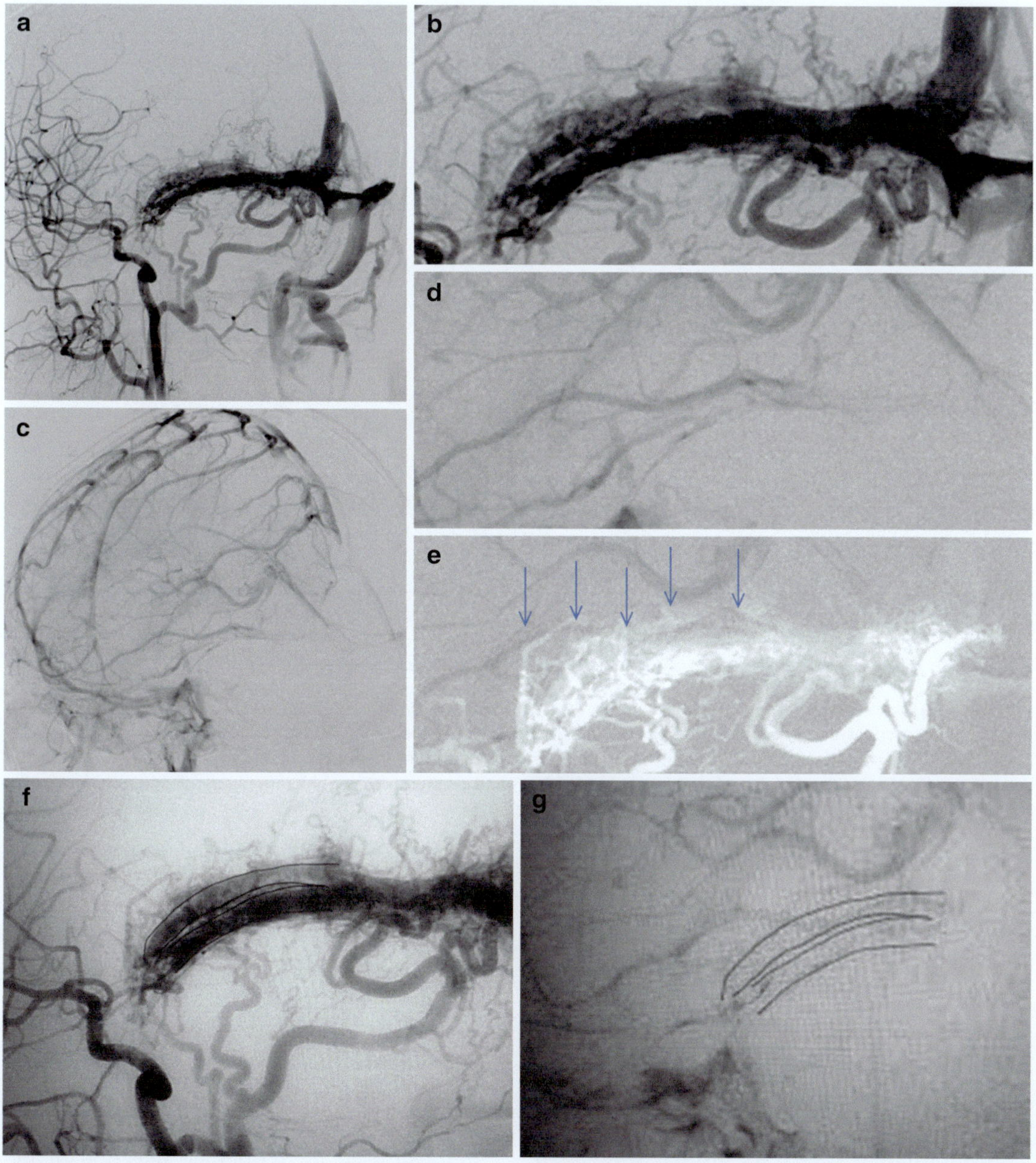

Fig. 62.2 (**a**) Pre-procedure right CCA and (**b**) its magnified view revealed another separate venous channel superior and parallel to the right transverse sinus. (**c**) Venous phase of right CCA and (**d**) its magnified view reveal the vein of Labbe entering superior channel. Changing the mask (**e**) and using permanent pen marker (**f**, **g**), we confirmed that the vein of Labbe was entering the superior channel

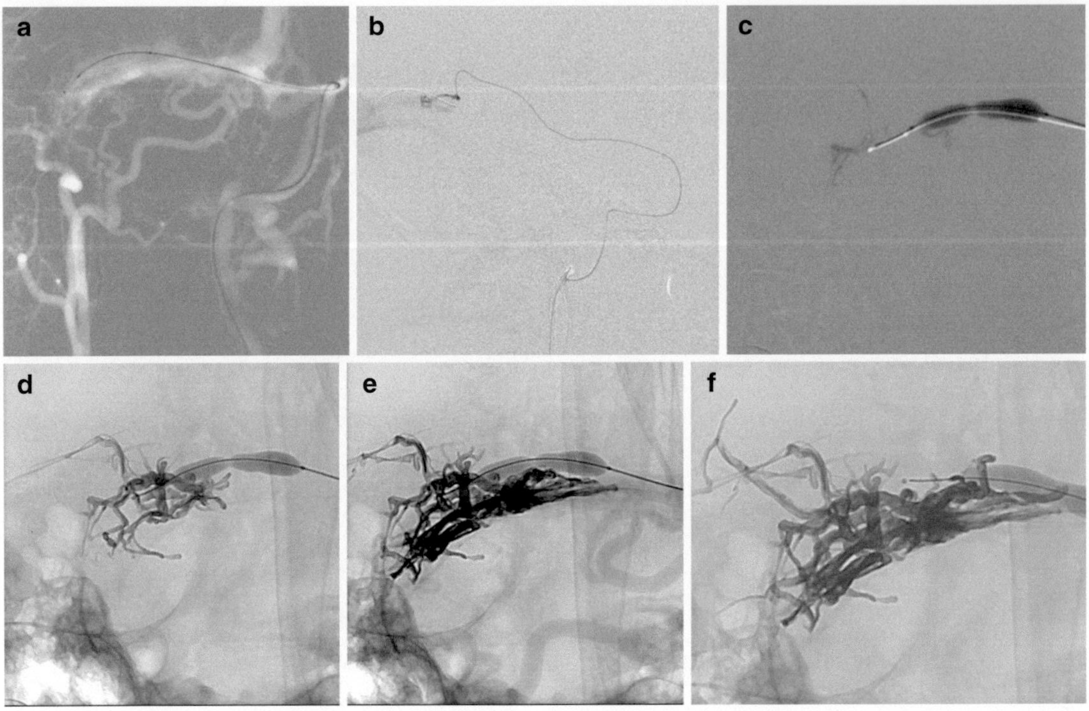

Fig. 62.3 (**a**) Scepter C balloon navigated into the superior channel to cover the opening of the vein of Labbe. Image (**b**) shows microcatheter angiogram after placing the microcatheter into the distal feeding branch of MMA. (**c–e**) Onyx embolization performed through microcatheter with balloon inflated. (**f**) To occlude fistula at the medial aspect supplied by left ECA feeders, balloon was placed more medially but still covering the vein of Labbe and further onyx embolization carried out

Tips and Tricks

1. Analysis of venous phase of angiogram is very important.
2. Analysis of various feeders of ECA is important; particularly one should look for if they join at the same segment of dural sinus.
3. One can try different techniques to assess the relationship between AV fistula, sinus, and normal vein draining into the involved sinus, e.g., we used lines drawn by permanent pen marker and changed the mask to confirm that the vein of Labbe is draining into the superior venous channel.
4. Balloon can be used to preserve the normal draining vein. A compliant balloon should be used as the diseased sinus has irregular shape and one may have to change the position of the balloon if required.
5. DMSO-compatible dual-lumen balloon can be also used for retrograde injection of the onyx for the management of the residual fistula as in this case.

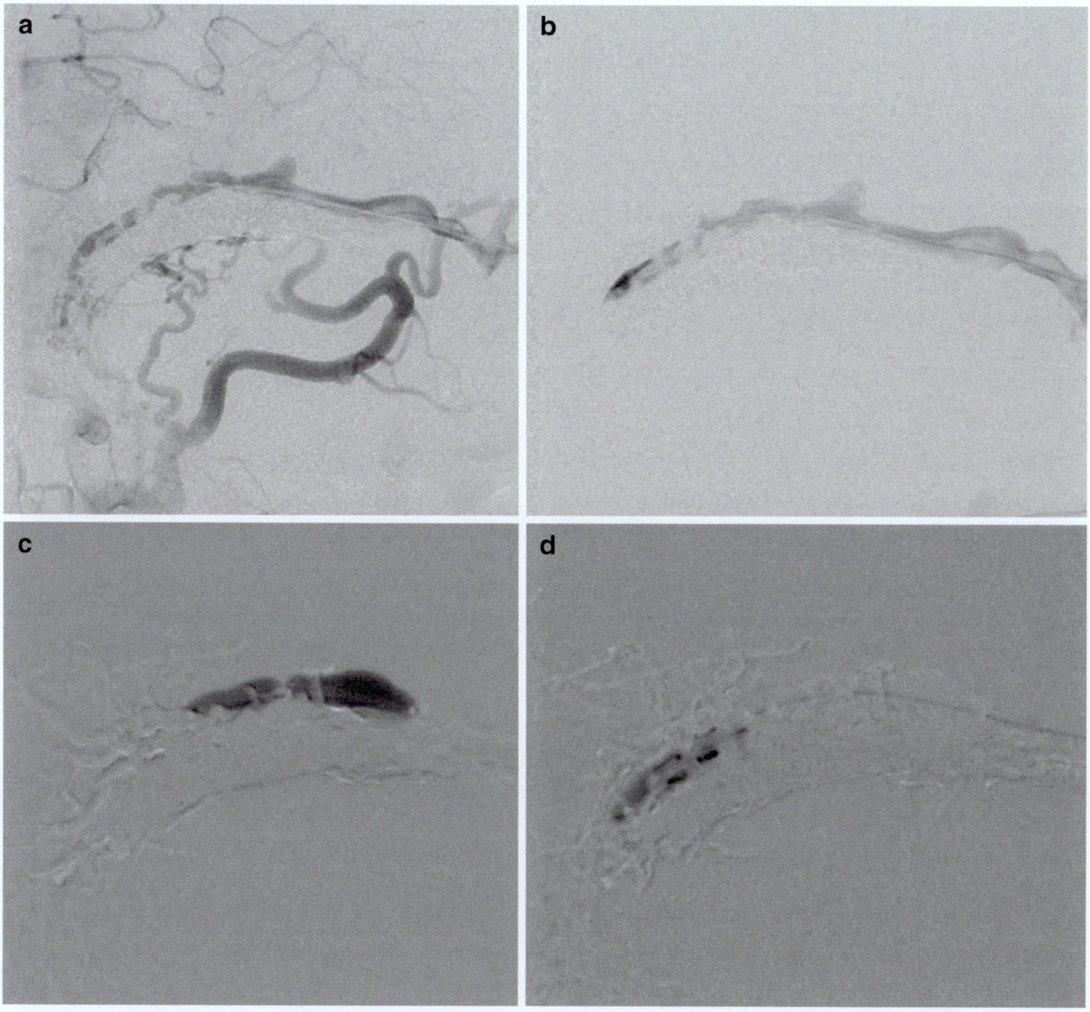

Fig. 62.4 (**a**) Right ECA angiogram AP view shows residual fistula at the lateral aspect of the sinus. (**b**) Injection through the lumen of balloon catheter shows patent superior venous channel. (**c**) Balloon advanced into the lateral aspect of superior channel. (**d**) Onyx was injected through the lumen of the balloon catheter

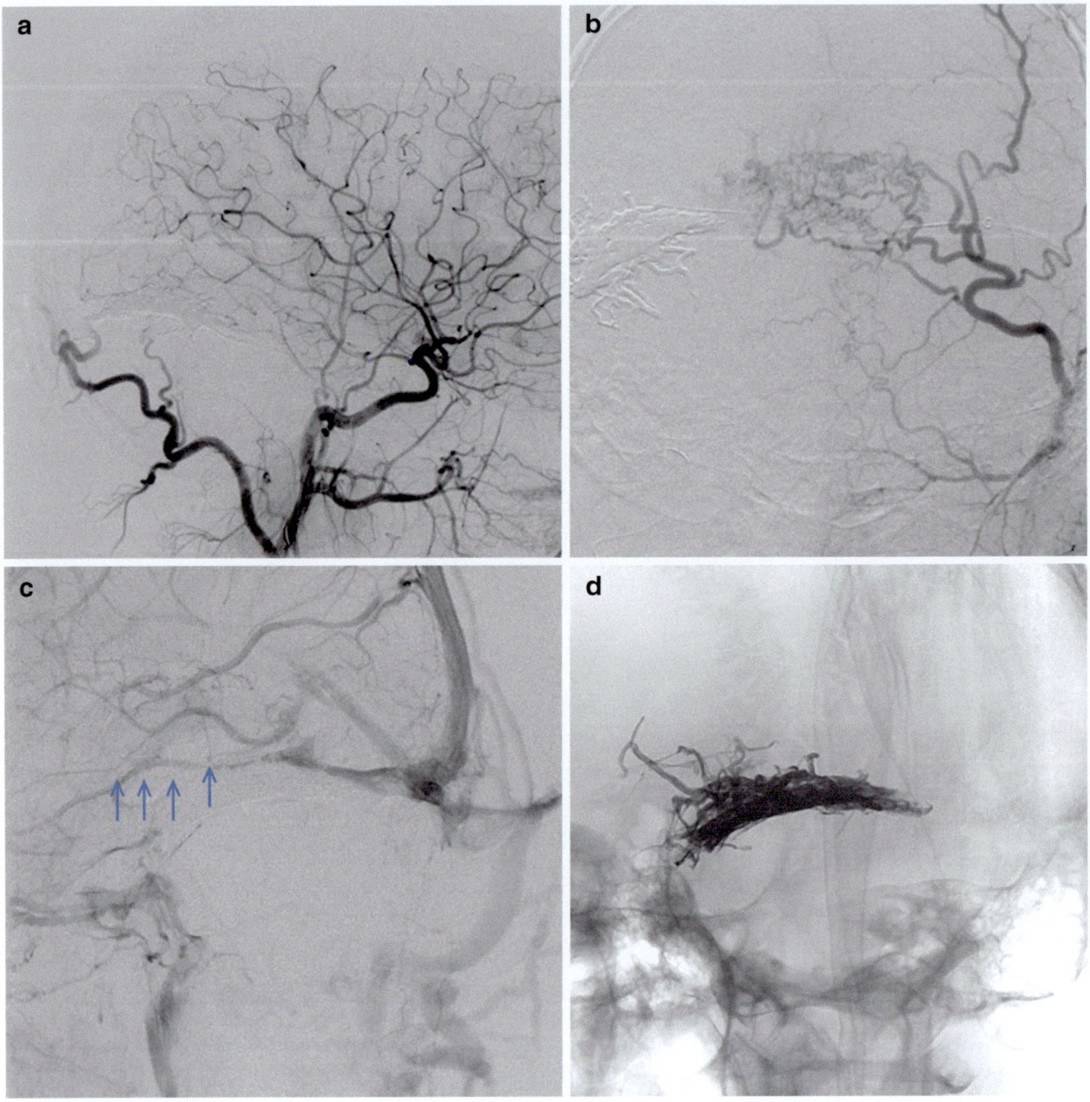

Fig. 62.5 (**a**, **b**) Post-procedure right CCA (**a**) and left ECA (**b**) angiograms show complete obliteration of the fistula. (**c**) Venous phase of post-procedure right CCA shows patent vein of Labbe. Image (**d**) shows final onyx cast

Suggested Reading

Shi ZS, Loh Y, Duckwiler GR, Jahan R, Vinuela F. Balloon-assisted transarterial embolization of intracranial dural arteriovenous fistulas. J Neurosurg. 2009;110:921–8.

Shi Z, Loh Y, Gonzalez N, et al. Flow control techniques for Onyx embolization of intracranial dural arteriovenous fistulae. J Neurointerv Surg. 2013;5:311–6.

Dural AVF with Venous Aneurysm Causing Mass Effect: Management Strategy

63

Vipul Gupta

Case

A 58-year-old male presented with progressively increasing headaches. CT scan revealed ventricular dilation (lateral and third ventricles) along with periventricular ooze. A hyperdense lesion was seen compressing upon dorsal midbrain (Fig. 63.1a, b). MRI brain revealed a large dilated vascular structure compressing upon the dorsal midbrain along with adjacent dilated vessels (Fig. 63.1c, d). It was causing compression of aqueduct with resultant hydrocephalus. DSA revealed a dural arteriovenous fistula fed by bilateral middle meningeal arteries (Fig. 63.1e, f). Aneurysmal dilation was seen in the draining vein. Trans-arterial onyx embolization was planned.

Issues

- Management of hydrocephalus.
- Probability of venous thrombosis due to sudden flow change after embolization and consequent exacerbation of mass effect.

V. Gupta
Neurointerventional Surgery, Stroke Unit, Artemis Agrim Institute of Neuroscience, Gurgaon, India
e-mail: vipul.gupta@artemishospitals.com

Management

The procedure was performed under general anaesthesia. Preparation for emergency external ventricular drain or shunt placement was done in the event of exacerbation of hydrocephalus. Bilateral trans-femoral arterial access was taken so that bilateral simultaneous carotid angiograms can be obtained. After placing 6F Chaperone guide catheter (MicroVention, Tustin, California, USA) in the distal right ECA, Marathon microcatheter (ev3 Inc., Irvine, California, USA) was navigated through the right middle meningeal artery to the site of fistula over a mirage microguidewire (ev3 Inc., Irvine, California, USA) (Fig. 63.2a, b). Thereafter, embolization was done with onyx as embolic material; care was taken to avoid onyx penetration into the large venous pouches (Fig. 63.2d, e). Once the proximal venous occlusion was achieved, retrograde reflux could be achieved into all the feeders, resulting in complete occlusion (Fig. 63.2f–i). Immediate DynaCT (Siemens, Erlangen, Germany) was performed which revealed contrast stasis in the venous pouches but no enlargement or increase in mass effect. The patient was extubated in intact clinical condition and was given low molecular weight heparin (Inj. Clexane 0.4 mL subcutaneously twice

V. Gupta et al. (eds.), *100 Interesting Case Studies in Neurointervention: Tips and Tricks*,
https://doi.org/10.1007/978-981-13-1346-2_63

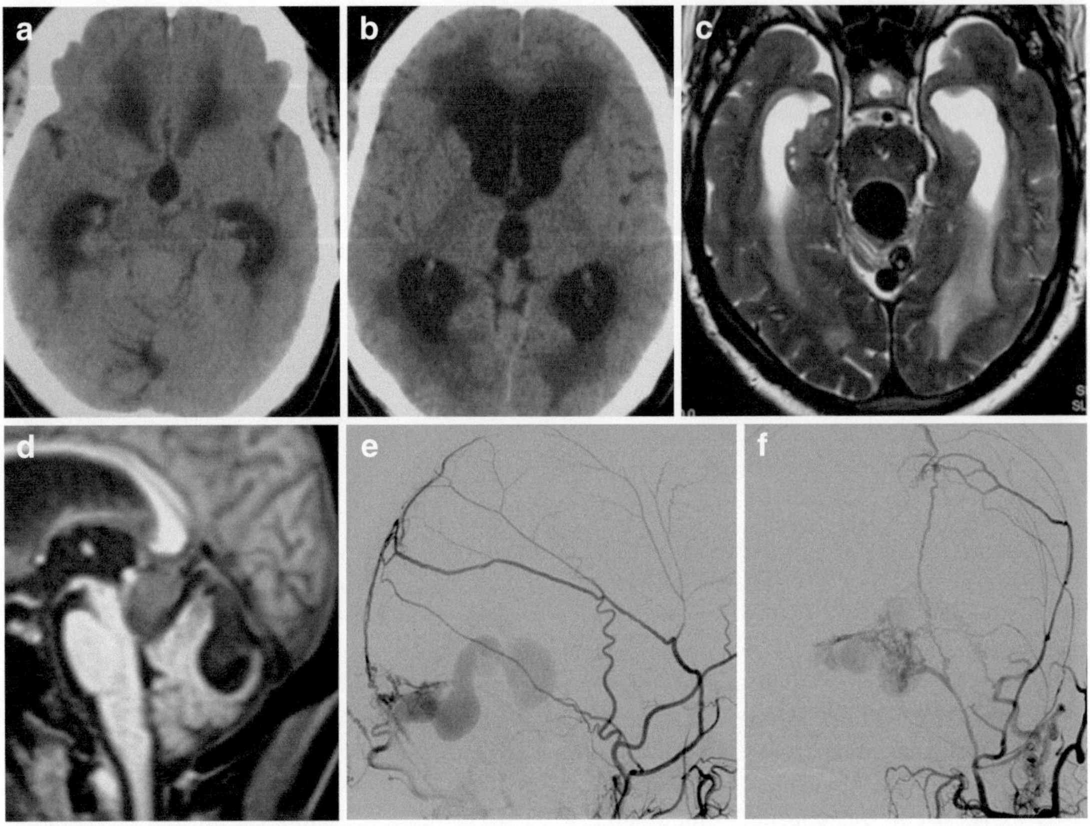

Fig. 63.1 (**a** and **b**) Non-contrast CT images showing dilated lateral and third ventricles with periventricular ooze. A hyperdense lesion is seen compressing the dorsal midbrain. (**c** and **d**) T2-weighted (**c**) and sagittal T1-weighted (**d**) MR images show a large flow void in relation with posterior aspect of the midbrain causing mass effect. Flow voids are also seen in the region of superior vermis. (**e** and **f**) DSA images of right (**e**) and left (**f**) external carotid arteries showing a dural arteriovenous fistula fed by branches of bilateral middle meningeal arteries. Large venous pouch seen in the draining vein

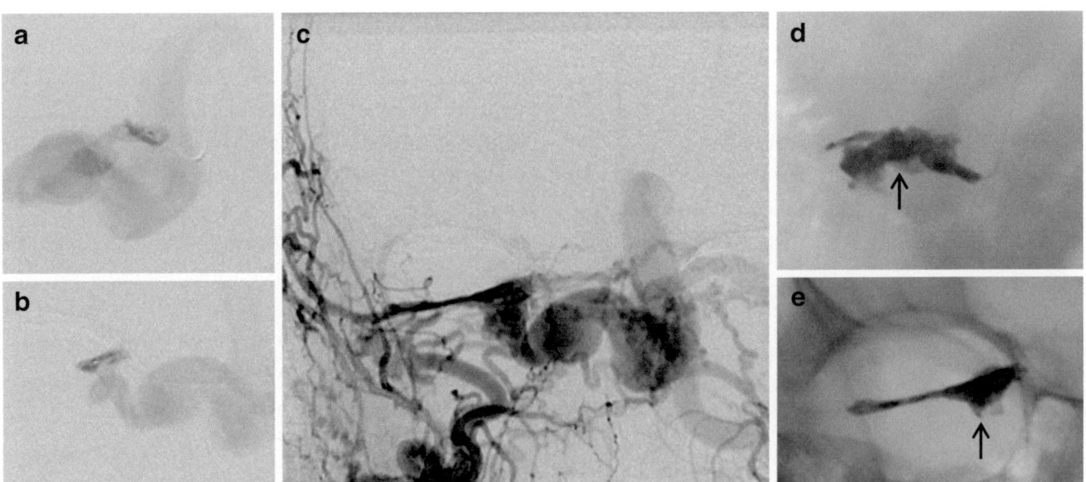

Fig. 63.2 (**a** and **b**) Microcatheter injection at site of fistula. (**c**) Bilateral simultaneous ECA injections show all the feeders and the fistula in entirety. (**d** and **e**) Initial onyx injection shows filling of the venous pouch (arrows) with reflux into the feeder artery. (**f** and **g**) Thereafter, onyx penetration was achieved into all the feeder vessels. (**h** and **i**) Bilateral ECA injections showing complete occlusion of the AVF

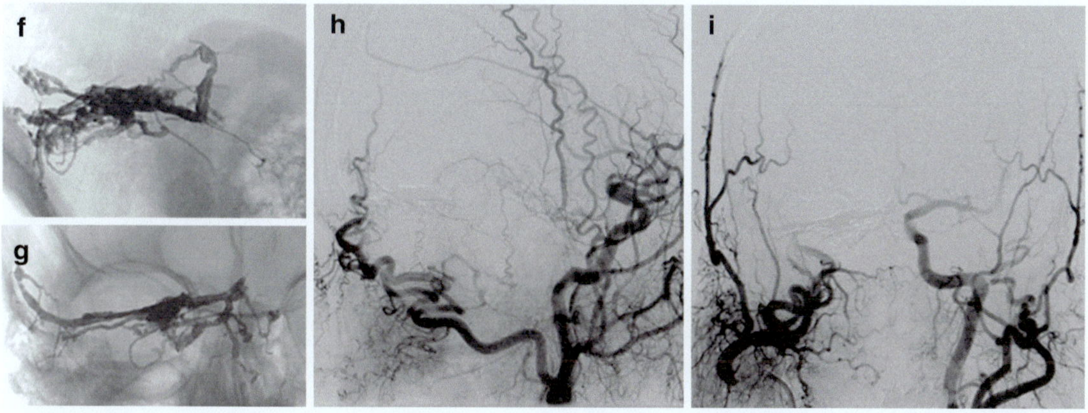

Fig. 63.2 (continued)

a day) for the next 3 days. Repeat CT brain revealed subtle decrease in size of venous dilations. Follow-up CT scan of the brain at 15-day post-embolization revealed remarkable shrinkage of veins with decrease in hydrocephalus (Fig. 63.3). Follow-up MRI at one and half years revealed thrombosed venous sac and resolution of the hydrocephalus (Fig. 63.4).

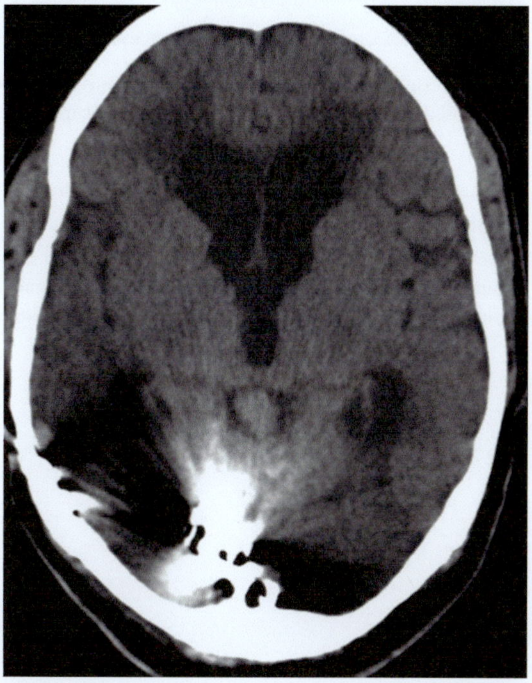

Fig. 63.3 Non-contrast CT brain on day 15 post-embolization showing significant shrinkage of venous pouch and reduction of the hydrocephalus

Tips and Tricks

1. In patients with large venous aneurysmal dilations associated with vascular malformations, proximal shunt occlusion leads to regression of the dilation and the mass effect.
2. All care should be taken in these cases that the embolization material remains proximal to the pouch.
3. If complete occlusion has been achieved, it is advisable to give heparin or equivalent so as to prevent progressive thrombosis in the dilated veins.

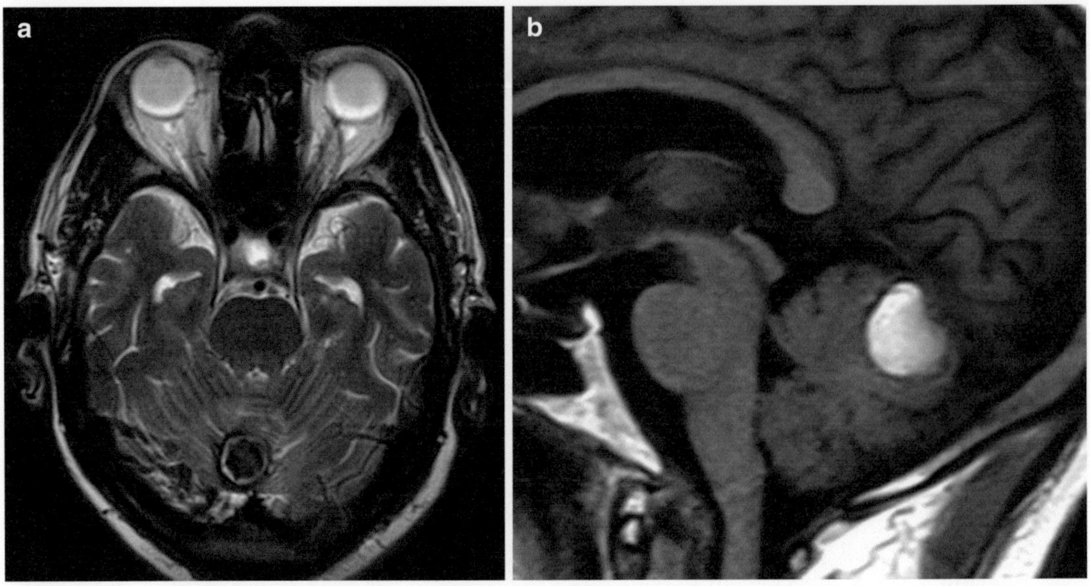

Fig. 63.4 (**a** and **b**) One and half year follow-up T2-weighted axial (**a**) and T1-weighted sagittal (**b**) MR images show thrombosed venous sac with resolution of hydrocephalus

Suggested Reading

Rammos S, Bortolotti C, Lanzino G. Endovascular management of intracranial dural arteriovenous fistulae. Neurosurg Clin N Am. 2014;25:539–49.

Dural AVF Draining into an Isolated Sac: Embolization Technique

64

Vipul Gupta

Case

A 38-year-old female presented with progressive headache followed by drowsiness and quadriparesis. At the time of presentation, she had papilloedema and her GCS was E3M4V2. The MRI revealed diffuse white matter edema along with dilated vessels in the subarachnoid space (Fig. 64.1a, b). Small areas of bleed were seen in the right occipital and frontal regions. Prominence of left transverse sinus was observed (Fig. 64.1c, d). Cerebral DSA revealed a high flow dural AVF with feeders from left middle meningeal and occipital arteries, the meningohypophyseal trunk of left ICA, and posterior meningeal branch of left posterior inferior cerebellar artery. It was draining into left sigmoid sinus and retrogradely into the straight sinus, superior sagittal sinus, and cortical and deep veins (Fig. 64.2a–d). There was a sharp kink in the left middle meningeal artery (MMA) (Fig. 64.2e). Both sigmoid sinuses were occluded. The case was planned for transarterial onyx embolization.

Issues

- Tight bend in the access artery posing a technical problem for navigation of microcatheter to the fistula site.
- As both sigmoid sinuses are occluded, transvenous route is not feasible.

Management

Procedure was performed under general anesthesia. A 6F long sheath (Cook medical, Bloomington, USA) was placed in left common carotid artery. Through the sheath, a 6F Envoy guiding catheter (Codman & Shurtleff, Inc., USA) was placed in left distal ECA. Pre-procedure left CCA angiogram showed that all feeders were entering a common venous sac just before joining the sigmoid sinus (Fig. 64.2f). After taking a road map, we tried to negotiate the tight bend in the left MMA with marathon microcatheter (ev3 Inc., Irvine, California, USA) over a curved tip mirage microguidewire. However, the microguidewire could not be advanced beyond the kink in the MMA. So we used Traxcess 0.014″ microguidewire (MicroVention, Tustin, California, USA) with a straight tip to negotiate the bend. Once the wire was distal, the marathon microcatheter was navigated to the fistula site over the wire (Fig. 64.3a–d). After confirming opti-

V. Gupta
Neurointerventional Surgery, Stroke Unit, Artemis Agrim Institute of Neuroscience, Gurgaon, India
e-mail: vipul.gupta@artemishospitals.com

V. Gupta et al. (eds.), *100 Interesting Case Studies in Neurointervention: Tips and Tricks*,
https://doi.org/10.1007/978-981-13-1346-2_64

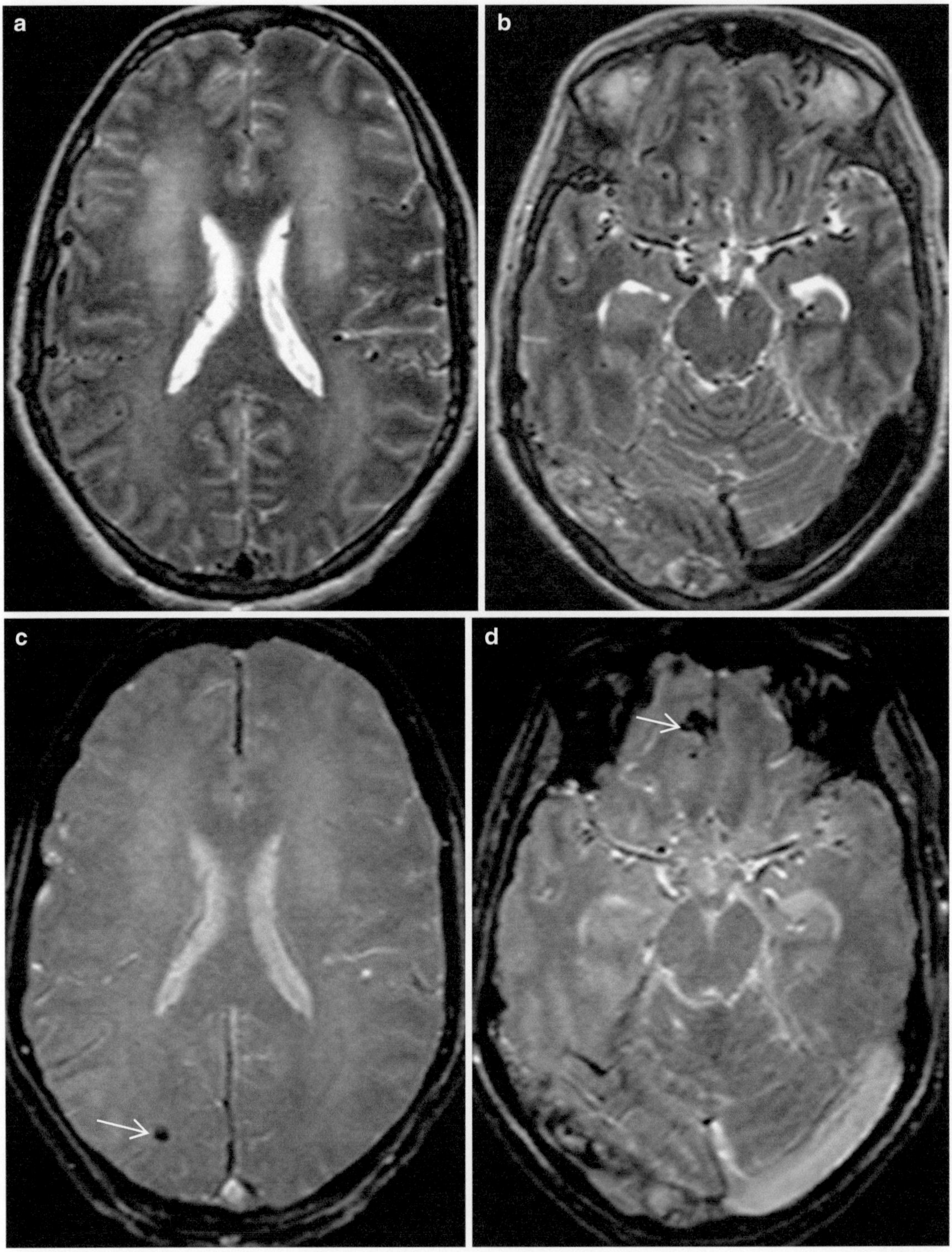

Fig. 64.1 (**a** and **b**) T2-weighted MR images reveal diffuse edema in white matter along with prominent flow voids in sulcal spaces. (**c** and **d**) Gradient echo images reveal small area of bleed (shown by arrow) in right occipital and frontal regions as well as dilated left transverse sinus

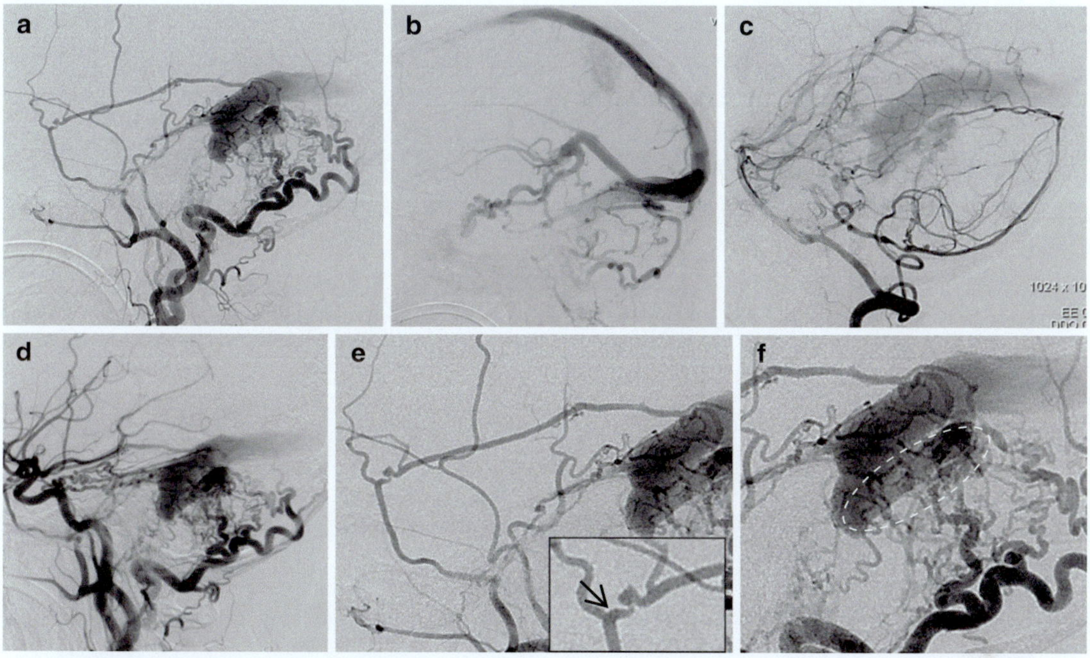

Fig. 64.2 (**a** and **b**) Left external carotid artery injection reveals a dural AVF draining into left sigmoid sinus and retrogradely into the straight sinus, into superior sagittal sinus, and into cortical and deep veins. Feeders were from middle meningeal and occipital arteries. (**c**) Left vertebral artery injection shows feeders from left posterior meningeal artery arising from posterior inferior cerebellar artery. (**d**) Left common carotid artery injection showing enlarged tentorial branches from left ICA feeding the AVF. (**e**) Left ECA injection shows a tight kink in the middle meningeal artery marked by arrow in the enlarged inset image. (**f**) Enlarged image of the fistula. All the feeders were converging onto a common sac (marked by dashed line) before joining the sigmoid sinus

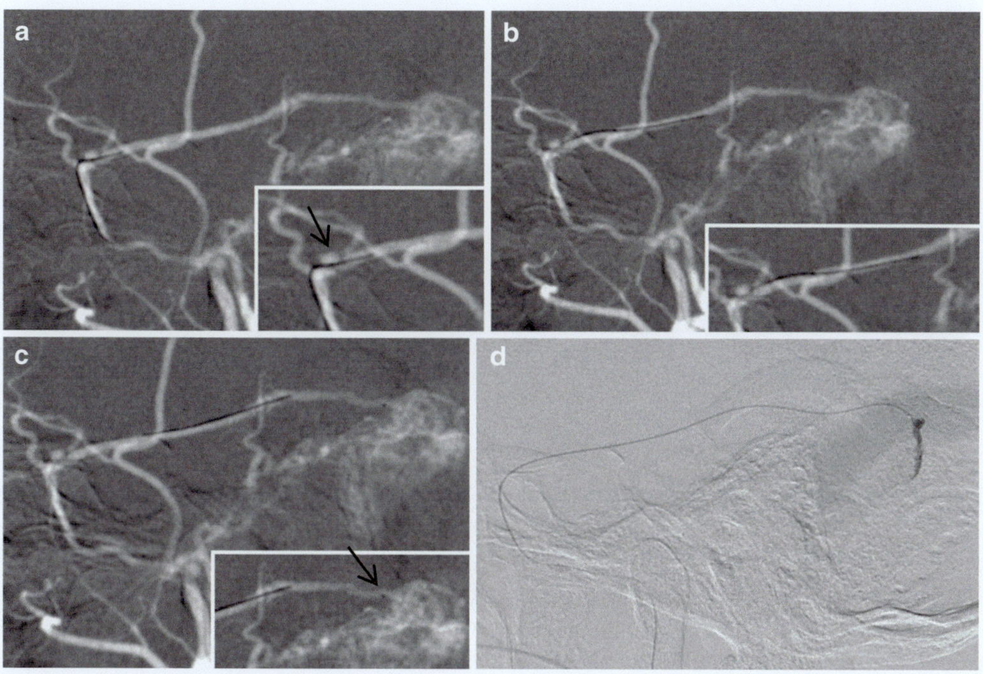

Fig. 64.3 (**a**) Roadmap image of a straight tip microguidewire being taken across the kink in the MMA. (**b**) Microcatheter taken across the kink over the wire. (**c**) With wire in the same position, microcatheter taken to a position adjacent to the fistula. (**d**) Microcatheter injection showing opacification of the AVF

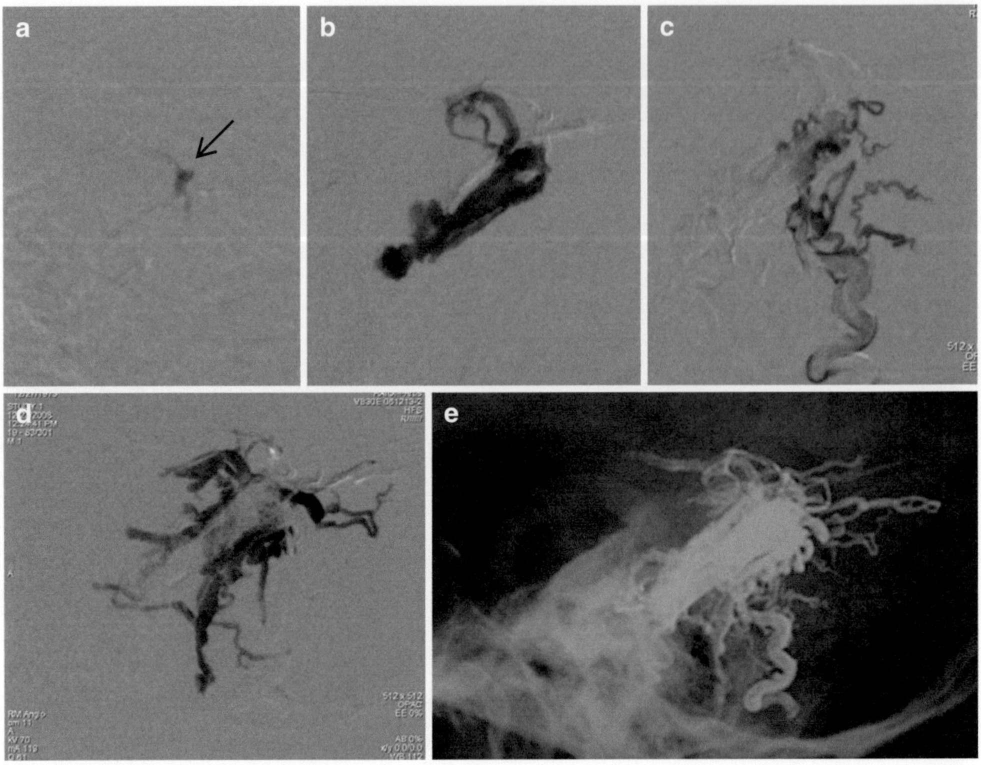

Fig. 64.4 Roadmap images showing onyx injection of the feeder (**a**) with a streak of material in the sac, filling of the venous sac (**b**) followed by retrograde filling of all the feeders (**c**, **d**). (**e**) Final onyx cast

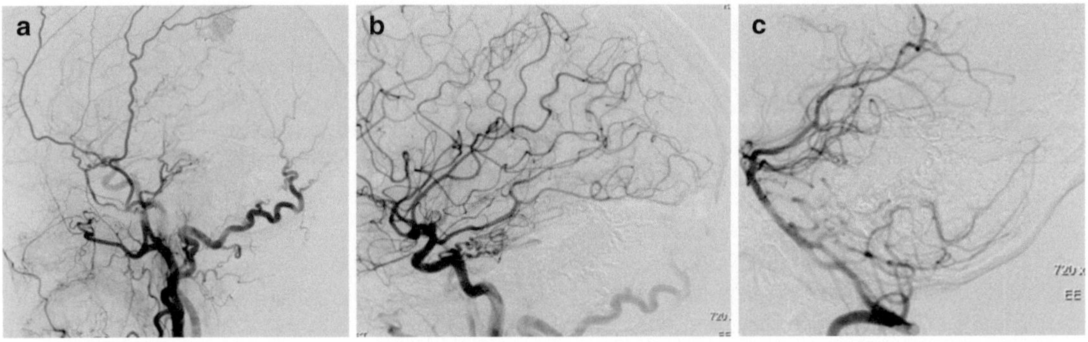

Fig. 64.5 Post-embolization angiograms of left ECA (**a**), left ICA (**b**), and left vertebral (**c**) arteries showing complete occlusion of the AVF

mal positioning of microcatheter, DMSO followed by onyx was injected with manual compression of the left CCA during initial phase (Fig. 64.4a, b). Once the venous sac was occluded (Fig. 64.4c–e). Post-procedure angiograms revealed complete occlusion of the dural AV fistula (Fig. 64.5). The patient was extubated in an intact clinical condition and was given low molecular weight heparin (Inj. Clexane 0.4 mL subcutaneously twice a day) for the next 2 days. She made uneventful recovery.

Tips and Tricks

1. The patient presented with progressive neurological deterioration with MRI findings suggestive of diffuse white matter edema; therefore, she required urgent treatment to avoid irreversible brain damage.
2. Middle meningeal artery (MMA) is generally thought to be the artery of choice for transarterial embolization of dural AVF as it has a relatively straight course; there is a better chance of reaching the site of fistula. However, the tight bend in the MMA can pose a technical difficulty while navigating softer tip microguidewires (like mirage). In such circumstances, a less stiff microguidewire (like Traxcess) with a straight tip can help in negotiating acute kinks in the access artery.
3. One should always try to identify the common venous segment where all feeders enter. Embolization of the common venous sac through access artery allows for retrograde filling of the rest of the feeders resulting into complete occlusion of the dural AVF.
4. Compression of CCA during initial phase of embolization prevents distal unintended migration of the onyx into normal sinus.
5. We prefer to give postoperative anticoagulation for 2–3 days to prevent development of dural sinus thrombosis due to altered hemodynamics as a result of closure of dural AV fistula.

Suggested Reading

Van Dijk JM, Willinsky RA. Venous congestive encephalopathy related to cranial dural arteriovenous fistulas. Neuroimaging Clin N Am. 2003;13:55–72.

Van Dijk JM, terBrugge KG, Willinsky RA, et al. Clinical course of cranial dural arteriovenous fistulas with long-term persistent cortical venous reflux. Stroke. 2002;33:1233–6.

65 Dural AVF Embolization-Tortuous Access: Wire Loop Technique

Vipul Gupta

Case

A 58-year-old male presented with sudden-onset weakness of the right lower limb. MRI revealed a small bleed adjacent to motor cortex. A large flow void was seen adjacent to the bleed along with multiple dilated serpiginous vessels in adjacent sulcal spaces (Fig. 65.1a). DSA revealed a dural arteriovenous fistula in the left frontoparietal region with feeders from bilateral middle meningeal and left superficial temporal arteries (Fig. 65.1b–f). Marked tortuosity of the feeder vessels and venous congestion was noticed. The case was planned for transarterial Onyx embolization.

Issues

- Placement of microcatheter across the tortuous access to the site of fistula.
- Complete occlusion of the fistula including feeders coming across the midline.

V. Gupta
Neurointerventional Surgery, Stroke Unit, Artemis Agrim Institute of Neuroscience, Gurgaon, India
e-mail: vipul.gupta@artemishospitals.com

Management

Procedure was performed under general anaesthesia. A 6F long sheath (Cook Medical, Bloomington, USA) was placed in left common carotid artery. Through the sheath, 5F chaperon guiding catheter (MicroVention, Tustin, California, USA) was placed in left ECA. Another diagnostic catheter was placed in right ECA. Marathon microcatheter (ev3 Inc., Irvine, California, USA) was navigated over a mirage microguidewire (ev3 Inc., Irvine, California, USA). A small sharp curve was given to the wire tip (Fig. 65.2a–e); this helped in forming a loop at distal end of the wire. The loop easily deflected at the turns and facilitated navigation across the multiple turns. A stepwise approach was taken; after the microwire was navigated distally for a certain distance, the microcatheter was advanced to enable pushing the wire further ahead. The technique enabled microcatheter placement close to the site of fistula (Fig. 65.3a). Embolization was performed (Fig. 65.3b–d), and Onyx penetration into the common draining vein resulted in complete occlusion of the fistula (Fig. 65.3e, f). Right ECA injection could be done through the diagnostic catheter to confirm the occlusion of the fistula before withdrawal of microcatheter. Patient made uneventful recovery.

V. Gupta et al. (eds.), *100 Interesting Case Studies in Neurointervention: Tips and Tricks*,
https://doi.org/10.1007/978-981-13-1346-2_65

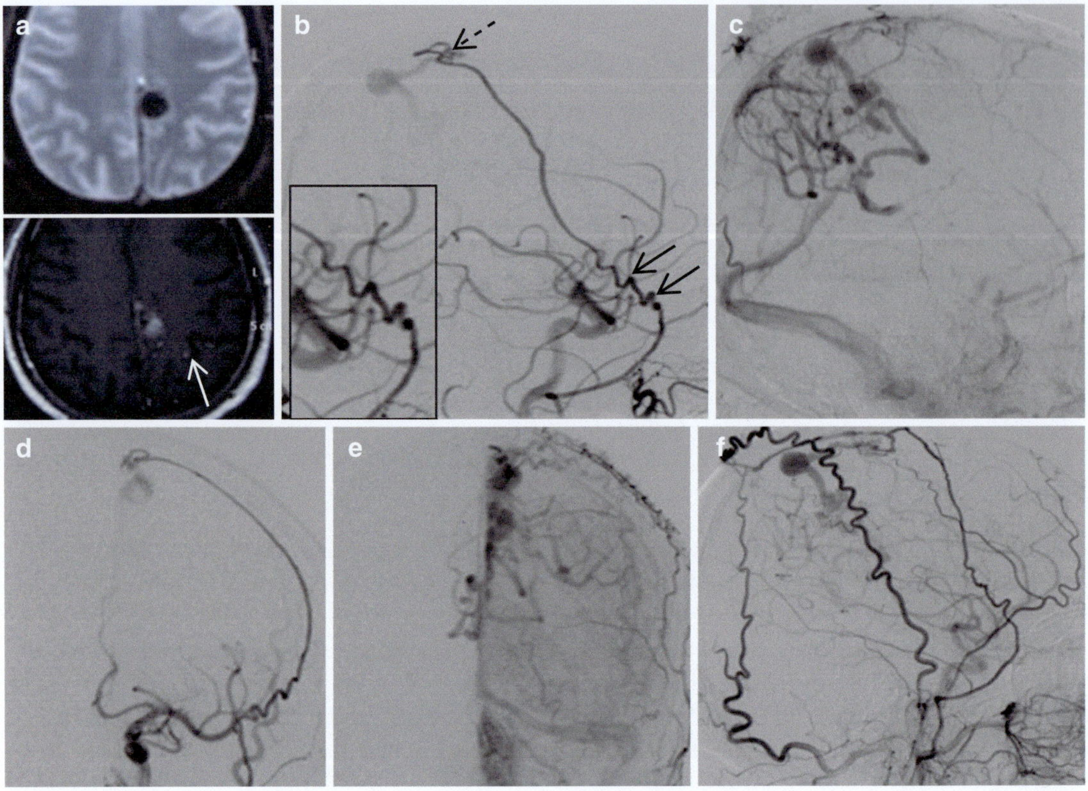

Fig. 65.1 (**a**) T2- and T1-weighted MR images show a small bleed in left posterior frontal region. Dilated vascular structures noted in T1WI (arrows), indicating a vascular malformation. (**b** and **c**) DSA images of right ECA injection show a dural AVF fed by middle meningeal artery. Marked cortical venous congestion seen in venous phase (**c**). Marked tortuosity of the feeding artery was seen (arrows). (**d** and **e**) AP view of left ECA injection. (**f**) Lateral view of left ECA injection revealing tortuous feeders from left MMA and superficial temporal artery

Tips and Tricks

1. Wire loop technique is useful in negotiating sharp vascular loops; the loop at the distal end of the wire gets deflected at the turns when you push on the wire and allows for catheterization of tortuous feeding artery with relative ease.
2. Microcatheter has to be advanced stepwise along with the wire to give support to the wire.
3. Park the guiding catheter as distally as possible to enable better force transmission to the microcatheter. During microcatheter placement, the guiding tip should be under view. A long sheath offers better support and stable guiding catheter position.
4. All attempts should be made to reach the site of fistula; changing to a new microguidewire helps in later stages.
5. Occlusion of the common segment of vein using Onyx results in closure of all the feeders.

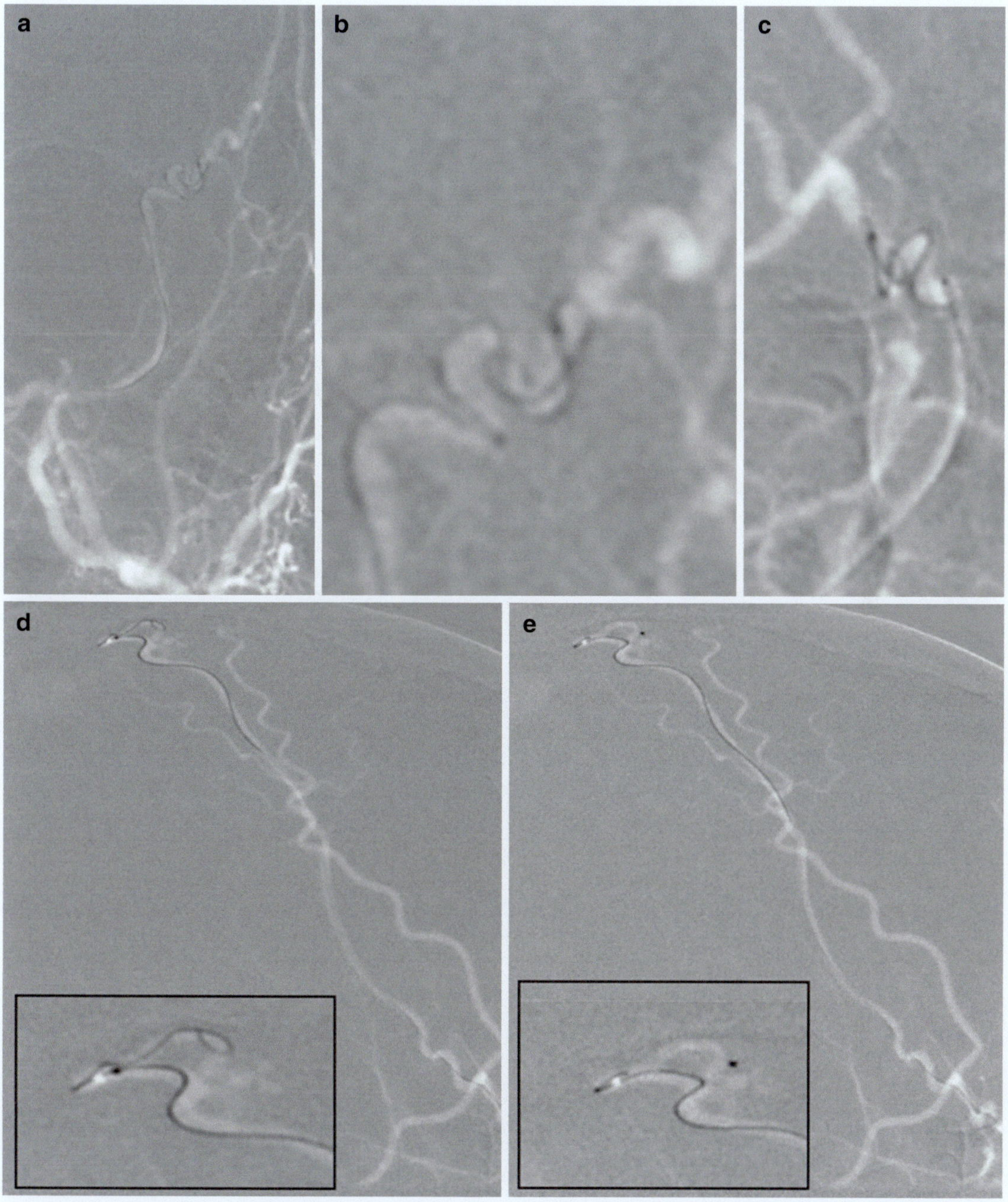

Fig. 65.2 (**a**) Roadmap image showing catheterization of left ECA feeder. (**b** and **c**) Magnified roadmap images in AP (**b**), and lateral (**c**) views show the loop of wire being used to negotiate the vascular loops. (**d**) Microcatheter navigation across the distal tight turn in the feeding artery; again a loop at the tip of the wire helped in taking the turn. (**e**) Final microcatheter position at the site of fistula

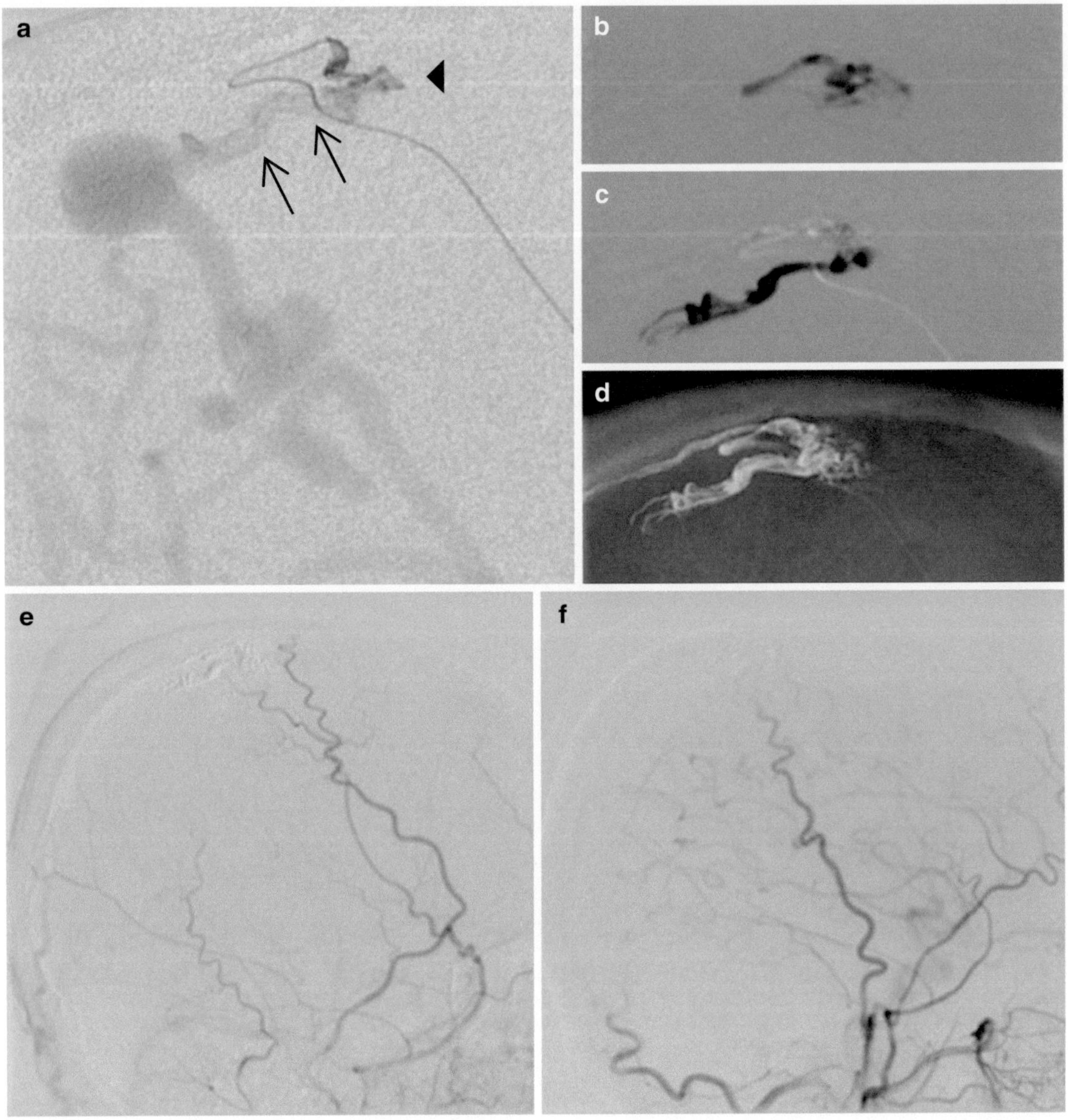

Fig. 65.3 (**a**) Microcatheter injection showing the fistula (arrow head) and the draining vein (arrows). (**b**) Onyx injection with partial filling of fistula and reflux into feeding artery. (**c**) Further injection with a new roadmap showing Onyx penetration into the vein. (**d**) Final Onyx cast. (**e** and **f**) Left (**e**) and right (**f**) ECA injections showing complete occlusion of the fistula

Suggested Reading

Hu YC, Newman CB, Dashti SR, et al. Cranial dural arteriovenous fistula: transarterial Onyx embolization experience and technical nuances. J Neurointervent Surg. 2011;3:5–13.

Transvenous Onyx Embolization of the Dural AVF

66

Vipul Gupta

Case

A 65-year-old man presented with a single episode of seizure. Plain CT scan head (Fig. 66.1a) revealed a small focal haemorrhage in the left high frontal region. Cerebral angiography revealed Borden type 3 dural AV fistula with dilated frontal cortical vein supplied by multiple tiny feeders from both ophthalmic arteries and draining into superior sagittal sinus (Fig. 66.1b–e).

Issues

- Dural AV fistula opening directly into the subarachnoid vein needs urgent treatment as there is high propensity for haemorrhage.
- Transarterial embolization via ophthalmic artery is not safe due to small feeders from the ophthalmic artery and high probability of reflux and occlusion of central retinal artery.
- For transvenous embolization, microcatheter should be navigated close to the fistula as there is a high chance of reflux onto the microcatheter.

V. Gupta
Neurointerventional Surgery, Stroke Unit, Artemis Agrim Institute of Neuroscience, Gurgaon, India
e-mail: vipul.gupta@artemishospitals.com

Management

As transarterial route was not feasible, we decided to perform transvenous Onyx embolization. Procedure was performed under general anaesthesia with bilateral common femoral arterial and right common femoral venous accesses. Bilateral arterial access was taken so that simultaneous bilateral CCA angiogram can be done. A 6F-long sheath (Raabe Modification, Cook Medical, Bloomington, USA) was placed in the proximal right internal jugular vein, and then a Neuron 6F guide catheter (Penumbra, Alameda, California, USA) was advanced into the posterior superior sagittal sinus (Fig. 66.2a). Following this, under roadmap guidance, Sonic 1.2 F microcatheter (Balt Extrusion, Montmorency, France) with 2.5 cm detachable tip was navigated over hybrid 007 microwire (Balt Extrusion, Montmorency, France) into the involved frontal cortical vein as close to the fistula as possible (Fig. 66.2b, c). After confirming the optimal microcatheter tip position, Onyx-34 was injected under biplane blank roadmap guidance, and adequate penetration into the segment of vein harbouring the fistula was achieved (Fig. 66.2d, e).

Post-procedure simultaneous bilateral CCA angiogram revealed complete obliteration of the fistula (Fig. 66.3a, b).

V. Gupta et al. (eds.), *100 Interesting Case Studies in Neurointervention: Tips and Tricks*,
https://doi.org/10.1007/978-981-13-1346-2_66

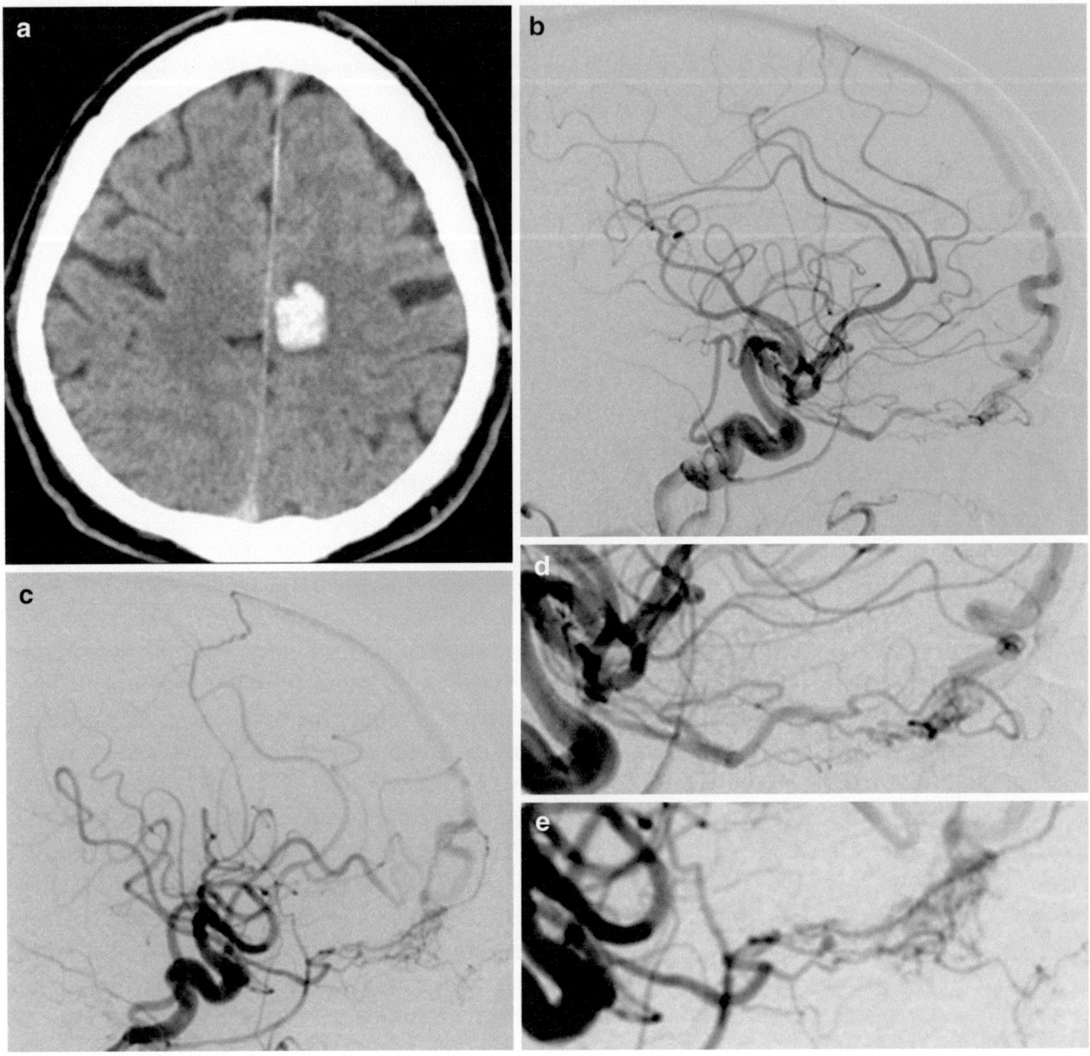

Fig. 66.1 (**a**) Plain CT brain shows focal haematoma in the left frontal lobe. (**b** and **c**) Right and left CCA angiograms show Borden type 3 dural AV fistula at dilated frontal cortical vein supplied by multiple tiny feeders from both ophthalmic arteries and draining into the superior sagittal sinus. (**d** and **e**) Show magnified views of the fistula on right and left CCA injection, respectively

Tips and Tricks

1. Transarterial embolization of dural AV fistula may not be feasible when the feeders are small. In these instances, a transvenous approach can be undertaken as one is usually able to navigate the microcatheter to the fistula site and therefore achieve complete obliteration.
2. As detailed above, microcatheter tip should be navigated close to the fistula as there is the possibility of reflux onto the microcatheter with venous approach as we are attempting retrograde penetration of the Onyx. For this reason, microcatheter with long detachable tip and Onyx-34 instead of Onyx-18 are advisable. Nowadays, microcatheters with detachable tip as long as 5 cm are available.

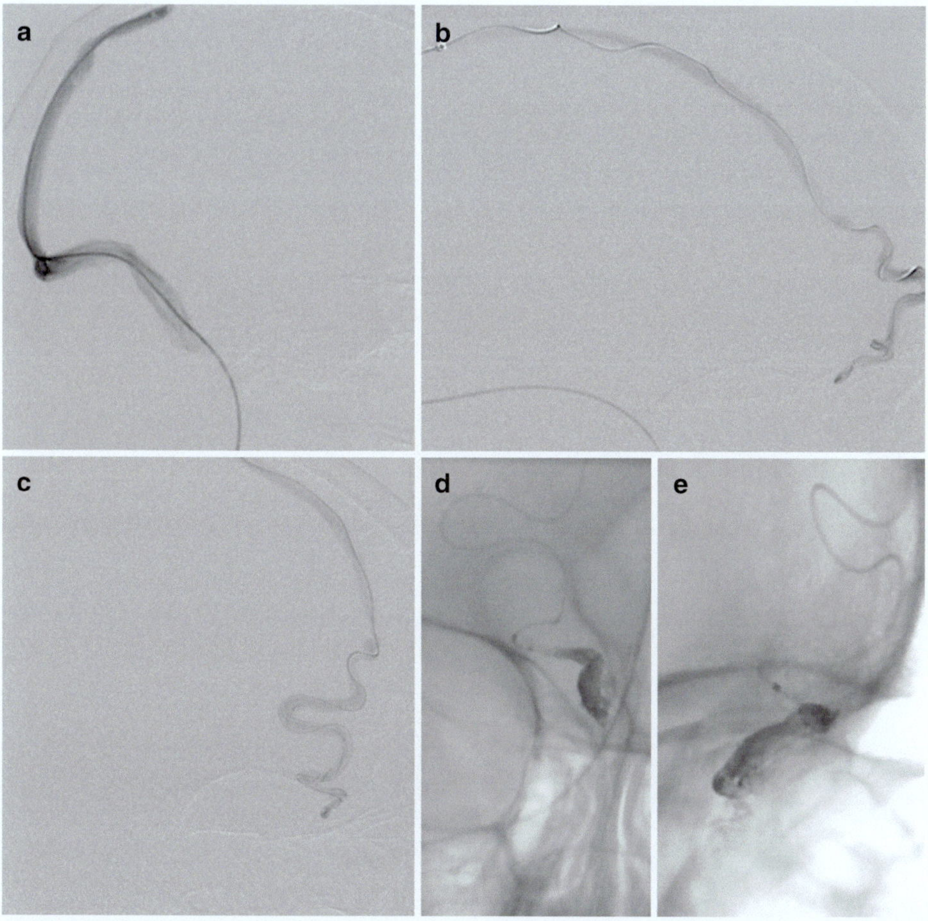

Fig. 66.2 (**a**) Shows Neuron 6F guide catheter placed in the posterior superior sagittal sinus. (**b**) Under roadmap guidance, microcatheter was positioned into the involved frontal cortical vein as close to the fistula as possible. (**c**) Shows microcatheter angiogram. (**d** and **e**) Show Onyx cast in AP and lateral views

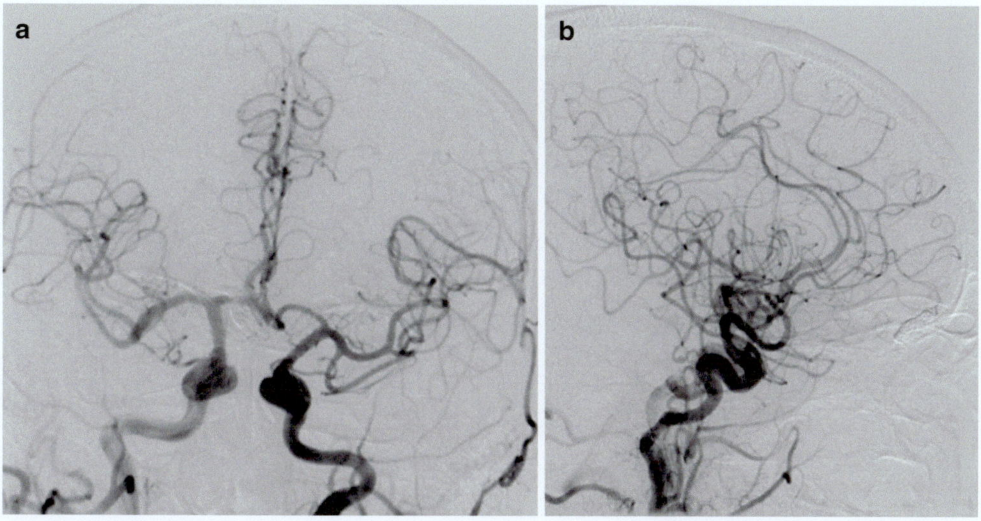

Fig. 66.3 (**a** and **b**) Bilateral CCA angiograms in AP (**a**) and lateral projections (**b**) demonstrating complete obliteration of the dural AV fistula

Suggested Reading

Defreyne L, Vanlangenhove P, Vandekerckhove T, et al. Transvenous embolization of a dural arteriovenous fistula of the anterior cranial fossa: preliminary results. Am J Neuroradiol. 2000;21:761–5.

Spiotta AM, Hawk H, Kellogg RT, Turner RD, Chaudry MI, Turk AS. Transfemoral venous approach for Onyx embolization of anterior fossa dural arteriovenous fistulae. J Neurointerv Surg. 2014;6(3):195–9.

Dural AVF with Progressive Edema and Mass Effect

67

Rajsrinivas Parthasarathy and Vipul Gupta

Case

A 51-year-old diabetic and hypertensive male presented with a 1 month history of progressive headache and blurred vision. His initial MRI brain (Fig. 67.1) revealed a small right temporal lobe hematoma with extensive surrounding edema involving the right temporal lobe and extending into the posterior frontal and the parieto-occipital region. MRI and MRV revealed right transverse sinus thrombosis along with multiple dilated serpiginous venous channels in the right temporal lobe. On interval repeat imaging (Fig. 67.2), there was further progression in the edema with mass effect resulting in the effacement of the right lateral ventricle, sphenoidal, and operculo-insular parts of the Sylvian cistern and the crural cistern. There was midline shift of approximately 5 mm along with early uncal herniation. Cerebral angiography (Fig. 67.3) revealed a right Borden type 3 tentorial dural AV fistula with feeders from the petrosal branch of the middle meningeal artery, transosseous branch of the occipital artery, and the neuromeningeal division of the ascending pharyngeal artery. The feeder from the petrosal branch of the middle meningeal artery was diminutive in caliber as compared to the other feeders. The venous drainage was redirected through pial cortical vein into the superior sagittal sinus. There was no forward flow through the right transverse sinus. Another small pial AVM nidus was seen in the right temporal lobe with feeders from the inferior division of the right MCA and venous outflow redirected through the cortical vein into the superior sagittal sinus.

Issue

- Understanding the pathophysiological basis for the nature and progressive increase in surrounding edema.
- Determining the most appropriate management strategy in this patient.

Management

The progressive increase in edema was disproportionate to the hematoma size and cannot be explained by isolated right transverse sinus thrombosis. There were multiple dilated venous channels suggestive of venous hypertension, and the venous outflow from the fistulous connection was redirected through cortical veins into the superior sagittal sinus. One can infer from the

R. Parthasarathy
Vascular Neurology and Neurointerventional Surgery, Artemis Agrim Institute of Neuroscience, Gurgaon, India

V. Gupta (✉)
Neurointerventional Surgery, Stroke Unit, Artemis Agrim Institute of Neuroscience, Gurgaon, India
e-mail: vipul.gupta@artemishospitals.com

V. Gupta et al. (eds.), *100 Interesting Case Studies in Neurointervention: Tips and Tricks*,
https://doi.org/10.1007/978-981-13-1346-2_67

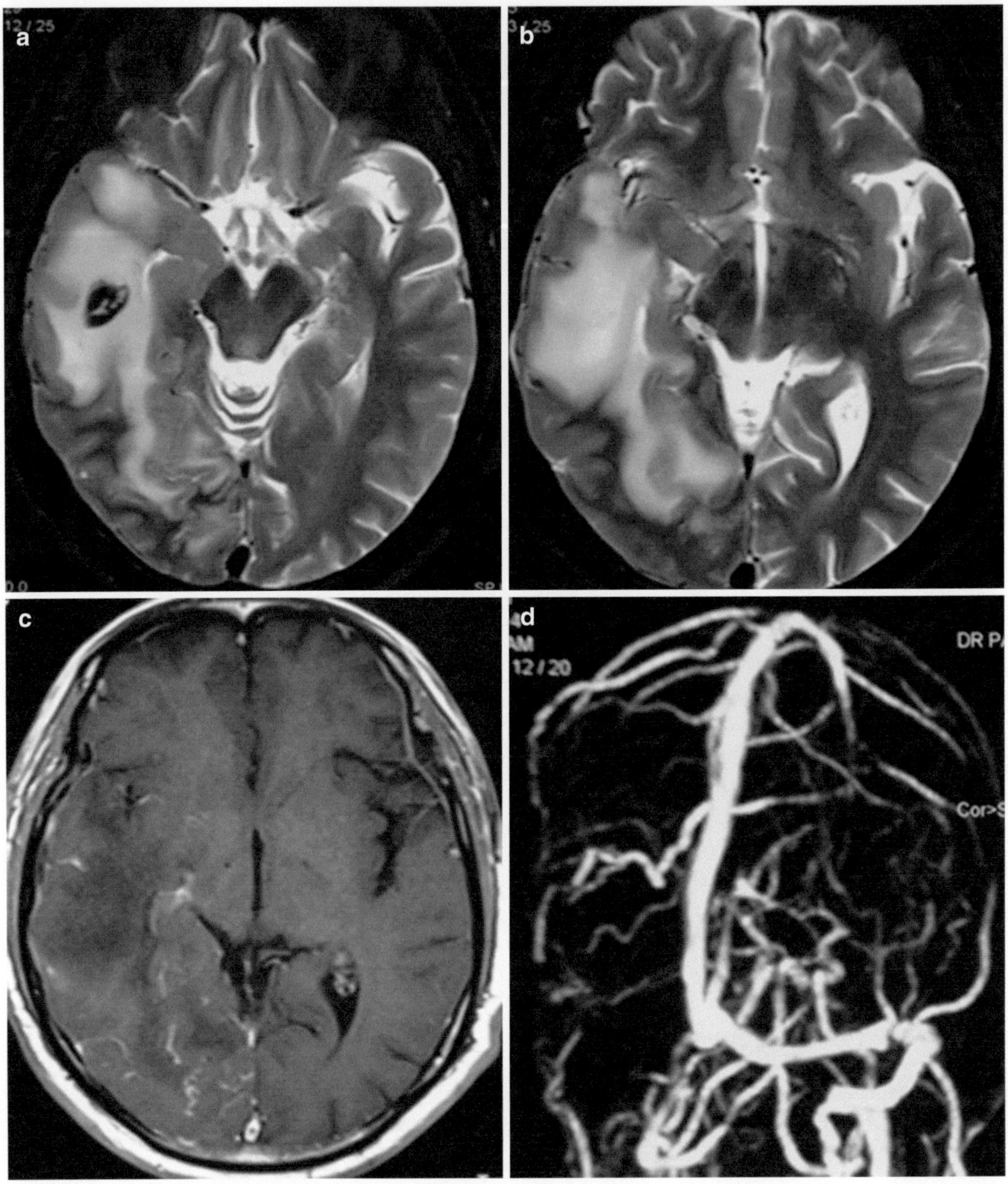

Fig. 67.1 (**a** and **b**) T2-W images show edema in the right temporo-occipital region with small hypointensity in the right temporal lobe suggestive of bleeding. (**c**) Post-contrast T1-W image shows serpiginous enhancement in sulcal spaces. (**d**) MR venography shows occlusion of right transverse and sigmoid sinuses

above that the edema is likely to be vasogenic in origin secondary to venous hypertension and the likely etiology for the progressive increase in swelling is a worsening in the grade of the dural AV fistula. Therefore, it was determined that early treatment of the dural AV fistula is the most appropriate next step in the management of this patient.

The procedure was performed via right trans-femoral route under general anesthesia. The

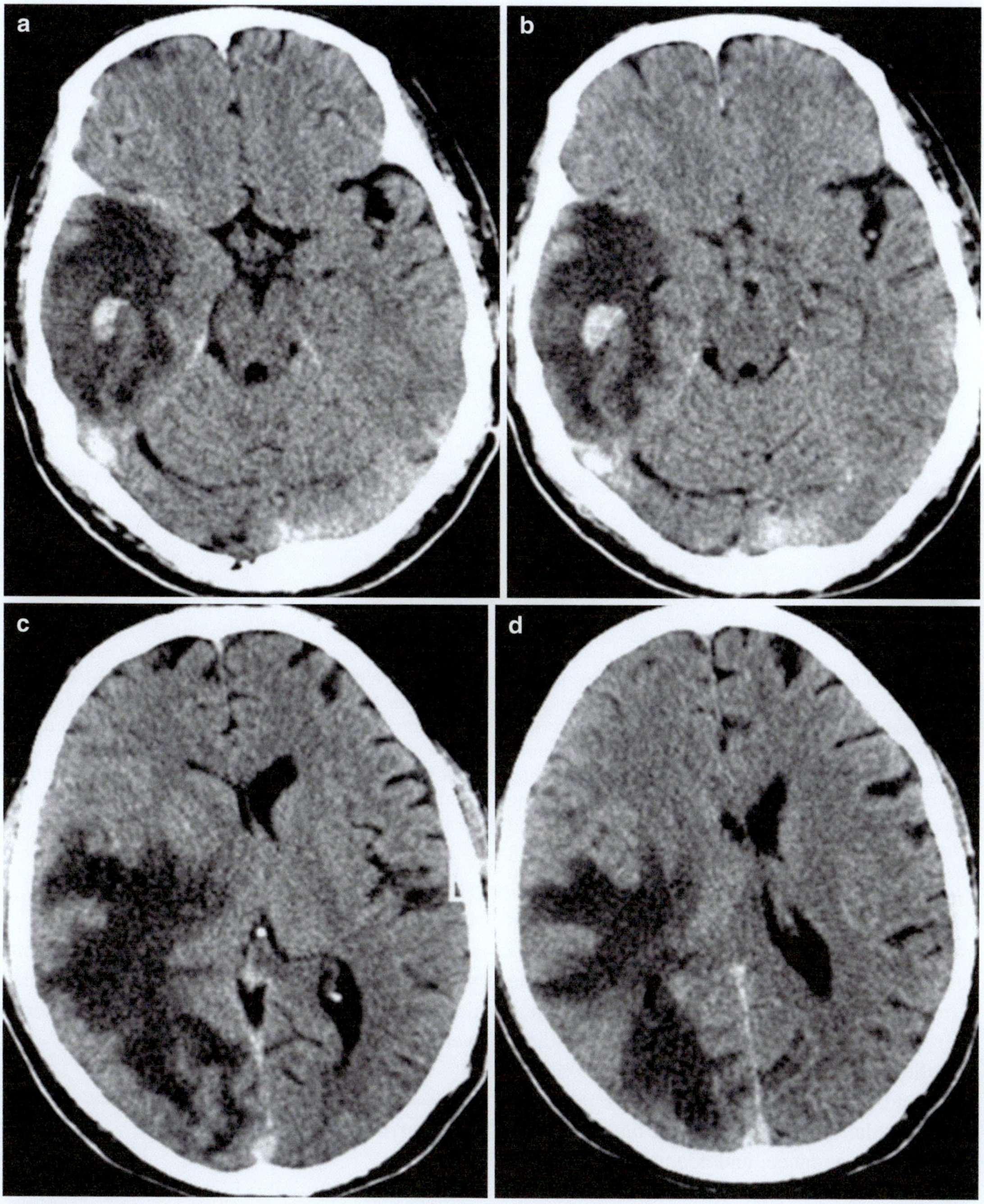

Fig. 67.2 (**a–d**) Repeat plain CT of the brain showed interval increase in the edema in the right temporo-occipital lobe with compression of the right lateral ventricle, midline shift to left side, and incipient right uncal herniation

feeder from the petrosal branch of the middle meningeal artery was diminutive in caliber as compared to the transosseous occipital and the ascending pharyngeal artery feeders. The petrosal division of middle meningeal artery however had a relatively linear course as compared to the other feeders and was therefore considered to be the feeder wherein distal navigation and

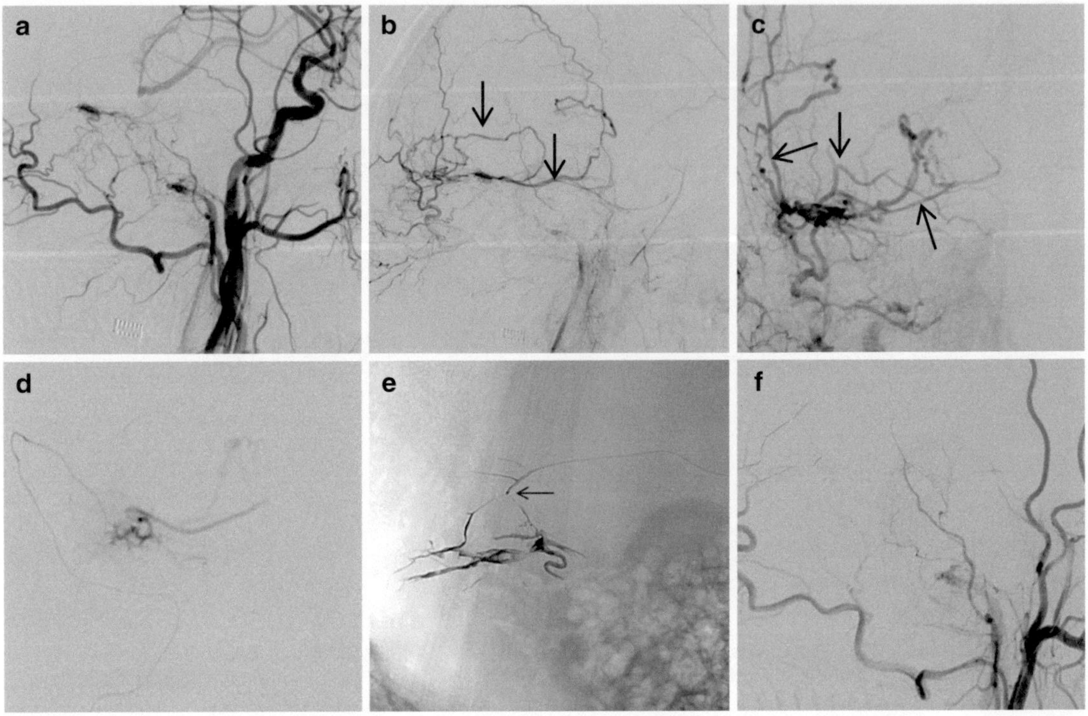

Fig. 67.3 (**a**) Right CCA angiogram lateral view reveals right transverse sinus dural AV fistula with feeders from the petrosal branch of the middle meningeal artery, transosseous branches of the occipital artery, and the neuromeningeal division of the ascending pharyngeal artery. Also noted is dural AV fistula of jugular bulb supplied by jugular division of the ascending pharyngeal artery. (**b** and **c**) Lateral and AP views of right ECA angiogram reveal extensive cortical venous reflux (arrows) with no forward flow in the right transverse sinus. (**d**) Microcatheter angiogram from MMA branch demonstrates dural AV fistula and cortical venous reflux. (**e**) Onyx cast with tip of microcatheter showed by arrow. (**f**) Post-embolization right ECA angiogram shows complete obliteration of the tentorial dural AV fistula with persistent opacification of the dural AV fistula of jugular bulb which was not treated

microcatheter maneuverability would be at its best. Henceforth, selective catheterization of the petrosal division of the right middle meningeal artery was done using Marathon 1.5 F (Covidien, Mansfield, MA) and Mirage 0.008″ (Covidien, Mansfield, MA) microguidewire. Once proximal to the fistula, Onyx was injected under biplane fluoroscopic guidance, and adequate penetration into the venous end of the fistula was achieved. Post-embolization angiogram revealed almost complete occlusion of the fistula (Fig. 67.3d–f). Small persistent shunt seen at the level of jugular bulb being fed by branch of ascending pharyngeal trunk; since it was draining antegrade without cortical reflux, it was spared.

MRI brain done at an interval of 3 weeks post procedure revealed significant reduction in the vasogenic edema. There was no mass effect with resolution of the midline shift and uncal herniation. The right lateral ventricle and the cisterns were normal in caliber.

Tips and Tricks

1. Dural sinus thrombosis commonly presents as brain hemorrhage that is associated with extensive edema. Recognizing an associated dural AVF can be critical for optimal management.
2. Progressive increase in vasogenic edema disproportionate to hematoma size suggests a worsening of intracranial venous hypertension due to the dural AV fistula. Understanding

the pathophysiological basis and early as opposed to delayed intervention is indicated in this group of patients.

3. Selective catheterization of the middle meningeal artery feeder is to be attempted first as better microcatheter maneuverability permits for navigating the catheter close to the nidus. This in turn allows for forming an occlusive plug of Onyx, thereby enabling better forward penetration of the embolic material.
4. Heating the Onyx allows for better forward penetration especially in low-flow malformations.

Suggested Reading

Fincher EF. Arteriovenous fistula between the middle meningeal artery and the greater petrosal sinus; case report. Ann Surg. 1951;133:886–8.

McConnell KA, Tjoumakaris SI, Allen J, et al. Neuroendovascular management of dural arteriovenous malformations. Neurosurg Clin N Am. 2009;20:431–9.

Narayanan S. Endovascular management of intracranial dural arteriovenous fistulas. Neurol Clin. 2010;28:899–911.

68 Dural AVF Embolization Using Proximal Balloon Catheter Occlusion Technique

Vipul Gupta

Case

A 48-year-old male presented with recurrent headaches associated with blurring of vision. Clinical examination was unremarkable. MRI of the brain revealed dilated vessels in sulcal spaces of right temporoparietal region. No evidence of parenchymal changes was seen (Fig. 68.1a, b). Cerebral DSA was performed via transfemoral route which revealed dural AVF in right temporal region with feeders from right middle meningeal and occipital arteries. Drainage was through dilated cortical veins into the superior sagittal and transverse sinuses. Cortical venous drainage carries significant risk of bleeding, and therefore it was decided to treat the malformation by embolization (Fig. 68.1d–f).

Issues

- One of the potential issues was the high risk of migration of Onyx into the cortical vein as the fistula appeared to be of high flow.
- The middle meningeal artery feeder was extremely dilated due to the high flow. Henceforth, creating a plug with Onyx can be challenging, and one would expect that reflux over the microcatheter for a long length can occur.

V. Gupta
Neurointerventional Surgery, Stroke Unit, Artemis Agrim Institute of Neuroscience, Gurgaon, India
e-mail: vipul.gupta@artemishospitals.com

Management

The procedure was performed under general anesthesia. A guiding catheter (Chaperone 5F) was placed in right ECA. A balloon catheter (Scepter XC 4 × 11, MicroVention, Inc.) was navigated into the right middle meningeal feeder over a microguidewire (Traxcess 0.014′, MicroVention, Inc.) (Fig. 68.1). The tip of the balloon catheter was placed near the site of fistula (Fig. 68.2a, b). Injection through the wire lumen (Fig. 68.2c, d) revealed high-flow fistula. The balloon was inflated under roadmap guidance (Fig. 68.2e) to completely occlude the feeding artery (Fig. 68.2f). Thereafter, Onyx injection was performed under blank road map. Due to the inflated balloon, no reflux was seen in the feeder vessel, and rapid penetration into the malformation and into the stem of the draining vein was achieved (Fig. 68.3a, b). Finally complete penetration onto the stem of the draining was seen, with reflux into the other feeders from right occipital and meningeal arteries, and the catheter was removed after deflating the balloon. Final angiogram revealed complete occlusion of the AVF. Patient made uneventful recovery.

V. Gupta et al. (eds.), *100 Interesting Case Studies in Neurointervention: Tips and Tricks*,
https://doi.org/10.1007/978-981-13-1346-2_68

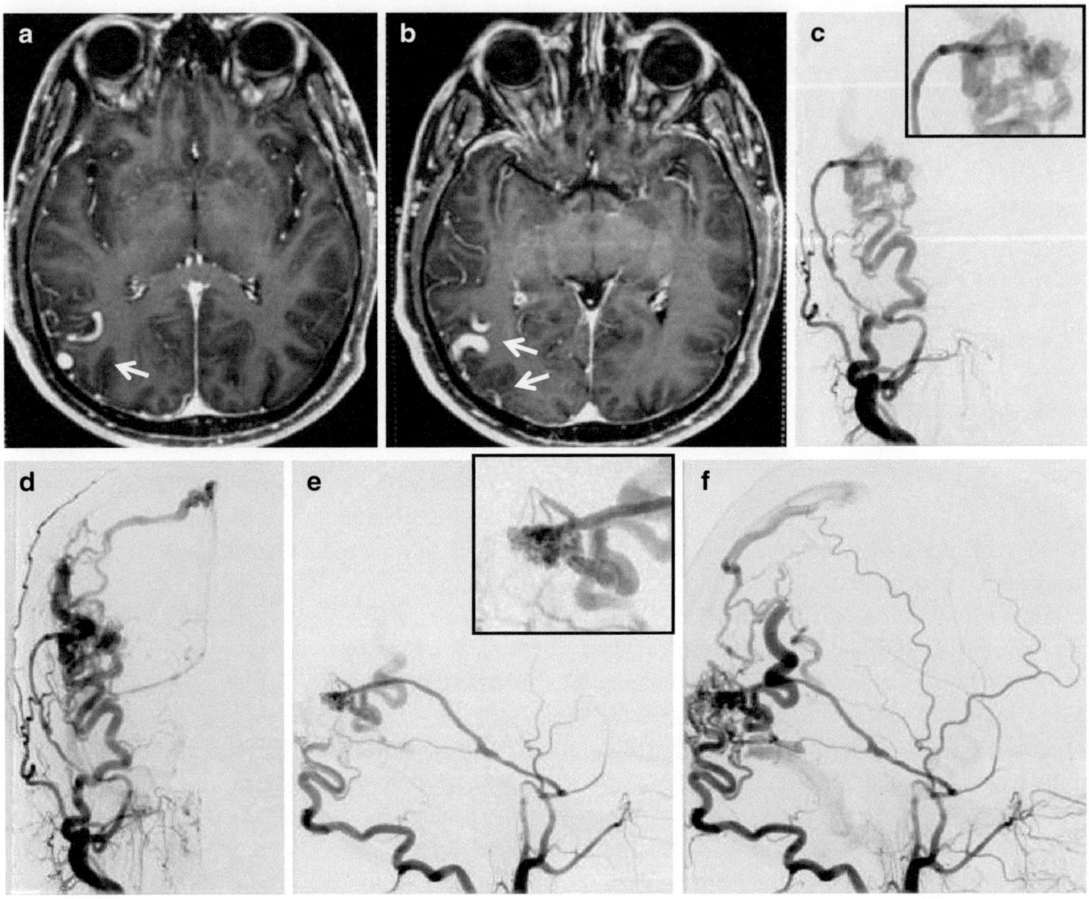

Fig. 68.1 (**a** and **b**) T1-weighted contrast-enhanced images reveal tortuous dilated vessels in right temporoparietal region. (**c**–**f**) Right ECA AP (**c**, **d**) and lateral (**e**, **f**) view revealed a dural AVF with feeders from right middle meningeal and occipital arteries, draining into cortical venous system and thereafter into the superior sagittal and transverse sinuses

Tips and Tricks

1. In high-flow malformations, Onyx injection can be injected through an onyx compatible double-lumen balloon catheter such as the scepter balloon.
2. Balloon inflation results in slowing of flow and therefore offers better control of the embolization material.
3. The balloon also prevents reflux of Onyx onto the parent vessel; this helps to avoid the time taken to form the plug with Onyx.

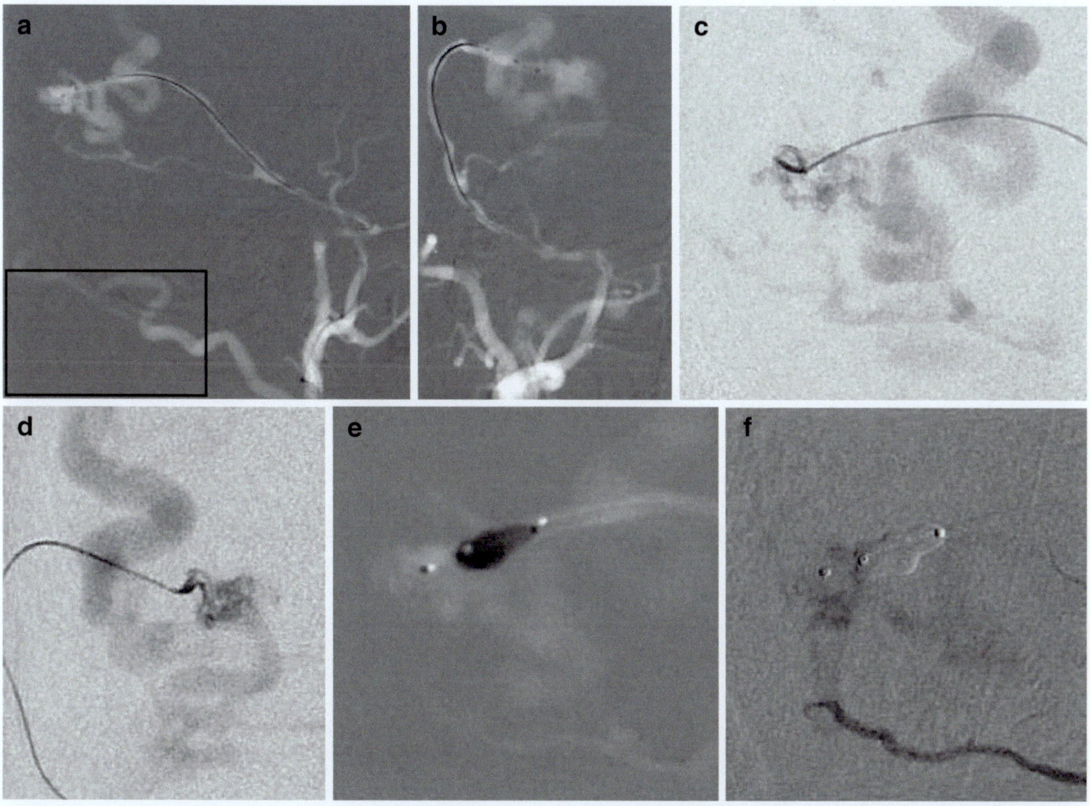

Fig. 68.2 (**a**, **b**) Roadmap images in lateral (**a**) and AP (**b**) view show the Scepter balloon catheter was placed over a microguidewire at the site of fistula. (**c**, **d**) Injection through the balloon catheter revealed a high-flow AVF. (**e**) Under road map, guidance balloon was inflated to occlude the feeding artery. (**f**) Injection through the guiding catheter confirmed complete occlusion of the middle meningeal branch; opacification of fistula is seen through other feeder vessels

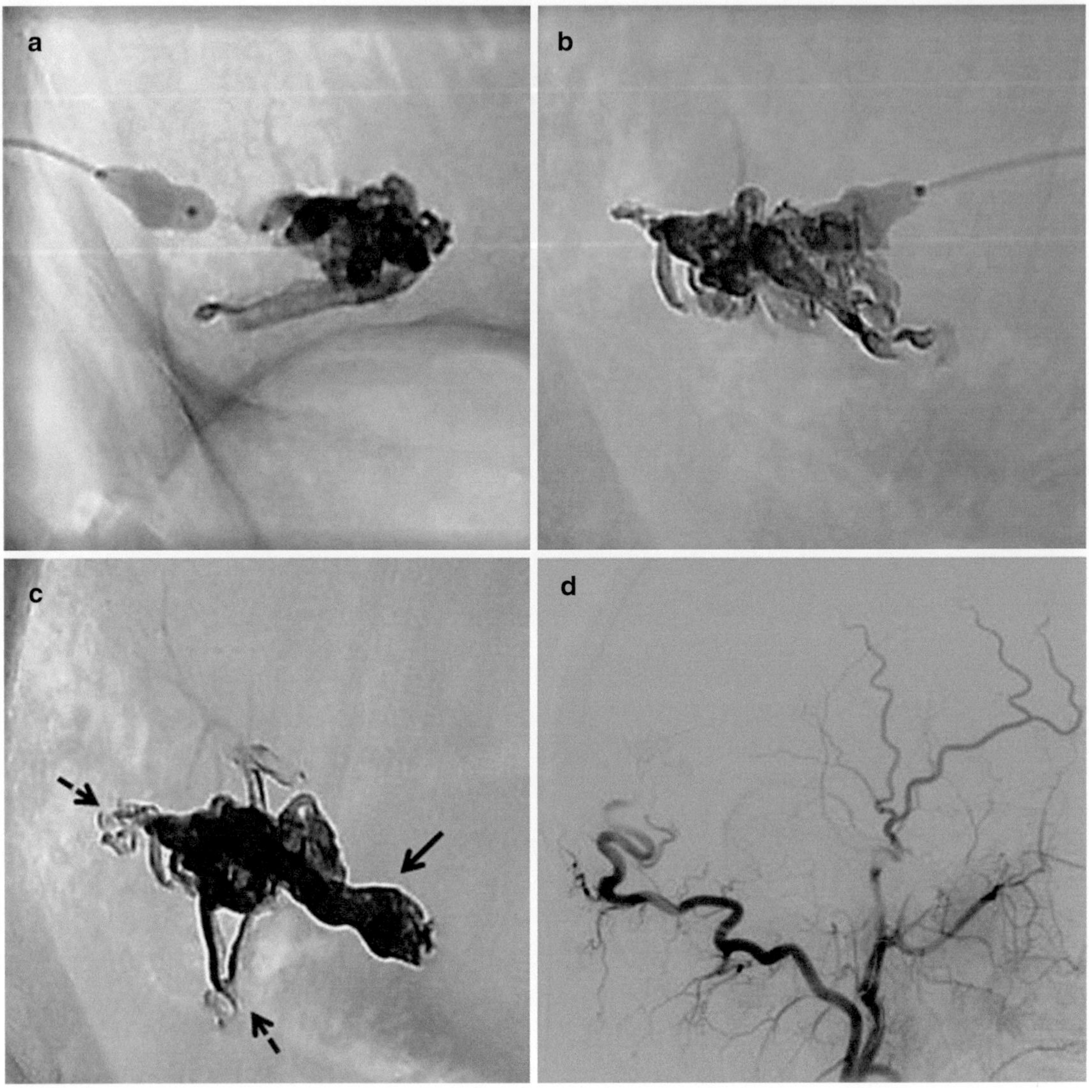

Fig. 68.3 (**a**, **b**) Onyx injection through the wire lumen of the balloon catheter. Note the lack of reflux in the parent vessel due to the inflated balloon. (**c**) Final Onyx cast, with complete occlusion of the fistula vein (arrow) as well as reflux of embolization material into all of the arterial feeders (dashed arrows). (**d**) Fistula is not seen anymore

Suggested Reading

Kim ST, et al. Onyx embolization of dural arteriovenous fistula, using Scepter C balloon catheter: a case report. Neurointervention. 2013;8(2):110–4.

Orozco LD, et al. Transarterial balloon assisted Onyx embolization of pericallosal arteriovenous malformations. J Neurointerv Surg. 2013;5(4):e18.

Small Cerebral AVM: Onyx Embolization

69

Vipul Gupta

Case

A 21-year-old male presented with sudden severe headache. CT and MRI revealed a small cerebral hematoma in the left parietal region. DSA was done 6 weeks after the hemorrhage. A small AVM was seen in left parietal region with feeder from parietal branch of left PCA (Fig. 69.1a, b). The draining vein was joining the superior sagittal sinus.

Issues

- Management strategy for the small AVM. In view of its size and location, it was considered amenable for surgery, embolization, and radiosurgery.
- With the history of hemorrhage, surgery or embolization leading to early occlusion was preferable. As there was a single feeder to this cortical AVM, there was high probability of complete occlusion with Onyx embolization.
- Ensuring complete occlusion during embolization and preventing bleeding during or after the intervention.

V. Gupta
Neurointerventional Surgery, Stroke Unit, Artemis Agrim Institute of Neuroscience, Gurgaon, India
e-mail: vipul.gupta@artemishospitals.com

Management

Embolization with Onyx was planned. The procedure was performed under general anesthesia. The guiding catheter was placed in left vertebral artery. Sonic 1.2 F (Balt, Balt Extrusion, Montmorency, France) microcatheter was navigated over microguidewire Mirage 0.008 microwire (ev3 Inc., Plymouth) to achieve an intra-nidal position of the microcatheter tip (Fig. 69.2a). The catheter was flushed with normal saline. DMSO was injected to fill the dead space of the microcatheter. Thereafter, Onyx was injected under roadmap guidance. A magnified view was used for visualization of the embolic material. The initial injection of Onyx resulted in penetration of the feeder and part of nidus (Fig. 69.2b). Angiogram revealed apparent complete occlusion of the fistula. Since Onyx hadn't penetrated whole of the nidus, embolization was continued. Further Onyx injection refluxed into parent vessel and thereafter penetrated the draining vein (Fig. 69.2d). The injection was continued until complete penetration of nidus (Fig. 69.2e) and perinidal vascular network (Fig. 69.2f, 69.3a, b) was achieved. At each stage a new road map was taken to clearly visualize the flow of embolic material. The total injection time was 17 min. The effect of heparin was reversed with protamine, and the microcatheter was detached by giving a gentle tug. Angio-CT did not reveal any

V. Gupta et al. (eds.), *100 Interesting Case Studies in Neurointervention: Tips and Tricks*,
https://doi.org/10.1007/978-981-13-1346-2_69

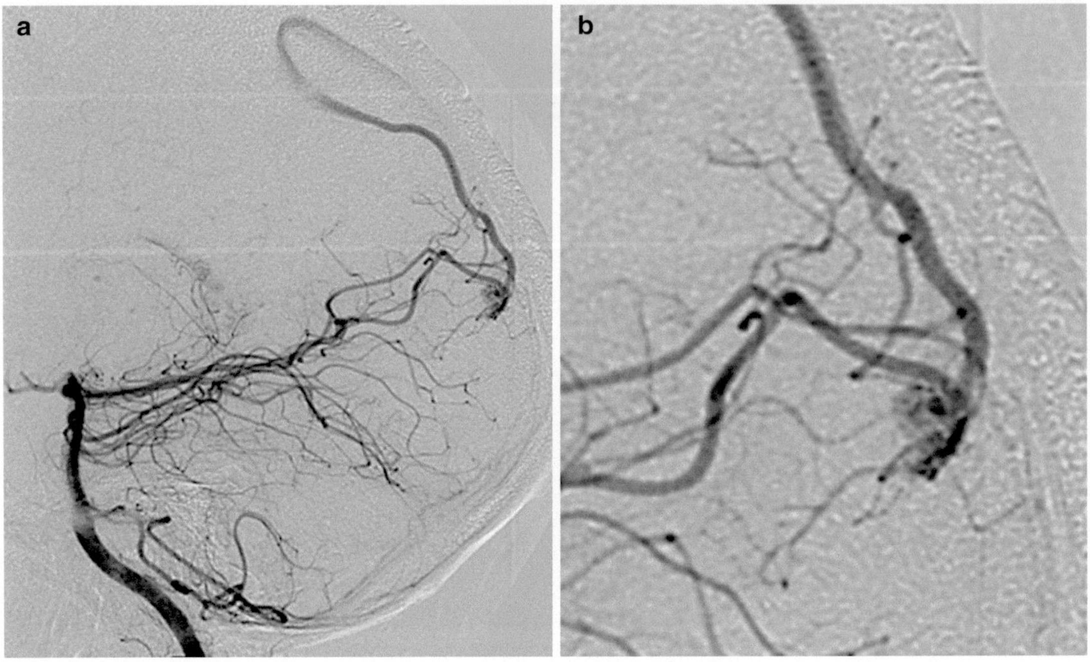

Fig. 69.1 (**a**) DSA image with vertebral injection revealing a small AVM in the parieto-occipital region. (**b**) Magnified image of the AVM

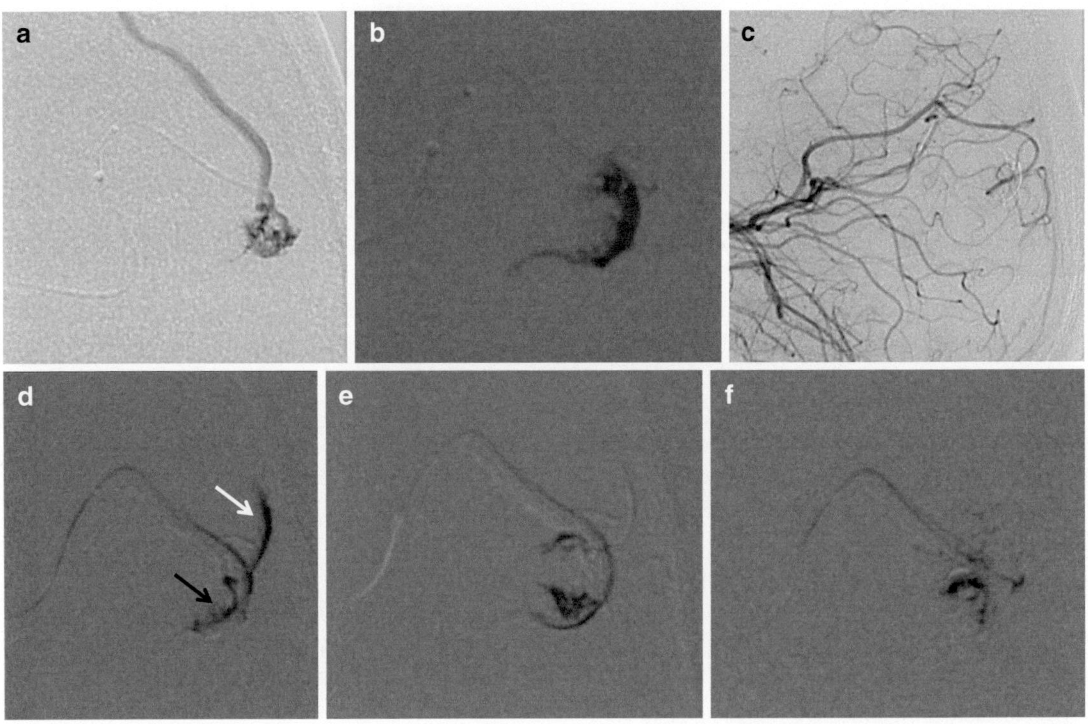

Fig. 69.2 (**a**) Microcatheter injection in the nidus. (**b**) Initial Onyx injection with partial penetration into the AVM. (**c**) DSA run showing apparent complete occlusion of the AVM. (**d–f**) Further Onyx injection. (**d**) Onyx penetration onto nidus, draining vein (*white arrow*) with reflux in parent artery (*black arrow*). (**e**) Penetration in the nidus. (**f**) Penetration into adjacent vascular network

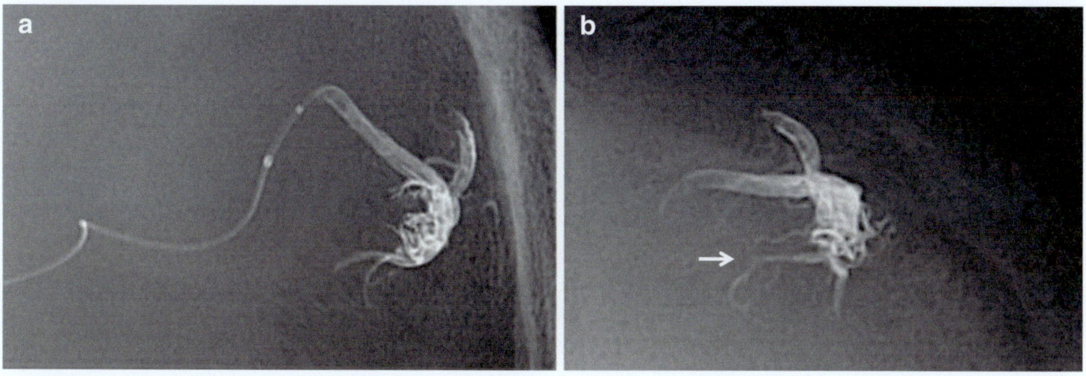

Fig. 69.3 (**a** and **b**) Show native images showing the Onyx cast. Note that the whole of nidus has been occluded by the embolization material (as compared to image 1**b**). Adjacent network (*arrow*, **b**) which may be very small feeders not appreciated on pre-embolization DSA has been well penetrated

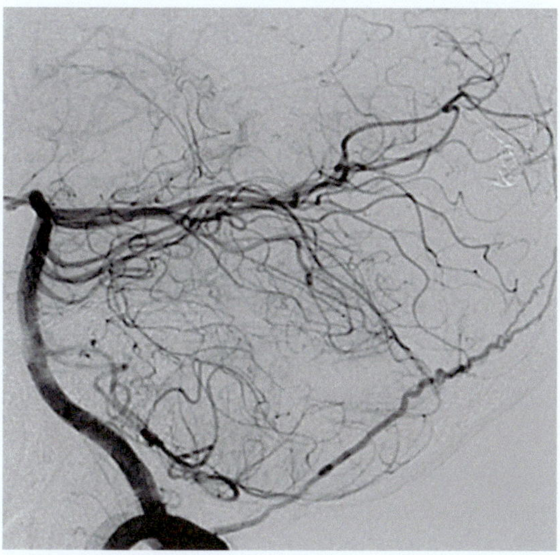

Fig. 69.4 Post-embolization image showing complete occlusion with preservation of normal arteries

fresh bleeding. Immediate post procedure cerebral angiography revealed complete occlusion of the nidus (Fig. 69.4). The mean arterial blood pressure was kept slightly lower than normal and the patient was extubated the next day, and was neurologically intact. The mean arterial blood pressure was kept slightly lower than normal during this period. Follow-up angiogram at 6 months did not reveal any recurrence of the AVM (Figs. 69.3 and 69.4).

Tips and Tricks

1. Every effort should be made to penetrate the complete nidal network during embolization of AVMs. Angiographic occlusion may be noted once the feeding artery is embolized; if the procedure is stopped at this stage, there is a high chance of recanalization of the part of nidus which has not been penetrated by the embolic material.
2. There may be perinidal vascularity that may not be seen on the DSA images. This may represent minute feeder vessels to the AVM. One should aim to penetrate the perinidal vascular network to prevent recurrence. Very small residual nidus fed by these small feeders may result in post-embolization bleeding particularly if the draining vein is occluded.
3. High-resolution fluoroscopy is critical for embolization using Onyx, and we prefer to perform under high magnification during the procedure.

Suggested Reading

van Rooija WJ, Sluzewskia M, Beuteb GN. Brain AVM embolization with Onyx. Am J Neuroradiol. 2007;28:172–7.

70 Cerebral Hematoma with a Micro-AVM: Intra-Arterial DynaCT Angiography-Guided Surgical Excision

Vipul Gupta

Case

A 16-year-old boy presented with sudden-onset severe headache along with right hemiplegia. His level of consciousness was intact. CT scan revealed a hematoma in left posterior frontal region (Fig. 70.1a). DSA revealed a fine network of vessels fed by slightly enlarged cortical branch of left MCA (Fig. 70.1b). Very small aneurysm (white arrow in Fig. 70.1b, c) was seen in the upper part of the abnormal vascularity with a barely discernable draining vein from inferior aspect of the network. Micro-AVM was suspected along with a pseudoaneurysm.

Issues

- Management of a small AVM in an eloquent region of the brain.
- In view of the associated aneurysm, early occlusion of the AVM is desirable to prevent rebleeding.
- Because of very small feeding artery, it was considered not amenable for intra-arterial embolization.
- Such a small AVM could be difficult to localize during surgery. Secondly, surgical excision could result in further injury in the motor cortex region.

Management

Intra-arterial DynaCT angiography was performed with intra-arterial injection of contrast after placing a diagnostic catheter in the proximal ICA (Fig. 70.2a–c). A DynaCT dataset (rotational dataset of CT projections) was acquired using a flat-panel monitor angiography suite (Artis Zee with DynaCT; Siemens, Erlangen, Germany) and the 20s DCT Head 70 kv program. Multiplanar reconstructions were generated with a dedicated workstation (Leonardo model, Siemens). This three-dimensional protocol includes the injection of 18 mL Omnipaque contrast medium mixed with 42 mL normal saline through a power injection syringe. A continuous contrast injection at 1 cc/s was performed during the entire 19-s image acquisition and 3-s X-ray delay. The DynaCT was performed with 0.4° increments, 512 matrix algorithm, 200° total angle, and approximately 30 frames/s, for a total of 496 projections.

Intra-arterial DynaCT angiography clearly demonstrated the small AVM in all the planes. The malformation stretched along the postero-medial aspect of hematoma. The aneurysm

V. Gupta
Neurointerventional Surgery, Stroke Unit, Artemis Agrim Institute of Neuroscience, Gurgaon, India
e-mail: vipul.gupta@artemishospitals.com

V. Gupta et al. (eds.), *100 Interesting Case Studies in Neurointervention: Tips and Tricks*,
https://doi.org/10.1007/978-981-13-1346-2_70

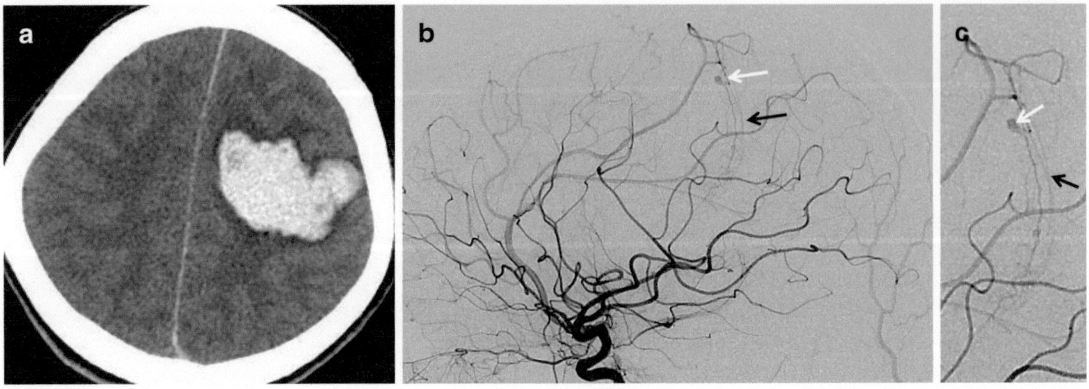

Fig. 70.1 (**a**) CT scan image showing left frontal hematoma. (**b**) DSA with intra-arterial injection in left ICA showing a leash of vessels in left parietal region with a small aneurysmal dilatation (white arrow). (**c**) Magnified view of abnormal region in image **b**, clearly showing the abnormal vascularity

could be localized (arrow, Fig. 70.2a), and the draining vein was noted to originate from the inferior aspect of nidus (lower arrow, Fig. 70.2b, c). The DynaCT angiography images could be transferred to image guidance system in the operation theater. Surgical excision of the AVM along with hematoma was performed under general anesthesia. The nidus could be localized on the basis of the DynaCT angiographic images facilitating the surgery. Follow-up angiography did not reveal any residual AVM. On follow-up, patient had partial recovery of his motor deficits.

Tips and Tricks

1. Very small AVMs associated with large hematomas may not be readily apparent. DSA images should be carefully scrutinized for abnormal vessels and early draining vein. Intra-arterial DynaCT angiography may help in confirming the presence of AVM in the wall of the hematoma.
2. Intra-arterial DynaCT angiography is very useful to determine the location of AVM nidus relative to the hematoma.
3. The spatial resolution of intra-arterial DynaCT angiography is more than conventional CT scanner, and it can be performed along with the DSA in cases with cerebral AVMs.
4. Intra-arterial DynaCT angiography images can be used in image guidance system during surgery. This helps in localization of AVM in relation with the hematoma and normal parenchyma.

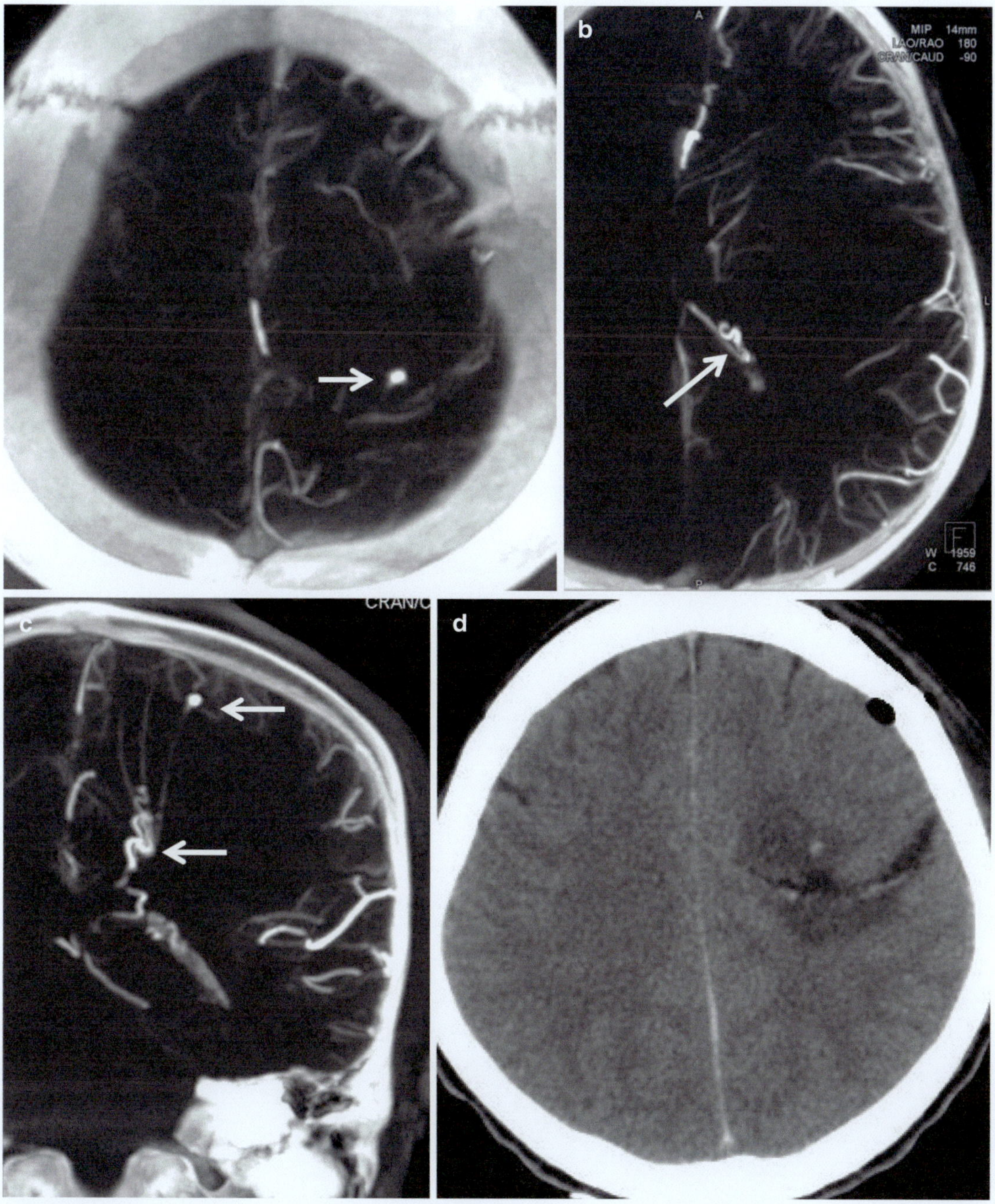

Fig. 70.2 (**a**–**c**) DynaCT angiography images with intra-arterial injection of contrast. (**a**) The small aneurysm seen in posterior aspect of hematoma. (**b**) Small network of vessels leading to a dilated vein. (**c**) Coronal image showing entire malformation in profile including the aneurysm (upper arrow) and the draining vein (lower arrow). (**d**) Postoperative CT with complete excision of the hematoma

Suggested Reading

Gupta V, Chugh M, Walia BS, Vaishya S, Jha AN. Use of CT angiography for anatomic localization of arteriovenous malformation Nidal components. Am J Neuroradiol. 2008;29(10):1837–40.

Mossa-Basha M, Chen J, Gandhi D. Imaging of cerebral arteriovenous malformations and dural arteriovenous fistulas. Neurosurg Clin N Am. 2012;23(1):27–42.

AVM with Haematoma: Embolization and Surgery in Single Session

71

Vipul Gupta

Case

A 24-year-old male presented with severe headache. He was drowsy but arousable and followed verbal commands. He didn't have any focal deficits. CT scan revealed large right frontal haematoma with midline shift (Fig. 71.1a). DSA revealed a moderate-sized AVM with feeders from right ACA and MCA cortical branches (Fig. 71.1b) with venous drainage into superior sagittal sinus.

Issues

- Management considerations include surgical excision and endovascular embolization followed by surgery and radiosurgery.
- Timing of the procedure.

Management

Endovascular embolization followed by surgical excision was considered the most appropriate management strategy. Patient was given general anaesthesia in the angiography suite. A guiding catheter (6F Envoy, Codman & Shurtleff, Inc., USA) was placed in left ICA. A microcatheter with detachable tip (Sonic 1.2 F, Balt Extrusion, Montmorency, France) was placed in a feeder from left ACA, and the AVM was embolized using Onyx (Fig. 71.1c). Post-embolization angiogram showed more than 90% occlusion of the AVM with small patchy residual component (Fig. 71.1d). Post-embolization DynaCT did not reveal any fresh haemorrhage. Patient was shifted to the operating theatre, and surgical excision of AVM along with the haematoma was performed. Surgery was uneventful with blood loss of less than 150 mL. Postoperative CT revealed complete excision of haematoma with decrease in mass effect (Fig. 71.1e). Patient was extubated in intact clinical condition. He made complete recovery, and follow-up angiogram did not reveal any residual AVM (Fig. 71.1f).

V. Gupta
Neurointerventional Surgery, Stroke Unit, Artemis Agrim Institute of Neuroscience, Gurgaon, India
e-mail: vipul.gupta@artemishospitals.com

Tips and Tricks

1. The risk of a repeat rupture is higher when an AVM has bled. We prefer to perform surgery or embolization in such cases to achieve early occlusion. Radiosurgery is reserved for malformations that are not amenable to other methods of treatment and for residual AVM after surgery or embolization.
2. In this patient, we decided to perform embolization followed by surgery. Embolization prior to surgery facilitates surgical excision

V. Gupta et al. (eds.), *100 Interesting Case Studies in Neurointervention: Tips and Tricks*,
https://doi.org/10.1007/978-981-13-1346-2_71

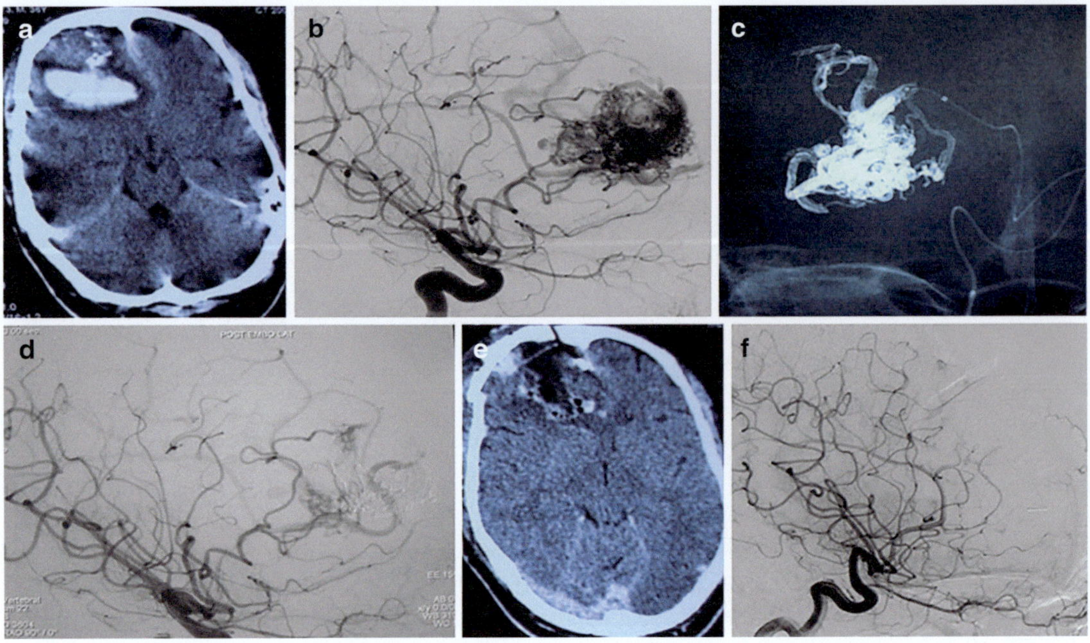

Fig. 71.1 (**a**) CT scan showing right frontal haematoma with mass effect. (**b**) Right ICA angiogram reveals AVM with feeders from right ACA and MCA. (**c**) Onyx embolization with a detachable tip microcatheter. (**d**) Post-embolization DSA shows small residual AVM. (**e**) Post-embolization CT after excision of AVM and haematoma. (**f**) Follow-up angiogram showing complete obliteration of the AVM

with reduced incidence of complications. We prefer to perform both the procedures in the same session under general anaesthesia with surgery being performed soon after the embolization. This reduces the risk of post-embolization haematoma since the entire malformation is excised soon after the embolization. The combined approach ensures early complete occlusion of the AVM and evacuation of the haematoma.

3. We always perform DynaCT after the embolization to determine if haemorrhage occurred during the intervention.
4. Surgeons usually find it easier to manipulate the AVM after embolization with Onyx as compared to glue.

Suggested Reading

van Rooij WJ, Jacobs S, Sluzewski M, et al. Endovascular treatment of ruptured brain AVMs in the acute phase of hemorrhage. Am J Neuroradiol. 2012;33(6):1162–6.

Cerebral Hematoma with AVM: Intra-Arterial DynaCT Angiography-Guided Targeted Embolization and Balloon-Assisted Catheterization

72

Vipul Gupta

Case

A 40-year-old female presented with sudden-onset severe headache. CT scan revealed callosal bleed. DSA showed an AVM with intranidal/perinidal aneurysm (white arrow). A venous aneurysm (black arrows) was also seen associated with a small fistula with the feeder from the lenticulostriate artery (Fig. 72.1).

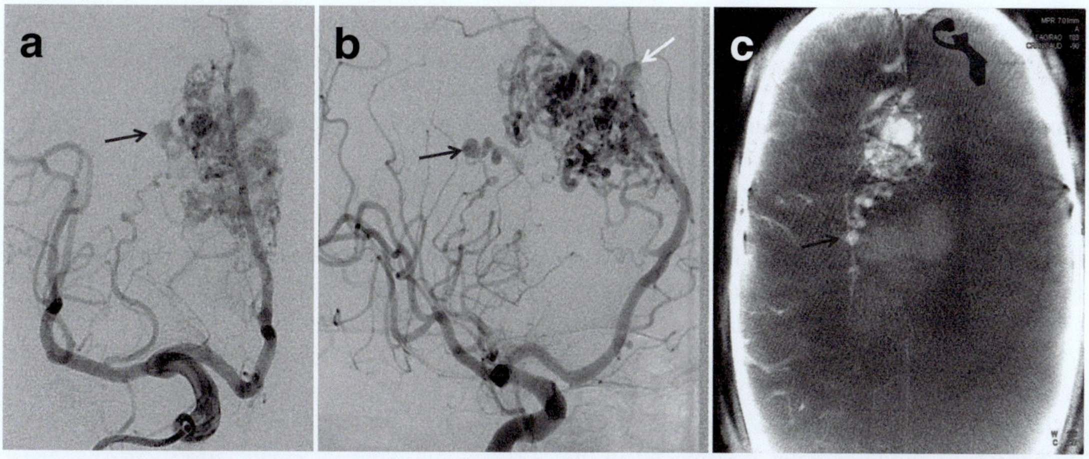

Fig. 72.1 (**a** and **b**) DSA AP and oblique views showing the AVM with intranidal/perinidal aneurysms (white arrow). A venous aneurysm (black arrows) was seen associated with a small fistula with the feeder from lenticulostriate artery. (**c**) Intra-arterial DynaCT angiography with intra-arterial contrast injection image showing bleed in corpus callosum with an aneurysm in the wall of the hematoma

V. Gupta
Neurointerventional Surgery, Stroke Unit,
Artemis Agrim Institute of Neuroscience,
Gurgaon, India
e-mail: vipul.gupta@artemishospitals.com

V. Gupta et al. (eds.), *100 Interesting Case Studies in Neurointervention: Tips and Tricks*,
https://doi.org/10.1007/978-981-13-1346-2_72

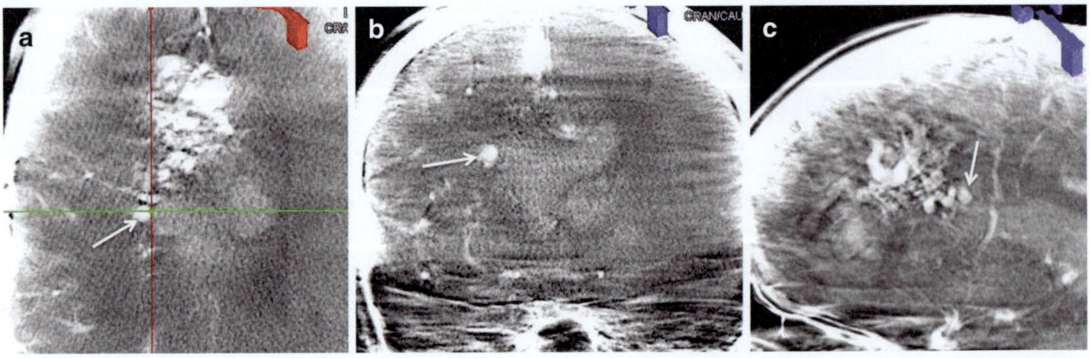

Fig. 72.2 Axial (**a**), coronal (**b**), and sagittal (**c**) reconstructions reveal that the aneurysm was located in the wall of the hematoma in all the three planes, indicating it to be the most probable site of bleeding

Issues

- Determining the weak spot: is it the nidal or the venous aneurysm that has bled?
- Catheterizing the lenticulostriate artery that has reverse origin from the M1 MCA.

Management

Procedure was performed under GA. Intra-arterial DynaCT angiography was performed with intra-arterial injection of contrast after placing a diagnostic catheter in the proximal ICA (Fig. 72.2a–c). Intra-arterial DynaCT angiography clearly demonstrated that the venous aneurysm and not the nidal aneurysm is the likely cause for bleeding. This was evident by the close correlation between the venous aneurysm to the hematoma wall in all planes (Fig. 72.2). A guide catheter was placed in the right petrous ICA. Following that, the Magic microcatheter 1.2 FM (Balt Inc.) was taken over a Hybrid 0.007′ microwire. Due to the reverse origin of the lenticulostriate artery, it was anticipated that catheterizing the perforator can be challenging. A double-lumen balloon was inflated beyond the origin of the lenticulostriate artery to provide the necessary support for the glue microcatheter. The microcatheter could not be navigated distally, and therefore dilute glue 25% was used to embolize the venous aneurysm (Fig. 72.3). Post-procedure DynaCT revealed glue cast in the venous aneurysm (Fig. 72.4). The venous aneurysm was not visualized on DSA runs. The patient made near-complete recovery.

Tips and Tricks

1. Intra-arterial DynaCT angiography is very useful to determine spatial relation of AVM nidus to the hematoma. Due to the high spatial resolution, the relationship of the weak spot (aneurysm) to the hematoma wall can be determined with certainty.
2. Catheterizing a small artery arising in a reverse fashion from a larger artery can be extremely challenging. One can consider using a balloon to serve as a temporary scaffold for the glue microcatheter while catheterizing the lenticulostriate artery.

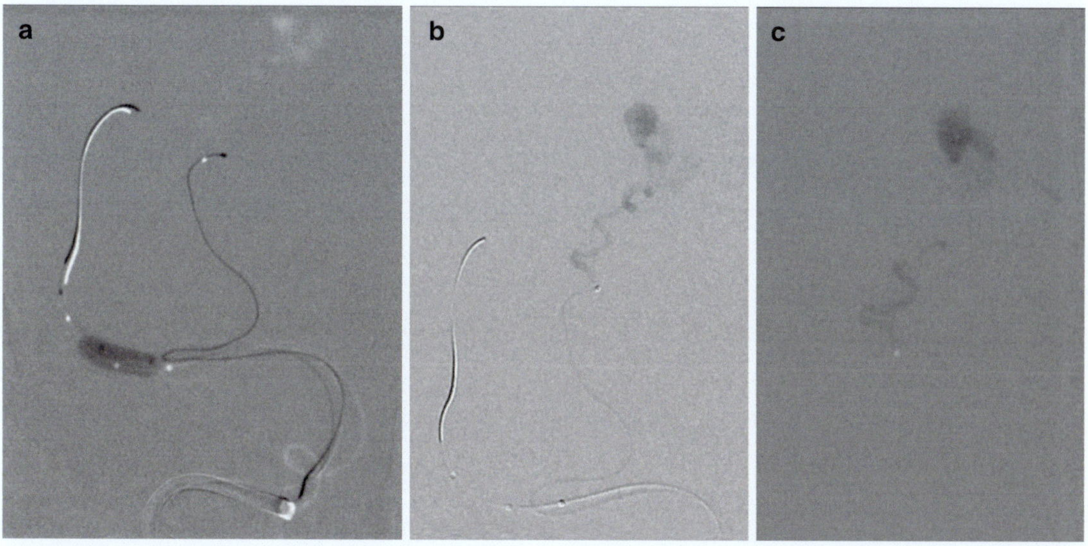

Fig. 72.3 (**a**) Road map image showing inflated balloon in the MCA just beyond the origin of the lenticulostriate feeder. The microcatheter has been placed in the feeder with the support of the balloon. (**b**) Microcatheter injection showing the small fistula with venous aneurysm. (**c**) Road map image showing the glue cast

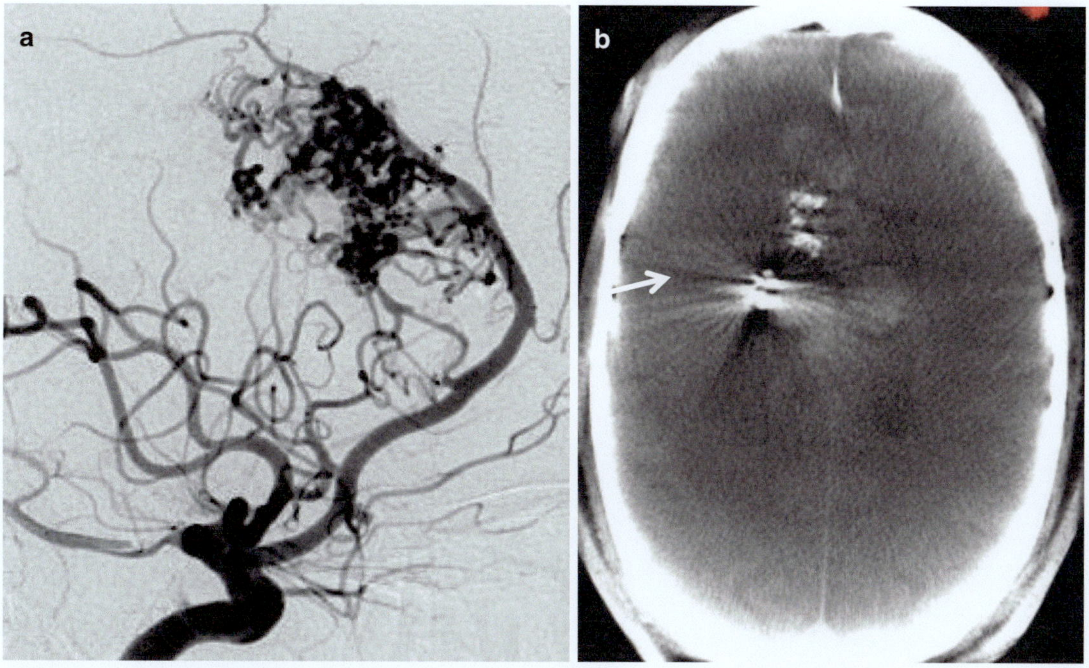

Fig. 72.4 (**a**) Post-embolization DSA showing complete occlusion of the aneurysm. (**b**) Post-embolization DynaCT image confirming the glue cast (shown by arrow) in the aneurysm

Suggested Reading

Gupta V, Chugh M, Walia BS, Vaishya S, Jha AN. Use of CT angiography for anatomic localization of arteriovenous malformation Nidal components. Am J Neuroradiol. 2008;29(10):1837–40.

Mossa-Basha M, Chen J, Gandhi D. Imaging of cerebral arteriovenous malformations and dural arteriovenous fistulas. Neurosurg Clin N Am. 2012;23(1):27–42.

High-Flow Pial AVF: Safety Considerations—Detachable Tip Microcatheter and Proximal Balloon Occlusion Technique

73

Aviraj Deshmukh, Rajsrinivas Parthasarathy, and Vipul Gupta

Case

A 27-year-old female presented with headache of 6 months duration. NCCT head revealed high density, extra-axial large vascular sacs in right parieto-occipital region (Fig. 73.1a). DSA showed a very high-flow single-hole pial fistula with large venous sacs, fed by cortical branch of the inferior division of right middle cerebral artery and draining into superior sagittal sinus (Fig. 73.1b, c).

Issues

1. Difficulty in controlling embolic material in high-flow fistula; the risk of distal migration of material is a cause for concern.
2. Treatment options considered were:
   (a) High concentration glue alone.
   (b) Coils followed by glue.
   (c) Proximal occlusion with balloon with glue embolization.
   (d) Onyx with/without balloon.
3. Risk of hyperperfusion bleeding after the procedure.

Management

Procedure was performed via right transfemoral route under general anaesthesia. 6 F, 70-cm-long sheath (Rabbe, Cook) was used. A 6 F80 cm guiding catheter (Neuron, Penumbra Inc.) was placed in right cavernous ICA. At the outset, two microcatheters were used in an attempt to form a stable coil mass by means of interlocking. Due to the extremely high flow, a stable cage could not be formed (Fig. 73.2a).

As a fallback strategy, to reduce the flow, a transform balloon (Stryker, 7 × 15 mm) over a microwire (014′ synchro, Stryker Neurovascular) was navigated to the distal part of MCA feeder and inflated. However, DSA run revealed rapid filling of the fistula through collaterals despite balloon occlusion of the feeder (Fig. 73.2b). Henceforth, the balloon was repositioned in proximal M1 MCA to achieve flow reduction in both MCA branches (Fig. 73.2c, d). Despite that, coils were not stable due to brisk flow in the fistula.

Strategy was changed, and it was planned to use glue for embolization with proximal MCA occlusion with balloon. Apollo microcather

A. Deshmukh
Neurointerventional Surgery, Artemis Agrim Institute of Neuroscience, Gurgaon, India

R. Parthasarathy
Vascular Neurology and Neurointerventional Surgery, Artemis Agrim Institute of Neuroscience, Gurgaon, India

V. Gupta (✉)
Neurointerventional Surgery, Stroke Unit, Artemis Agrim Institute of Neuroscience, Gurgaon, India
e-mail: vipul.gupta@artemishospitals.com

V. Gupta et al. (eds.), *100 Interesting Case Studies in Neurointervention: Tips and Tricks*,
https://doi.org/10.1007/978-981-13-1346-2_73

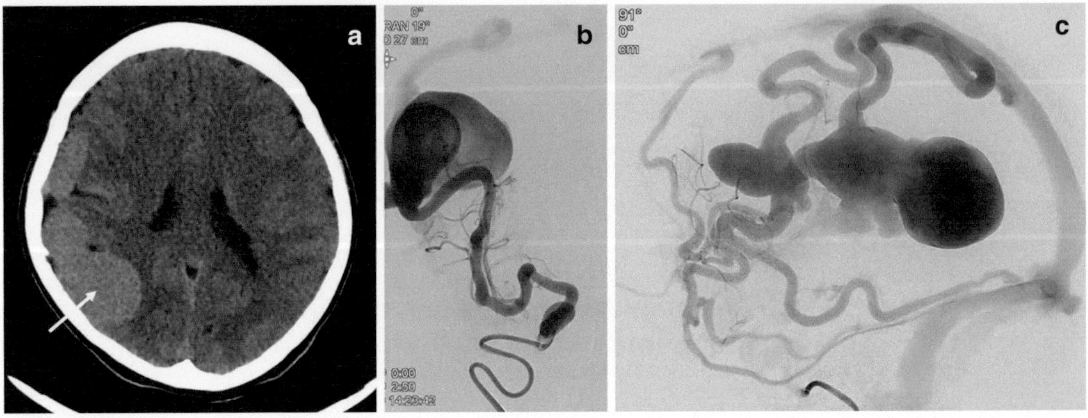

Fig. 73.1 (**a**) Dilated venous sacs on ncct brain. (**b**) Right ica injection revealed a very high flow single hole pial av fistula with large venous sacs , fed by cortical branch of inferior division of MCA. (**c**) Extensive venous congestion & drainage into the superior sagittal sinus

(1.5 F, 3 cm detachable tip) was positioned in a feeder branch with tip abutting the wall of the feeder artery to achieve better control of the glue. High concentration (80% glue, *N*-butyl cyanoacrylate) glue was used to reduce the risk of distal migration of glue into the venous sinuses.

Glue was injected under DSA run. Initial rapid injection allows for layering along the wall of the feeder artery. Following that the rate of injection is slowed to obtain penetration of the fistulous site with typical cauliflower-like appearance (Fig. 73.3a–f). Reflux on to the microcatheter was noted, and injection was stopped. The balloon was deflated, and DSA run revealed a slow-flow residual fistula. Further glue injection was undertaken with deflated balloon; glue penetration of the fistula was noted. Post-procedure run revealed stasis in venous sacs with some filling of the sacs from small tiny vessels which are likely to represent secondary angiogenetic vessels (Fig. 73.4a, b). Post-procedure NCCT head revealed no evidence of haemorrhage (Fig. 73.4c). DSA was repeated again on Day 3 post procedure. It revealed complete cure of the fistula without any residual filling of the sacs (Fig. 73.5a, b).

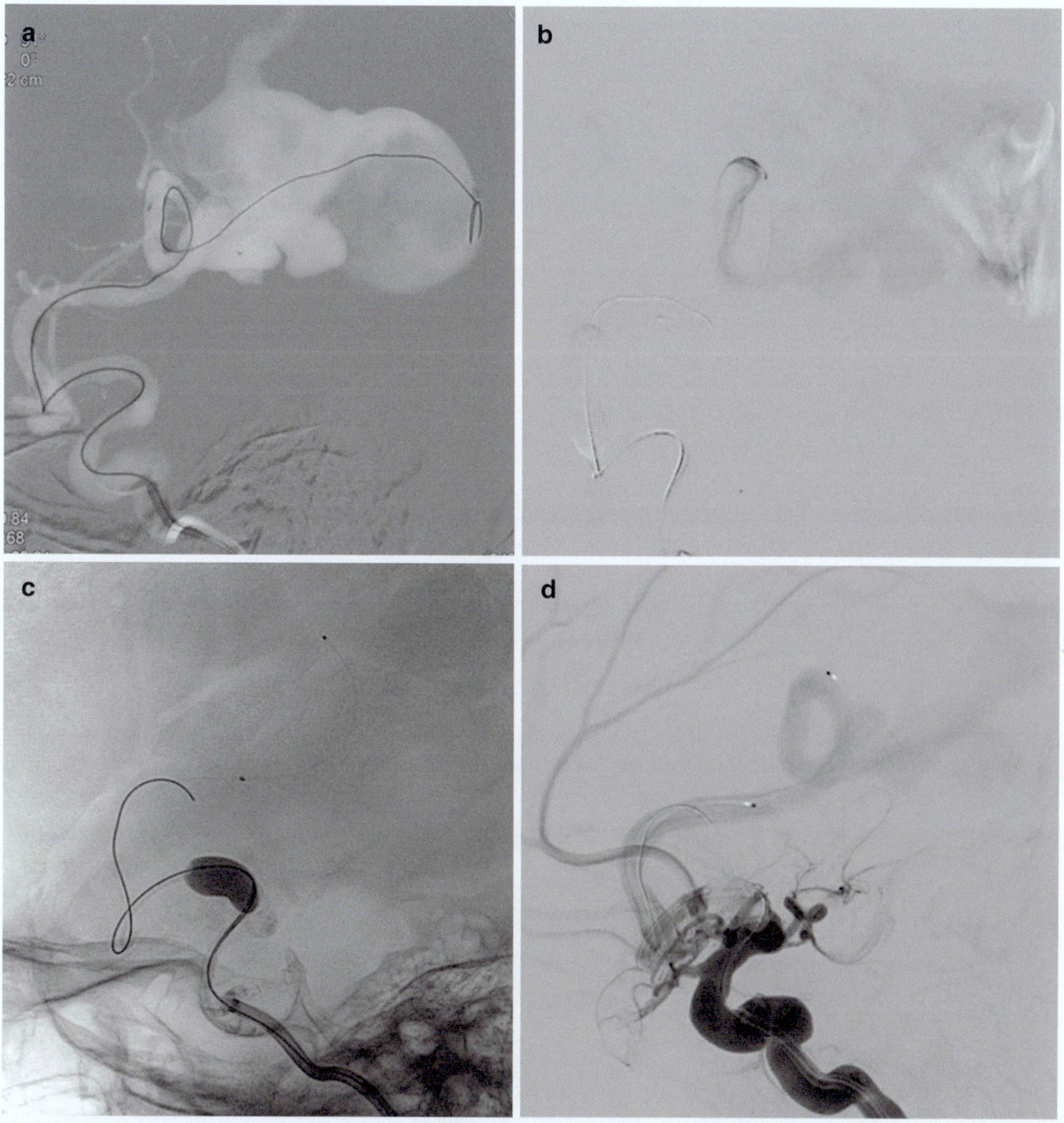

Fig. 73.2 (**a**) Distal migration of the loop due to high flow; note two microcatheters in place to attempt dual microcatheter technique. (**c**) Balloon placement in the main MCA trunk. (**b**, **d**) Flow assessment with inflated balloon and detachable tip microcatheter

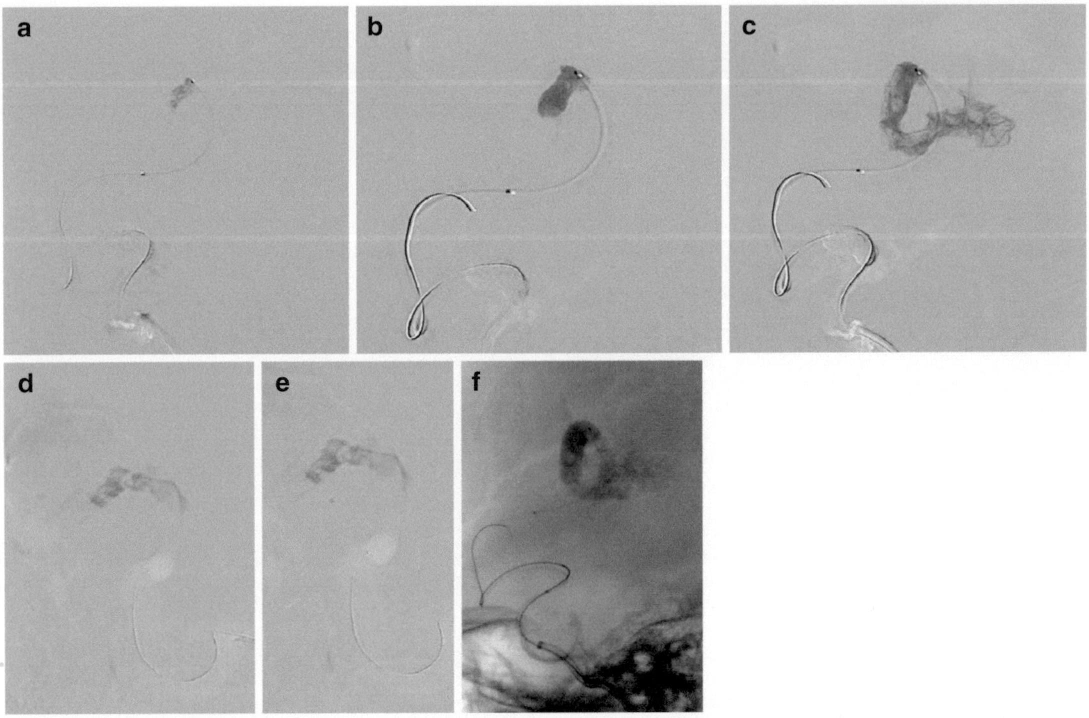

Fig. 73.3 (**a**-**f**) Initial rapid injection allows for layering along the wall of the feeder artery. Following that, the rate of injection is slowed to obtain penetration of the fistulous site with typical cauliflower-like appearance

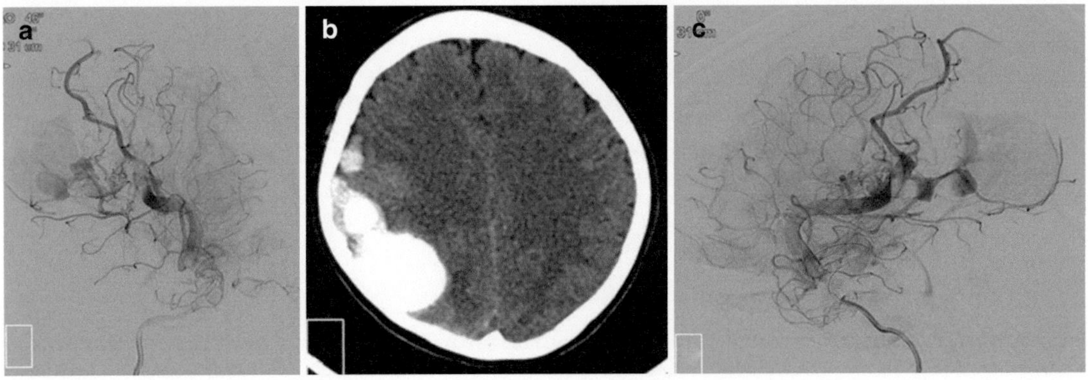

Fig. 73.4 Post-procedure run revealed stasis in venous sacs with some filling of the sacs from small tiny vessels which are likely to represent secondary angiogenetic vessels (**a** and **b**). Post-procedure NCCT head revealed no evidence of haemorrhage (**c**)

Tips and Tricks

1. It is always difficult to control the glue in embolization of high-flow fistula. There is always a risk of distal embolization of the material into the venous system in such cases, leading to venous thrombosis. Considerable operator experience is required in such cases for controlling the glue.
2. Strategic poisoning of the balloon in the proximal part of MCA helped us to achieve maximum reduction in the flow of the fistula.

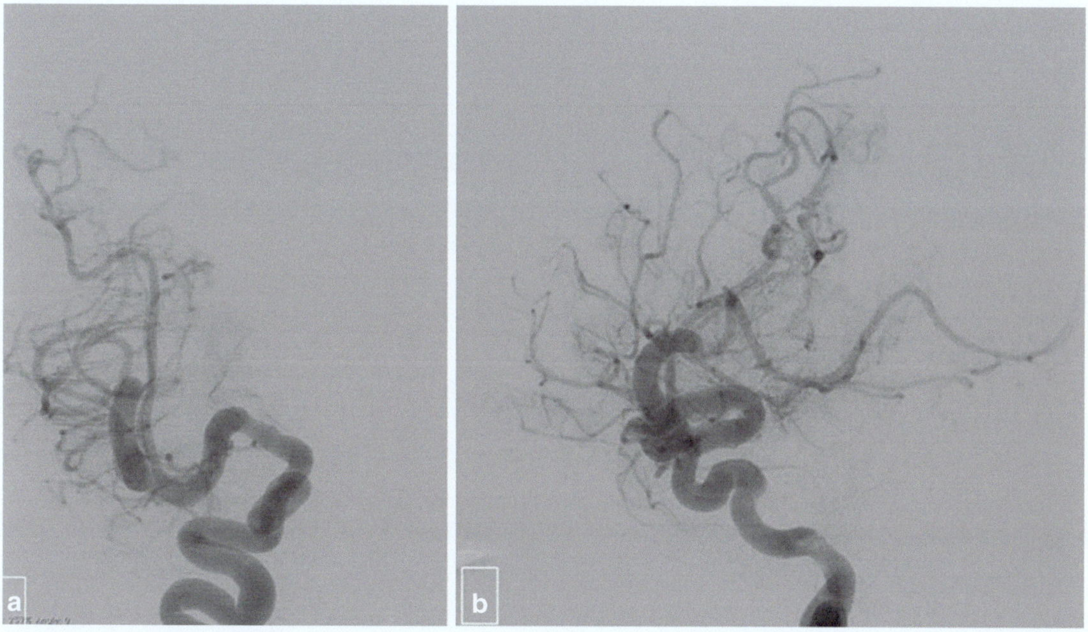

Fig. 73.5 DSA was repeated again on Day 3 post procedure. It revealed complete cure of the fistula without any residual filling of the sacs (**a** and **b**)

3. Microcatheter positioning with tip abutting the wall of the feeder vessel helped us to control the glue. Initial injection is fast to achieve layering followed by slow injection to achieve penetration.
4. Detachable tip microcatheter gave us a time for deflation of the balloon and removal of the microcatheter. It also provided us margin for retrograde filling of the feeder so that complete penetration of the fistula was achieved.
5. Small residual feeders in the wall usually gets thrombosed with time once fistulous site is completely embolized.

Suggested Reading

Limaye US, et al. Endovascular management of intracranial pial arterio-venous fistulas. Neurol India. 2004;52:87–90.

Paramasivam S, et al. Development, clinical presentation and endovascular management of congenital intracranial pial arteriovenous fistulas. J Neurointerv Surg. 2013;5(3):184–90. https://doi.org/10.1136/neurintsurg-2011-010241.

Acutely Ruptured Arteriovenous Malformation (AVM) with Venous Aneurysm: En Passage Feeder—Endovascular Strategy

74

Aviraj Deshmukh, Rajsrinivas Parthasarathy, and Vipul Gupta

Case

An eighteen year old male patient presented to the emergency room with headache, nausea and vomiting, and left hemianopia. CT showed right occipitotemporal hematoma (Fig. 74.1a, b). DSA was done which revealed patchy, compressed AVM nidus with multiple small feeders from the temporal branch of the right PCA and drainage into the right transverse sinus, along with evidence of venous aneurysm (Fig. 74.2c, d).

Issues

1. Urgency of treatment of AVM in acute phase due to the presence of intra-nidal venous aneurysm.
2. Compressed AVM nidus due to the presence of hematoma leading to difficulty in delineating AVM anatomy.
3. Possible presence of en passage feeders from the temporal branch of PCA.

Management

Procedure was performed via right transfemoral route under general anesthesia. 6 Fr guiding Envoy was placed in the right vertebral artery and advanced up to V2 segment of the right vertebral artery. 3D angiography was done to delineate the AVM anatomy, which revealed at least three small AVM feeders arising from the temporal branch of PCA (Fig. 74.3a, b). 3D surface-shaded display allowed for better visualization of AVM nidus and its feeders (Fig. 74.3c, d). In these views road map was taken, and Apollo microcatheter (1.5F, 165 cm, Covidien) with 3 cm detachable tip was navigated over Mirage micro-guidewire (008, 200 cm, Covidien) into the temporal branch of the right PCA. Super-selective microcatheter run showed multiple small feeders arising from the artery, and distal artery showed to and fro flow, suggesting the possibility of its en passage nature (Fig. 74.4a). Microcatheter was slightly withdrawn from its distal position so as to have enough length of catheter for adequate plug formation and penetration into the feeders (Fig. 74.4b). Onyx 18 was injected under fluoroscopic guidance, and penetration of AVM feeders was achieved (Fig. 74.5a).

A. Deshmukh
Neurointerventional Surgery, Artemis Agrim Institute of Neuroscience, Gurgaon, India

R. Parthasarathy
Vascular Neurology and Neurointerventional Surgery, Artemis Agrim Institute of Neuroscience, Gurgaon, India

V. Gupta (✉)
Neurointerventional Surgery, Stroke Unit, Artemis Agrim Institute of Neuroscience, Gurgaon, India
e-mail: vipul.gupta@artemishospitals.com

V. Gupta et al. (eds.), *100 Interesting Case Studies in Neurointervention: Tips and Tricks*,
https://doi.org/10.1007/978-981-13-1346-2_74

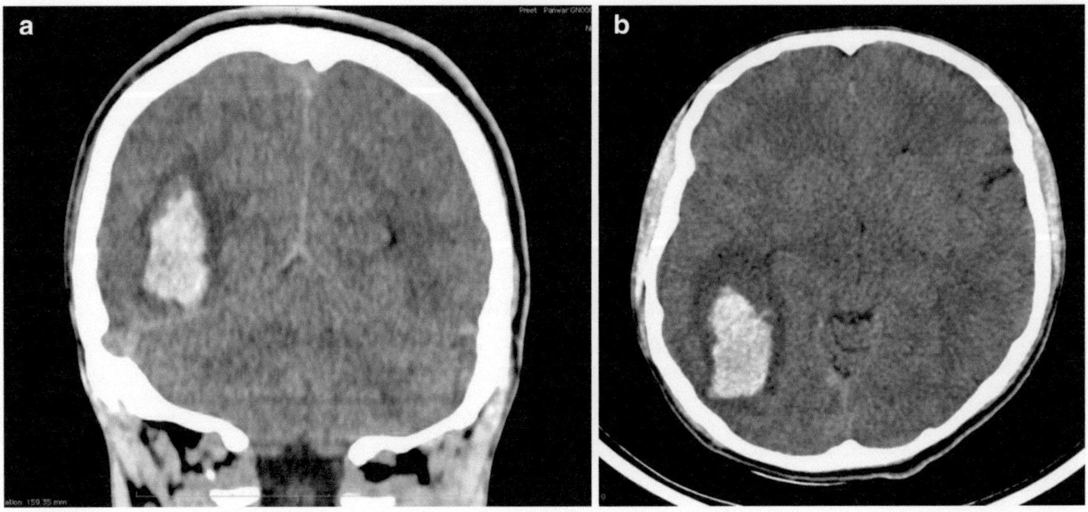

Fig. 74.1 (**a** and **b**) CT brain and right occipitoparietal bleed

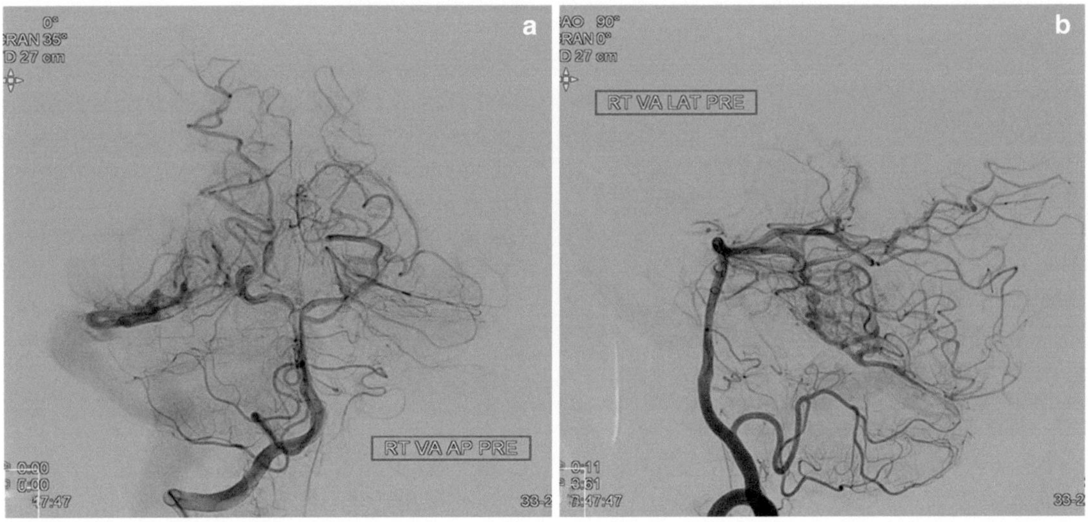

Fig. 74.2 (**a** and **b**) AP and lat angiogram, showing patchy, compressed AVM nidus with small multiple feeders from the temporal branch of the right PCA and drainage into the right transverse sinus

DSA run was taken which showed collateral filling of the AVM from other temporal branches which were not visible previously on DSA as well as 3D angiography (Fig. 74.5b). Hence, Onyx embolization was continued. After multiple attempts of Onyx plug formation, forward flow of Onyx into the temporal branch of PCA was seen, confirming its en passage nature. Onyx embolization was stopped temporarily to avoid further penetration into the en passage artery. On further injection, progressive filling of AVM nidus and its feeders was achieved along with filling of venous aneurysm (Fig. 74.6a, b). Post-procedure DSA run showed complete obliteration of AVM feeder and its nidus (Fig. 74.7a, b). Post-procedure neurological evaluation of the patient did not reveal any new neurological deficit. CT did not reveal any obvious new infarctions.

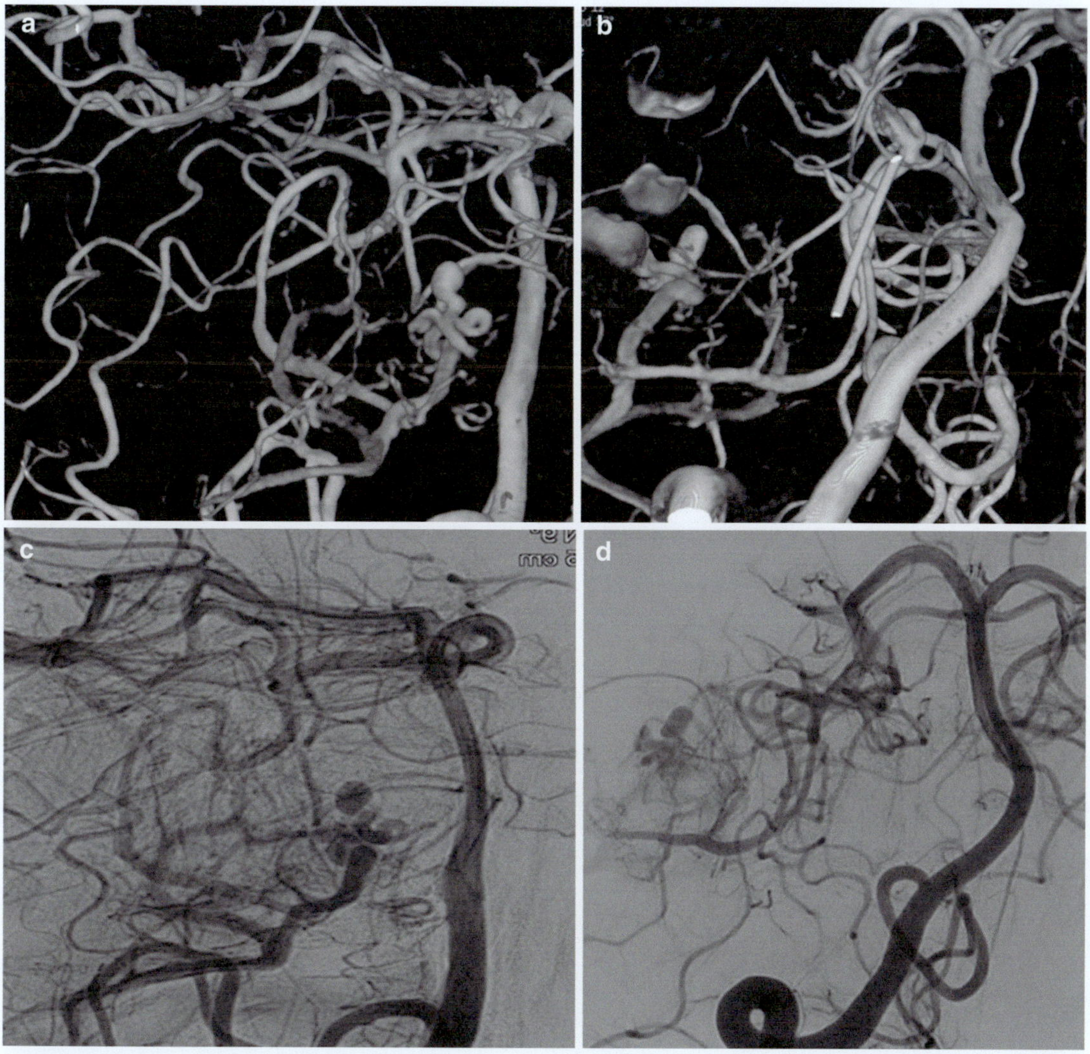

Fig. 74.3 (**a–d**) 3D angiogram with corresponding 2D angiogram, depicting AVM nidus along with intra-nidal aneurysm and at least three small feeders from the temporal branch of PCA

Tips and Tricks

1. Presence of intra-nidal aneurysm warrants early treatment of AVM in the acute phase.
2. 3D angiography can give useful information in cases of AVM, when anatomy is not completely discernible on DSA.
3. Careful microcatheter positioning is important to achieve adequate nidal penetration.
4. In author's experience, in medial temporal AVM, temporal branch of PCA usually gives en passage feeders to the AVM. In such circumstances, one should hold back from penetrating distally into the en passage feeder; however, with proximal occlusion, the flow in the distal vascular bed will be taken over by collateral feeders.
5. Collateral feeders to the AVM may be visible only when primary feeders are occluded. Therefore, permanent AVM cure can be achieved only when complete nidal penetration is attained.

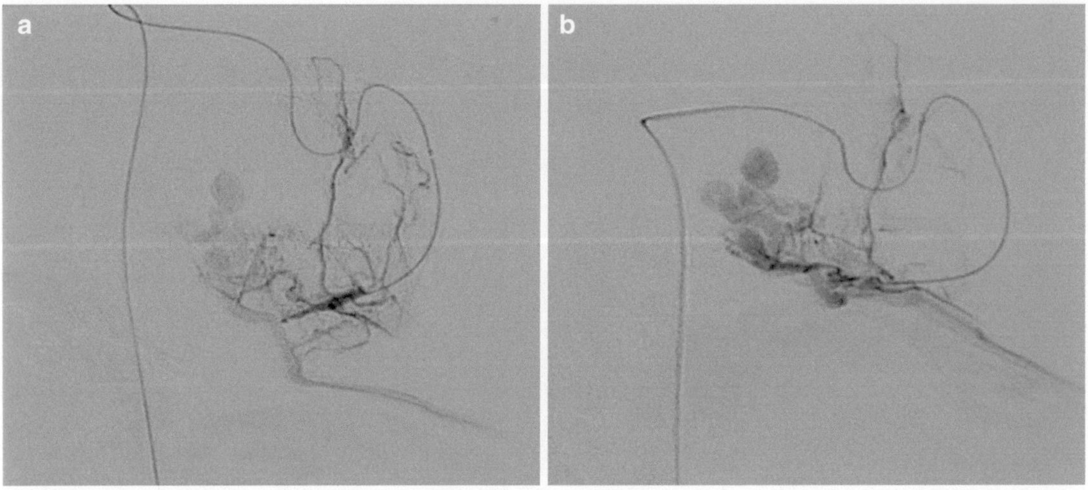

Fig. 74.4 (**a**) Microcatheter run from its distal position in the temporal branch of PCA, showing sudden cutoff of the artery with inadequate filling of the AVM nidus and intra-nidal aneurysm. (**b**) Microcatheter run after proximal withdrawal of the catheter, showing appropriate filling of the AVM nidus along with intra-nidal aneurysm

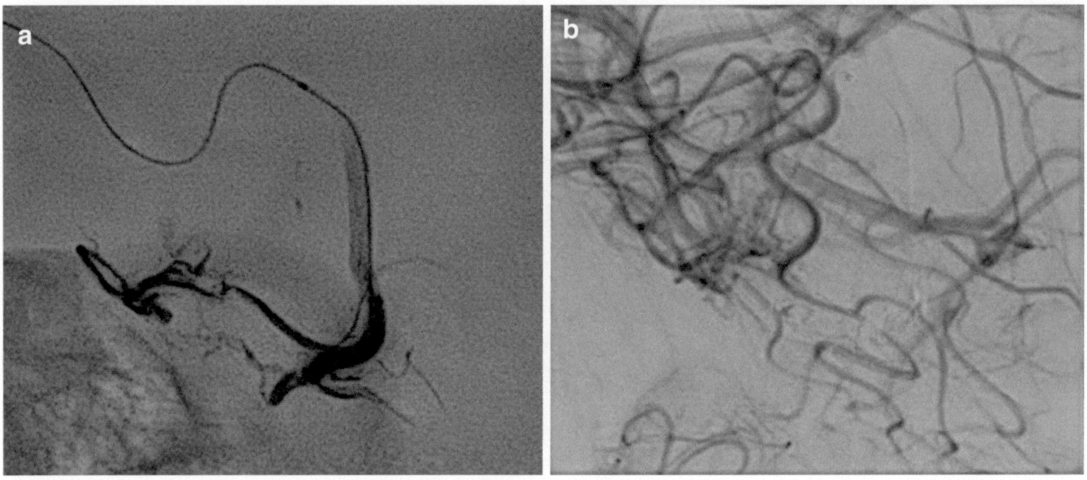

Fig. 74.5 (**a**) Onyx cast after initial embolization, showing filling of AVM feeders along with the part of the nidus. (**b**) Postembolization run showing filling of the AVM from collaterals which were not visualized previously on 2D and 3D angiogram

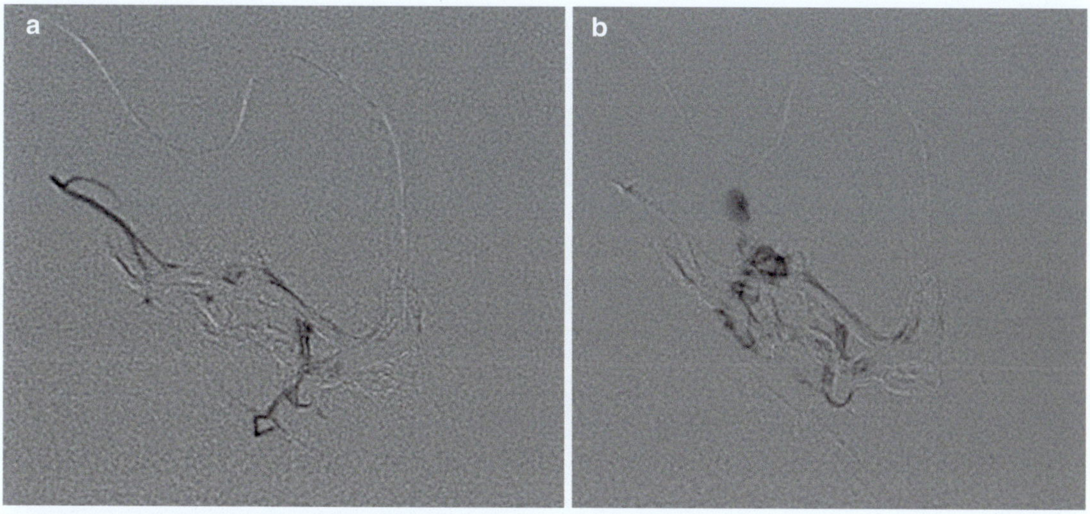

Fig. 74.6 (**a** and **b**) Onyx penetration into AVM nidus and intra-nidal aneurysm

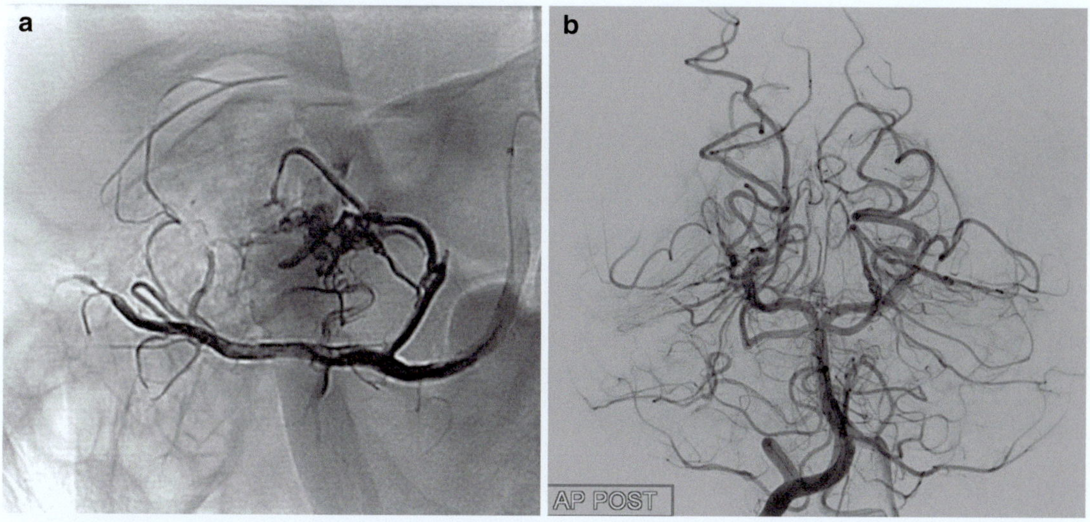

Fig. 74.7 (**a**) Final Onyx cast after completion of the procedure. (**b**) Post-procedure DSA run showed obliteration of the AVM nidus and intra-nidal aneurysm

Suggested Reading

Krings T, et al. Partial "targeted" embolisation of brain arteriovenous malformations. Eur Radiol. 2010;20(11): 2723–31.

Cerebral AVM Embolization: Postoperative Bleeding Due to Draining Vein Occlusion – Part 1

75

Vipul Gupta

Case

A 48-year-old male presented with sudden onset of severe headache followed by drowsiness. CT scan revealed hemorrhage in the right peritrigonal region with intraventricular extension. Lobulated hyperdense mass with specks of calcification highly suggestive of dilated vascular channels was noted (Fig. 75.1a, b). DSA revealed arteriovenous malformation in right parieto-occipital region with feeders from right PCA and MCA and draining into straight and superior sagittal sinus. Multiple venous aneurysms were seen (Fig. 75.1c–e).

Issues

- Occlusion of high-flow fistulas without occluding the draining vein.
- Patient needed urgent external ventricular drainage in view of increasing drowsiness and hydrocephalus; however, there was risk of rupture of the intraventricular venous aneurysms.

V. Gupta
Neurointerventional Surgery, Stroke Unit,
Artemis Agrim Institute of Neuroscience,
Gurgaon, India
e-mail: vipul.gupta@artemishospitals.com

Management

The management strategy was as follows: to first achieve partial flow reduction by occluding the high-flow arteriovenous fistulae followed by EVD insertion. The procedure was performed under general anesthesia. A guiding catheter was placed in right vertebral artery. A microcatheter (Magic 1.2 FM over a Mirage wire) was navigated into a large high-flow AVF arising from right PCA (Fig. 75.1f). The fistula was embolized (Fig. 75.1g) using high-concentration glue (n-butyl-2-cyanoacrylate diluted to 80% lipiodol). A second fistula was then catheterized (Fig. 75.2a). During glue injection, the glue was seen to go into the draining vein to the junction of the vein with superior sagittal sinus (Fig. 75.2b–f). As glue migrated into the draining vein, the other arteriovenous fistulae were also embolized (Fig. 75.3a), and almost complete occlusion of the AVM was achieved on vertebral artery injections. ICA injection revealed residual malformation fed by right MCA feeders; however, this component appeared to be diffuse with low flow and therefore was not embolized (Fig. 75.3b–e). Patient was maintained under general anesthesia with strict monitoring and control of blood pressure. The heparin effect was reversed with protamine, and an EVD was performed soon after the procedure, and this resulted in decompression of the ventricles (Fig. 75.3f). However, after few hours the patient deteriorated, and

V. Gupta et al. (eds.), *100 Interesting Case Studies in Neurointervention: Tips and Tricks*,
https://doi.org/10.1007/978-981-13-1346-2_75

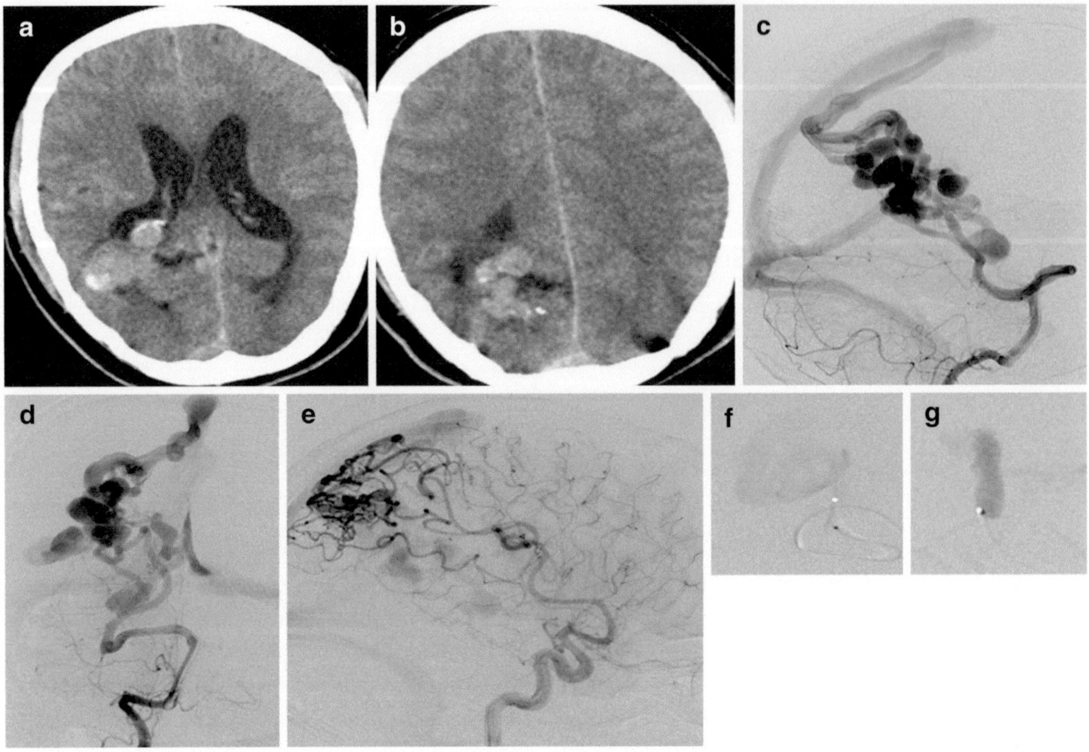

Fig. 75.1 (**a** and **b**) CT scan images (non-contrast) showing hemorrhage in right periventricular region with intraventricular extension and secondary hydrocephalus. Dilated vascular channels are seen in right parietal region. (**c** and **d**) Right vertebral angiogram shows an AVM with feeders from right PCA and multiple venous aneurysms. (**e**) Right ICA injection shows small feeders from right MCA cortical branches. (**f**) Microcatheter injection shows a high-flow fistula. (**g**) Glue embolization of the fistula

repeat CT revealed fresh parenchymal, intraventricular, and subarachnoid hemorrhage. Patient died after a prolonged stay in hospital (Fig. 75.4).

Tips and Tricks

1. In the presence of high-flow fistulae with venous angiopathy, glue can migrate into the veins and tends to get lodged at site of venous stenosis/narrowing. This can result in sudden increase in intranidal pressure, leading to rupture of the AVM.
2. If inadvertent venous occlusion occurred, it is advisable to reverse the heparin and lower the blood pressure to decrease the probability of AVM rupture.
3. In the cases of iatrogenic venous occlusion, we prefer to embolize the residual AVM as much as possible in order to decrease the intranidal pressure. In retrospect, embolization of the feeders from right MCA could have averted the repeat hemorrhage.
4. Immediate surgery to excise the AVM nidus post-embolization is an alternative strategy to prevent repeat hemorrhage.

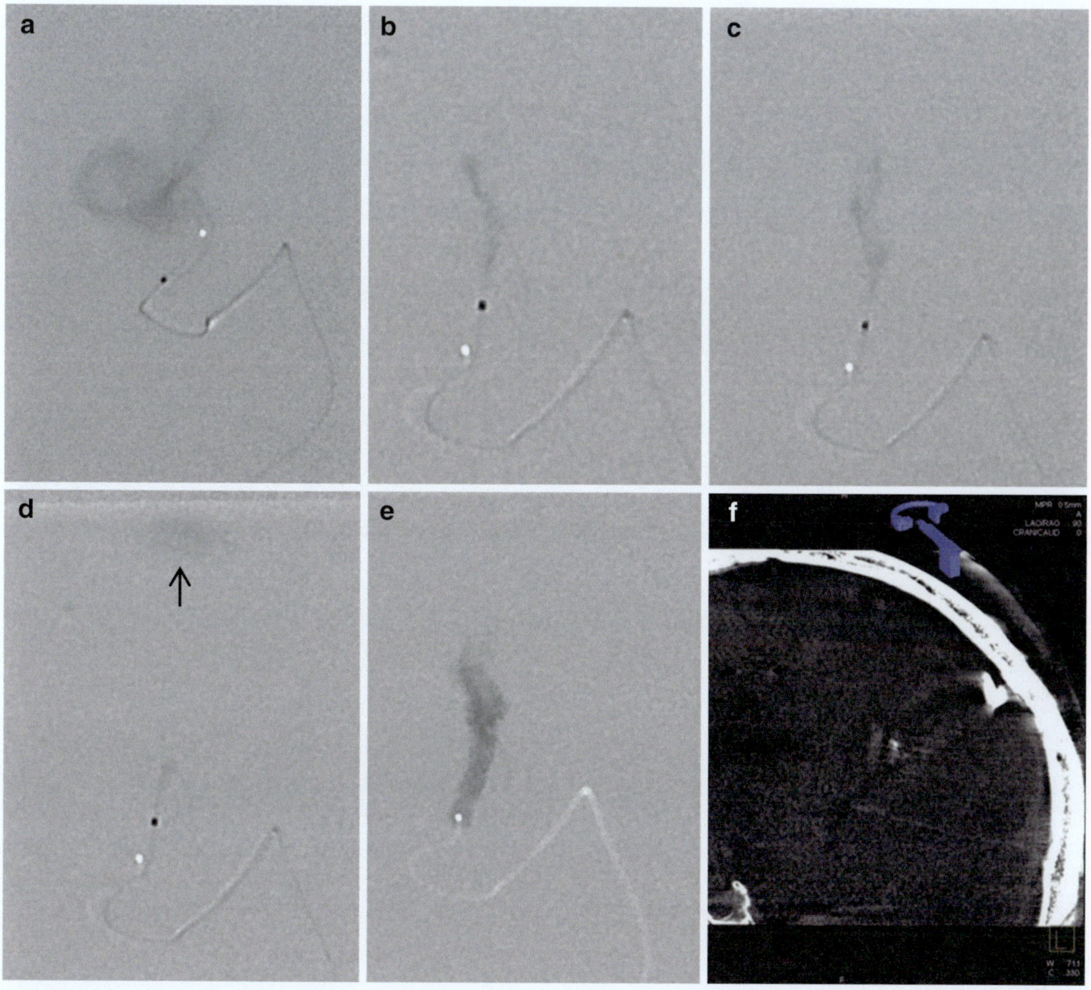

Fig. 75.2 (**a**) Microcatheter injection in another fistula. (**b–e**) Sequential DSA images of glue injection. (**b** and **c**) Initial whiff of glue. (**d**) The mass of glue fragmented and went to the distal segment of draining vein (arrow). (**e**) Final glue cast. (**f**) Angio-CT image showing dense mass of glue at junction of draining vein and superior sagittal sinus

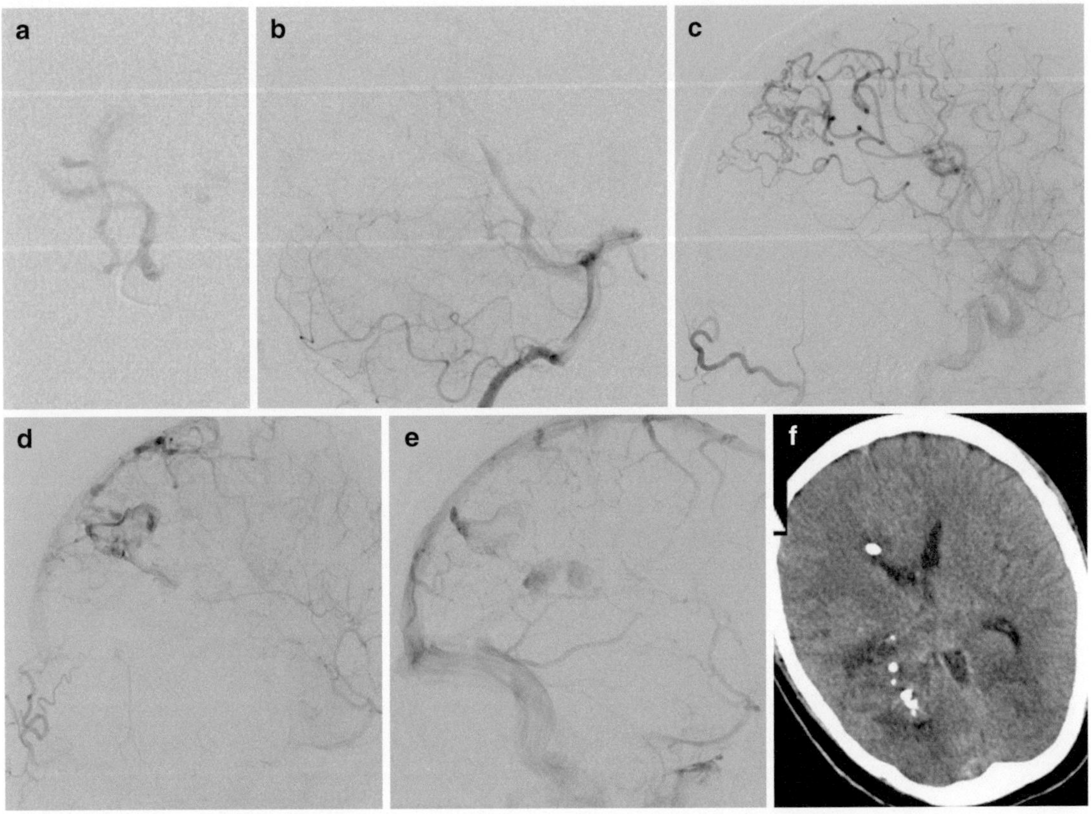

Fig. 75.3 (**a**) Glue cast from third injection. (**b**) Vertebral artery injection almost complete occlusion from AVFs. (**c–e**) ICA injection residual AVM draining through small venous channels. The main draining vein as seen in pre-embolization angiogram is not visualized. (**f**) Post-embolization CT after placement of ventricular catheter doesn't show any fresh bleeding

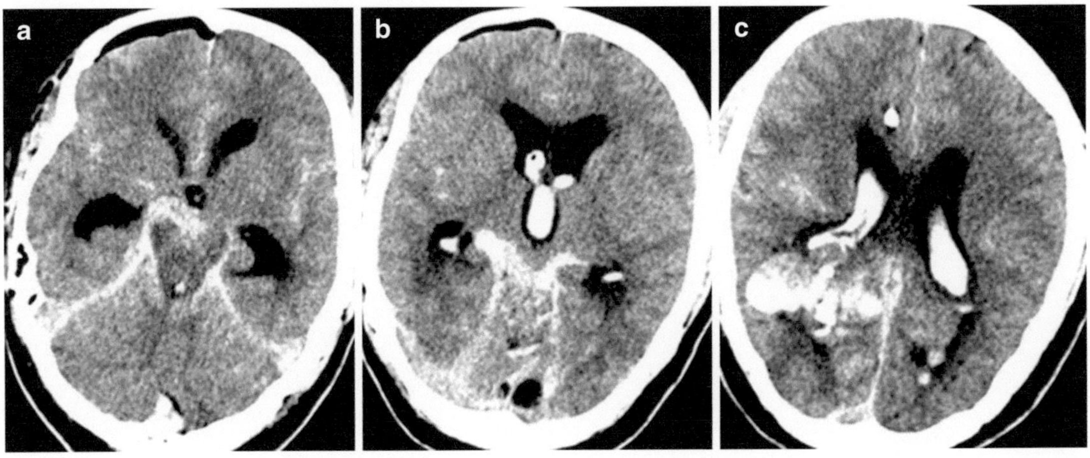

Fig. 75.4 CT scan images showing fresh parenchymal, intraventricular, and subarachnoid hemorrhage

Suggested Reading

Andreou A, Ioannidis I, Nasis N. Transarterial balloon-assisted glue embolization of high-flow arteriovenous fistulas. Neuroradiology. 2008;50:267–72. [PubMed].

Cerebral AVM Embolization: Postoperative Bleed Due to Draining Vein Occlusion—2

76

Vipul Gupta

Case

A 28-year-old female presented with severe headache associated with blurring of vision. CT scan revealed hematoma in left peri-trigonal region with intraventricular extension (Fig. 76.1a). DSA (Fig. 76.1b–f) revealed an AVM in left temporo-occipital region with feeders from left PCA and draining into the straight sinus. Multiple intra- and perinidal aneurysms were seen.

Issues

In view of multiple peri- and intranidal aneurysms, it was advisable to perform early occlusion of the AVM and the associated aneurysms.

Since normal arterial branches were seen to arise adjacent to the AVM nidus, it was considered not appropriate to use onyx as embolization material.

Management

The management strategy was to undertake partial glue (*n*-butyl 2-cyanoacrylate) embolization of the AVM and the associated aneurysms followed by radiosurgery for the residual nidus. Under general anesthesia, a guiding catheter was placed in left vertebral artery. A microcatheter (Magic 1.2 FM) was navigated to intranidal location and embolization was performed with 60% glue (Fig. 76.2a, b); however, adequate nidal penetration was not achieved (Fig. 76.2b). Therefore, another feeder was catheterized (Fig. 76.2c) and embolized with dilute glue (20%) with the hope of achieving better nidal penetration. However, during the glue injection, migration of glue to the venous side into the vein of Galen and the proximal straight sinus was noted (Fig. 76.2d). Guiding catheter injection revealed residual AVM nidus with complete occlusion of the deep venous drainage. A small cortical vein was noted draining the residual malformation. The effect of heparin was reversed with protamine, and a low mean arterial blood pressure was targeted (Fig. 76.3a, b). As the primary venous outlet was occluded, the residual feeders were catheterized (Fig. 76.3c–e) and embolized with glue. Final angiogram revealed near-complete occlusion of the AVM (Fig. 76.4a–c). Glue cast on native images showing migration into the draining vein and dyna CT post procedure showed no ICH immediate post oper-

V. Gupta
Neurointerventional Surgery, Stroke Unit,
Artemis Agrim Institute of Neuroscience,
Gurgaon, India
e-mail: vipul.gupta@artemishospitals.com

V. Gupta et al. (eds.), *100 Interesting Case Studies in Neurointervention: Tips and Tricks*,
https://doi.org/10.1007/978-981-13-1346-2_76

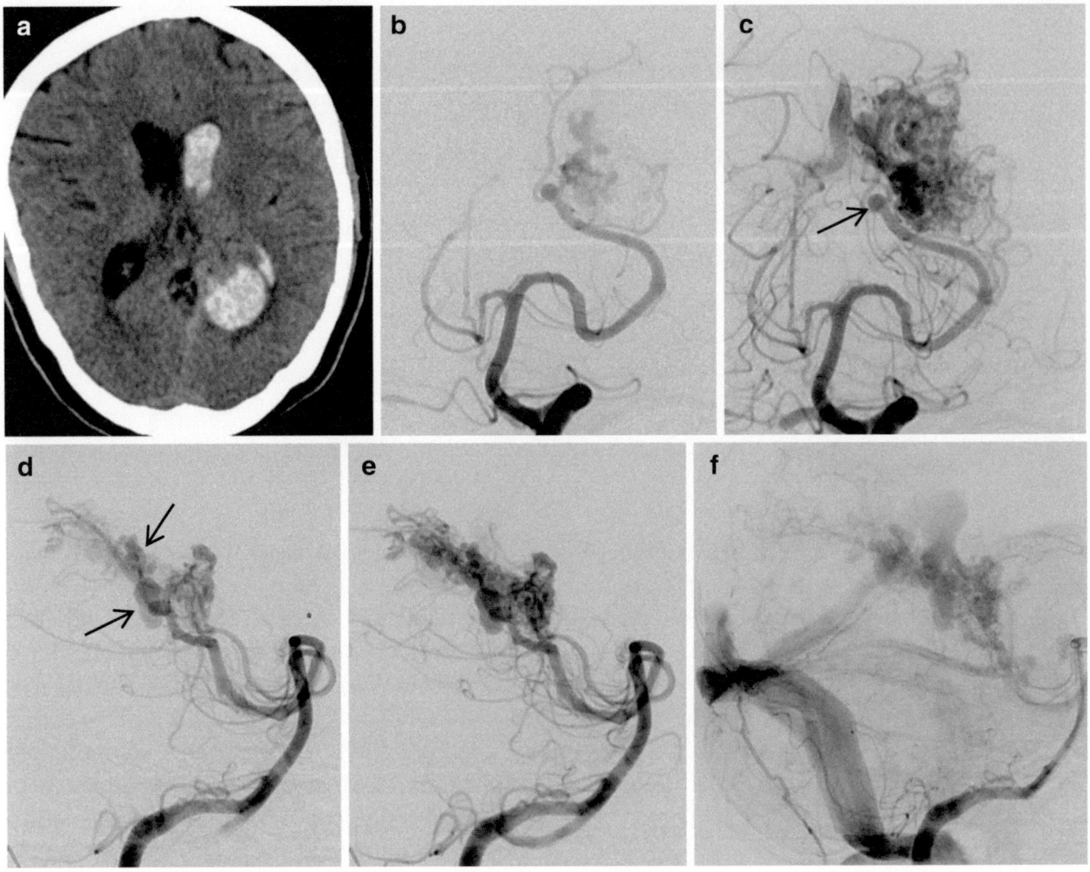

Fig. 76.1 (**a**) CT scan image showing a hematoma in left peri-trigonal region with intraventricular extension. (**b** and **c**) (AP views) and (**c**–**f**) (lateral view)—left vertebral angiogram reveals an AVM in left temporo-occipital region with feeders from left PCA draining via vein of Galen into the straight sinus. Multiple peri- and intranidal aneurysms could be seen (arrows)

ative period. Nidal rebleed was anticipated; therefore, the vascular neurosurgery team was consulted regarding excision of the malformation. In view of deep location of the AVM, surgery was not considered to be advisable. Therefore, the patient was maintained under anesthesia and mean arterial blood pressure was kept low. An EVD was placed so as to have control over intracranial pressure in the event of a repeat bleed. Patient was extubated 76-h post-procedure with careful monitoring of blood pressure during the weaning off process; any sudden increase in blood pressure could result in bleed. Daily CT scans were performed during the period she was maintained under general anesthesia. Patient did not suffer from any untoward event, and the EVD catheter was removed after a few days. Follow-up angiogram after 3 months revealed a small residual AVM which was treated by radiosurgery.

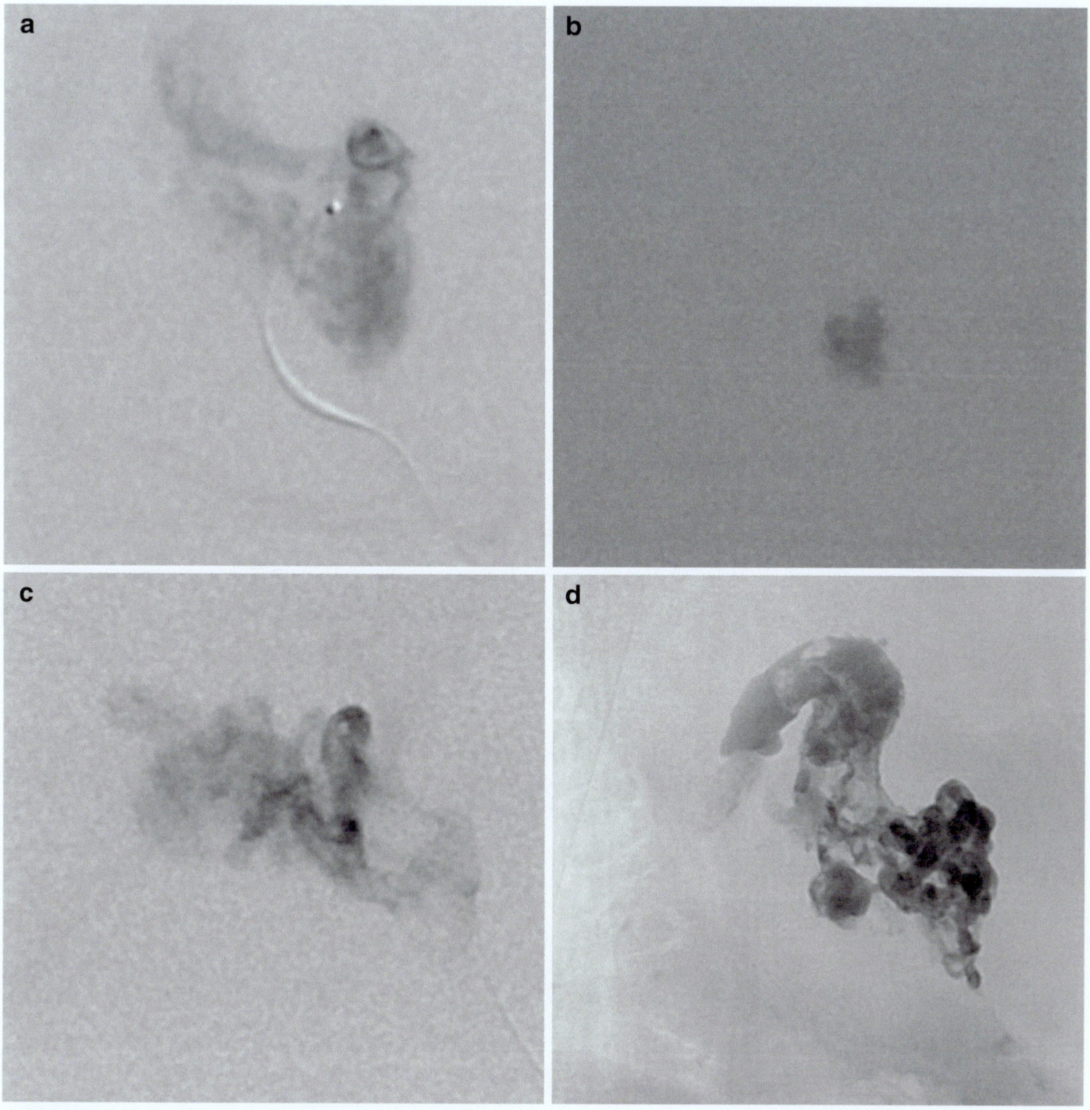

Fig. 76.2 (**a**) Microcatheter injection showing AVM nidus. (**b**) Glue cast with inadequate penetration into the nidus. (**c**) Placement of second microcatheter. (**d**) Glue cast in nidus as well as vein of Galen and straight sinus

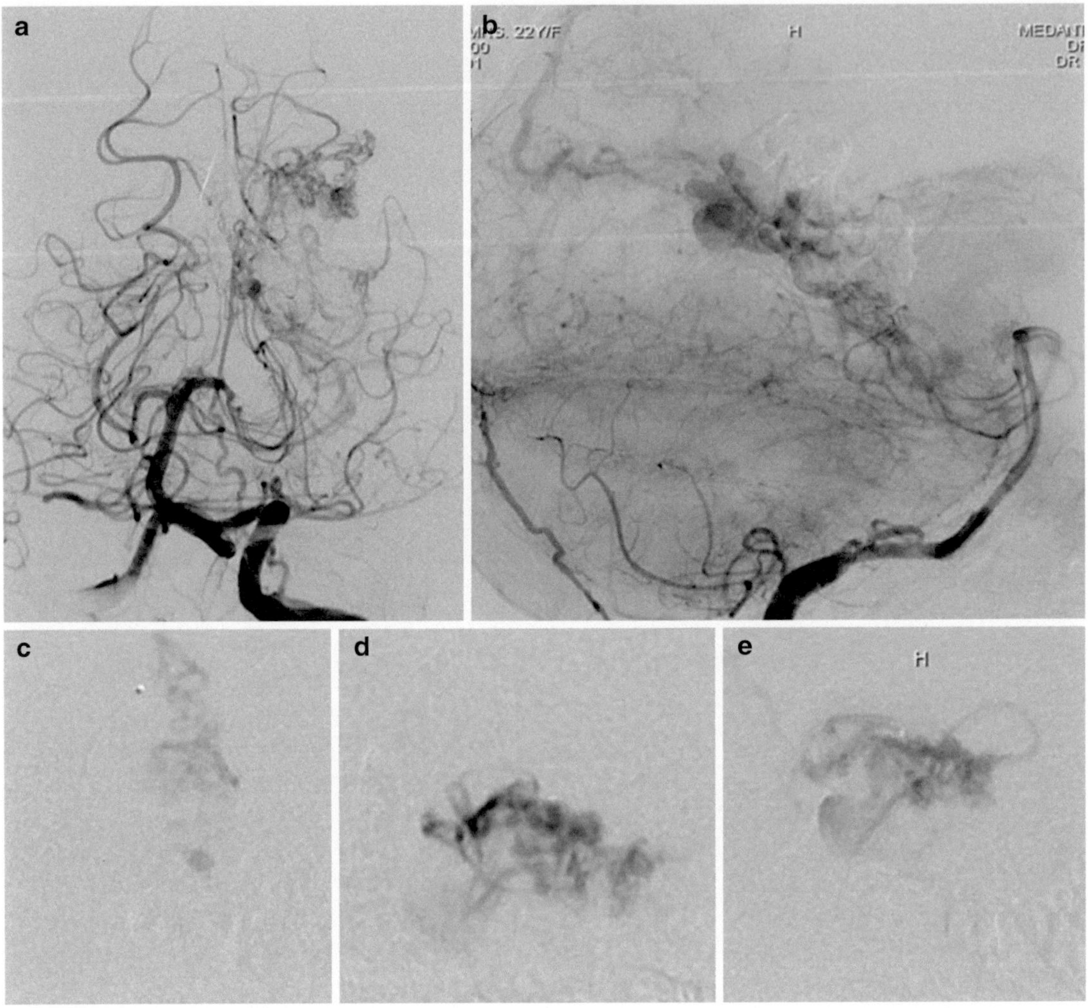

Fig. 76.3 (**a** and **b**) AP (**a**) and lateral (**b**) views showing residual AVM with a small cortical draining vein. Straight sinus is no longer visualized. (**c**–**e**) Microcatheter injections in residual feeders

Tips and Tricks

1. In the event of accidental occlusion of the primary draining vein, reduce and maintain a low mean arterial pressure in an attempt to reduce intranidal pressure. Further, reverse the effect of heparin to reduce the chances of repeat intracranial hemorrhage.
2. Every attempt should be made to embolize as much of the AVM nidus as possible as this would result in reduction of the intranidal pressure.
3. We prefer to keep the patients with high risk of post-embolization bleeding under general anesthesia and lower mean arterial blood pressure. An EVD catheter would enable monitoring intracranial pressure and would allow for reduction of intracranial pressure in the event of repeat intracranial hemorrhage.
4. Stringent measures should be taken to keep the blood pressure low and avoid any increase during extubation.
5. Post-embolization residual nidal excision with hematoma removal should be considered in all with high risk of post-embolization rebleed.

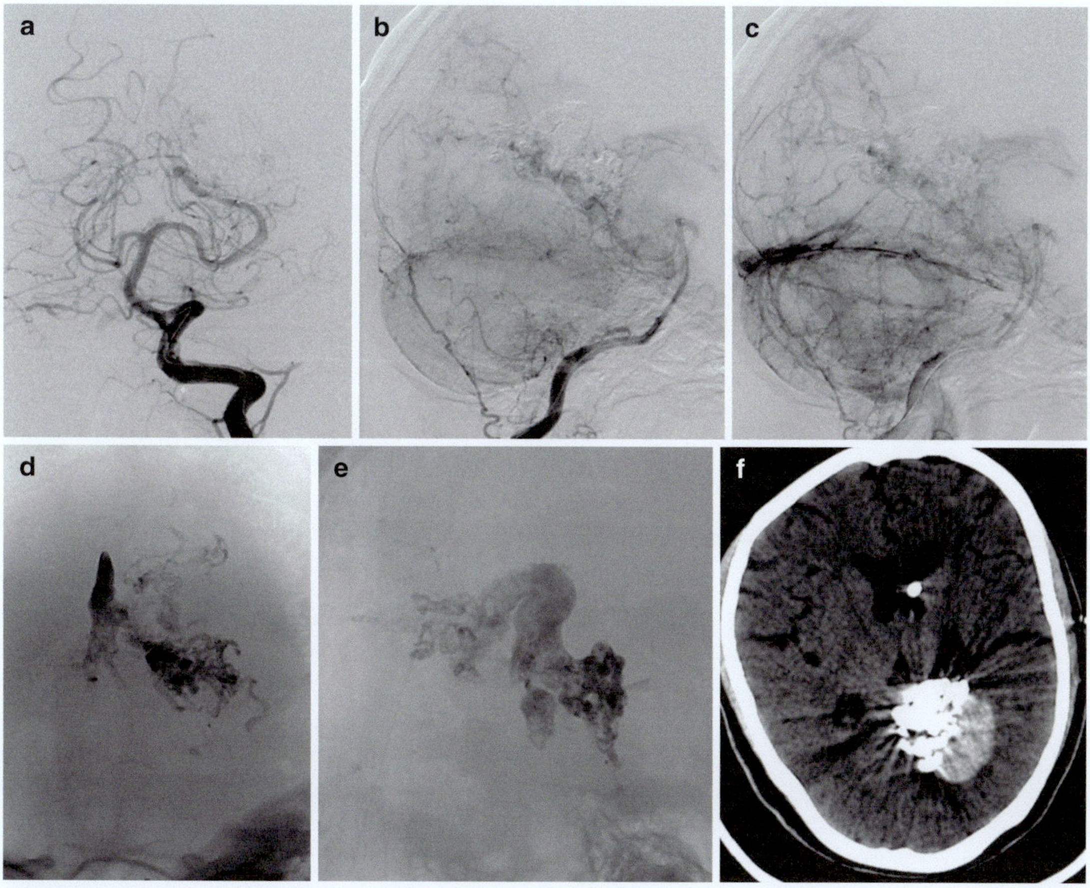

Fig. 76.4 (**a–c**) AP (**a**) and lateral (**b**, **c**) views of post-embolization angiogram showing almost complete occlusion of the AVM. (**d**, **e**) The glue cast. (**f**) Post-embolization CT does not show any fresh bleed. EVD tube is seen in left frontal horn

Suggested Reading

Andreou A, Ioannidis I, Nasis N. Transarterial balloon-assisted glue embolization of high-flow arteriovenous fistulas. Neuroradiology. 2008;50:267–72. [PubMed].

77 Vein of Galen Aneurysmal Malformation: Emergency Embolization for Cardiac Failure

Rajsrinivas Parthasarathy and Vipul Gupta

Case

A 2-month-old female baby presented with severe congestive cardiac failure and was diagnosed with vein of Galen aneurysmal malformation. She needed ventilator support for managing the cardiorespiratory failure before being transferred to our center. On admission to our center, she had transient anuria secondary to prerenal acute renal failure with an elevated urea and normal creatinine, normal liver functions, and severe congestive heart failure causing respiratory failure needing ventilatory support. Echocardiography revealed flow reversal in the descending thoracic aorta, pulmonary artery hypertension, atrial septal defect, and shift of interventricular septum to the left. Ultrasound abdomen did not reveal hepatomegaly. She had an isolated convulsion, and the MRI of the brain did not show any evidence of encephalomalacia or ventriculomegaly. The Bicêtre neonatal evaluation score (BNES) was 9 (cardiac, 1; cerebral, 2; respiratory, 1; hepatic, 3; renal, 2). Cardiorespiratory failure was refractory to medical management needing ventilation, and with a BNES of 9, a decision to treat was undertaken.

R. Parthasarathy (✉)
Vascular Neurology and Neurointerventional Surgery, Artemis Agrim Institute of Neuroscience, Gurgaon, India

V. Gupta
Neurointerventional Surgery, Stroke Unit, Artemis Agrim Institute of Neuroscience, Gurgaon, India
e-mail: vipul.gupta@artemishospitals.com

Issues

1. Determinants for early as opposed to late intervention in infants with VGAM
2. Minimizing the radiation and contrast exposure
3. Technical challenge of using low-profile catheter system in such small child

Management

Procedure was performed under general anesthesia. A 4F sheath was used to cannulate the femoral artery. A 4F diagnostic catheter (MPA, Cook medical, Bloomington, USA) was used to perform the cerebral angiography. Care was taken to use minimal dye, and catheter aspiration was performed after each dye injection. Cerebral angiography revealed a choroidal-type VGAM with feeders from anterior and posterior choroidal arteries and choroidal branches from the ACA and the thalamoperforators (Fig. 77.1a–d). The transverse and sigmoid sinuses were of normal caliber without evidence of hypoplasia, and there was no jugular bulb stenosis. Cavernous capture of the Sylvian vein was not seen, and there was no supra- or infratentorial pial reflux. The DSA

V. Gupta et al. (eds.), *100 Interesting Case Studies in Neurointervention: Tips and Tricks*,
https://doi.org/10.1007/978-981-13-1346-2_77

image was itself used for navigating the microcatheter by using the fluoro-fade technology, thereby avoiding administering more dye for road map acquisition. Glue embolization was performed using Marathon 1.5 F (ev3 Inc., Irvine, California, USA) microcatheter using 80% glue, and four fistulas were closed. Approximately 30% of the nidus was obliterated in the first session. However, the need for ventilation persisted and henceforth a second session was undertaken after 3 days. Using the same techniques, a 50% reduction in AVM nidus was achieved with stabilization in the cardiorespiratory status (Fig. 77.2a–d).

Tips and Tricks

1. Congestive cardiac failure is the most common presenting feature of choroidal-type VGAM in the neonatal period. Hydrodynamic disorders are uncommon in the neonatal period and occur later in infancy.
2. Bicêtre neonatal evaluation score (BNES), a holistic 21-point scoring system that encompasses a systematic evaluation of five organ systems (cardiac, cerebral, respiratory, renal, and hepatic), acts as a primary determinant for timing of intervention. A BNES <8 is a contraindication for treatment because of poor prognosis in spite of multiple attempts at treatment. Emergency treatment is indicated when the score is between 8 and 12. Neonates and infants with a score >12 are initiated on maximal medical therapy, and interventional management is delayed until 5 months of age. Indications for early treatment when the BNES score is high are (a) heart failure refractory to medical therapy, (b) rapid increase in head circumference, (c) preclinical MRI evidence of intraventricular hyper-pressure, and (d) significant developmental delay (>20% below normal).
3. Cardiac evaluation should include assessment of (a) pulmonary artery hypertension, (b) presence of ASD/PDA, and (c) excursion of interventricular septum into the cavity of the left ventricle and flow reversal in the descending thoracic aorta. All of the above echocardiographic findings were seen in our patient. Cardiac poor prognostic indicators included supra-systemic pulmonary artery pressure, significant interventricular septum excursion to the left, and descending aorta diastolic flow reversal. Mortality was higher in the group of patients with the above findings.
4. Endovascular sessions are usually staged and performed every 3–6 months with the first session planned for at 5 months. Earlier treatment can be performed for the abovementioned indications. Both diagnostic angiography and therapeutics are performed in the same session to minimize contrast usage and avoid repeat general anesthesia. Judicial use of contrast that is less toxic to the kidneys is advisable.
5. Femoral puncture can be a particularly challenging endeavor in emaciated babies and is advisable to have experienced pediatric intervention team input. A 4F short sheath is used to cannulate the femoral artery. Catheterization of the feeding artery could potentially be done without the use of a guiding catheter. One can use the DSA image for guidance by fluoro-fade technology, thereby avoiding contrast injection for road map acquisition. After every dye injection, catheter can be aspirated to remove the dye form the lumen (dead space) of the catheter.
6. Angiographic description should include the type of VGAM (choroidal vs mural), arterial feeders, and the venous drainage. The key features to be determined are (a) the presence of proximal choroidal vein drainage, (b) pial venous reflux, (c) superior petrosal sinus drainage of the infratentorial veins, and (d) cavernous capture of the Sylvian vein. Proximal choroidal vein drainage precludes embolization from the venous end and also predisposes to intraventricular hemorrhage. Pial venous reflux both supra- and infratentorial reflects on venous hypertension secondary to hypoplastic transverse and sigmoid sinuses when the primitive occipital and marginal sinus regresses and jugular bulb dysmaturation and stenosis secondary to skull base maturation. Cavernous capture of the Sylvian vein provides for an alternate route for venous drainage resulting in decrease in the venous hypertension and transient stabilization of symptoms. None of the above red flags were seen in our patient.

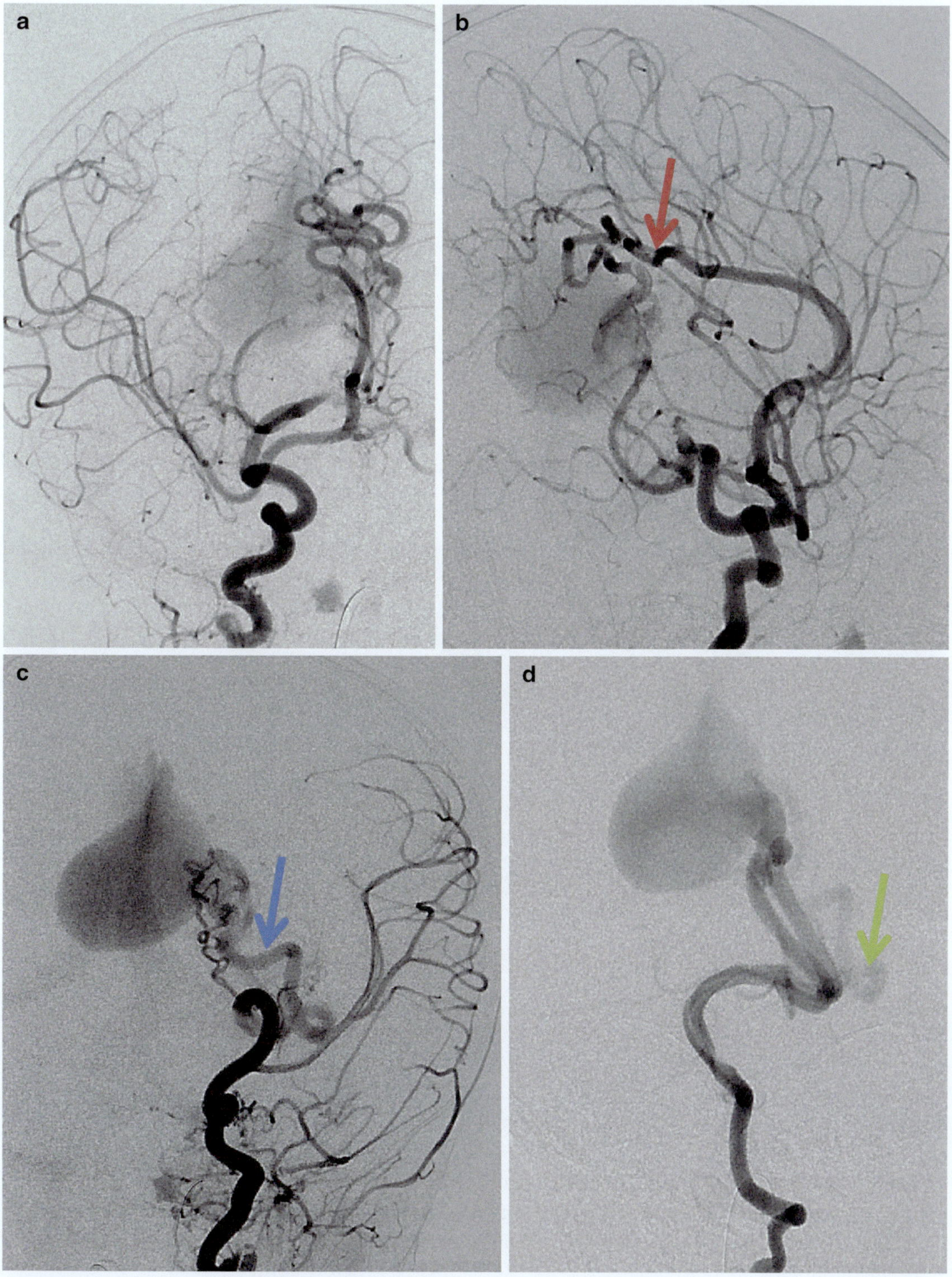

Fig. 77.1 Cerebral angiography demonstrated choroidal type of vein of Galen malformation. (**a**) Right ICA AP and (**b**) lateral view showing arterial feeders from the right anterior choroidal artery and anterior cerebral artery (red arrow). (**c**) Left ICA AP view demonstrates feeders from the left anterior choroidal artery and left posterior choroidal artery (blue arrow). (**d**) Left vertebral AP view showing left posterior choroidal artery feeders and left PCA feeders (green arrow)

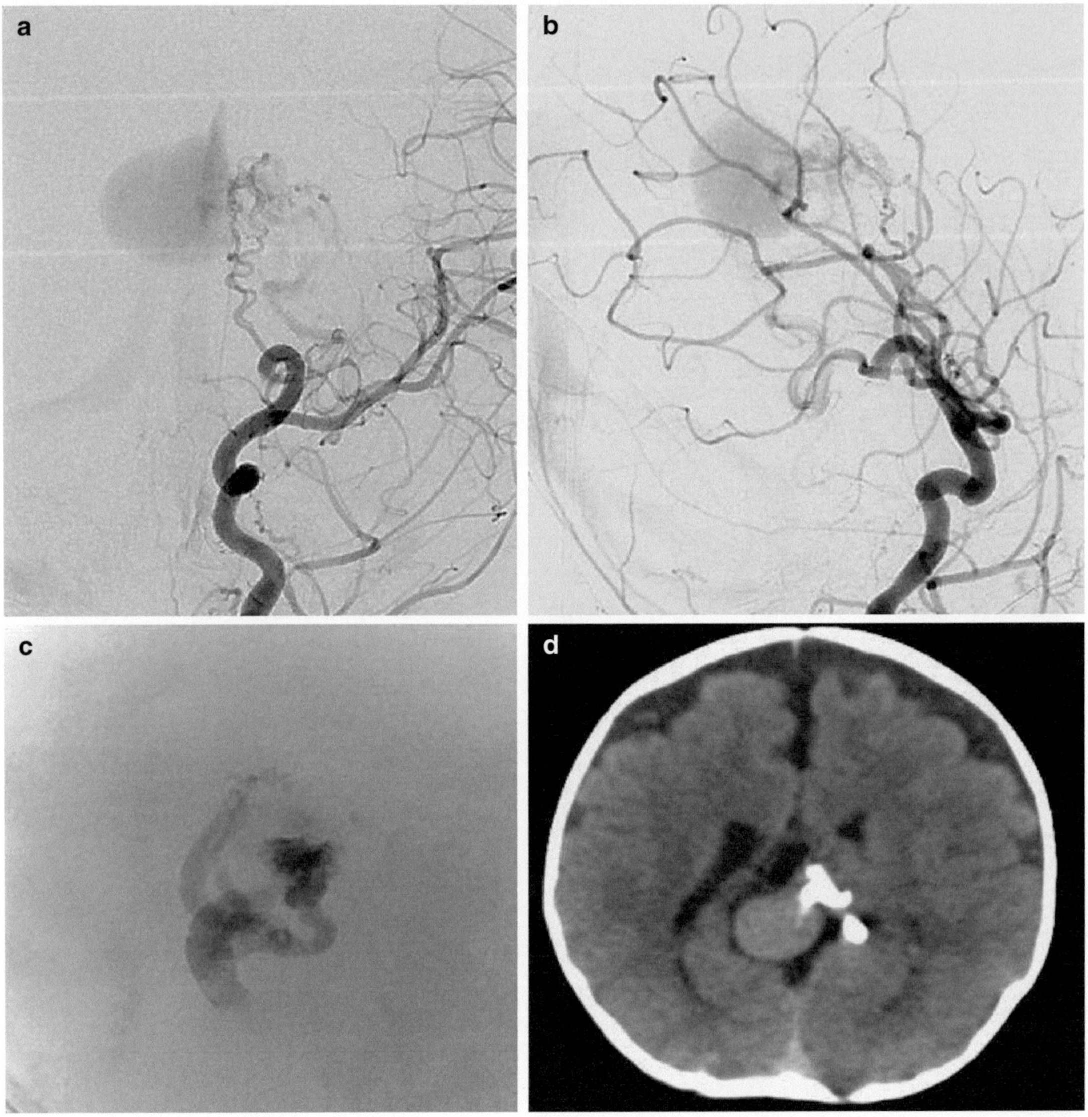

Fig. 77.2 (**a**) Left ICA AP and (**b**) lateral view after two sessions. There is marked reduction in the flow of the fistula. (**c**) Final glue cast. (**d**) Post-procedure CT head shows reduction in the size of the venous sac

Pearls

1. Angiographic red flags include supra- and infratentorial pial reflux, transverse and sigmoid hypoplasia, and jugular bulb dysmaturation.
2. Maximal medical therapy to delay intervention until 5 months of age.
3. Emergent intervention when BNES 8–12, heart failure refractory to medical therapy, rapid increase in head circumference, preclinical MRI evidence of intraventricular hyperpressure, and significant developmental delay (>20% below normal).
4. Experienced pediatric cardiology input to manage hyperdynamic cardiac failure.

Suggested Reading

Bhattacharya JJ, Thammaroj J. Vein of galen malformations. J Neurol Neurosurg Psychiatry. 2003;74:I42–4.

Jones BV, et al. Vein of Galen aneurysmal malformation: diagnosis and treatment of 13 children with extended clinical follow-up. Am J Neuroradiol. 2002;23(10):1717–24.

78 Cerebral Proliferative Angiopathy: Differentiation from Arteriovenous Malformation (AVM)

Vipul Gupta

Case

An 18-year-old male presented with recurrent headaches and two episodes of seizures. On examination, he had no neurological deficits. Contrast-enhanced CT scan of brain revealed a markedly enhancing lesion in right frontal region (Fig. 78.1a, b). No mass effect was seen. MRI revealed a diffuse network of flow voids in parenchymal and subarachnoid space (Fig. 78.1c–f). The dilated vascular spaces seemed to be interspersed with normal brain parenchyma. DSA was performed which revealed a densely enhancing vascular spaces in the frontal region (Fig. 78.2a–d). The arteries in the region were mildly dilated, but no dominant feeder could be seen. There was early venous filling, but relative to the size of the lesion, veins were few and mildly dilated. No evidence of any arteriovenous fistula was seen.

Issue

To determine the nature of the lesion and management options.

Management

Patient was treated by antiepileptics.

V. Gupta
Neurointerventional Surgery, Stroke Unit,
Artemis Agrim Institute of Neuroscience,
Gurgaon, India
e-mail: vipul.gupta@artemishospitals.com

V. Gupta et al. (eds.), *100 Interesting Case Studies in Neurointervention: Tips and Tricks*,
https://doi.org/10.1007/978-981-13-1346-2_78

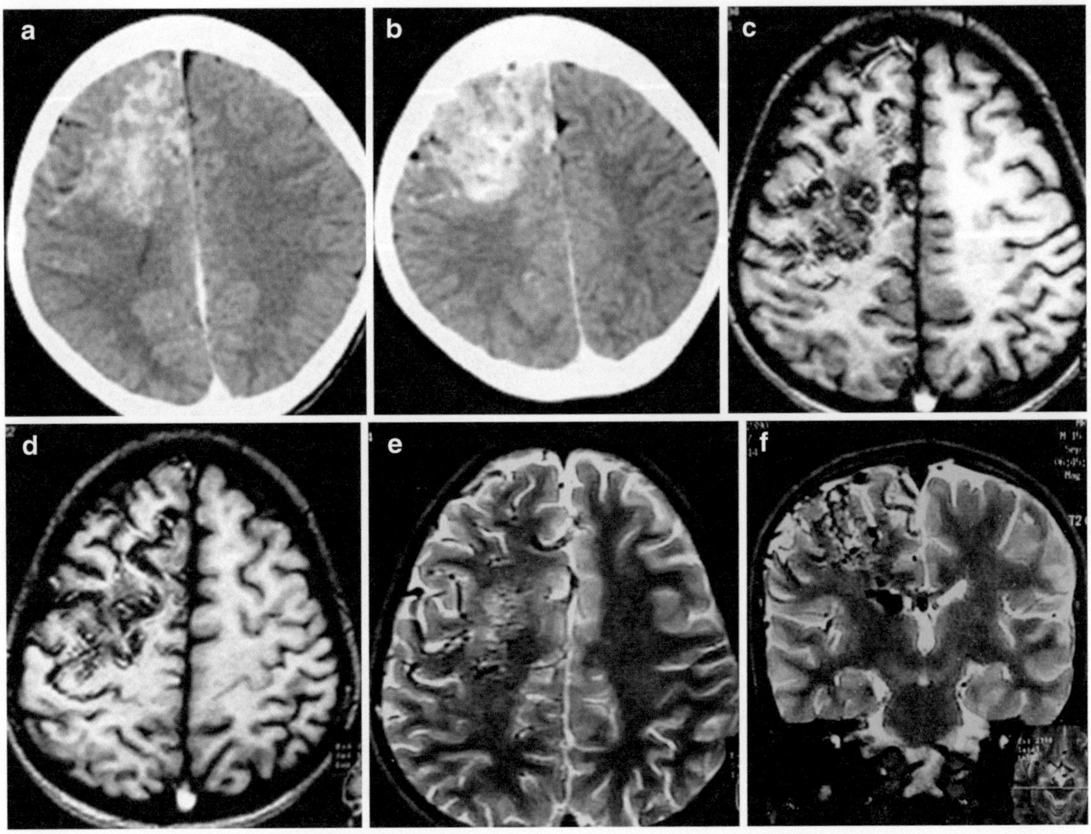

Fig. 78.1 (**a** and **b**) Contrast-enhanced CT scan images reveal diffuse enhancement in right frontal region. (**c** and **d**) T1-weighted as well as (**e** and **f**) T2-weighted MR images reveal scattered flow voids in right frontal region interspersed with cerebral parenchyma

Tips and Tricks

1. The appearance of diffuse network of vessels interspersed with normal parenchyma and relative lack of AV shunting as compared to size of the lesion with small arteries and few draining veins were against the diagnosis of an AVM.
2. The features are diagnostic of "cerebral proliferative angiopathy."
3. This is an entity different from cerebral AVM and is probably related to tissue ischemia and secondary diffuse angiogenesis.
4. As the lesion is intermixed with normal parenchyma, any intervention is likely to result in tissue injury and possible deficits. Therefore, we prefer to treat these lesions symptomatically with antiepileptics. Low rates of bleed are seen in these cases.

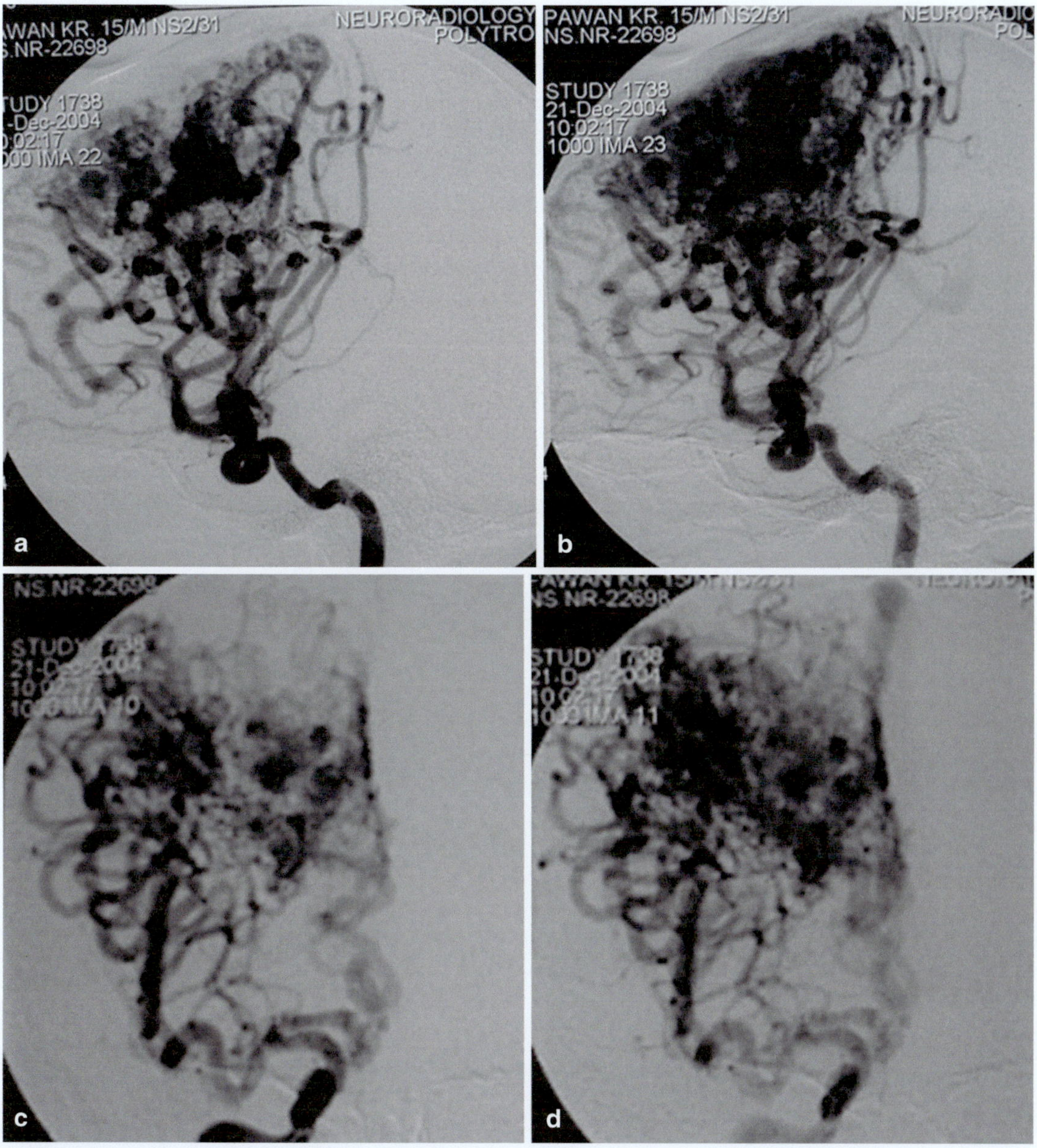

Fig. 78.2 Right ICA angiogram in lateral (**a**, **b**) and AP (**c**, **d**) views reveal a diffuse enhancing network in frontal region. Although it gives the appearance of an AVM nidus, there is relatively small size of feeding arteries and relative paucity of veins as compared to size of the lesion

Suggested Reading

Lasjaunias PL, Landrieu P, Rodesch G, et al. Cerebral proliferative angiopathy: clinical and angiographic description of an entity different from cerebral AVMs. Stroke. 2008;39(3):878–85.

79 Spinal Arteriovenous Fistula from Anterior Spinal Artery: Embolization Technique

Vipul Gupta

Case

A 28-year-old Nigerian lady presented with a 4-year history of gradually progressive weakness and numbness involving both lower limbs and urinary frequency. Examination revealed a spastic paraparesis with a pyramidal pattern of weakness and a sensory level corresponding to D9 level. MRI revealed edema in lower dorsal cord (Fig. 79.1). Dilated tortuous flow voids were seen particularly anterior to the cord. Spinal angiogram revealed an enlarged radiculo-medullary artery arising from right D9 level and feeding the arteriovenous fistula at D9–D10 levels (Fig. 79.1a). Delayed run showed a venous aneurysm and a descending vein (Fig. 79.1b). Another feeder was seen from left 12th intercostal artery and ascending to the same level of the fistula (Fig. 79.2c–e). In view of the anterior midline location of both the feeding arteries, the central vertical segments represented anterior spinal artery. The branch arising from ASA and feeding the AVF represented enlarged sulco-commissural artery.

V. Gupta
Neurointerventional Surgery, Stroke Unit, Artemis Agrim Institute of Neuroscience, Gurgaon, India
e-mail: vipul.gupta@artemishospitals.com

Issues

- Embolization of the spinal AVF while preserving the anterior spinal artery
- Understanding the angio-architecture of AVM to perform the embolization

Management

The procedure was performed under GA. Injection with high frame rate was taken from both the feeders (Fig. 79.3a, b). Both the feeders converged to supply the same fistula. The plan was to enter the single common channel and embolize the fistula while preserving the ASA. The microcatheter was navigated from the left D12 intercostal artery because of the less acute angle with the feeding vessel (Fig. 79.3).

The microcatheter (Marathon 1.5 F, ev3 Neurovascular, Irvine, CA) was navigated deep into the feeding artery using micro-guidewires (Mirage 0.008, ev3 Neurovascular, Irvine, CA; Hybrid 0.008, Balt, Montmorency, France). Microcatheter injection revealed fistulas that were draining into single common venous channel. At least two fistulas were visualized with no evidence of intervening nidus network. In view of the high flow, it was decided to use 80% glue (*n*-butyl 2-cyanoacrylate diluted with lipiodol).

Care was taken during the glue injection to close the feeders and the fistulas while preserving

V. Gupta et al. (eds.), *100 Interesting Case Studies in Neurointervention: Tips and Tricks*, https://doi.org/10.1007/978-981-13-1346-2_79

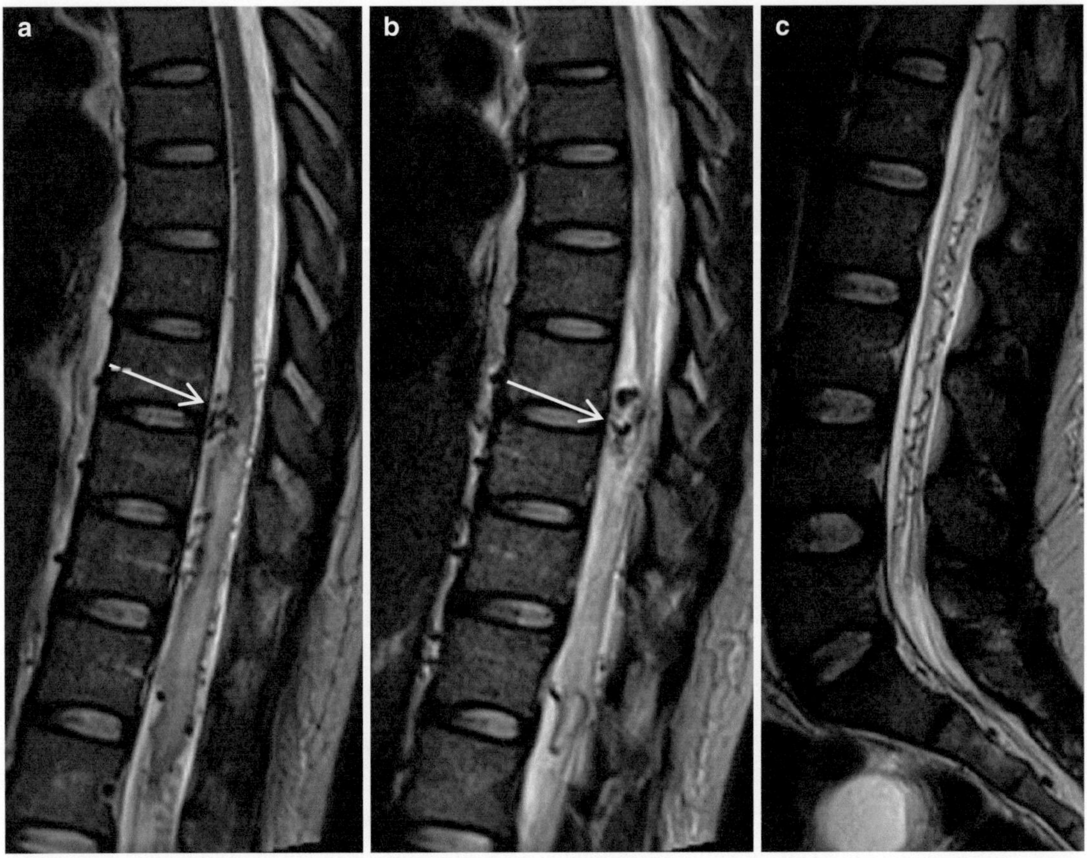

Fig. 79.1 (**a** and **b**) Sagittal T2-weighted images show multiple prominent flow voids in the lower dorsal and in lumbar region particularly anterior to the cord (arrow, **b**); flow void seen at the level of the conus (**c**)

the anterior spinal access by stopping the glue injection as soon as it refluxed over the microcatheter tip (Fig. 79.3). Post-embolization angiogram of left 12th segmental artery revealed no evidence of any residual arteriovenous fistula. Retrograde filling of the feeders from the right 9th intercostal was seen, confirming the initial analysis that both the feeders supplied the common final channel to feed the AVF. The stump of the feeder was well visualized in the angiogram. Postoperative angio-CT (DynaCT, Siemens German) was performed which revealed the glue cast in the feeders as well both the limbs of AVF, with some of the glue in the veins as well (Fig. 79.4).

Patient did not have any complications related to the procedure. She had progressive improvement in her neurological deficits over next few months, and at 3 months, the patient had 4/5 power in both lower limbs and was walking without support.

Tip and Tricks

1. It is important to recognize an anterior spinal artery feeder in spinal arteriovenous malformations. Look at the native view; if the feeder takes a hairpin bend in the midline of the spinal canal, it indicates probable anterior spinal artery feeder and can be confirmed by looking at the lateral views in which the anterior spinal artery feeders lies in the anterior part of spinal canal.
2. It is important to understand the angioarchitecture of the spinal AVM before embolizing or performing surgery. It is also useful to look at those images in the

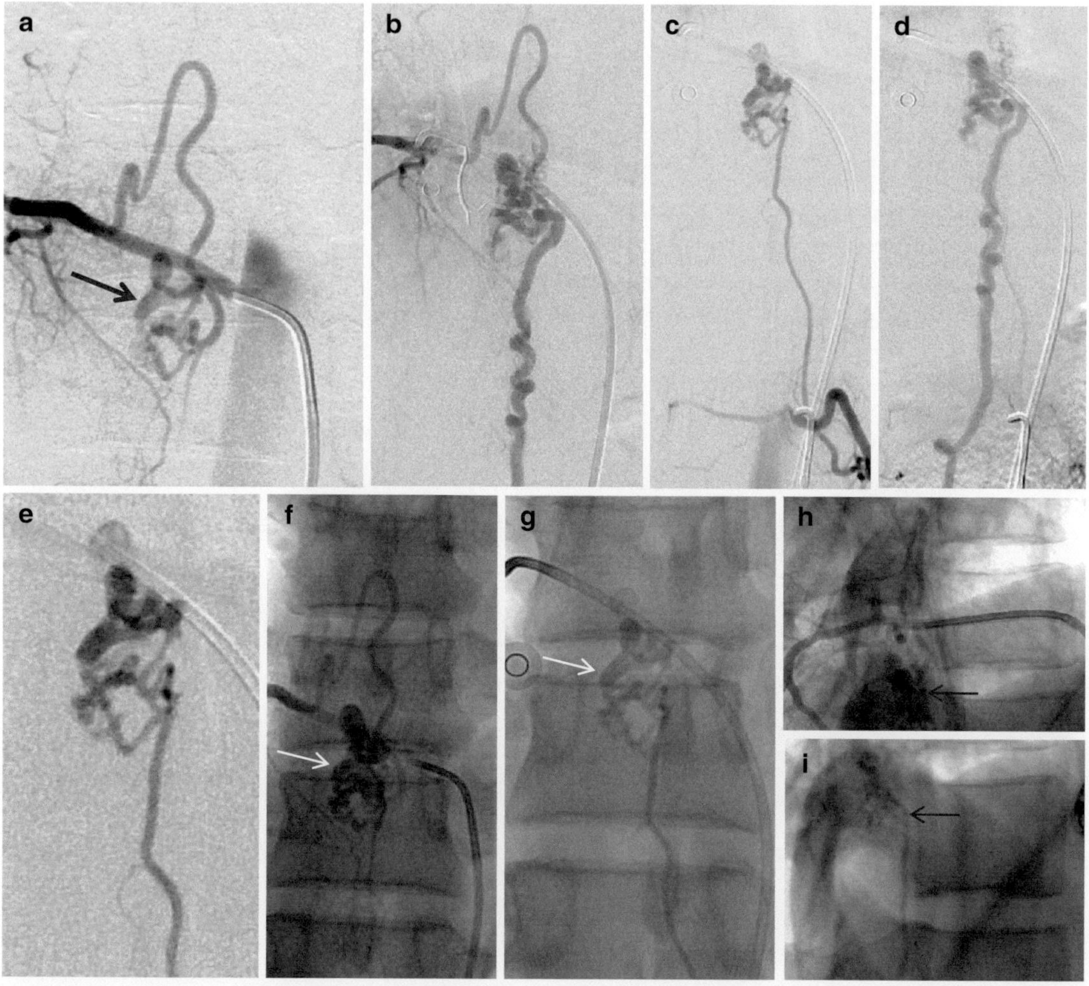

Fig. 79.2 (**a** and **b**) Right ninth intercostal artery injection shows an arteriovenous fistula along with venous aneurysms and single draining vein. (**c**–**e**) Right 12th intercostal artery injection showing filling of the same AVF. As seen in Fig. (**e**), the AVF filling from the 12th intercostal artery injection is same as from the upper (Fig. **a**, ninth intercostal) injection. (**f**–**i**)—(**f** and **g**) shows AP view of native images from 9th intercostal (**f**) and 12th intercostal (**g**) injections which show that AVF is located in midline at 9th to 10th dorsal level. The feedings arteries are in midline and the ninth intercostal feeder forms a hairpin bend in midline. (**h**) and (**i**) Native images in lateral view show that AVF is located in anterior part of spinal canal. Analysis of these angiographic findings confirm that the AVF is located at 9th to 10th dorsal level fed from anterior spinal axis and the same fistula fills from both the feeders

native view so that one can understand the location of various parts of the AVM being filled by different feeders and relationship to each other by seeing them in the background of the bony images. In our case, the understanding that both the feeders were converging to feed the same arteriovenous fistula was immensely useful in planning the embolization.

3. It is important to preserve anterior spinal axis in cases with feeders arising from the anterior spinal artery. Anterior spinal artery is usually in the midline anterior to the cord. From the ASA, sulco-commissural arteries arise which usually ascend posterosuperiorly to supply the cord or in cases of AVM to supply the vascular malformation. If one can selectively enter the enlarged sulco-commissural branch and

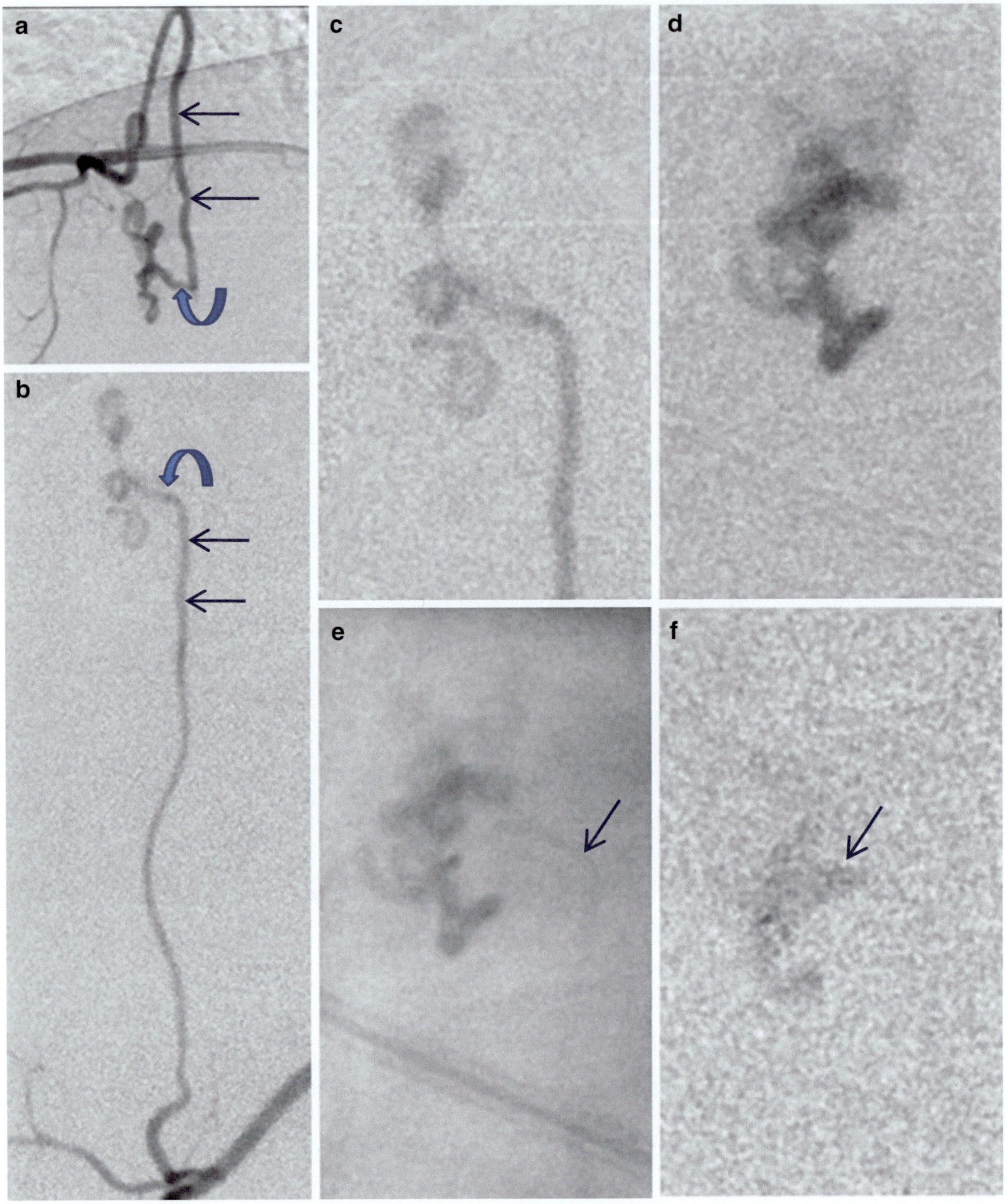

Fig. 79.3 Embolization procedure (**a** and **b**). Early frames of right ninth intercostal (**a**) and 12th intercostal injection (**b**) show that both feeders converge to a common feeder channel (curved arrows). This is likely to represent enlarged sulco-commissural artery, while the main channels (arrows) represent enlarged anterior spinal axis. It was vital to preserve the anterior spinal artery. Notice that the angle between main artery and this branch is less acute in the 12th intercostal artery feeder. (**c**) Enlarged view of (**b**) shows AVF very well. (**d**) Microcatheter injection reveals the fistula. The catheter was placed from lower 12th IC feeder due to more convenient angle between the spinal axis and sulco-commissural feeder. (**e**) Native images of microcatheter injection show the angle (arrow) where it enters the branch from main spinal axis, which tells us the absolute limit of glue reflux. (**f**) Glue cast shows that there has been no reflux into the main spinal artery

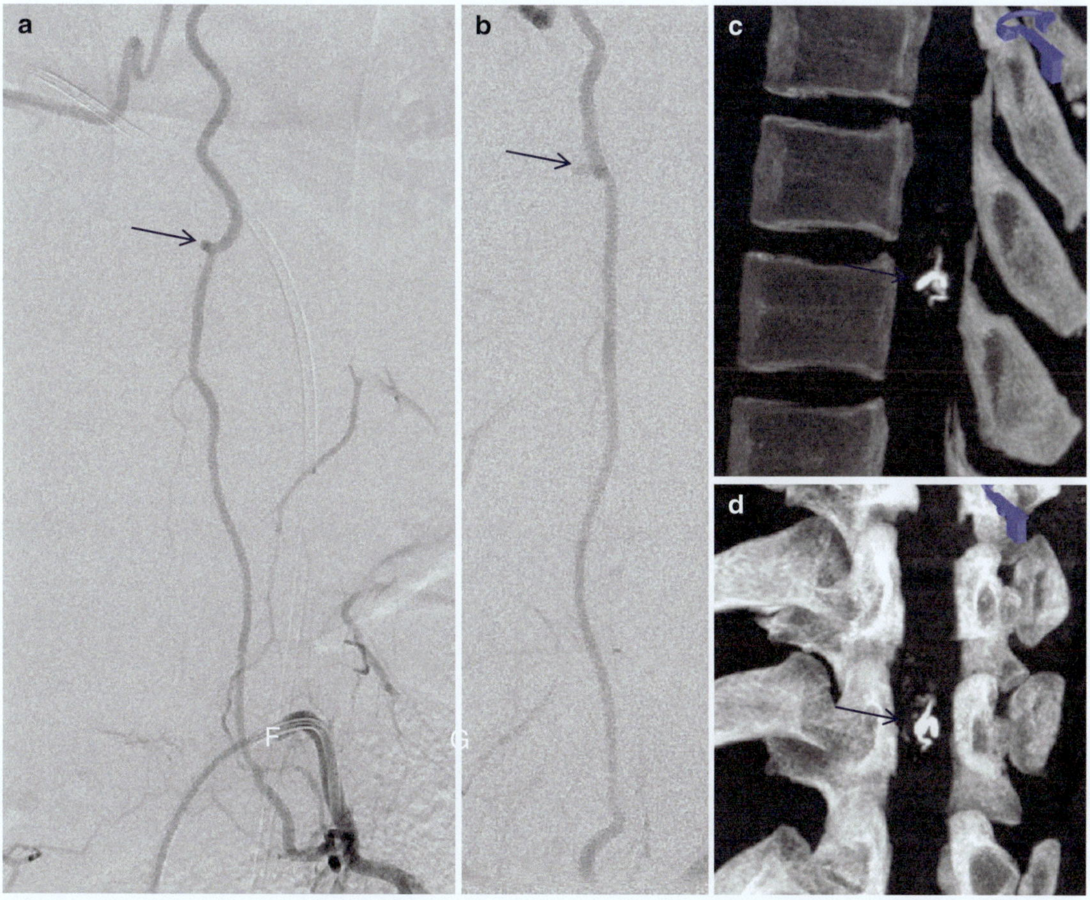

Fig. 79.4 (**a** and **b**) Injection from left 12th intercostal artery reveals complete occlusion of the AVF with preservation of anterior spinal axis. Notice antegrade flow into the right ninth intercostal artery. Arrow indicates the stump of occluded feeder. (**c** and **d**) Angio-CT image of glue cast

embolize through it while preserving the anterior spinal axis, one is unlikely to cause clinical complication.

4. As shown in Fig. 79.3, careful evaluation of the angio-architecture was important in understanding the junction between ASA and the feeder which was an enlarged sulco-commissural artery. It is crucial to have a mental picture to decide the allowable extent of glue reflux on to the microcatheter and all precautions should be taken not to let it come back to the ASA which can lead to devastating consequences.
5. Angio-CT is sometimes useful to visualize the glue cast that may be not be visualized in fluoroscopy or DSA images.
6. Embolization can be performed using a DSA run instead of the road map in cases of high-flow fistula in which high concentration of glue is used.

Suggested Reading

Andres RH, Barth A, Guzman R, Remonda L, El-Koussy M, Seiler RW, Widmer HR, Schroth G. Endovascular and surgical treatment of spinal dural arteriovenous fistulas. Neuroradiology. 2008;50:869–76.

Willinsky R, terBrugge K, Montanera W, et al. Spinal epidural arteriovenous fistulas: arterial and venous approaches to embolization. AJNR Am J Neuroradiol. 1993;14:812–7.

Spinal Dural Arteriovenous Fistula (AVF)

80

Vipul Gupta

Case

A 50-year-old man presented with a history of numbness in both lower limbs and associated urine and fecal incontinence for 6 months. There was no history of trauma. MRI scan showed multiple flow voids in the lower cervical and dorsal spine along with cord edema in the lower thoracic cord suggestive of a vascular malformation (Fig. 80.1). Spinal angiography demonstrated spinal dural AV fistula at L4–L5 levels with arterial feeders from the lateral sacral branches (Fig. 80.2).

Issues

1. Multiple small tortuous feeders

Management

A small 11-cm-long 5F sheath (Cordis) was used to access the right femoral artery. Following this a 5F diagnostic catheter (Cook) was positioned in the left internal iliac artery. The diagnostic catheter acts as a guiding catheter. Following this, a Marathon 1.5F microcatheter (ev3 Neurovascular, Irvine, CA) over a Mirage 0.008 micro-guidewire (ev3 Neurovascular, Irvine, CA) was placed as distal as possible. Due to the ultra-narrow caliber of the feeders and tortuosity, it was not possible to navigate the microcatheter till the fistula site (Fig. 80.3).

Once the microcatheter was positioned as distal as possible in the feeding artery, the fistula was embolized using 15% glue (mixed with lipiodol). The glue penetrated into the venous side obliterating the fistula (Fig. 80.4).

Patient made good clinical recovery with significant improvement over a period of 6 months.

V. Gupta
Neurointerventional Surgery, Stroke Unit, Artemis Agrim Institute of Neuroscience, Gurgaon, India
e-mail: vipul.gupta@artemishospitals.com

Tips and Tricks

1. The aim of treatment in spinal dural fistula is to obliterate the draining vein.
2. A proximal arterial occlusion will lead to a transient improvement of symptoms; however, the fistula is prone to recur from collaterals.
3. A slow continuous injection of much dilute glue (15% glue and 85% lipiodol) has a higher chance of reaching the draining vein and obliterating the fistula.
4. In cases of suspected spinal fistula, complete spinal and cranial angiogram is essential as the feeding arteries can be superior or inferior to the fistulous segment.
5. Use of flow guided microcatheter is highly recommended.

V. Gupta et al. (eds.), *100 Interesting Case Studies in Neurointervention: Tips and Tricks*,
https://doi.org/10.1007/978-981-13-1346-2_80

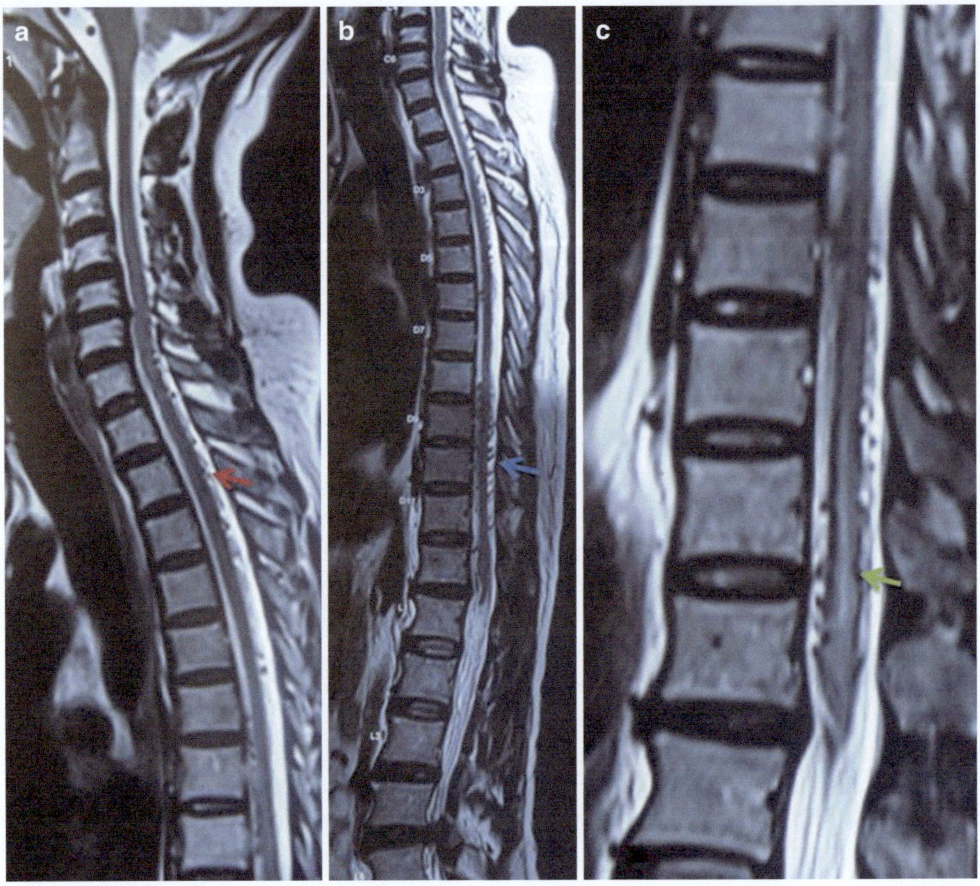

Fig. 80.1 MRI spine shows multiple flow voids in the lower cervical and upper dorsal spine (**a**) (red arrow) and in the lower dorsal spine (**b**) (blue arrow). (**c**) Marked edema in the lower thoracic cord (green arrow)

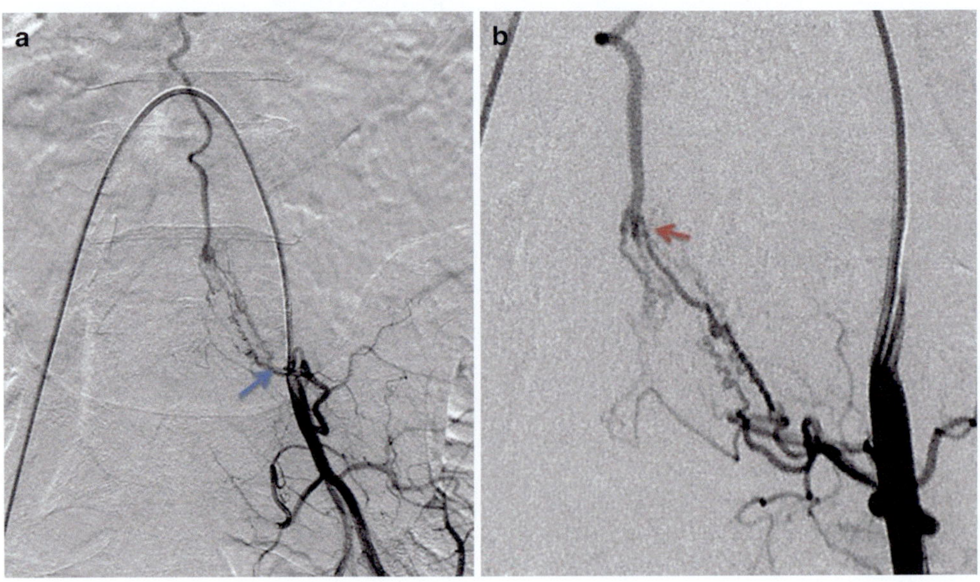

Fig. 80.2 Spinal angiography demonstrated spinal dural AV fistula at L4–L5 levels with arterial feeders from the lateral sacral branches (**a**) (blue arrow). (**b**) Magnified view demonstrating multiple tortuous feeders and site of the fistula (red arrow)

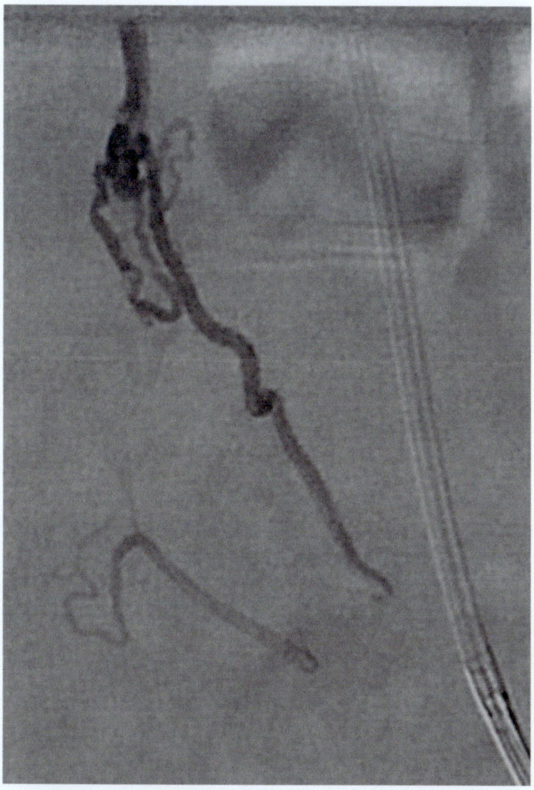

Fig. 80.3 Super-selective microcatheter injection demonstrating the fistula

Suggested Reading

Andres RH, Barth A, Guzman R, Remonda L, El-Koussy M, Seiler RW, Widmer HR, Schroth G. Endovascular and surgical treatment of spinal dural arteriovenous fistulas. Neuroradiology. 2008;50:869–76.

Willinsky R, terBrugge K, Montanera W, et al. Spinal epidural arteriovenous fistulas: arterial and venous approaches to embolization. AJNR Am J Neuroradiol. 1993;14:812–7.

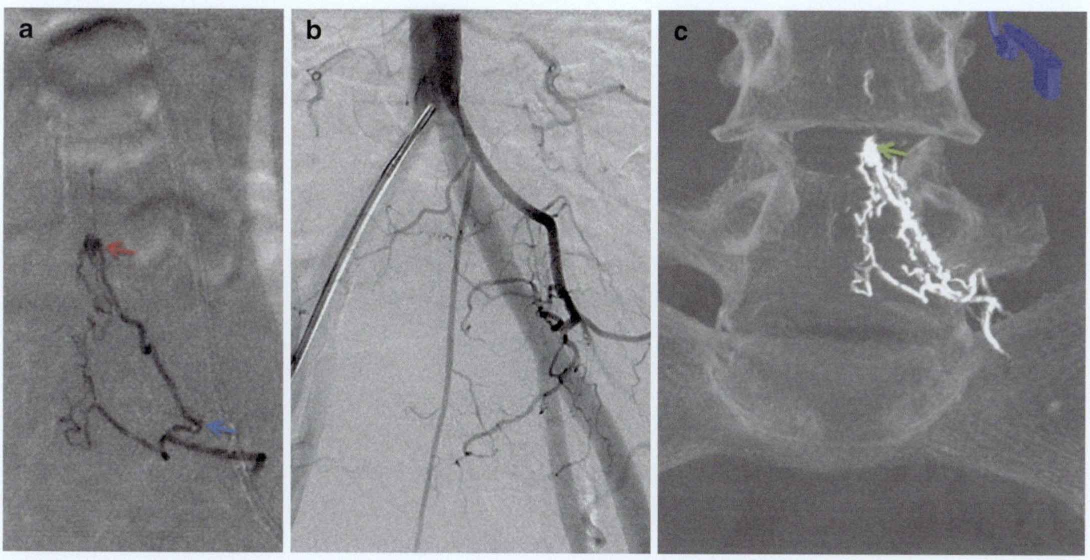

Fig. 80.4 (**a**) The fistula was embolized using much diluted glue (15%). The blue arrow marks the microcatheter position, while the red arrow marks the entry of glue into the proximal draining vein. (**b**) Post-embolization angiogram demonstrates complete obliteration of the fistula. (**c**) Post-procedure DynaCT (angiographic CT) demonstrated the complete glue cast and more importantly, the obliteration of the vein (green arrow)

Part III

Stroke and Carotid Disease

Acute Mechanical Thrombectomy Using Stent Retriever with Balloon Guide Catheter: Proximal Flow Arrest and Reversal

81

Ajit S. Puri, Aviraj Deshmukh, and Rajsrinivas Parthasarathy

Case

A 71-year-old male presented with right hemiplegia and global aphasia of 4 h duration. On admission the NIHSS was 25. On multimodal imaging, he was noted to have terminal ICA occlusion with small infarct core size. Direct mechanical thrombectomy was planned as IV tpa was contraindicated in view of recent myocardial infarction (Figs. 81.1, 81.2, 81.3, and 81.4).

Issues

1. General vs local anesthesia
2. Risk of migration of clot to distal and new territories
3. Avoiding cannulation of perforator branch while crossing the clot, and therefore, the risk of perforation
4. Rapid and first-pass reperfusion

Management

Patient was uncooperative with high NIHSS score, and henceforth, procedure was done under general anesthesia. An 8F short sheath was introduced through right femoral artery. Then, 8F balloon guide catheter (BGC) was navigated to the proximal left ICA origin. Initial run showed occlusion at the ophthalmic segment of ICA (Fig. 81.1). A 014′ microwire (Traxcess, Microvention, Tustin, California, USA) was used along with stent delivery straight-tip microcatheter (XT 27, Stryker Neurovascular). A tight loop at the tip of the wire was used to traverse the clot. The XT 27 microcatheter was then advanced over the wire across the clot. A Trevo stent 4 × 30 mm was deployed using "push and fluff" technique (Fig. 81.2). There was minimal antegrade flow (Fig. 81.3). Four-minute interval time was given for the entrapment of the clot into the stent. BGC catheter was then inflated with 50% contrast. Suction force was employed with aspiration through a 60 CC syringe. The stent along with the clot was pulled back into the guiding catheter. Vigorous aspiration was done once again after stent retrieval, as there are chances of clot detach-

A. S. Puri (✉)
Radiology, and Neurosurgery,
Division of Neurointerventional Surgery,
Neurointerventional Fellowship Program,
University of Massachusetts Medical Center,
Worcester, MA, USA
e-mail: ajit.puri@umassmemorial.org

A. Deshmukh
Neurointerventional Surgery, Artemis Agrim Institute of Neuroscience, Gurgaon, India

R. Parthasarathy
Vascular Neurology and Neurointerventional Surgery,
Artemis Agrim Institute of Neuroscience,
Gurgaon, India

V. Gupta et al. (eds.), *100 Interesting Case Studies in Neurointervention: Tips and Tricks*,
https://doi.org/10.1007/978-981-13-1346-2_81

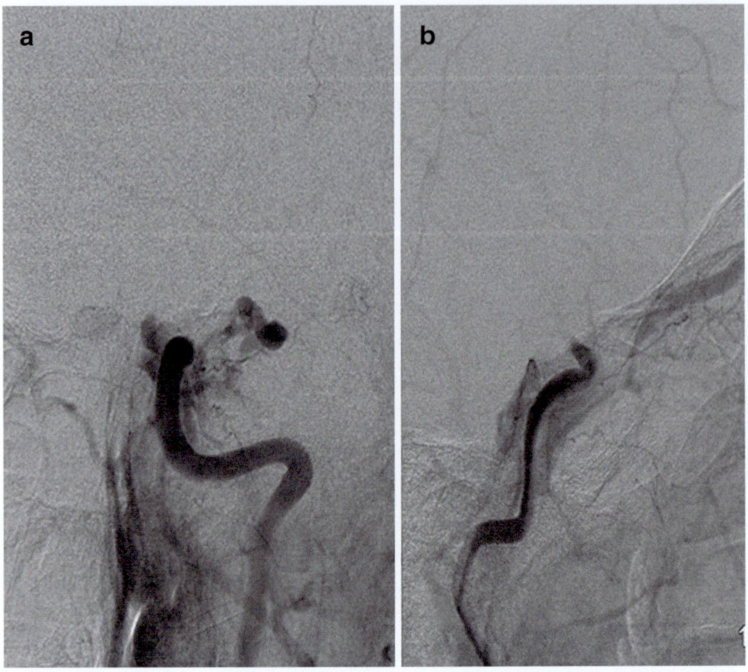

Fig. 81.1 Frontal (**a**) and lateral (**b**) angiogram of the left ICA shows stasis and occlusion at the ophthalmic segment

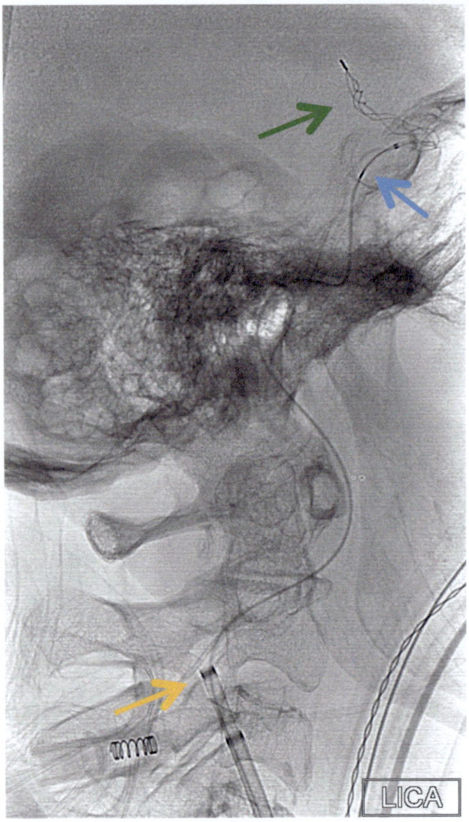

Fig. 81.2 The set-up includes a 8F balloon guide catheter (orange arrow), microcatheter was stent-retriever delivery (blue arrow) and the stent-retriever (green arrow)

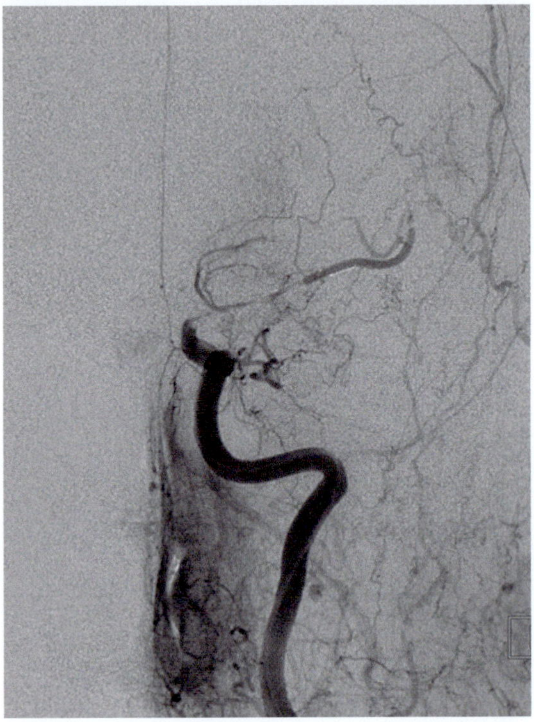

Fig. 81.3 Frontal angiogram after stent retriever deployment shows minimal flow through the left MCA

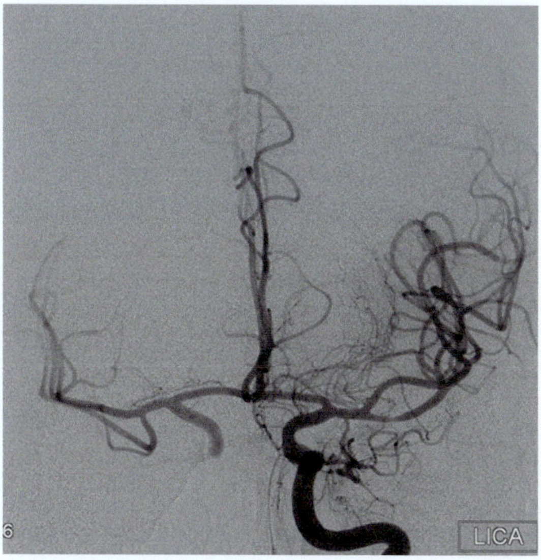

Fig. 81.4 Frontal angiogram after retrieval of the clot shows TICI 3 recanalization with minimal spasm in the inferior division of the left MCA

ment during stent retrieval. Post procedure angiogram revealed TICI 3 reperfusion in ICA with minimal spasm in the inferior division of the left MCA (Fig. 81.4). NIHSS score at discharge was 2 with MRS score of 1. MRS at 90 days was 0.

Tips and Tricks

1. Use balloon guide catheter for proximal flow arrest, and reversal of flow can be achieved by manual/mechanical suction through the side port during stent retrieval to avoid distal embolization.
2. Loop at the wire tip helps avoid inadvertent canalization of perforator branches and subsequent risk of wire perforation.
3. Usually the clot burden in ICA occlusion is high; henceforth, use a long stent to adequately cover the clot and a large diameter stent to allow for greater radical strength that helps with better engagement of the clot.
4. Partially resheath the proximal end of the stent during retrieval to avoid chances of stent detachment during retrieval in case of detachable stents.
5. Use the Push and fluff technique. First, unsheath the distal aspect of the stent. The stent expands and forms an anchor to the arterial wall. Then, push the stent out so that catheter retracts on its own. Following that, push both catheter and stent to fluff it open. Push and fluff technique improves wall opposition and clot engagement and therefore higher chances of first-pass reperfusion, lower number of passes, and improved rates of recanalization.
6. Vigorous aspiration after stent retrieval is necessary as there are chances of clot detachment during retrieval

Suggested Reading

Bush CK, et al. endovascular treatment with stent-retriever devices for acute ischemic stroke: a meta-analysis of randomized controlled trials. PLoS One. 2016;11(1):e0147287.

Haussen D, et al. Optimizating clot retrieval in acute stroke: the push and fluff technique for closed-cell stentriever. Stroke. 2015;46(10):2838–42.

82 ADAPT Technique for Stroke Thrombectomy

Ajit S. Puri, Aviraj Deshmukh, and Rajsrinivas Parthasarathy

Case 1

An 88-year-old male patient with wake-up stroke had left hemiplegia and hemineglect on examination and an admission NIHSS of 17. Angiography (CTA) showed right MCA occlusion.

Issues

Navigating the large lumen suction catheter distally to the site of clot across the tortuous ICA
Preventing distal embolization of clot

A. S. Puri (✉)
Radiology, and Neurosurgery,
Division of Neurointerventional Surgery,
Neurointerventional Fellowship Program,
University of Massachusetts Medical Center,
Worcester, MA, USA
e-mail: ajit.puri@umassmemorial.org

A. Deshmukh
Neurointerventional Surgery, Artemis Agrim Institute of Neuroscience, Gurgaon, India

R. Parthasarathy
Vascular Neurology and Neurointerventional Surgery,
Artemis Agrim Institute of Neuroscience,
Gurgaon, India

Management

Procedure was done under local anesthesia. An 8F short sheath was used along with 6F Neuron Max (Penumbra Inc) for good distal support. Neuron Max was advanced to the distal cervical ICA. Initial run revealed a right M1 MCA occlusion (Fig. 82.1a). A 5 Max ACE catheter was then coaxially advanced over the 014 microwire and XT 27 microcatheter (Stryker Neurovascular). Clot was traversed with microwire and not the microcatheter, to avoid risk of distal embolization. Once the distal end of 5 Max ace catheter is adequately positioned just proximal of the clot in right M1 MCA (Fig. 82.1b), microwire-microcatheter system was removed and aspiration catheter attached to the mechanical aspiration pump (Penumbra aspiration pump). Aspiration was turned on, and good blood flow was noted in the tubing. The suction catheter was slowly advanced further to engage the clot. Absence of blood flow in the system was noted at this point, which is an indicator of engagement of clot. At this point, catheter is advanced by 1–2 mm for solid engagement of the thrombus. Aspiration was maintained for 2 min and then slowly removed under constant aspiration. Vigorous aspiration of the sheath was done once again so as to remove any fragmented particles of the clot. Post-aspiration run revealed complete recanalization (TICI 3 score) of middle cerebral artery (Fig. 82.1c). NIHSS on discharge was 1 with MRS of 0. On 90-day follow-up, NIHSS was 0.

V. Gupta et al. (eds.), *100 Interesting Case Studies in Neurointervention: Tips and Tricks*,
https://doi.org/10.1007/978-981-13-1346-2_82

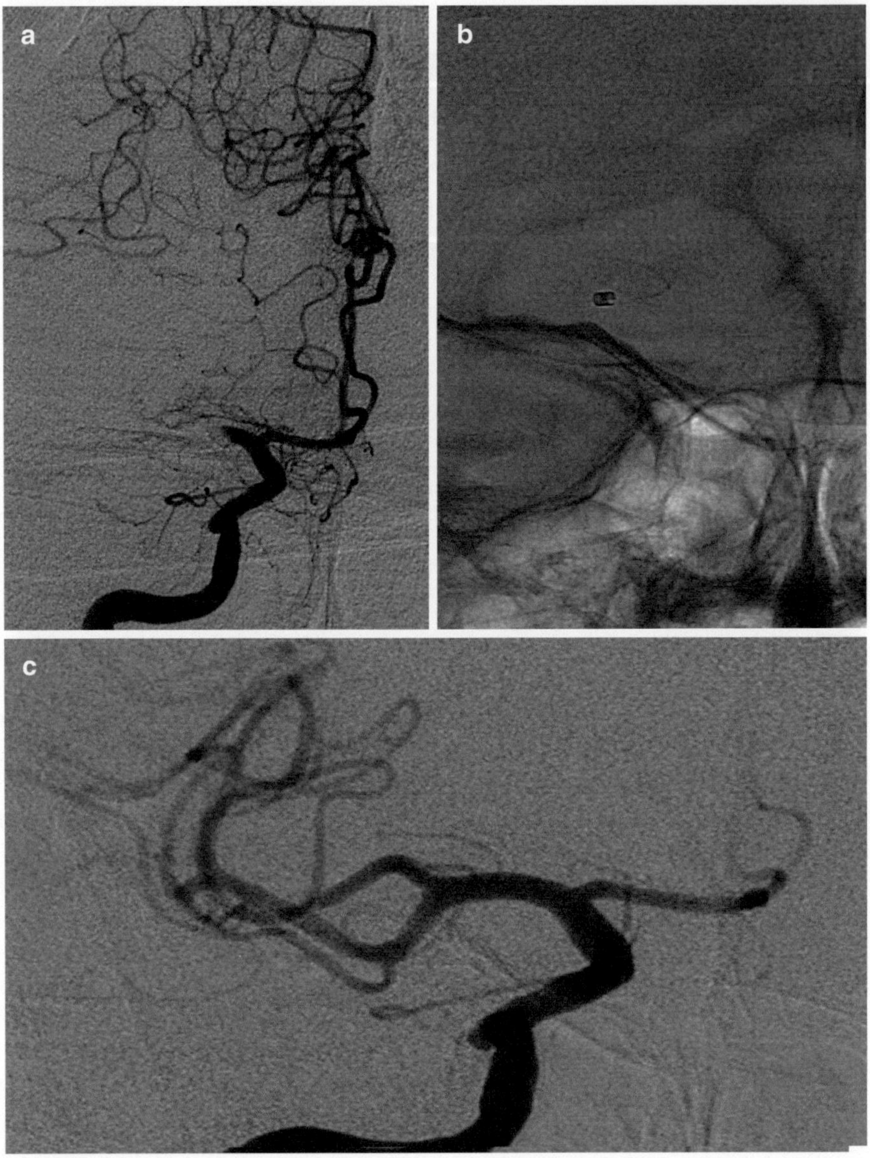

Fig. 82.1 (**a**) Frontal angiogram of the right ICA shows a proximal right MCA occlusion. (**b**) Aspiration catheter tip in right MCA. (**c**) Post-thrombectomy frontal angiogram shows complete recanalization

Case 2

A 65-year-old male with CAD, atrial fibrillation on anticoagulation presented with quadriparesis and somnolence. CTA was suggestive of basilar occlusion.

Management

An 8F Neuron Max was positioned into distal part of V2 segment of vertebral artery. Initial run revealed a mid basilar trunk occlusion (Fig. 82.2a). A 5 Max catheter along with

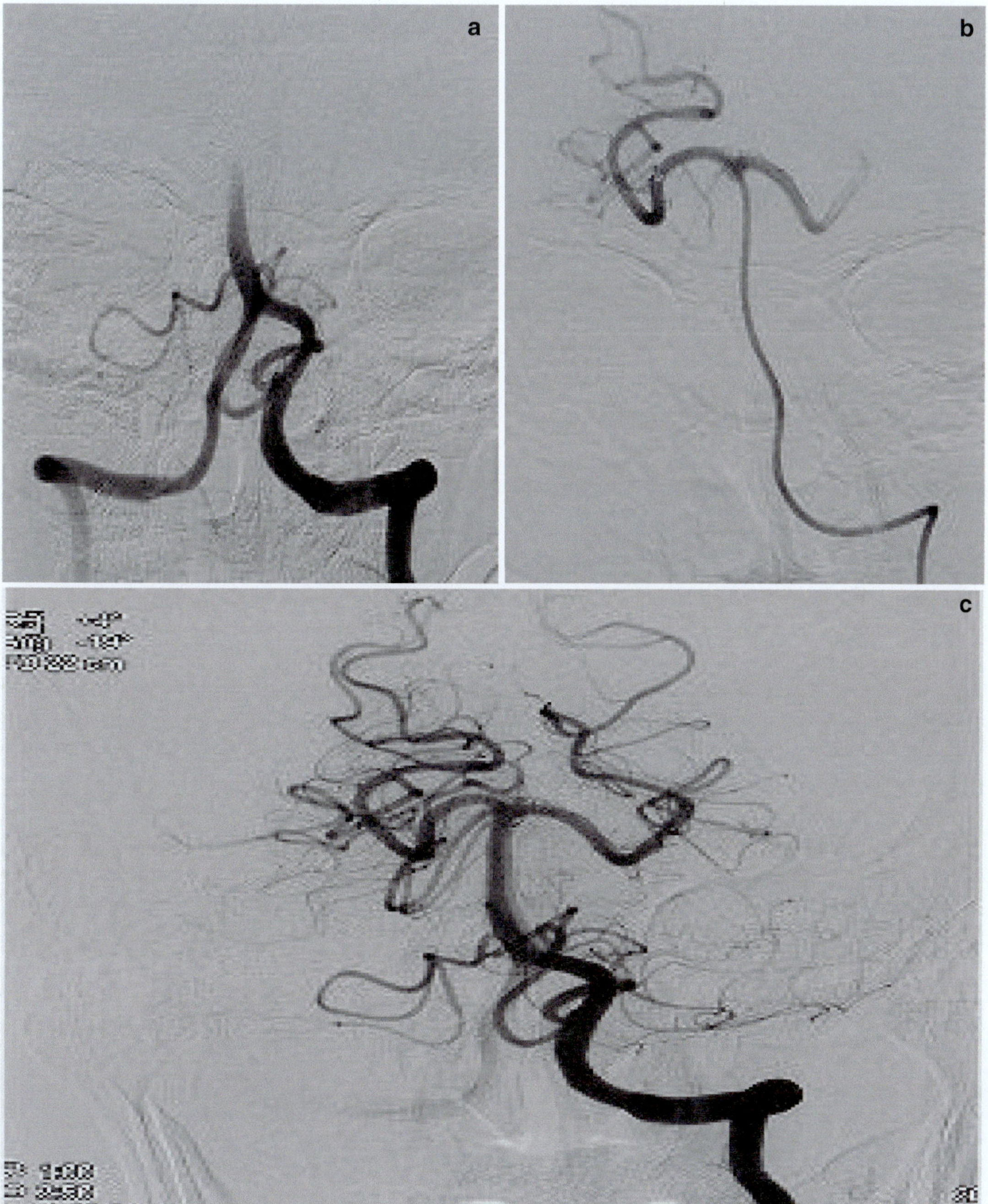

Fig. 82.2 (**a**) Left vertebral angiogram shows mid-top of the basilar occlusion. (**b**) Suction catheter has been advanced into the right P1–P2 PCA under constant aspiration. (**c**) Follow-up angiogram shows complete recanalization

microwire-microcatheter was advanced to the distal part of basilar artery and aspiration was initiated as mentioned above (Fig. 82.2b). Post-aspiration angiogram revealed good flow in bilateral PCA (Fig. 82.2c). Patient improved post-procedure and discharged with NIHSS of 3 and MRS of 1. On 90-day follow-up, NIHSS was 1 and MRS 0.

Tips and Tricks

1. Always select the largest caliber aspiration catheter in order to maximize the suction force that can be delivered at the distal end of the catheter.
2. An 8F Neuron Max sheath is navigated as distally as possible into the cervical/petrous segment of internal carotid artery or distal V2 segment of vertebral artery to provide the necessary support to navigate the aspiration catheter into the intracranial arteries.
3. We prefer using 0.014′ microwire with 0.027′ microcatheter to coaxially advance 5 Max catheter, as 027′ catheter provides better support to navigate the intermediate catheter.
4. In cases where there is tortuosity in ICA or vertebral artery, 5 Max catheter can be coaxially advanced over 3 Max along with microwire-microcatheter system.
5. Always cross clot only with the microwire. Avoid using microcatheter to cross the clot to avoid distal displacement of the clot.
6. Continuous aspiration with aspiration pump can be applied safely for up to 4 min.

Suggested Reading

Stapleton CJ, et al. A direct aspiration first-pass technique vs Stentriever thrombectomy in emergent large vessel intracranial occlusions. J Neurosurg. 2017:1–8.

Turk AS, et al. ADAPT FAST study: a direct aspiration first pass technique for acute stroke thrombectomy. J Neurointerv Surg. 2014;6(4):260–4.

Solumbra Technique

83

Ajit S. Puri, Aviraj Deshmukh,
and Rajsrinivas Parthasarathy

Case

A 53-year-old male patient with left UL and LL weakness had a NIHSS score of 8. The ASPECTS score and the collateral score were favorable. The frontal right ICA angiogram shows a right M1 MCA occlusion.

Issues

1. Can be considered as a rescue technique when there is failure of either direct aspiration or stentriever-based mechanical thrombectomy
2. Navigating the large lumen suction catheter distally to the site of clot across the tortuous ICA or vertebral artery

A. S. Puri (✉)
Radiology, and Neurosurgery,
Division of Neurointerventional Surgery,
Neurointerventional Fellowship Program,
University of Massachusetts Medical Center,
Worcester, MA, USA
e-mail: ajit.puri@umassmemorial.org

A. Deshmukh
Neurointerventional Surgery, Artemis Agrim Institute of Neuroscience, Gurgaon, India

R. Parthasarathy
Vascular Neurology and Neurointerventional Surgery,
Artemis Agrim Institute of Neuroscience,
Gurgaon, India

Management

Procedure was done under local anesthesia. An 8F short sheath was used along with Neuron Max. Neuron Max (Penumbra Inc.) was advanced to the cervical ICA. Initial angiography revealed right M1 MCA occlusion (Fig. 83.1a). A 5 Max (Penumbra Inc.) was used as an aspiration catheter. It was coaxially advanced across the tortuous bend of ICA over 3 Max and 0.014′ microwire up to M1 part of MCA just proximal to the thrombus. Curved wire along with microcatheter (Prowler 0.021′) was slowly advanced across the clot. Wire was removed. Microcatheter run was taken to confirm the position. A Trevo 4 x 30 mm was then introduced through the microcatheter, and stent was then deployed using push and fluff technique. Once deployed, the microcatheter was removed (Fig. 83.1b). The 5 Max was connected to the aspiration system. The stent with clot is pulled back into the Intermediate catheter until resistance is noted. The system as whole is then retrieved into the Neuron Max under suction. Once the intermediate catheter is removed, strong suction is applied to the Neuron Max to aspirate any fragmented clot. Post-procedure angiogram revealed TICI 3 flow in right MCA (Fig. 83.1c). Patient improved completely over the next 2–3 days. NIHSS at discharge was 0.

V. Gupta et al. (eds.), *100 Interesting Case Studies in Neurointervention: Tips and Tricks*,
https://doi.org/10.1007/978-981-13-1346-2_83

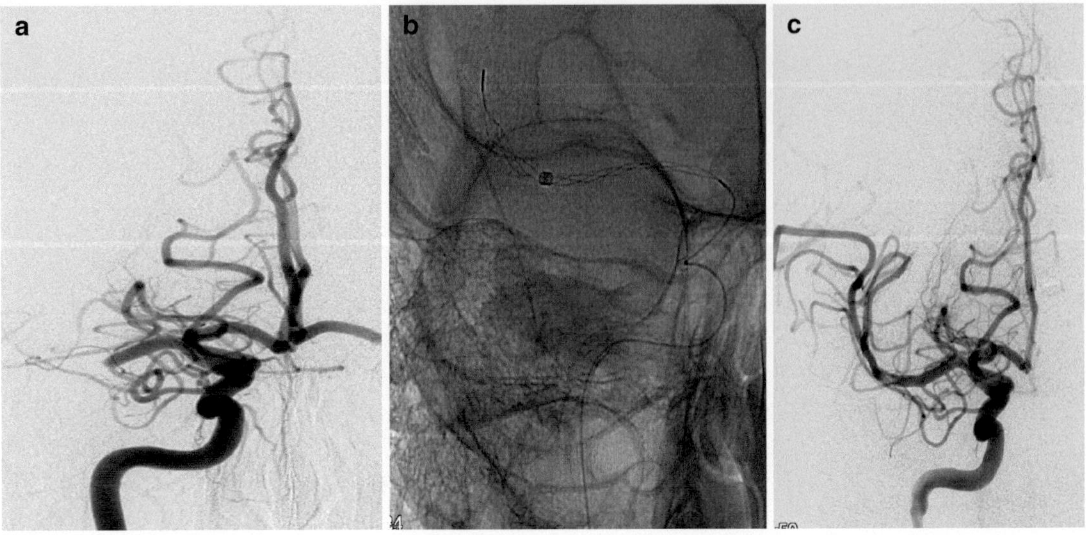

Fig. 83.1 (**a**) R MCA occlusion, (**b**) stent partly deployed, intermediate catheter till the proximal end of the clot, and (**c**) TICI3 flow achieved

Tips and Tricks

1. Solumbra technique is particularly helpful when there is failure of either direct aspiration or stent retriever technique alone. This is particularly true when the clot burden is large or if the clot is a hard clot.
2. Use of aspiration catheter along with stent increases the rates of reperfusion with less chance of distal embolization.
3. In patients with tortuous ICA or vertebral artery, deployed stent acts as an anchor to advance aspiration catheter across the bend.

Suggested Reading

Delgado Almandoz JE, et al. Comparison of clinical outcomes in patients with acute ischemic strokes treated with mechanical thrombectomy using either Solumbra or ADAPT techniques. J Neurointerv Surg. 2016;8(11):1123–8.

Aspiration Retriever Technique in Stroke (ARTS)

84

Ajit S. Puri and Rajsrinivas Parthasarathy

Case

An 83-year-old female presented with acute onset right-sided weakness and facial droop. Intravenous t-PA was administered at outside hospital. The patient was transferred to our center, and as patient had persistent deficit (NIHSS 27) and repeat imaging showed left M1 MCA occlusion, mechanical thrombectomy was undertaken (Fig. 84.1a, b).

A. S. Puri (✉)
Radiology, and Neurosurgery,
Division of Neurointerventional Surgery,
Neurointerventional Fellowship Program,
University of Massachusetts Medical Center,
Worcester, MA, USA
e-mail: ajit.puri@umassmemorial.org

R. Parthasarathy
Vascular Neurology and Neurointerventional Surgery,
Artemis Agrim Institute of Neuroscience,
Gurgaon, India

Issues

- Distal embolism into new (ACA) territory resulting in impairment of collateral flow
- Distal embolism in MCA territory
- Safely navigating a large-bore catheter proximal to the clot and avoiding dissection while navigating through tortuous anatomy
- Rapid reperfusion

Management

Procedure was performed under general anesthesia. An 8F short sheath was inserted into the right femoral artery. Following that, a balloon guide MERCI 8F (BGC) was parked in the proximal left cervical ICA. Thereafter, Penumbra 5 MAX (Penumbra Inc.) was taken over a Rebar 27 microcatheter (ev3, Irvine, USA), proximal to the clot. The clot was traversed with the wire, following which the microcatheter was advanced beyond the clot. A loop at the tip of the wire was used to traverse the clot to avoid entry into perforator/side branches. Stentriever, Solitaire 4 × 40 mm stent (ev3, Irvine, USA), was then deployed across the clot. Initial unsheathing allowed the distal end of the stent to open and anchor to the wall of the artery. Thereafter, the stent was pushed out while maintaining forward tension in the microcatheter to ensure adequate opening of the stent. The microcatheter was

V. Gupta et al. (eds.), *100 Interesting Case Studies in Neurointervention: Tips and Tricks*,
https://doi.org/10.1007/978-981-13-1346-2_84

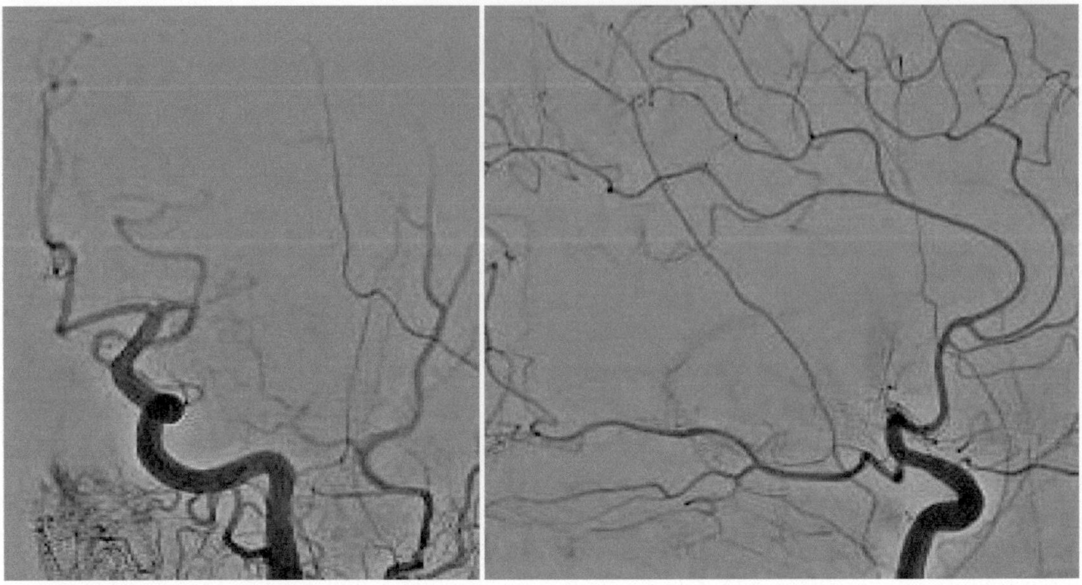

Fig. 84.1 Left ICA injection shows occluded left M1 MCA

removed. After 4 min, the BGC was inflated to achieve proximal flow arrest, and the intermediate catheter was attached to the aspiration pump. The stentriever was retracted into the intermediate guide catheter until resistance was noted. Following that, the system as a whole was removed, and the balloon guide catheter was aspirated (steps described in Fig. 84.2 cartoon). TICI 3 recanalization was achieved (Fig. 84.3). Patient had a mRS of 1 at 90 days.

Tips and Tricks

1. Balloon guides are large-bore catheters; henceforth, one should be careful while navigating the catheter across a bend in the ICA. Severe spasm and dissections are not uncommon, and the authors would suggest taking the BGC coaxially over a 5 F catheter.
2. Navigating a large-bore catheter across the cavernous bend to the site of the clot can be challenging particularly in tortuous anatomy.
3. Steps to consider in a sequential manner if unable to navigate the large-bore catheter to the MCA.
   (a) 0.014′ microwire, 0.027′ microcatheter (rebar 27; XT 27; velocity 0.025′), 5 MAX Penumbra (coaxial).
   (b) Deploy the stent across the clot. This gives the necessary anchorage to take the 5 MAX up.
   (c) 0.014′ microwire, 0.017′ microcatheter, 3 MAX, and 5 MAX coaxial system
   (d) 0.014′ wire, 0.021′ microcatheter, 0.038 DAC, and 5 MAX.
4. BGC should be adequately inflated to achieve flow arrest. Negative suction through a 60 cc syringe should be applied through the side port while aspirating through the intermediate catheter.

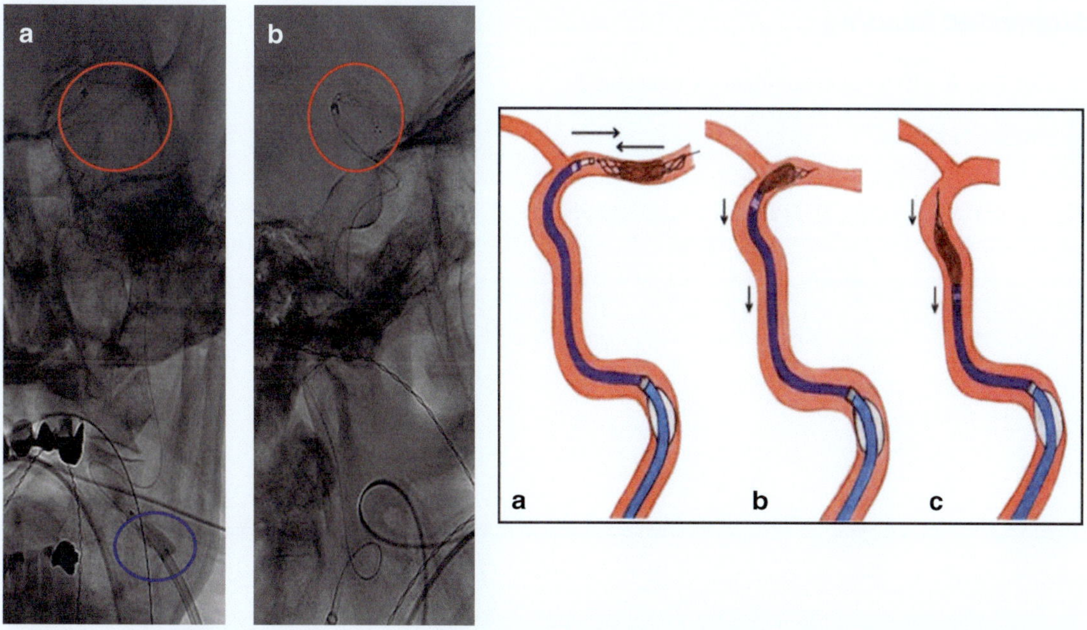

Fig. 84.2 (**a**) Inflated balloon guide (blue circle); (**a**, **b**) Penumbra 5 MAX proximal to the clot with the stent deployed. (Cartoon: *a*) Balloon guide in the proximal ICA; stentriever deployed across the clot; note microcatheter proximal to the clot. *b*) Microcatheter removed, the Penumbra 5 MAX is connected to the suction pump, and the stent is pulled back into the 5 MAX until resistance is noted. *c*) Stent with clot pulled out)

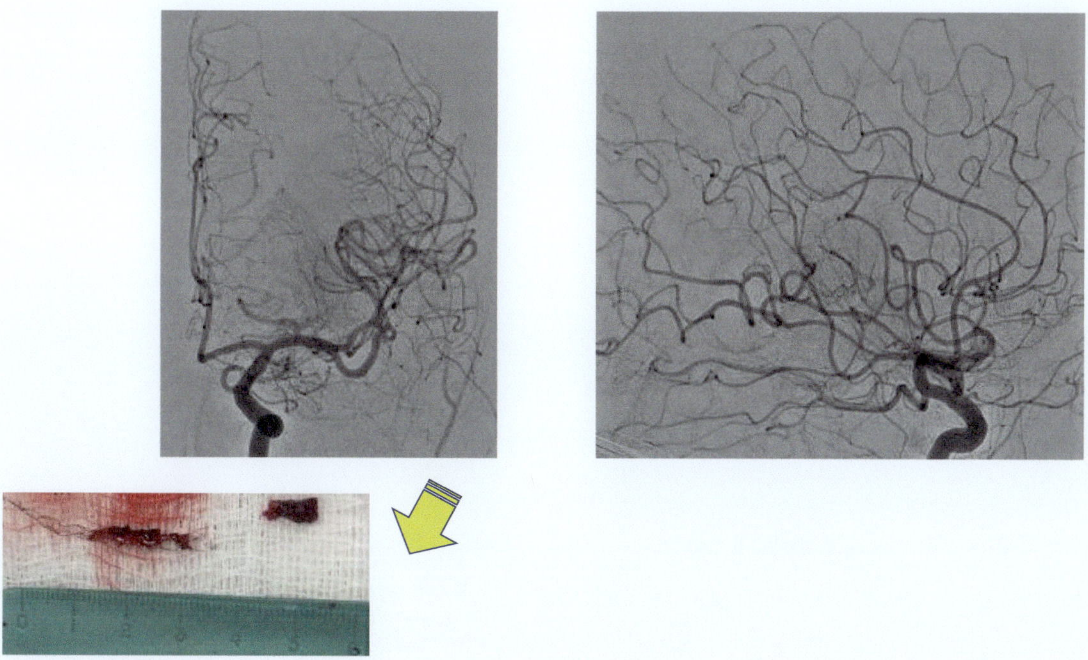

Fig. 84.3 TICI 3 reperfusion; clot noted in the retrieved stent

Suggested Reading

Massari F, et al. ARTS (aspiration-retriever technique for stroke): initial clinical experience. Interv Neuroradiol. 2016;22(3):325–32.

Terminal ICA Occlusion: The Utility of 6 mm × 30 mm Retrievable Stents

85

Mohammed A. Almekhlafi and Mayank Goyal

Case

An 81-year-old woman presented to the emergency with left-sided weakness of 2 h duration. The NIHSS score was 17; the ASPECTS score was 10, and CT angiogram confirmed the presence of right intracranial ICA occlusion but patent anterior and middle cerebral arteries. The patient was started on IV tPA and then transferred to the angiography suite.

Issue

1. The large clot burden may make it challenging to achieve successful reperfusion.
2. The inability to visualize the ICA branches during microwire navigation significantly increases the procedural risks, e.g., perforation of small branches as the ACh artery.

Management

An 8-French balloon guide catheter was advanced over a diagnostic catheter into the mid right internal carotid artery. DSA in frontal and lateral projections were obtained (Fig. 85.1a and b).

Direct manual suction through the guide catheter did not yield any thrombi. Subsequently, a microcatheter/wire assembly was carefully advanced into the right MCA. From that position, we first deployed a 4 × 40 mm Solitaire stent (Covidien, Irvine, USA), but no flow was noted (Fig. 85.2). The stent was retrieved but did not yield any thrombi, and no reperfusion was achieved. After that, a 6 × 30 mm Solitaire stent (Covidien, Irvine, USA) was deployed, and forward flow was noted. Therefore, the stent was left in place for about 3 min and then pulled out using standard technique under manual suction with a 60-cc syringe. A large clot was obtained, and check angiogram after that showed full recanalization with reperfusion of the right ICA territory with no evidence of distal embolization.

M. A. Almekhlafi (✉)
Department of Neurology, Faculty of Medicine, King Abdulaziz University, Jeddah, Saudi Arabia
e-mail: malmekhlafi@kau.edu.sa

M. Goyal
Department of Radiology, Seaman Family MR Research Centre, Foothills Medical Centre, Calgary, AB, Canada
e-mail: mgoyal@ucalgary.ca

V. Gupta et al. (eds.), *100 Interesting Case Studies in Neurointervention: Tips and Tricks*,
https://doi.org/10.1007/978-981-13-1346-2_85

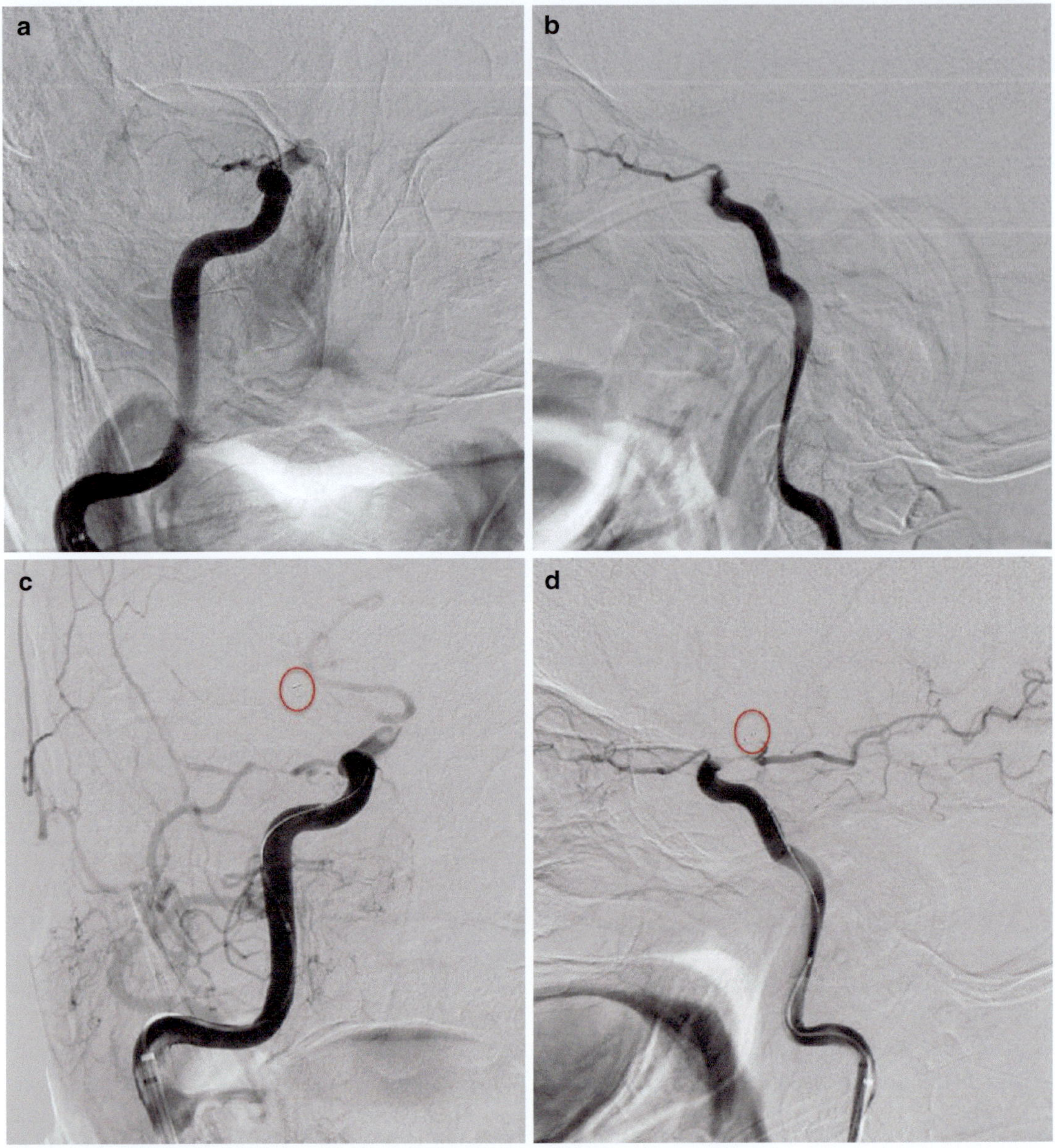

Fig. 85.1 (**a**, **b**) Angiographic images showing the occluded terminal segment of the right internal carotid artery with no opacification of the artery beyond the ophthalmic branch. (**c**, **d**) Images while the 4 × 40 mm Solitaire stent (circle point the stent markers) was deployed showing no bypass effect. The posterior communicating artery was filling

Tips and Tricks

1. In cases with an isolated distal ICA occlusion, the use of a large diameter stent can be a handy "tip" to obviate the need for multiple deployments and to secure successful recanalization.
2. Given the stent diameter, it can be challenging to push the stent through the usual 0.021″ microcatheters.

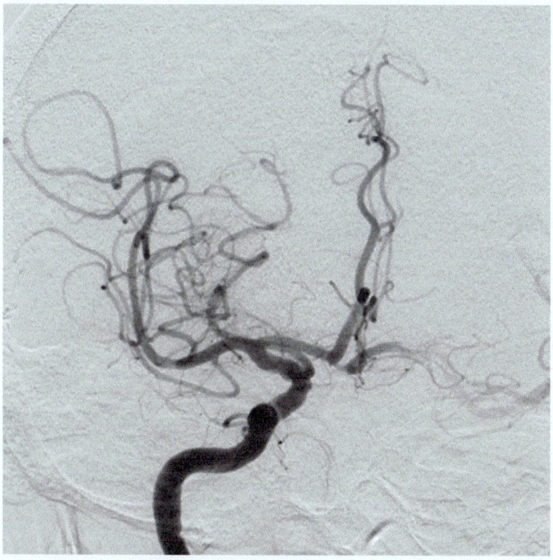

Fig. 85.2 Final angiographic images showing full recanalization of the distal ICA with complete reperfusion of the target territory

Suggested Reading

Bush CK, et al. Endovascular treatment with stent-retriever devices for acute ischemic stroke: a meta-analysis of randomized controlled trials. PLoS One. 2016;11(1):e0147287.

Haussen D, et al. Optimizating clot retrieval in acute stroke: the push and fluff technique for closed-cell stentrievers. Stroke. 2015;46(10):2838–42.

Atherosclerotic BA Occlusion: The Need to Detach the Stents

86

Mohammed A. Almekhlafi and Mayank Goyal

Case

A 67-year-old woman presented with decreased level of consciousness and left-sided weakness. NCCT Brain showed a hyperdense basilar artery and CT angiogram confirmed the presence of a proximal basilar artery occlusion. There was moderate atherosclerotic narrowing at the origin of both vertebral arteries. She was started on IV tPA and then transferred for endovascular therapy.

Issue

Occlusion of the basilar artery carries high morbidity and mortality risks. In addition to difficulties related to obtaining access, achieving recanalization can be especially difficult in patients with acute occlusion with underlying chronic atherosclerotic stenosis. Those patients are at a high risk of reocclusion after successful recanalization if the area of stenosis was left untreated.

Management

A 6-French guiding catheter was advanced into the distal V2 segment of the right vertebral artery. Check angiogram confirmed the basilar occlusion with only filling of the right PICA (Fig. 86.1a, b).

A microcatheter/wire combination crossed the occlusion, and a 5 × 40 mm Solitaire stent was deployed. Check angiogram showed recanalization of the basilar artery with a residual stenosis of the right vertebrobasilar junction (Fig. 86.2, arrow) and a distal occlusion of the left PCA that was too distal for mechanical intervention (Fig. 86.2, arrow head).

The VB junction stenosis was felt to be high risk, and a repeat angiogram showed interval complete reocclusion of the basilar artery. Therefore, permanent deployment of the Solitaire stent across the stenosis was decided. A DynaCT was performed on the angiography table which ruled out intracranial hemorrhage. The patient was then loaded with IA abciximab, and the Solitaire stent was deployed and detached. Check images confirmed restoration of the flow with recanalization of the left PCA, but a new right PCA occlusion was noted. Repeat delayed images confirmed the patency of the BA (Fig. 86.3). Check runs from the right ICA showed good MCA/PCA collaterals. Therefore, no intervention was felt necessary for the right PCA occlusion.

M. A. Almekhlafi (✉)
Department of Neurology, Faculty of Medicine, King Abdulaziz University, Jeddah, Saudi Arabia
e-mail: malmekhlafi@kau.edu.sa

M. Goyal
Department of Radiology, Seaman Family MR Research Centre, Foothills Medical Centre, Calgary, AB, Canada
e-mail: mgoyal@ucalgary.ca

V. Gupta et al. (eds.), *100 Interesting Case Studies in Neurointervention: Tips and Tricks*,
https://doi.org/10.1007/978-981-13-1346-2_86

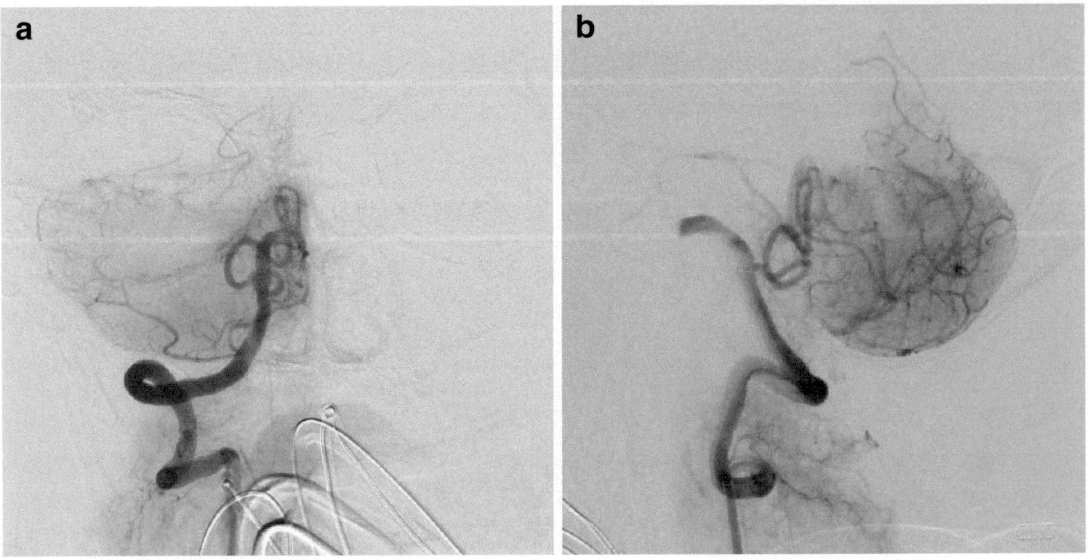

Fig. 86.1 Initial angiographic images showing occlusion of the proximal basilar artery with no filling of the right VA beyond its PICA branch in the frontal (**a**) and lateral planes (**b**)

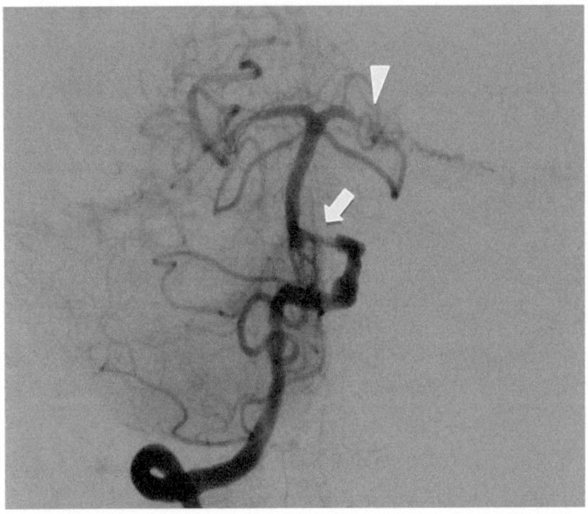

Fig. 86.2 Angiographic images following Solitaire deployment showing recanalization of the basilar artery revealing stenosis at the proximal basilar artery (arrow) and residual distal occlusion of the left PCA (arrow head)

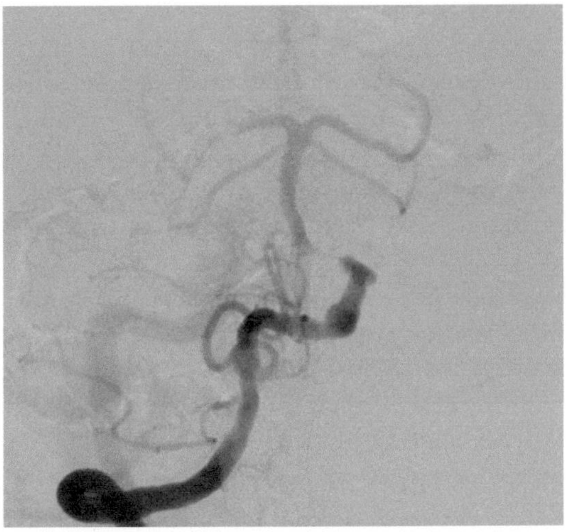

Fig. 86.3 Final images showing full recanalization of the BA after Solitaire stent detachment

Tips and Tricks

1. In cases where acute arterial occlusion on top of atherosclerotic narrowing is suspected, delayed repeat angiographic runs are advised even if complete recanalization of the occluded segment is achieved to check for recurrent occlusion.
2. If recurrent occlusion is observed, permanently detaching the Solitaire stent is a viable option as repeated deployments carry the risk of vascular injury or the accidental detachment of the stent.
3. Antiplatelet agents via a nasogastric tube or the parenteral route can been administered prior to stent detachment. However, a DynaCT to rule out intracranial hemorrhage is advised prior to administering these agents.

Suggested Reading

Chong BW, et al. Thrombolysis, angioplasty and stenting of acute basilar artery occlusion in an octogenarian. Radiol Case Rep. 2008;3(2):157.
Yeung TJ, et al. Endovascular revascularization for basilar artery occlusion. Interv Neurol. 2015;3(1):31–40.

87 Anterior Cerebral Artery Branch Occlusion

Mohammed A. Almekhlafi and Mayank Goyal

Case

A 58-year-old woman presented with global aphasia and right hemiparesis shortly after she woke up. CT angiogram showed left A2-ACA occlusion (Fig. 87.1a, b). The patient was treated with IV tPA and then transferred for endovascular intervention. Diagnostic runs showed persistent occlusion of the ACA. An incidental aneurysm of the right PCom was noted (Fig. 87.1c, d).

Issue

Occlusion of distal arteries, like A2 segment of anterior cerebral artery, can be challenging to reach with the stroke assembly. In addition, the small size of these arteries can limit the devices that can be safely used. The presence of an unruptured aneurysm en route to the occlusion makes it essential to weigh the procedure's risk vs. benefit.

Management

Through an 8-Fr balloon-guiding catheter, a Prowler Select Plus microcatheter was carefully navigated over a 0.016″ microwire into the left ACA and through the occlusion site (Fig. 87.2a). From that position, a 3 × 30 mm Solitaire stent was deployed (Fig. 87.2b). The stent was then pulled out, and final angiogram showed complete recanalization of the anterior cerebral artery.

Tips and Tricks

1. Reaching distal arterial beds with 0.021 microcatheters can be challenging.
2. When retrievable stents are deployed in distal or tortuous arteries, resheathing the stent fully or partially can aid in preventing accidental stent detachment.
3. Endothelial/vessel wall injury is less likely with smaller diameter stents.

M. A. Almekhlafi (✉)
Department of Neurology, Faculty of Medicine, King Abdulaziz University, Jeddah, Saudi Arabia
e-mail: malmekhlafi@kau.edu.sa

M. Goyal
Department of Radiology, Seaman Family MR Research Centre, Foothills Medical Centre, Calgary, AB, Canada
e-mail: mgoyal@ucalgary.ca

V. Gupta et al. (eds.), *100 Interesting Case Studies in Neurointervention: Tips and Tricks*,
https://doi.org/10.1007/978-981-13-1346-2_87

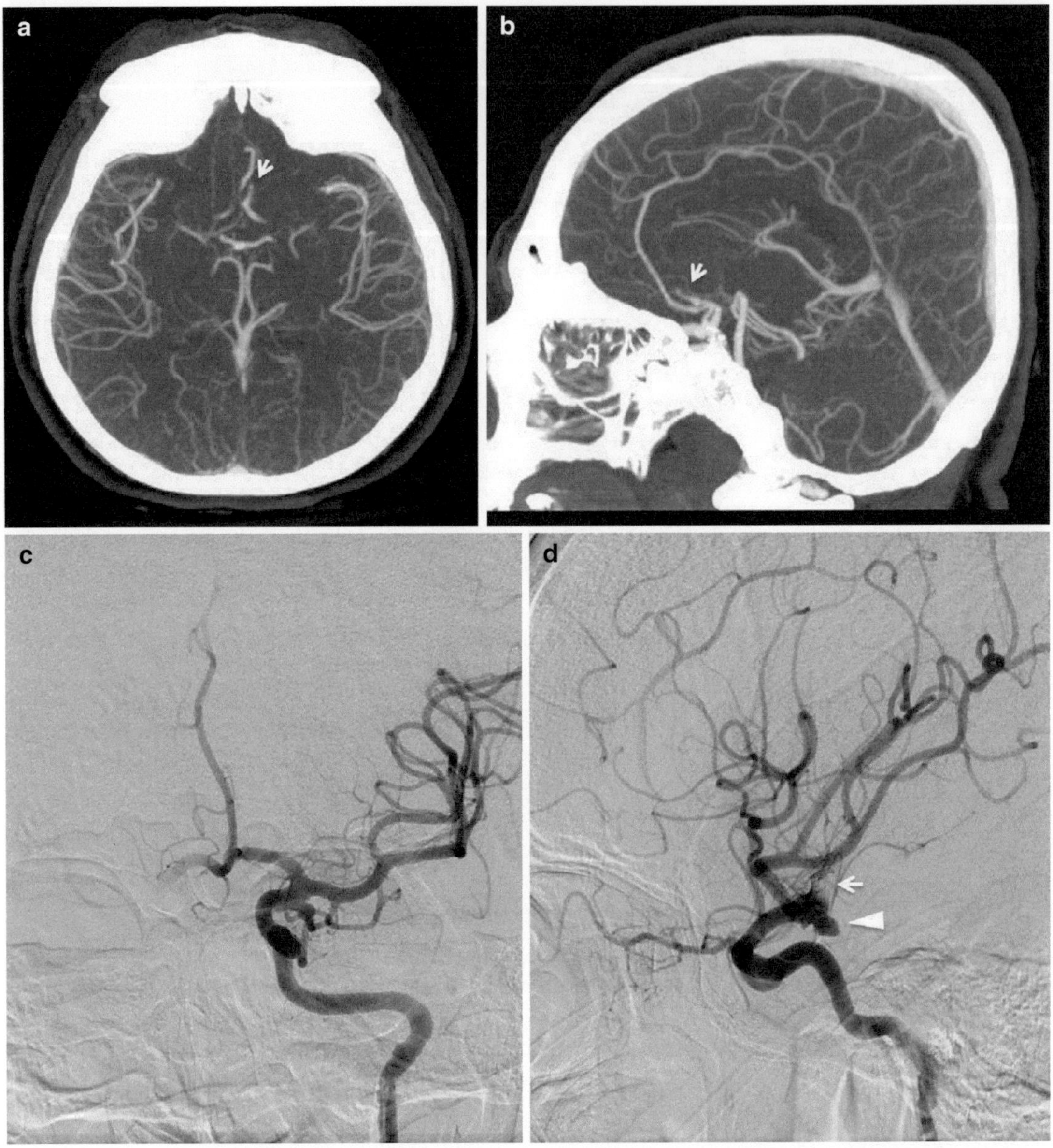

Fig. 87.1 Baseline CTA showing occlusion of the left A2-ACA (arrow) in the axial (**a**) and sagittal (**b**) planes. Initial angiographic images show only filling of the right ACA but not the left in the frontal plane (**c**), and in the lateral plane, the site of occlusion is seen (arrow) as well as the incidental PCom aneurysm (arrow head) (**d**)

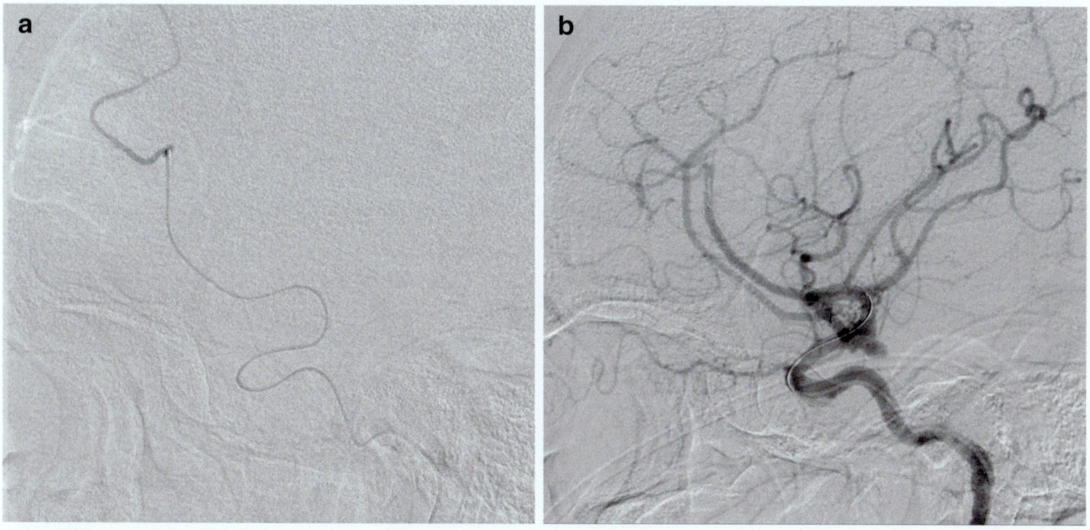

Fig. 87.2 Microcatheter run confirming the appropriate positioning distal to the thrombus (**a**). Angiographic images after and during the stent deployment showing anterograde filling of the left ACA with flow through and beyond the stent (**b**)

Suggested Reading

Dorn F, et al. Mechanical thrombectomy of M2-occlusion. J Stroke Cerebrovasc Dis. 2015;24(7):1465–70.

Pfaff J, et al. Mechanical thrombectomy of distal occlusions in the anterior cerebral artery: recanalization rates, periprocedural complications, and clinical outcome. AJNR Am J Neuroradiol. 2016;37(4):673–8.

Stroke in Evolution Due to Critical MCA Stenosis

88

Mohammed A. Almekhlafi and Mayank Goyal

Case

An 82-year-old man presented with a right MCA clinical syndrome that started almost 24 h prior to his presentation. CT angiogram showed a near complete occlusive narrowing of the distal right M1. An acute MRI brain showed critical hypoperfusion of the right MCA territory with minimal core on DWI (Fig. 88.1). He was referred for delayed reperfusion therapy.

Issue

This patient had symptoms onset beyond the conventional treatment window. However, he had evidence of clinical–radiographic mismatch (severe clinical deficit not explained by the DWI lesion). This was more in favor of atherosclerotic narrowing with unstable plaque vs. a nonocclusive thrombus. In such circumstances, the tissue window is more relevant than the time window.

Management

He was loaded with ASA and clopidogrel in anticipation of possible stenting. The angiographic runs showed near complete occlusion of the distal right M1-MCA with very slow filling of both M2 branches (Fig. 88.2). The area of narrowing was believed to represent an atherosclerotic critical stenosis, and permanent stent detachment was decided.

Under road map guidance, a Prowler select plus microcatheter was advanced over a Transcend Platinum wire across the stenotic segment into an M2 branch. A check run through the microcatheter confirmed the appropriate landing zone for the stent. From there, a 3 × 30 mm Solitaire stent was deployed from the proximal M2 branch to the proximal right M1-MCA. This immediately resulted in significant improvement of the right hemispheric flow (Fig. 88.3). The stent was successfully detached after that. Check angiogram showed good anterograde flow intracranially with no distal emboli. The patient had significant clinical improvement.

M. A. Almekhlafi (✉)
Department of Neurology, Faculty of Medicine, King Abdulaziz University, Jeddah, Saudi Arabia
e-mail: malmekhlafi@kau.edu.sa

M. Goyal
Department of Radiology, Seaman Family MR Research Centre, Foothills Medical Centre, Calgary, AB, Canada
e-mail: mgoyal@ucalgary.ca

V. Gupta et al. (eds.), *100 Interesting Case Studies in Neurointervention: Tips and Tricks*,
https://doi.org/10.1007/978-981-13-1346-2_88

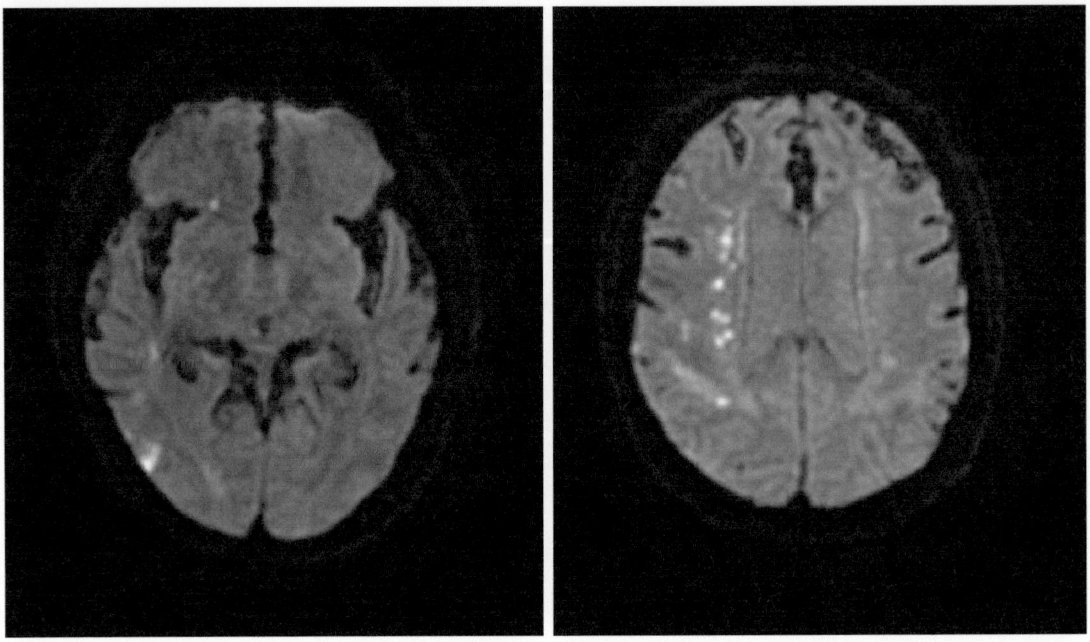

Fig. 88.1 Acute diffusion-weighted MRI showing small areas of scattered cortical restricted diffusion and in the deep white matter

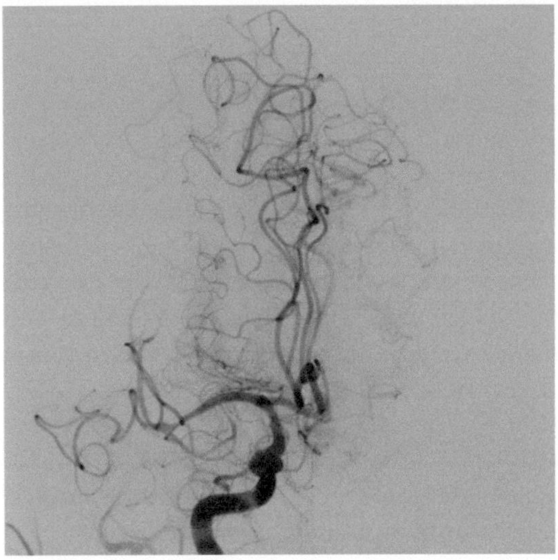

Fig. 88.2 Initial angiographic run showing tapering and narrowing of the right distal middle cerebral artery with slow flow in the M2 branches as can be seen in the delayed M2 filling relative to the ACA

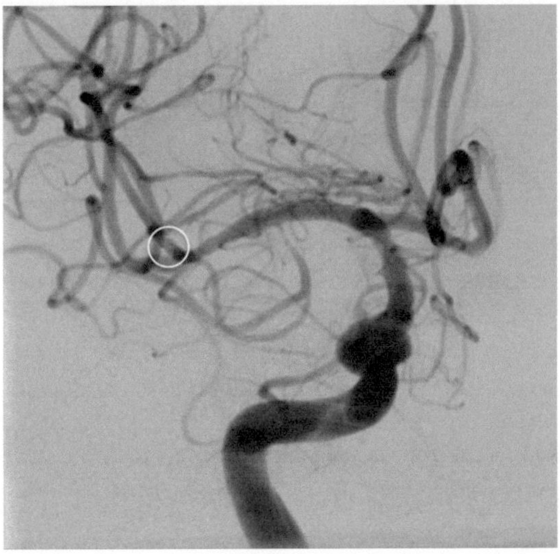

Fig. 88.3 Final angiographic run showing restoration of normal flow through the stent (circle) and the MCA branches

Tips and Tricks

1. A tissue-based paradigm can be used to extend the treatment window in carefully selected patients.
2. Pre-planning the procedure to use detachable stent is important when atherosclerotic narrowing is suspected as the underlying mechanism.

Suggested Reading

Ansari S, et al. Intracranial stents for treatment of acute ischemic stroke: evolution and current status. World Neurosurg. 2011;76(6 Suppl):S24–34.

Xavier AR, et al. Safety and efficacy of intracranial stenting for acute ischemic stroke beyond 8 h of symptom onset. J Neurointerv Surg. 2012;4(2):94–100.

89 Intracranial Atherosclerotic Disease (ICAD): Submaximal Angioplasty

Srinivasan Paramasivam

Case

A 58-year-old male with past medical history of DM, HTN, and hyperlipidemia on treatment presented with left eye visual obscurations since morning. She was initially seen by an ophthalmologist and was cleared of ocular pathology. Later in the day, he had confusion and difficulty in reading newspapers. He came to the hospital by around 8 PM as his confusion progressed. MRA revealed non-visualization of left ICA beyond bifurcation (Fig. 89.1a), and half an hour later he developed a complete left MCA syndrome with NIHSS of 22. Intravenous tPA was administered, and patient was transferred to the neurointerventional suite. The DSA revealed no flow in the ICA just distal to bifurcation (Fig. 89.1c). There is good collateral across the Acom to the left ACA (Fig. 89.1b).

Issues

1. Acutely symptomatic flow-limiting/occlusive intracranial stenosis

Management

The procedure was done under local anesthesia. A 6 Fr shuttle sheath was inserted into the right common femoral artery and DSA of right and left CCA was performed and the catheter is placed in the left CCA. DSA revealed no flow in the left ICA with good flow in the right ICA. There is good Acom with good flow in both ACAs. There is no flow visualized in the MCA. Selectively catheterization of left ICA with Excelsior XT 27 microcatheter over Synchro 2 standard microguide wire revealed critical narrowing of the left ICA. (Fig. 89.1d). Balloon angioplasty using Maverick Balloon of size 2 × 20 mm followed by 3 × 20 mm was performed. Following balloon angioplasty good anterograde flow was established (Fig. 89.1e, f). MRI of the brain performed few days later revealed multifocal patchy cortical infarcts (Fig. 89.2a–c), and MRA revealed good flow in the left ICA and MCA (Fig. 89.1g). The patient was managed with dual antiplatelets and high-dose statins. Follow-up angiogram done at 6 weeks revealed good flow in the left ICA and MCA (Fig. 89.2d–f). The patient continues to be symptom-free.

S. Paramasivam
Apollo Hospitals, Chennai, India
e-mail: kpvasan@hotmail.com

V. Gupta et al. (eds.), *100 Interesting Case Studies in Neurointervention: Tips and Tricks*,
https://doi.org/10.1007/978-981-13-1346-2_89

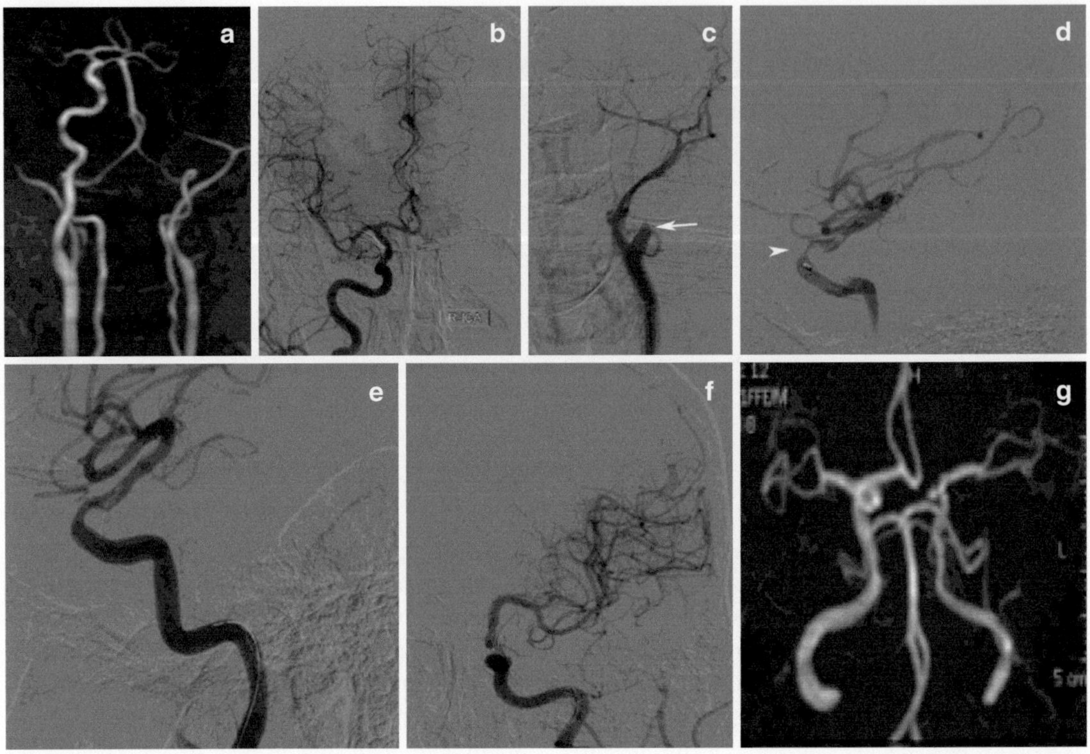

Fig. 89.1 (**a**) No flow in the left ICA beyond bifurcation in the MRA. DSA (**b** and **c**) show no flow in the left ICA and good flow in the right ICA and good flow across the Acom to both anterior cerebral arteries. Selective catheterization of left ICA using microcatheter was performed, and DSA at the ophthalmic segment reveal a critical narrowing of the left internal carotid artery (**d**). Submaximal balloon angioplasty was performed. Post angioplasty the flow to the left MCA was well established (**e** and **f**), and A1 segment was aplastic. Clinically the symptoms completely resolved. MRA done few days later revealed the re-establishment of flow in the left ICA and MCA (**g**)

Tips and Tricks

1. No flow in the ICA in acute stroke in general is due to distal occlusion of ICA. Gentle exploration of the ICA using microcatheter over microguidewire and super-selective angiogram is mandatory to understand the location and type of occlusion.
2. Intracranial atherosclerotic disease in the acute setting can be effectively managed by balloon angioplasty.
3. If angioplasty alone does not result in recanalization, one may consider stent deployment.

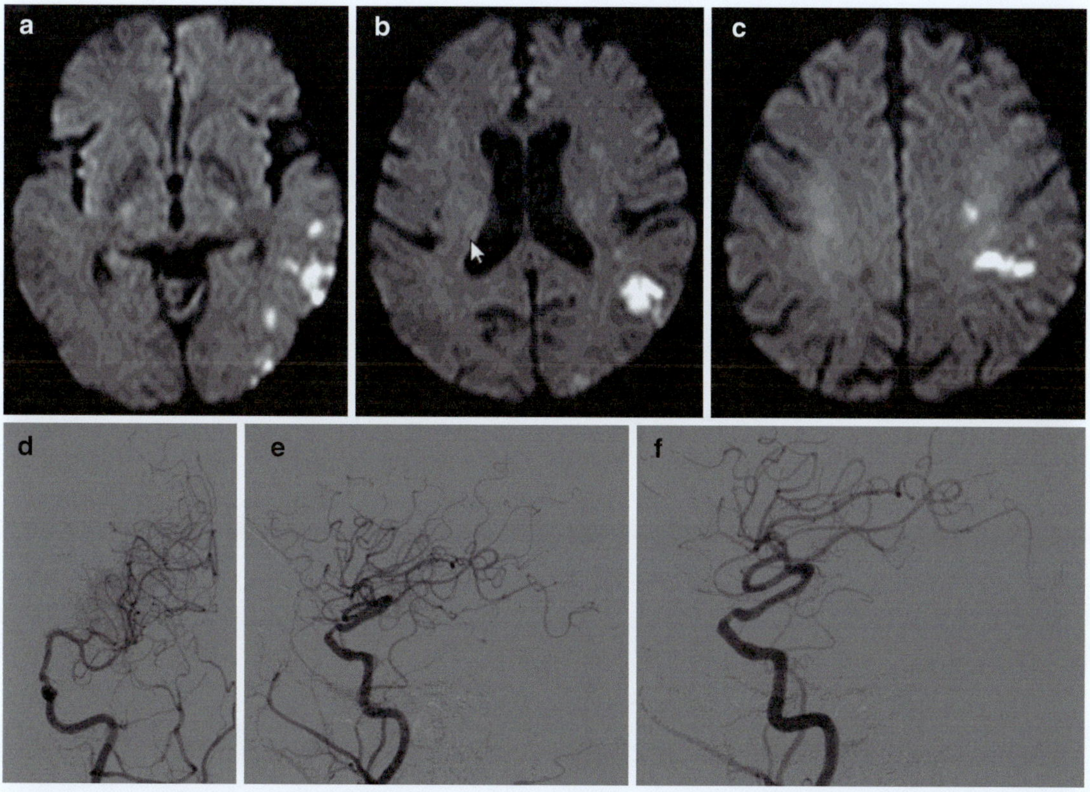

Fig. 89.2 Follow-up MRI done few days later revealed patchy cortical infarcts in the left MCA territory; however, a significant portion of left MCA territory is preserved (**a**–**c**). Patient was placed on dual antiplatelets and high-dose statins. Follow-up angiogram at 6 weeks revealed good flow in the left ICA with non-flow-limiting residual narrowing in the ophthalmic segment of ICA (**d**–**f**)

Suggested Reading

Connors JJ III, Wojak JC. Percutaneous transluminal angioplasty for intracranial atherosclerotic lesions: evolution of technique and short-term results. J Neurosurg. 1999;91:415–23. https://doi.org/10.3171/jns.1999.91.3.0415.

Dumont TM, Sonig A, et al. Submaximal angioplasty for symptomatic intracranial atherosclerosis: a prospective phase I study. J Neurosurg. 2016;125(4):964–71.

Marks MP, Wojak JC, Al-Ali F, Jayaraman M, Marcellus ML, Connors JJ, et al. Angioplasty for symptomatic intracranial stenosis: clinical outcome. Stroke. 2006;37:1016–20. https://doi.org/10.1161/01.STR.0000206142.03677.c2.

Tandem Occlusions (Antegrade First Technique with Stent)

90

Mohammed A. Almekhlafi and Mayank Goyal

Case

A 70-year-old male was admitted with 5 h duration of left-sided weakness. The NIHSS score was 17, and the patient had a tandem occlusion; there was a tight stenosis at the origin of the right ICA along with M1 MCA occlusion. There were good collaterals along with a small infarct core (Fig. 90.1).

Issues

- Anterograde versus retrograde approach
- Crossing the tight stenosis—Dotter method vs cross with microwire and microcatheter/balloon angioplasty
- Choice of hardware and when to use embolic protection device
- Antiplatelet regimen

Management

The procedure was performed under local anaesthesia. An anterograde approach was undertaken. An 8F short sheath was inserted in the right femoral artery. Following that, an 8F Neuron Max (Penumbra Inc.) was navigated to the distal right CCA. The tight stenosis was crossed with a 0.014′ Traxcess microwire. The microcatheter was then navigated beyond the stenosis; a microcatheter run was taken to confirm intraluminal location. Balloon angioplasty was performed with a 2.5 × 15 mm rapid exchange side port balloon. Following that a Xact 6–8 30 mm stent was deployed across the stenosis; post-stenting angioplasty was performed with a 4 × 20 mm rapid exchange balloon (Fig. 90.2). The wire access was maintained by attaching a docking wire, and the guiding catheter (6F DAC, Stryker Neurovascular) was taken across the stent and thrombectomy was performed by the stentriever technique. Loading dose of Ecosprin (300 mg) was administered through NG tube at the time of stent delivery. Post-procedure DynaCT showed small infarct in the basal ganglia; there was no evidence of haemorrhage. The patient was loaded with 600 mg of clopidogrel as there was no evidence of haemorrhage.

M. A. Almekhlafi (✉)
Department of Neurology, Faculty of Medicine, King Abdulaziz University, Jeddah, Saudi Arabia
e-mail: malmekhlafi@kau.edu.sa

M. Goyal
Department of Radiology, Seaman Family MR Research Centre, Foothills Medical Centre, Calgary, AB, Canada
e-mail: mgoyal@ucalgary.ca

V. Gupta et al. (eds.), *100 Interesting Case Studies in Neurointervention: Tips and Tricks*, https://doi.org/10.1007/978-981-13-1346-2_90

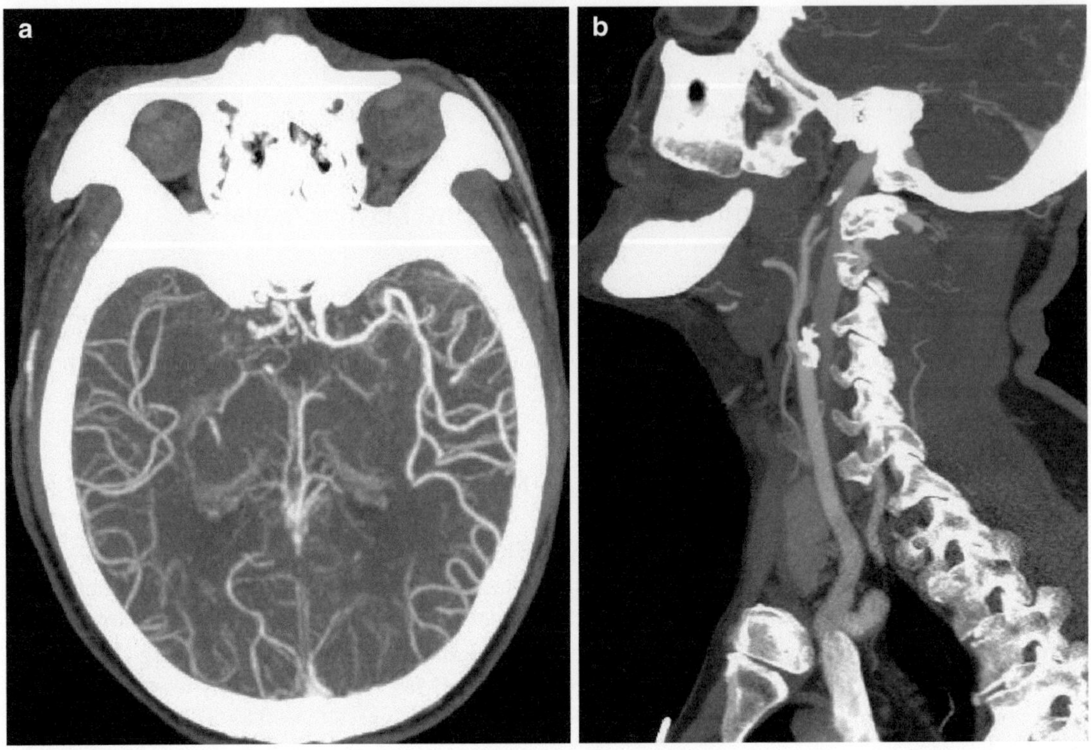

Fig. 90.1 (**a**) Right M1 occlusion. (**b**) Right ICA occlusion at bulb with wall calcification

Tips and Tricks

1. In the antegrade approach, the proximal stenosis is revascularised first. The key advantage of addressing the proximal lesion in a controlled manner is that it allows for taking a large bore catheter distally to manage the intracranial occlusion. However, this approach may lead to delay in brain reperfusion.
2. An 8F Neuron Max or 6F Shuttle is used as the inner diameter is compatible with both the Xact stent and Protégé Stent delivery systems. A Merci balloon guide will not allow the stent delivery systems to pass through. However, a 9f Cello or FlowGate (Stryker Neurovascular) balloon guide is compatible with the above delivery systems.
3. Crossing the stenosis with a microwire and microcatheter allows for determining the patency of the distal artery, confirming the location (i.e. true lumen or not) and performing a balloon angioplasty.
4. A controlled dissection by means of balloon angioplasty is favoured over navigating a large bore catheter through the stenosis. The latter approach risks further plaque rupture and clot migration into new territory.
5. Embolic protection device may be considered in patients with distal M1 or M2 occlusions as any further embolisation can cause occlusion in a new territory or add to the clot burden.
6. A Traxcess 0.014′ wire can be used to cross the lesion as a docking wire can be attached to enable taking the guiding catheter across the stent. It is always useful to maintain wire access even after stent deployment as there is the risk of thrombotic occlusion of the stent in the acute stenting where patient has not received prior antiplatelet.

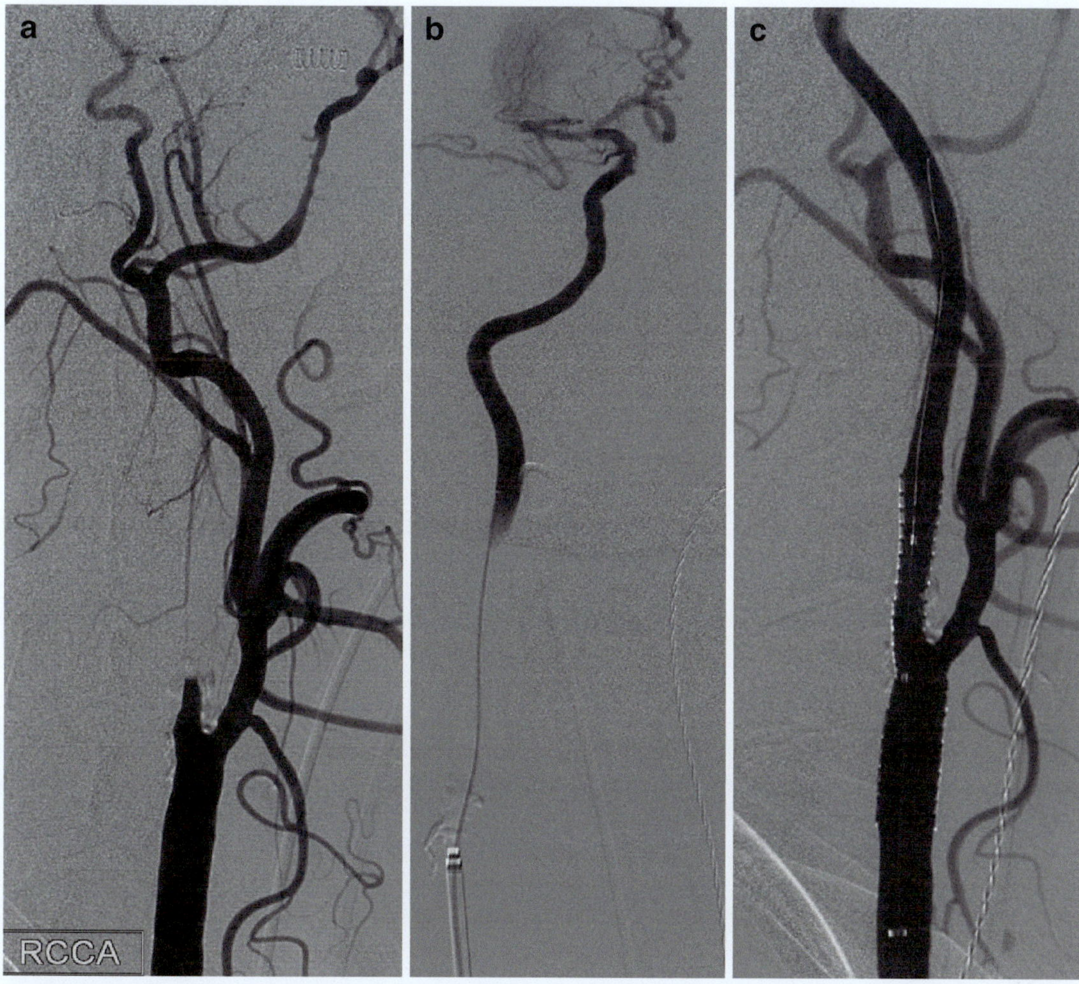

Fig. 90.2 Angiogram in the lateral plane confirms the carotid occlusion. (**a**) SL10 microcatheter with a Synchro wire was used to cross the lesion. (**b**) Microcatheter angiogram is used to confirm the true lumen and the distal MCA occlusion. (**c**) Exchange length Synchro wire was used, carotid stent was placed, and the guide catheter was advanced distal to the carotid stent. Thereafter, mechanical thrombectomy was performed

7. A 6F guiding catheter is navigated beyond the stent and mechanical thrombectomy performed with a stentriever. It is always advisable to take the guiding catheter distal to the stent to avoid dislodgement of the carotid stent by the Solitaire stent. As proximal flow arrest is not possible, there is the risk of embolism to distal or new territory.
8. To avoid any distal embolism, one may try ADAPT technique with a 5 MAX ACE catheter as first line.
9. Antiplatelet regimen should be individualised on a case-to-case basis. In general in a patient with a small core who has not received thrombolysis, loading dose of intravenous gp 2b/3a inhibitor is administered. A NCCT scan is done after 6 hours and if there is no evidence of hematoma, reperfusion injury or midline shift, dual antiplatelet loading is performed. On the other hand, if the patient had received thrombolysis, loading dose of gp 2b/3a inhibitor is administered; six hours later if the NCCT scan does not show any red flags, Aspirin loading is administered; 24 hours later if there are no adverse features on NCCT brain, clopidogrel loading is performed.

Suggested Reading

Marnat G, et al. Endovascular management of tandem occlusion stroke related to internal carotid artery dissection using a distal to proximal approach: insight from the RECOST study. AJNR Am J Neuroradiol. 2016;37(7):1281–8.

Spiotta AM, et al. Proximal to distal approach in the treatment of tandem occlusions causing an acute stroke. J Neurointerv Surg. 2015;7(3):164–9.

Intracranial Occlusion with Tandem Carotid Stenosis: Distal to Proximal Approach

91

Ajit S. Puri and Rajsrinivas Parthasarathy

Case

A 61-year-old man presented with right hemiplegia and aphasia. NIH stroke scale was 20. The ASPECTS score was 9, and CT angiogram showed occlusion at the origin of the left internal carotid artery and left M1–MCA occlusion. He was started on IV tPA and transferred for endovascular management.

Issue

Occlusion or stenosis of the internal carotid artery tandem to an intracranial occlusion is seen in over 20% of acute ischemic stroke cases. The optimal management of the carotid stenosis in this setting remains controversial. Options include stenting the carotid first followed by treating the intracranial occlusion or going through the occluded/stenotic segment to treat the intracranial occlusion first and then treat the carotid stenosis in the same setting or at an interval.

Management

A coaxial system of a 6-Fr Shuttle sheath over a 5 French Vert catheter was advanced into the midsection of the left common carotid artery. From that position, angiographic runs from the common carotid artery showed interval recanalization of the cervical ICA uncovering an underlying severe stenosis (Fig. 91.1a) and a tandem occlusion of the distal M1-MCA (Fig. 91.1b).

A Prowler Select Plus microcatheter was advanced beyond the MCA-occluded segment into one of the M2 branches. A 4 × 20 mm Solitaire stent was deployed, and on retrieval of the stent, complete reperfusion was achieved (Fig. 91.2).

Subsequently, through the Shuttle sheath, carotid stenting was performed after the placement of a distal protection device (Fig. 91.3).

Tips and Tricks

1. In cases with tandem cervical carotid and intracranial occlusions, dealing with the intracranial occlusion first is our preference to halt the progression of ischemia and to allow for blood flow to the brain through the carotid or Willisian collaterals.

A. S. Puri (✉)
Radiology, and Neurosurgery,
Division of Neurointerventional Surgery,
Neurointerventional Fellowship Program,
University of Massachusetts Medical Center,
Worcester, MA, USA
e-mail: ajit.puri@umassmemorial.org

R. Parthasarathy
Vascular Neurology and Neurointerventional Surgery,
Artemis Agrim Institute of Neuroscience,
Gurgaon, India

V. Gupta et al. (eds.), *100 Interesting Case Studies in Neurointervention: Tips and Tricks*,
https://doi.org/10.1007/978-981-13-1346-2_91

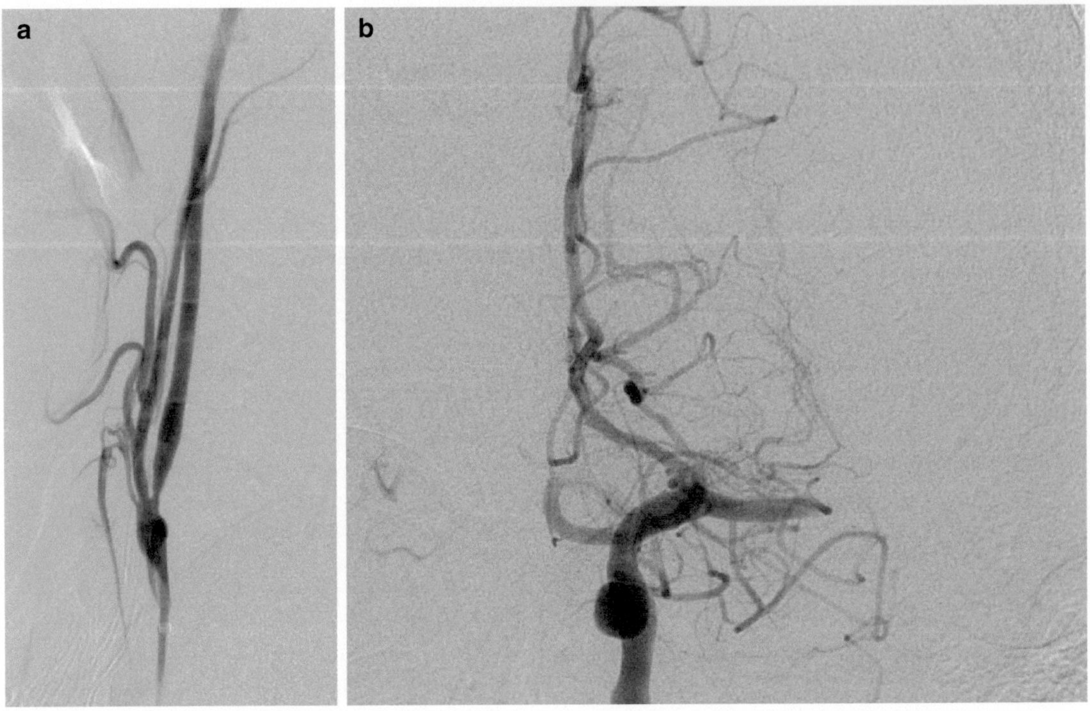

Fig. 91.1 Initial angiographic imaging from the left common carotid artery showing the severe stenosis in the origin of the left ICA (**a**) and the distal M1-MCA occlusion (**b**)

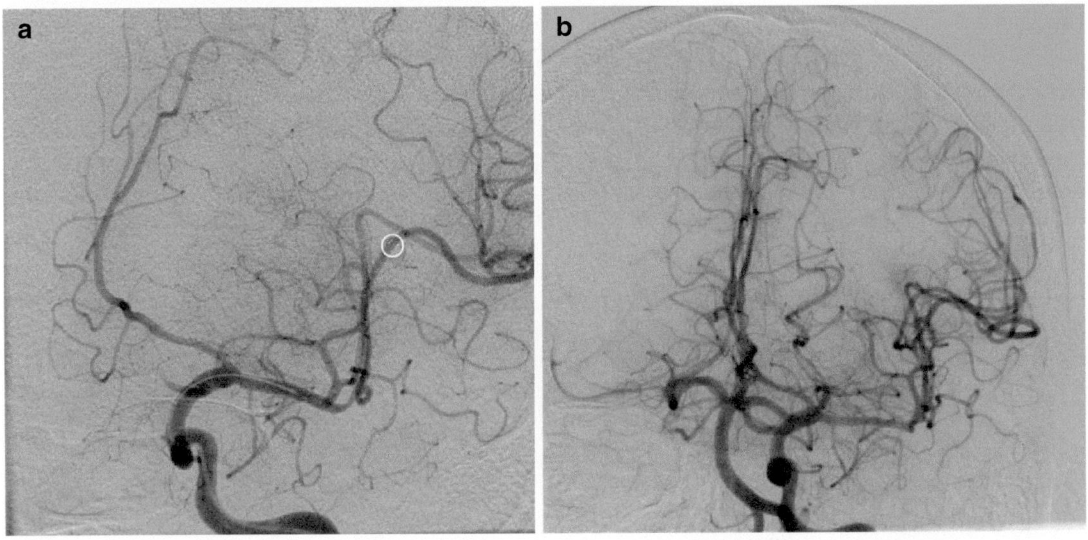

Fig. 91.2 Angiographic runs with the stent deployed (**a**, circle) and immediately following stent removal (**b**)

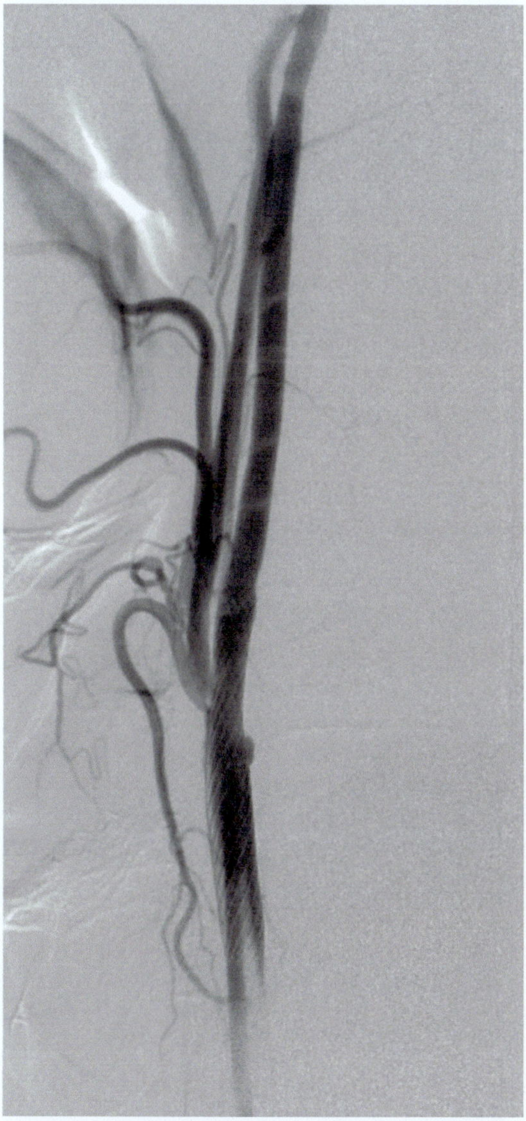

Fig. 91.3 Left common carotid angiography showing the stent placement with no residual stenosis

2. Occasionally, terminal intracranial carotid occlusion gives the picture of a tapering, flame-shaped, occlusion of the cervical carotid artery which is a flow-related phenomena but not a real occlusion. In these circumstances, manual suction using 60 cc syringe from the common carotid artery via a balloon-guide catheter can successfully debulk the thrombus, often converting a T/L-type terminal ICA occlusion into an M1 occlusion.
3. Interval stenting offers the advantage of avoiding loading doses of dual antiplatelets.
4. If stenting is considered in the same sitting, antiplatelet regimen should be individualized on a case-to-case basis. In general in a patient with a small core who has not received thrombolysis, loading dose of intravenous gp 2b/3a inhibitor is administered. A NCCT scan is done after 6 hours, and if there is no evidence of hematoma, reperfusion injury or midline shift, dual antiplatelet loading is performed. On the other hand, if the patient had received thrombolysis, loading dose of gp 2b/3a inhibitor is administered; six hours later if the NCCT scan does not show any red flags, Aspirin loading is administered; 24 hours later if there are no adverse features on NCCT brain, clopidogrel loading is performed.

Suggested Reading

Marnat G, et al. Endovascular management of tandem occlusion stroke related to internal carotid artery dissection using a distal to proximal approach: insight from the RECOST study. AJNR Am J Neuroradiol. 2016;37(7):1281–8.

Rangel-Castilla L, et al. Management of acute ischemic stroke due to tandem occlusion: should endovascular recanalization of the extracranial or intracranial occlusive lesion be done first? Neurosurg Focus. 2017;42(4):E16.

Spiotta AM, et al. Proximal to distal approach in the treatment of tandem occlusions causing an acute stroke. J Neurointerv Surg. 2015;7(3):164–9.

92 Intracranial Occlusion with Tandem Carotid Stenosis: Retained Filter

Rajsrinivas Parthasarathy and Vipul Gupta

Case

A 70-year-old diabetic and hypertensive presented at 2 h with right-sided weakness and speech disturbance. Examination revealed dense right-sided weakness and global aphasia adding up to a NIHSS score of 19. NCCT brain revealed a small core and hyperdense MCA (Fig. 91.1a–c). Tandem left ICA origin and M1 occlusion was noted on CTA.

Issue

Crossing proximal occlusion: dotters technique vs balloon angioplasty first followed by navigation of guiding catheter
Tandem occlusion: distal to proximal vs proximal to distal
Approach to occlusion of ICA post stenting

R. Parthasarathy (✉)
Vascular Neurology and Neurointerventional Surgery, Artemis Agrim Institute of Neuroscience, Gurgaon, India

V. Gupta
Neurointerventional Surgery, Stroke Unit, Artemis Agrim Institute of Neuroscience, Gurgaon, India
e-mail: vipul.gupta@artemishospitals.com

Management

A coaxial system of a 6-Fr Shuttle sheath over a 5 French Vert catheter was advanced into the midsection of the left common carotid artery. From that position, angiographic runs from the common carotid artery showed tight stenosis at the origin of the left ICA with no antegrade flow (Fig. 92.2a). The neuron-guiding catheter was advanced over a 0.035′ Terumo wire into the cervical ICA (Fig. 92.2b) (Dotters technique). The distal cervical ICA and the rest of the ICA segments were patent along with a M1-MCA occlusion (Fig. 92.2c, d). Stentriever thrombectomy was performed for the intracranial occlusion first. TICI 3 flow was established (Fig. 92.3a–d). Following that, microwire access was maintained by adding a docking wire to Traxcess 0.014′ microwire (Microvention. Inc) (Fig. 92.4a, b), and carotid artery stenting was performed with a distal protection device (Fig. 92.4c). Soon after filter device placement, thrombus formation was noted in the cervical ICA, in particular around the filter device (Fig. 92.4c, d). Moments after stenting, complete occlusion of the ICA from the origin was noted (Fig. 92.4e). Good collateral flow from ACOM and PCOM was noted (Fig. 92.5a, b). It was felt that there was significant clot burden in the ICA, and therefore, it was decided not retrieve the filter device. The filter device was cut at the groin (Fig. 92.5c, f). Post procedure NCCT showed no hemorrhage and no expansion in infarct. Patient made complete recovery.

V. Gupta et al. (eds.), *100 Interesting Case Studies in Neurointervention: Tips and Tricks*,
https://doi.org/10.1007/978-981-13-1346-2_92

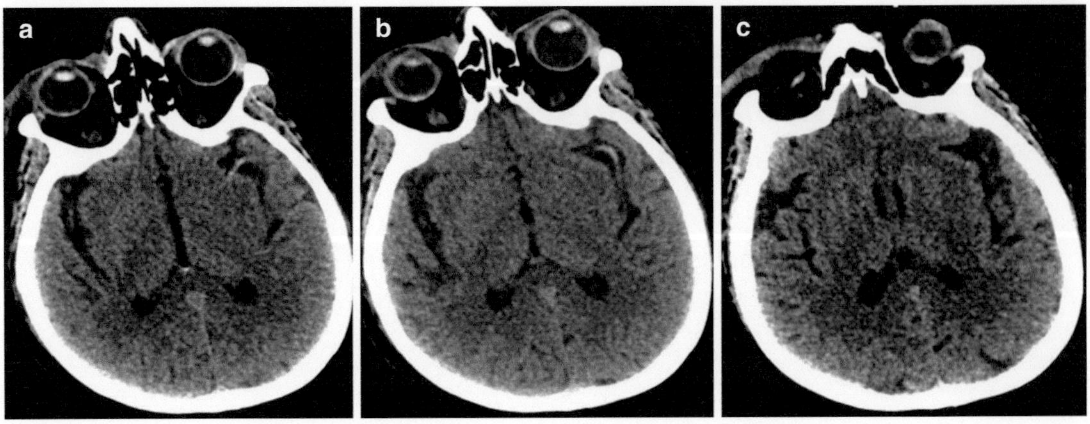

Fig. 92.1 (**a–c**), Noncontrast CT brain showing small core with a hyperdense middle cerebral artery

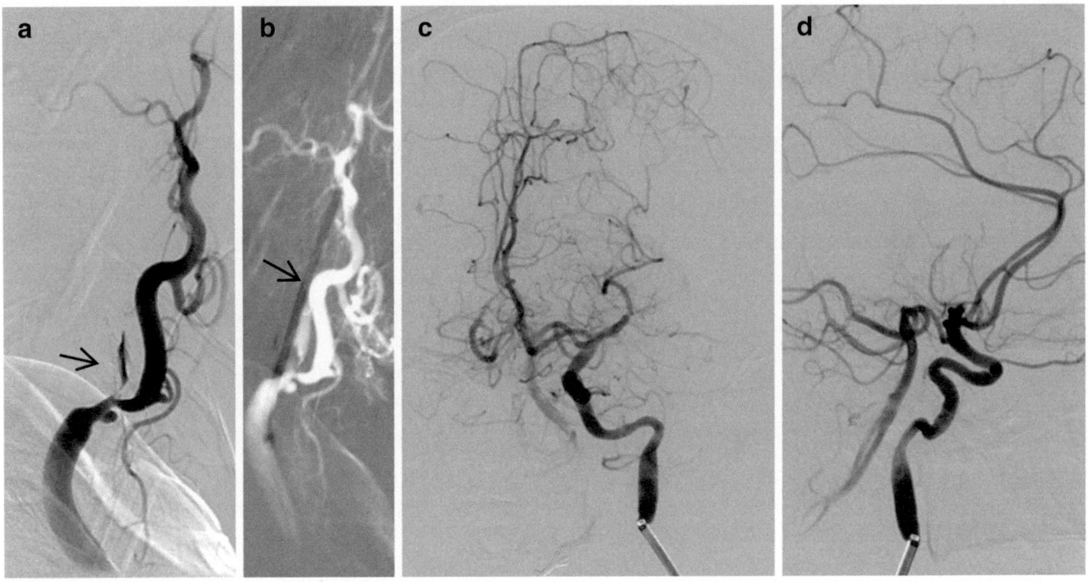

Fig. 92.2 (**a**) sheath run demonstrating a tight stenosis at the ICA origin with no significant antegrade flow (arrow), (**b**) 6F Neuron guiding catheter taken across the stenosis over a 0.035' terumo wire, (**c**, **d**) AP and lateral views showing occluded left M1 MCA with poor leptomeningeal collaterals

Tips and Tricks

1. In cases with tandem cervical carotid and intracranial occlusions, dealing with the intracranial occlusion first is our preference in order to halt the progression of ischemia and to allow for blood flow to the brain through the carotid or Willisian collaterals.
2. Navigating the proximal occlusion—Dotters' technique: The guiding catheter is advanced over a 0.035′ Terumo wire across the stenosis segment without prior angioplasty. Vigorous aspiration is done once in the cervical ICA. The diameter of the guiding catheter is large and fits snugly at the stenotic segment with no space around resulting in flow arrest. Stentriever thrombectomy is then undertaken.
3. One should carefully consider if emergent stenting is required; there is a higher chance of thrombus formation around the filter device and within the stent as patients are generally not primed with antiplatelet agents.

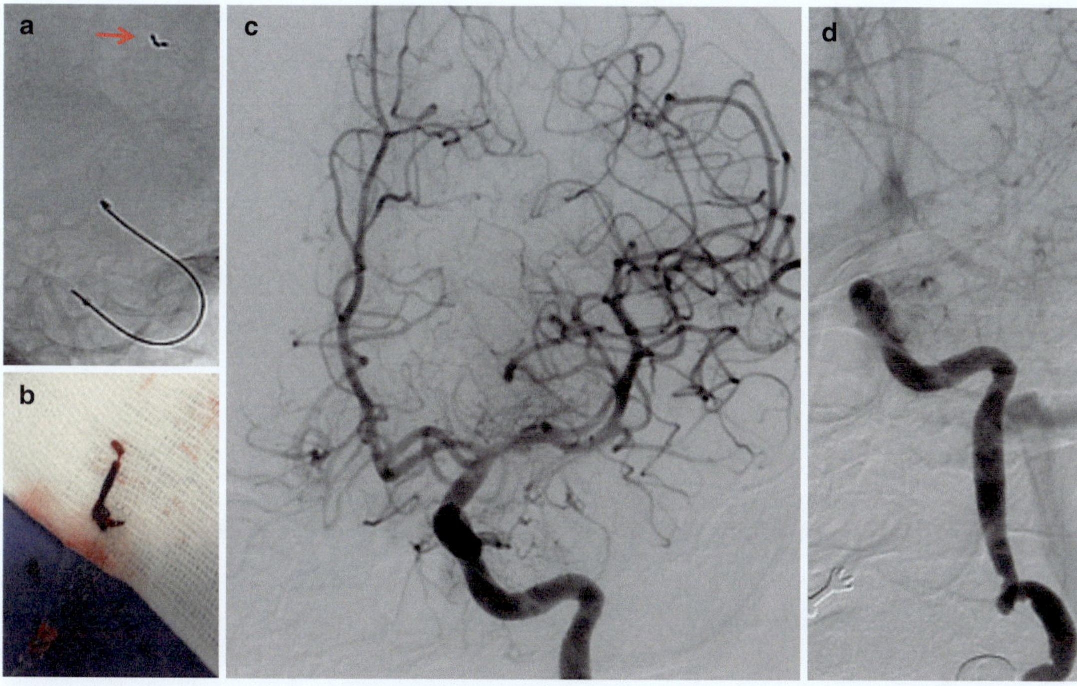

Fig. 92.3 (**a**) Solitaire 4x 40 mm stent deployed across the clot, (**b**) thrombus attached to the stent, (**c**) TICI 3 reperfusion, (**d**) stasis in the left ICA due to the proximal stenosis

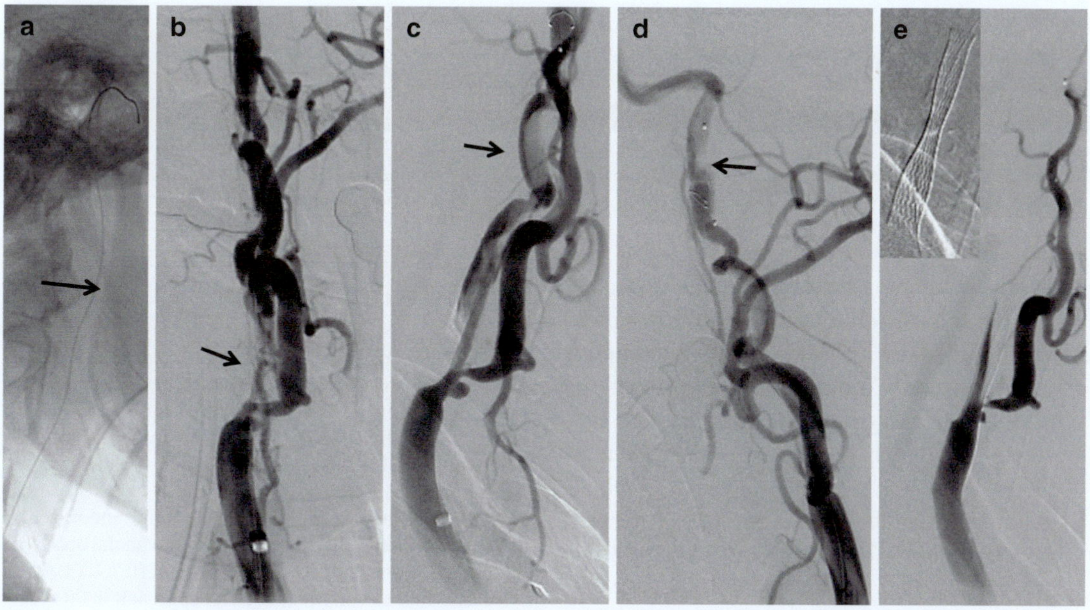

Fig. 92.4 (**a**) Wire access maintained by attaching a docking to the 0.014' traxcess microwire, (**b**) thrombus formation noted at site of stenosis, (**c**, **d**) stent deployed with distal protection device, note progressive thrombus formation around the filter and the cervical ICA, (**e**) occluded ICA from the origin with large clot burden, inset showing the stent in situ

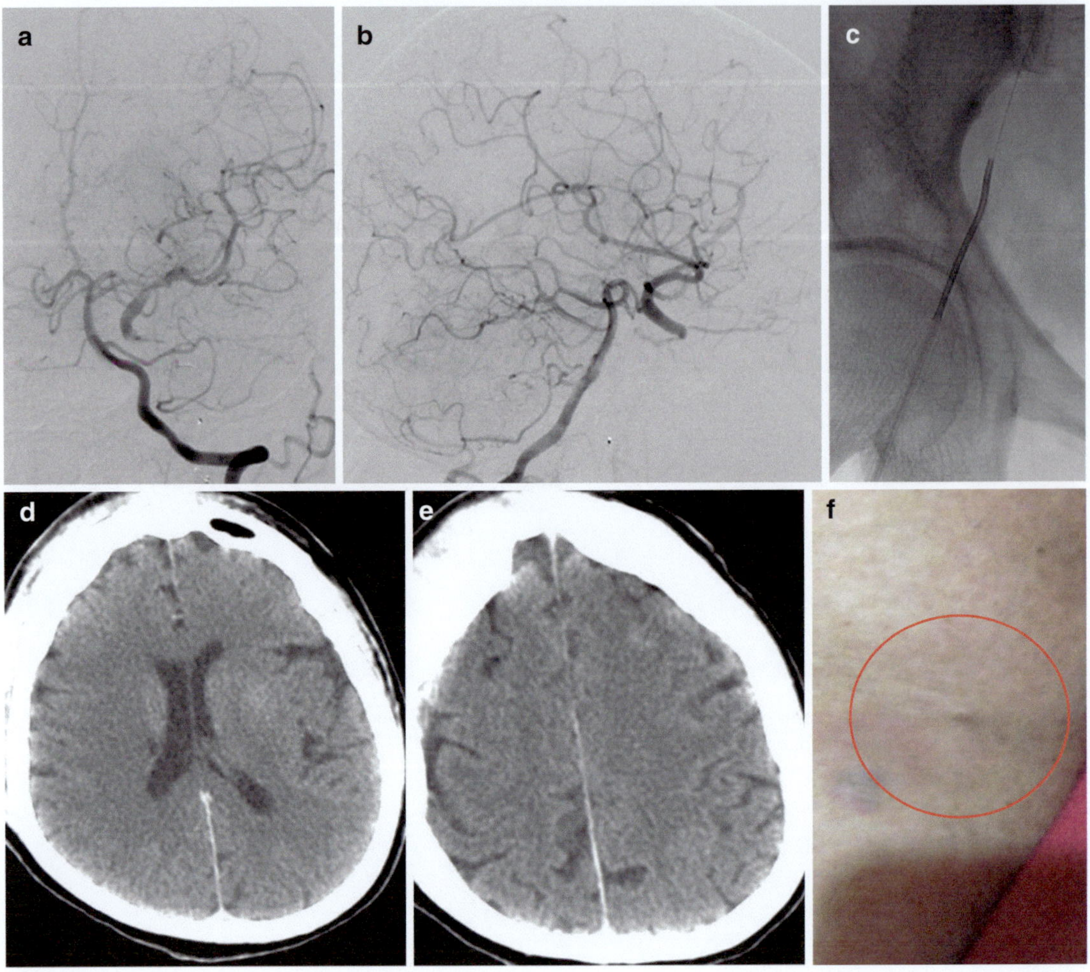

Fig. 92.5 (**a**, **b**) left vertebral artery injection reveals good PCOM subserving the left ICA territory, (**c**, **f**) filter wire cut at the groin, (**d**, **e**) post procedure dyna CT showing no hemorrhage and no new infarcts

4. In this case, progressive thrombus formation was noted in the left ICA. Initially the thrombus was around the filter; later, there was complete ICA occlusion. Collateral flow assessment was done. There was good ACOM and PCOM subserving the left ICA territory with no venous phase delay. Retrieving the filter risks embolization to distal territory. There was no forward flow in the ICA. Therefore, a decision to leave the filter in vivo was made, and the wire was cut at the groin. One may have to carefully consider the pros and cons of carotid revascularization when the intracranial flow is established through collaterals as attempting revascularization can potentially be detrimental.

Suggested Reading

Marnat G, et al. Endovascular management of tandem occlusion stroke related to internal carotid artery dissection using a distal to proximal approach: insight from the RECOST study. AJNR Am J Neuroradiol. 2016;37(7):1281–8.

Rangel-Castilla L, et al. Management of acute ischemic stroke due to tandem occlusion: should endovascular recanalization of the extracranial or intracranial occlusive lesion be done first? Neurosurg Focus. 2017;42(4):E16.

Spiotta AM, et al. Proximal to distal approach in the treatment of tandem occlusions causing an acute stroke. J Neurointerv Surg. 2015;7(3):164–9.

93 Acute ICA Dissection: Stent-Assisted Recanalization

Vipul Gupta and Rajsrinivas Parthasarathy

Case

A 48-year-old male presented with subarachnoid hemorrhage (Hunt and Hess Grade II, Fisher Grade III). Cerebral angiography revealed irregular broad-based projection from supraclinoid segment of the left internal carotid artery, suggesting a blister aneurysm (Fig. 93.1b). 3D rotational angiography was performed with a diagnostic catheter in ICA. Soon after the rotational run, patient had a seizure and became unconscious and had to be intubated. Repeat angiogram (Fig. 93.1d) revealed complete occlusion of left ICA with tapered margins giving rise to flame-like appearance, suggesting a possibility of dissection. AngioCT (DynaCT, Siemens, Germany) did not reveal any fresh intracranial hemorrhage.

Issues

1. Ischemic issue: management of acute ICA occlusion
2. Hemorrhagic issue: management of the blister aneurysm in this setting

Management

Patient's AngioCT did not reveal any fresh hemorrhage. The angiographic appearance of ICA suggested acute dissection, probably during rotational angiography. In view of this, it was decided to assess the collateral flow to left cerebral hemisphere. The right ICA angiogram (Fig. 93.2a) and left vertebral injections (not shown) did not reveal any of the communicating arteries. Thereafter it was decided to attempt to recanalize the left ICA. A 6F long sheath was placed in left CCA, and a microcatheter (Excelsior SL 10, Stryker Neurovascular, US) was navigated across the occlusion with help of microguidewire (Transend 14, Stryker Neurovascular). Microcatheter injections revealed patent intracranial ICA including the petrous ICA (Fig. 93.2b). The microcatheter was exchanged over a 300 cm exchange length microguidewire (Transend, Stryker neurovascular), and two overlapping self-expanding stents (XACT, Abbott, US) were placed in cervical ICA resulting in complete recanalization of ICA (Fig. 93.2c, d). Patient was given loading

V. Gupta (✉)
Neurointerventional Surgery, Stroke Unit,
Artemis Agrim Institute of Neuroscience,
Gurgaon, India
e-mail: vipul.gupta@artemishospitals.com

R. Parthasarathy
Vascular Neurology and Neurointerventional Surgery,
Artemis Agrim Institute of Neuroscience,
Gurgaon, India

V. Gupta et al. (eds.), *100 Interesting Case Studies in Neurointervention: Tips and Tricks*,
https://doi.org/10.1007/978-981-13-1346-2_93

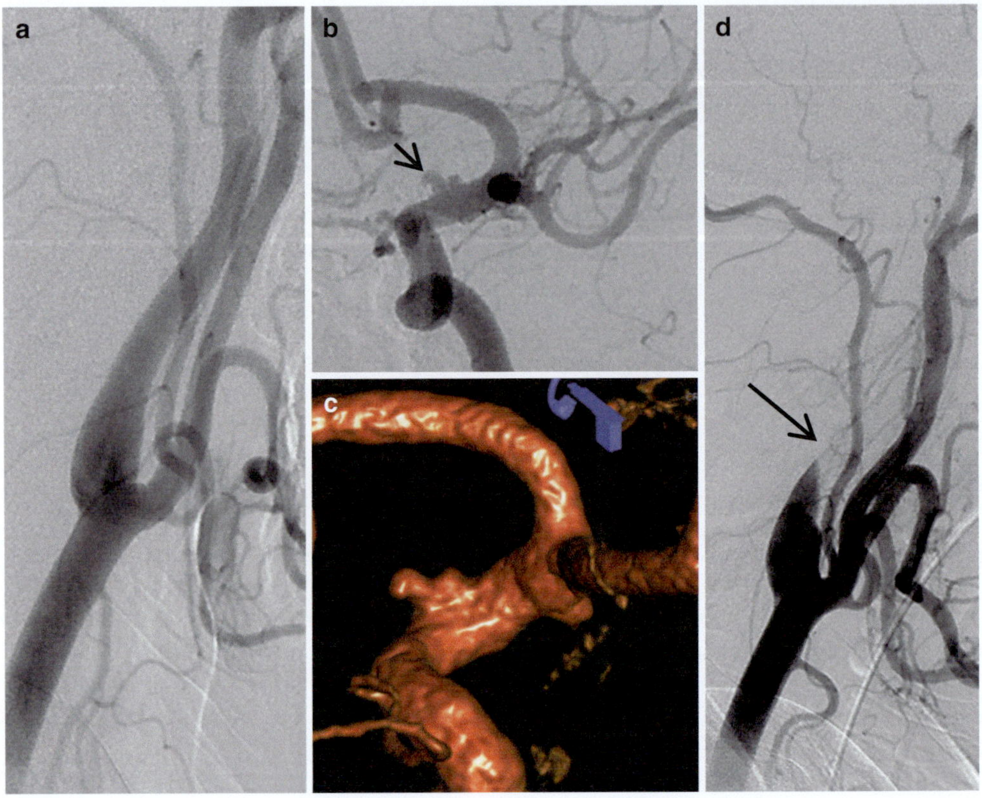

Fig. 93.1 (**a**) Left CCA injection showing a normal cervical ICA. (**b** and **c**) DSA (**b**) and 3D reconstructed image (**c**) showing a blister aneurysm in supraclinoid ICA (short arrow). (**d**) Angiogram done after patients' deterioration showing complete occlusion of ICA with a tapered occlusion (long arrow), suggesting possible dissection

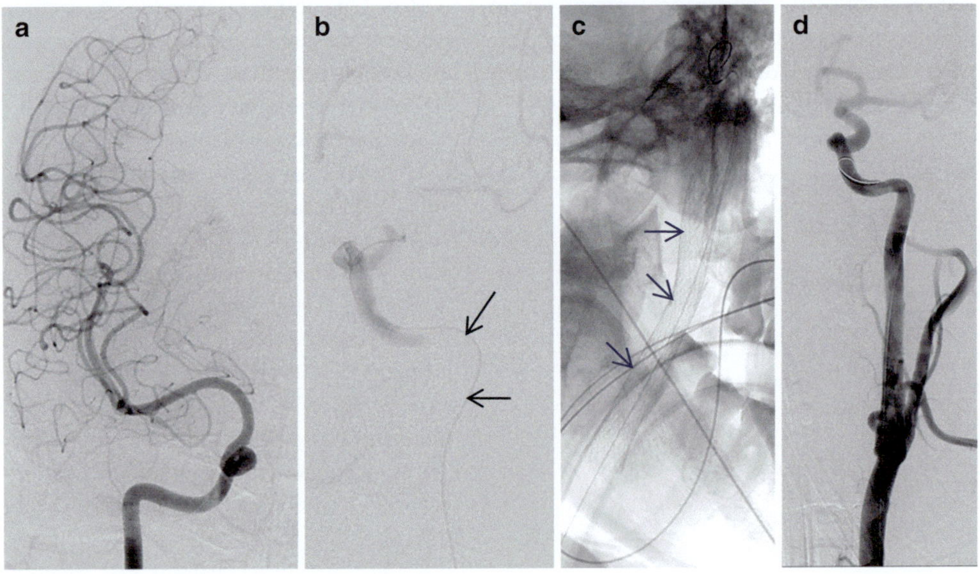

Fig. 93.2 (**a**) Right ICA angiogram shows hypoplastic/absent A1 segment of right ACA with no collateral flow to left side. (**b**) Microcatheter in left cavernous ICA shows patent ICA with retrograde flow into petrous segment. (**c**) Overlapping stents placed in left cervical ICA. (**d**) DSA after stenting showing patent ICA

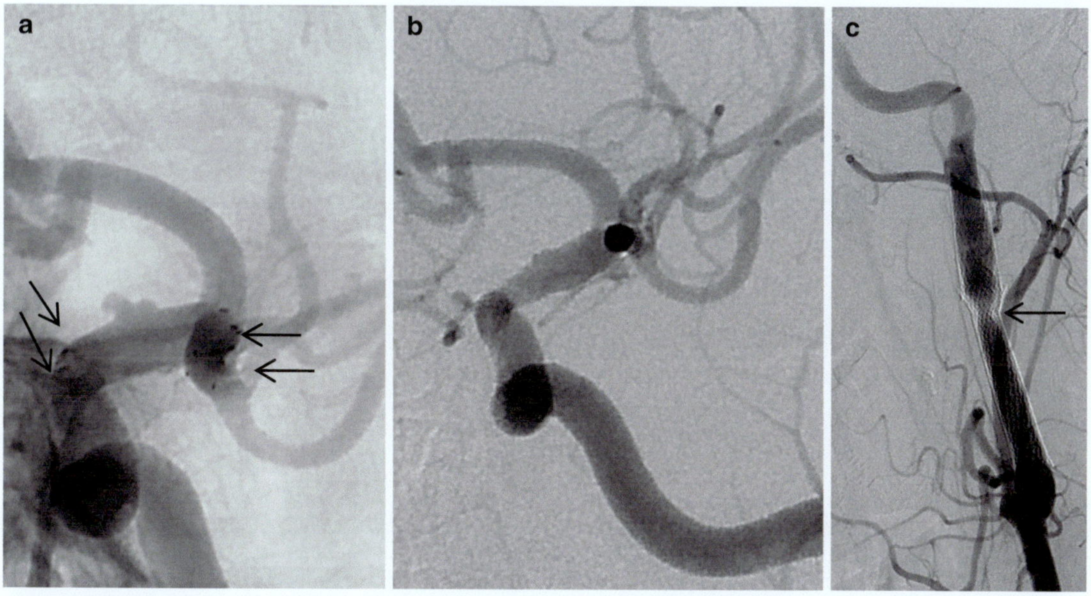

Fig. 93.3 (**a**) Overlapping stents placed across the blister aneurysm. (**b** and **c**) Follow-up after 6 months almost complete occlusion of the aneurysm (**b**) with mild stenosis in left cervical ICA (arrow)

dose of antiplatelet agents (Ecospirin 300 mg and Clopidogrel 450 mg) through Ryles tube. Since the antiplatelet agents had been given, it was imperative to treat the blister aneurysm. It was decided to place two overlapping stents (Enterprise, Codman Neurovascular, Johnson and Johnson, US) as shown in Fig. 93.3a. This was performed after placing a guiding catheter (Neuron, Penumbra, Alameda, California, USA) in the cervical ICA within the stents. Post stenting angiogram revealed mild stasis in the aneurysm (image not shown). Patient was observed for 30 min for any clot formation. Repeat CT did not show any fresh hemorrhage, and the patient was extubated in intact neurological condition. Follow-up DSA (Fig. 93.3b, c) revealed almost complete occlusion of aneurysm and moderate stenosis with in the stents in cervical ICA. Since patient was asymptomatic, it was decided not to perform further intervention.

Tips and Tricks

1. Catheter injections can result in ICA dissection. Usually these are nonocclusive and can be managed by anticoagulant or antiplatelet therapy. Rarely, the dissection can result in severe stenosis or occlusion, which may warrant recanalization.
2. It is prudent to assess for collateral circulation; if good cross flow is present, one may manage conservatively.
3. ICA dissections in cervical ICA usually start beyond the ICA origin and end in distal ICA, at junction of cervical and petrous segments. In these cases stents are necessary to recanalize and angioplasty is almost never successful. Dissections are usually easy to cross with a microguidewire, and after documenting the distal patent lumen stent placement can be done.

Suggested Reading

Fisher CM, Ojemann RG, Roberson GH. Spontaneous dissection of cervico-cerebral arteries. Can J NeurolSci. 1978;5(1):9–19.

Meling TR, Sorteberg A, Bakke SJ, Slettebo H, Hernesniemi J, Sorteberg W. Blood blister-like aneurysms of the internal carotid artery trunk causing subarachnoid hemorrhage: treatment and outcome. J Neurosurg. 2008;108:662–71.

Ogawa A, Suzuki M, Ogasawara K. Aneurysms at nonbranching sites in the surpaclinoid portion of the internal carotid artery: internal carotid artery trunk aneurysms. Neurosurgery. 2000;47:578–83. Discussion 583–586.

Ojemann RG, Fisher CM, Rich JC. Spontaneous dissecting aneurysm of the internal carotid artery. Stroke. 1972;3(4):434–40.

Pham MH, Rahme RJ, Arnaout O, et al. Endovascular stenting of extracranial carotid and vertebral artery dissections: a systematic review of the literature. Neurosurgery. 2011;68(4):856–66. [discussion:866].

Extensive Stent Reconstruction for Long-Segment Symptomatic Dissections

94

Ajit S. Puri and Rajsrinivas Parthasarathy

Case

A patient in her early 50s presented to the emergency department with a sudden onset of left-sided hemiplegia and neglect. The initial stroke scale was 16. CTA showed a right common carotid artery (CCA) occlusion close to its origin. An emergency MRI/MRA showed multiple small emboli in the right cerebral hemisphere with non-visualization of the right common and internal carotid arteries (Fig. 94.1a, b). Perfusion MRI showed a large penumbra on the right side (Fig. 94.1c, d). The patient was prepared for an emergency revascularization under general anesthesia.

Issue

Crossing long-segment dissection
Choice of stent particularly when one has to deliver it across the petrous bend
Antiplatelet agents' strategy

A. S. Puri (✉)
Radiology, and Neurosurgery,
Division of Neurointerventional Surgery,
Neurointerventional Fellowship Program,
University of Massachusetts Medical Center,
Worcester, MA, USA
e-mail: ajit.puri@umassmemorial.org

R. Parthasarathy
Vascular Neurology and Neurointerventional Surgery,
Artemis Agrim Institute of Neuroscience,
Gurgaon, India

Management

Procedure was performed under general anesthesia. An angiogram of the left ICA and posterior circulation demonstrated poor collaterals to the right hemisphere. A 6F shuttle guide catheter was placed in the proximal right CCA; an angiogram confirmed non-opacification of the proximal right CCA with filling defect in the lumen (Fig. 94.2a). The dissected segment was crossed with a microwire and a small caliber microcatheter (SL 10, Stryker neurovascular). Microcatheter injection confirmed location within the true lumen and helped with identifying the distal end of the pathology. Thereafter, multiple stents were deployed from a distal to proximal end over a 014″ microguidewire. A balloon-mounted stent was deployed across the petrous bend and following that self-expanding stents were deployed in telescoping fashion (Fig. 94.2). The final angiogram showed stent revascularization of the entire right CCA and ICA up to the petrous segment establishing a normal intracranial blood supply.

Tips and Tricks

1. Long-segment dissections can be particularly challenging to treat in tortuous anatomy.
2. A microcatheter along with a microwire with a tight loop at the tip can be used to cross the

V. Gupta et al. (eds.), *100 Interesting Case Studies in Neurointervention: Tips and Tricks*,
https://doi.org/10.1007/978-981-13-1346-2_94

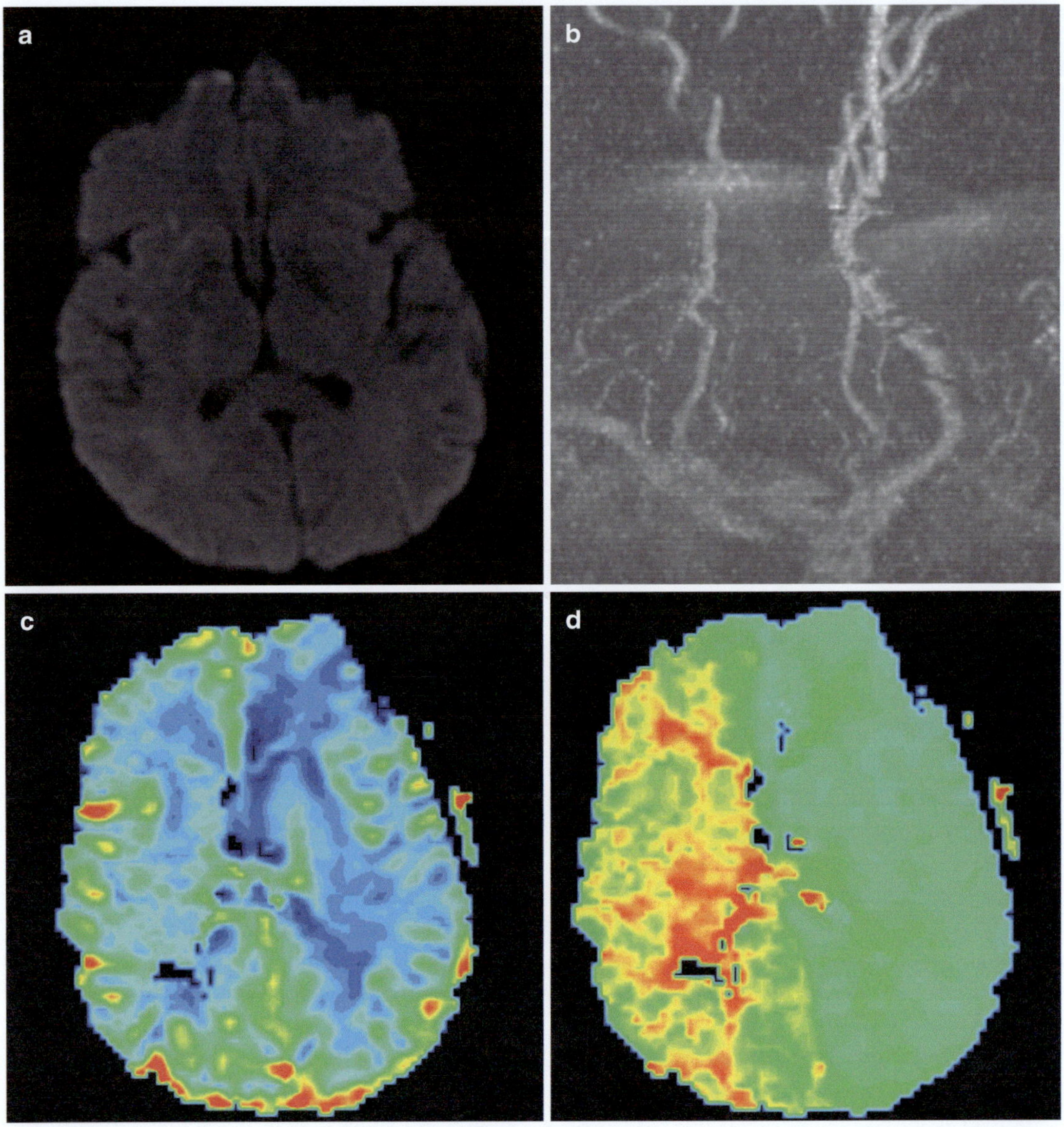

Fig. 94.1 An emergency MRI/MRA showed multiple small emboli in the right cerebral hemisphere with non-visualization of the right common and internal carotid arteries (**a**, **b**). Perfusion MRI showed a large penumbra on the right side (**c**, **d**)

dissected segment. A loop at the tip of the wire tends to stay within the true lumen.

3. Once the microcatheter is across, a microcatheter injection is taken to confirm intraluminal location and determine the distal end of the pathology in occlusive dissections.
4. When the dissection extends to the petrous segment, a stent that is less likely to kink at the petrous bend should be used.
5. The Enterprise (Codman Neurovascular) stent tends to ovalize and attenuate more than that of a Solitaire (Medtronic). However, both stents can potentially kink at 90° bend. With Solitaire, the advantage is that one can do a DynaCT post stent deployment to check for kinking and if noted can be partly or fully re-sheathed and deployed again.

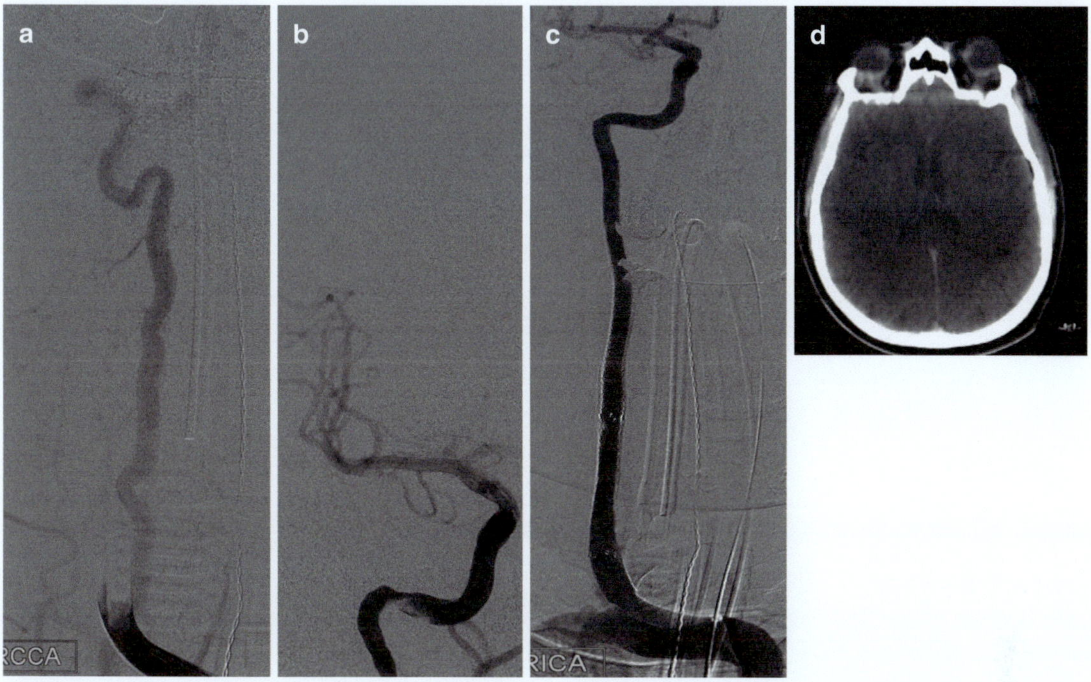

Fig. 94.2 (**a**) Injection from shuttle placed in the common carotid artery showing complete occlusion. (**b**) A microcatheter microwire combination is taken across the dissected vessel. Microcatheter injections are done once distal to dissected lumen. Using an exchange length wire, self-expanding, balloon expandable, and/or carotid stents are placed from distal to proximal fashion to cover the diseased segment. (**c**) Post-stent deployment complete reconstruction of the parent artery. (**d**) Post procedure NCCT—no large infarct or hemorrhage noted

6. To overcome the risk of kinking, one can use a balloon-mounted cardiac stent. Navigation may be difficult in tortuous cervical anatomy. However, the likelihood of kinking resulting in flow limitation is negligible as deployment is with balloon inflation. The authors prefer using a balloon-mounted stent at the petrous segment.
7. For long-segment dissections, one may use a wall stent in the straight segment as longer lengths are available in this stent category.
8. When the infarct core is small, one can load the patient with 300 mg Ecosprin on table; this should be followed with clopidogrel 300–600 mg immediate post procedure. Gp 2b/3a inhibitors should be administered if clot formation is noted during the procedure.

Suggested Reading

Cohen JE, et al. Emergent stenting to treat patients with carotid artery dissection. Stroke. 2003;34:e254–7.

Kadkhodayan Y, et al. Angioplasty and stenting in carotid dissection with or without associated pseudoaneurysm. Am J Neuroradiol. 2005;26(9):2328–35.

Carotid Stenosis with Thrombus

95

Vipul Gupta and Swati D. Chinchure

Case

A 44-year-old male, with history of tobacco chewing and hypercholesterolemia presented with sudden onset of inability to speak. MRI revealed multiple small acute infarcts in the left temporoparietal area (Fig. 95.1a). His speech improved partially in the next few days. CT angiogram revealed severe stenosis of left internal carotid artery (Fig. 95.1b). Cerebral DSA was performed. It revealed a severe sub-occlusive stenosis at the origin of the left internal carotid artery (Fig. 95.1b and blue arrow, c). A long filling defect was also seen extending from the plaque into the middle third of cervical portion of ICA (Fig. 95.1b and red arrows, c). This was suggestive of thrombus which is usually associated with plaque rupture.

Issue

Rupture of plaque can result in thrombus formation, and such free-floating thrombus associated with carotid stenosis can result in embolism and stroke. Carotid artery stenting in such cases is likely to be associated with thromboembolism.

Management

In view of the long length of clot, there was a possibility of embolism even if endarterectomy was attempted. The patient was treated by antiplatelet (Ecosprin 150 mg/day) agents as well as anticoagulant (low-molecular-weight heparin, Inj. Clexane 0.4 ml twice a day). Repeat CT angiography after 2 weeks of stroke revealed complete resolution of the thrombus. The anticoagulants were stopped, and double antiplatelet therapy was initiated (Ecosprin 150 mg/day, Clopidogrel 75 mg/day) with plan for stenting. DSA confirmed resolution of thrombus (Fig. 95.2a, b). Carotid artery stenting was performed. A protection device (SpiderFX, ev3 Inc, USA) was placed in the upper cervical ICA, and angioplasty was performed with a 2.5 mm balloon. Thereafter, stent placement was done (XACT, Abbott Vascular, USA) followed by angioplasty with a 4 mm balloon. Final angiogram revealed complete resolution of stenosis (Fig. 95.2c, d).

Tips and Tricks

1. One should carefully observe for any thrombus associated with carotid stenosis. This can be suspected on noninvasive vascular imaging,

V. Gupta (✉)
Neurointerventional Surgery, Stroke Unit, Artemis Agrim Institute of Neuroscience, Gurgaon, India
e-mail: vipul.gupta@artemishospitals.com

S. D. Chinchure
Medanta Institute of Neurosciences, Medanta Hospital, Vijay Nagar, Indore, India

V. Gupta et al. (eds.), *100 Interesting Case Studies in Neurointervention: Tips and Tricks*,
https://doi.org/10.1007/978-981-13-1346-2_95

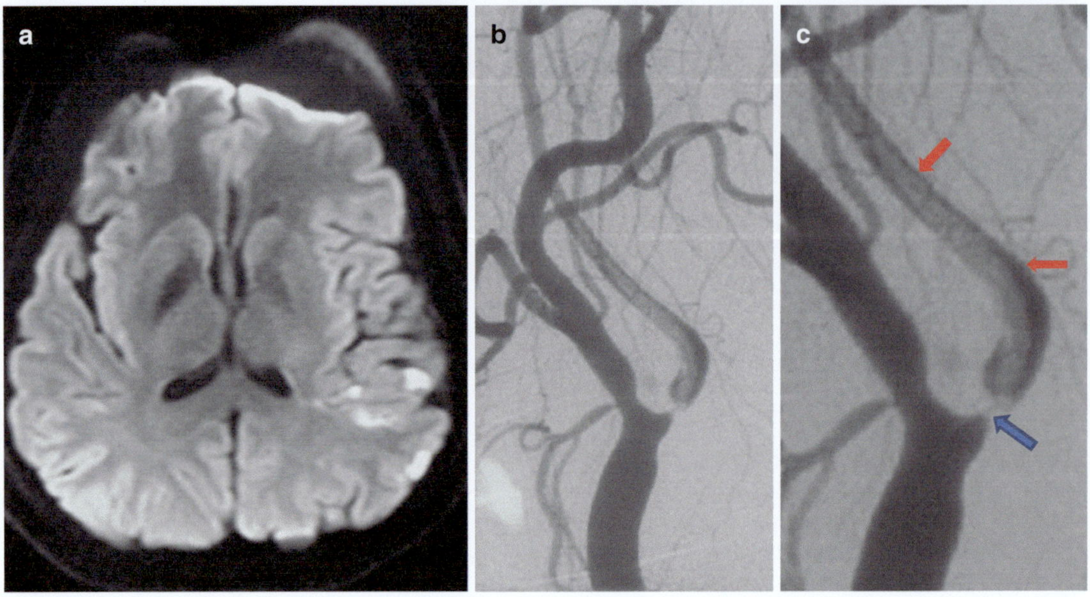

Fig. 95.1 (**a**) DWI image reveals small embolic infarctions in left temporoparietal area. (**b** and **c**) DSA images showing severe stenosis of left ICA (blue arrow, **c**) along with a long filling defect in left ICA (red arrows, **c**) suggestive of a thrombus

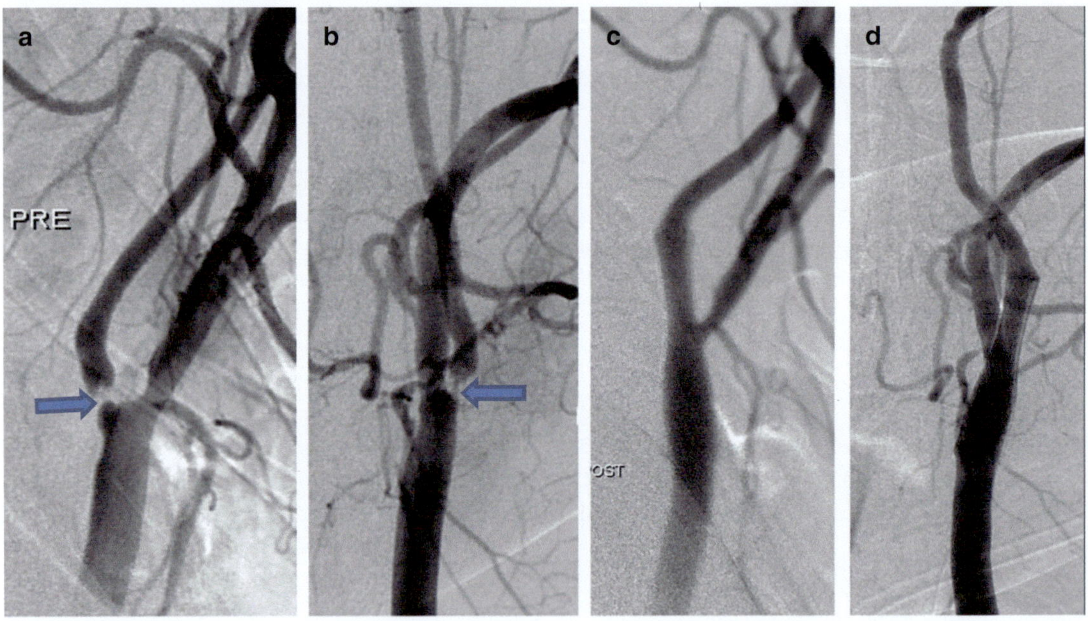

Fig. 95.2 (**a** and **b**) DSA images of left ICA showing severe stenosis of left ICA (blue arrows). The thrombus seen in the previous angiogram has resolved completely. (**c**) and (**d**) Angiogram after the stent procedure showing complete revascularization of the left ICA

and if need be, catheter angiography can be performed for confirmation. Small irregular filling defects can indicate fresh thrombus at the site of stenosis.

2. Free-floating thrombus associated with carotid stenosis has high risk of embolism and stroke. Carotid artery stenting in such cases is likely to be associated with thromboembolism and hence contraindicated. Carotid artery endarterectomy is preferable in such cases.
3. If endarterectomy is not possible/feasible, then patients should preferably be treated with anticoagulants. It is author's practice to give one antiplatelet agent (Ecosprin or Clopidogrel) along with heparin and to perform repeat imaging in 1–2 weeks. If the thrombus has resolved, stenting can be performed.

Suggested Reading

Sallustio F, et al. Floating carotid thrombus treated by intravenous heparin and endarterectomy. J Vasc Surg. 2011;53(2):489–91.

96 Difficult to Cross Carotid Stenosis: Microcatheter Exchange Technique

Vipul Gupta

Case

A 54-year-old male presented with transient weakness of the right hand lasting for 2 min. MRI did not reveal any parenchymal injury, but the MR angiography revealed severe stenosis with ulceration of left ICA. The case was planned for stenting procedure.

Issues

- To avoid plaque injury during crossing the ulcerated stenosis

Management

The procedure was planned under local anesthesia. A 6F long sheath (Flexor, Tuohy-Borst Side-Arm Introducer, Shuttle Select, Cook medical, Bloomington, USA) was placed in the left common carotid artery by coaxial technique using a long 5F Vert catheter (Cook medical, Bloomington, USA) and 0.035 in. Terumo guidewire. DSA revealed severe stenosis of the left ICA along with an ulceration (Fig. 96.1). An attempt was made to cross the stenosis with Traxcess 014 microguidewire (Microvention, Tustin, California, USA) to place the filter protection device (Spider Fx, ev3 Inc., Irvine, California, USA). However, due to the curve in the stenosis and presence of the ulceration at a bend in the stenotic area, the wire tip repeatedly entered the ulceration, and in spite of multiple attempts, it could not be taken across the stenotic segment (Fig. 96.2). The decision was taken to use a microcatheter to cross the lesion. The microcatheter tip was given slight curve at the tip and taken to the lower end of the stenosis. Thereafter, the wire with a curved tip could be torqued at the level of ulceration and was taken across the stenosis (Fig. 96.3a–e). The microcatheter was taken across the stenosis to upper cervical ICA and was withdrawn after placing Transend 014 exchange wire (Stryker Neurovascular, CA, USA) (Fig. 96.4a). The protection device was placed over the exchange wire into the cervical ICA (Fig. 96.4b). An angioplasty was done with 3 mm balloon followed by stent placement (XACT, Abbott Vascular, CA, USA). Post-dilatation was performed with a 4 mm coronary balloon (Fig. 96.4c) followed by retrieval of the filter device. Final angiogram revealed well-opposed stent with disappearance of the ulcer (Fig. 96.4d). Patient remained stable during the procedure, and postoperative course was uneventful.

V. Gupta
Neurointerventional Surgery, Stroke Unit, Artemis Agrim Institute of Neuroscience, Gurgaon, India
e-mail: vipul.gupta@artemishospitals.com

V. Gupta et al. (eds.), *100 Interesting Case Studies in Neurointervention: Tips and Tricks*,
https://doi.org/10.1007/978-981-13-1346-2_96

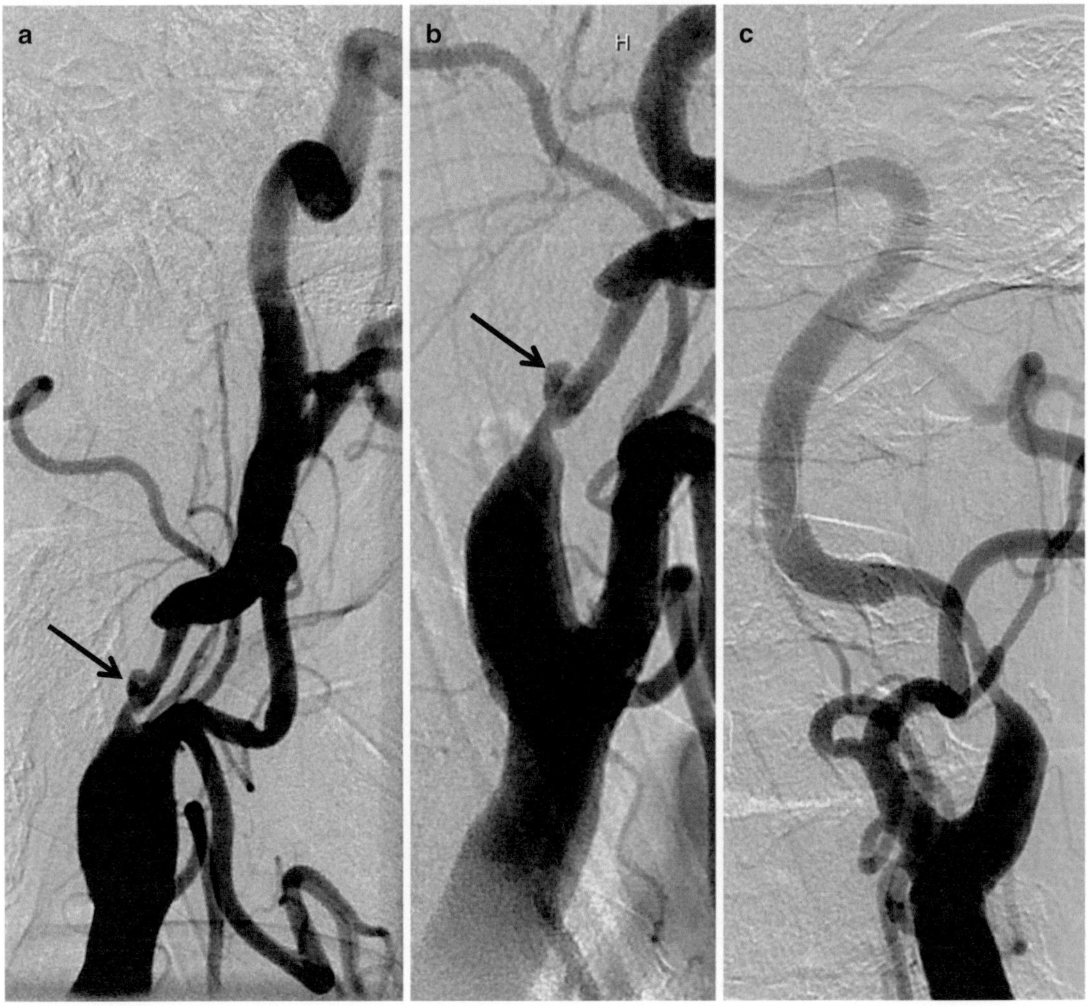

Fig. 96.1 (**a**) Left CCA angiogram (lateral view) reveals severe stenosis of left ICA. An ulcer is seen in the stenotic segment (arrow). (**b**) Magnified view of the stenotic segment profiling the ulcer (arrow). (**c**) Angiogram in oblique view showing the stenosis and mild tortuosity of cervical ICA

Tips and Tricks

1. In circumstances where there is a long segment of irregular lumen, it may be difficult to navigate the wire across the stenosis. Excessive manipulation, particularly in ulcerations as in our case, can lead to plaque injury and embolism.
2. In such a situation, it may be prudent to use a microcatheter to cross the lesion. The curve in the microcatheter can help in negotiating the curves and it helps in torqueing the wire in narrow tracks. After taking the microcatheter across the lesion, an exchange can be performed to place a filter device.
3. Our device of choice in this setting is a device like "Spider Fx" with which an independent wire can be used.
4. High-quality road map should be used to cross severe stenosis with ulcerations so as to avoid plaque injury.

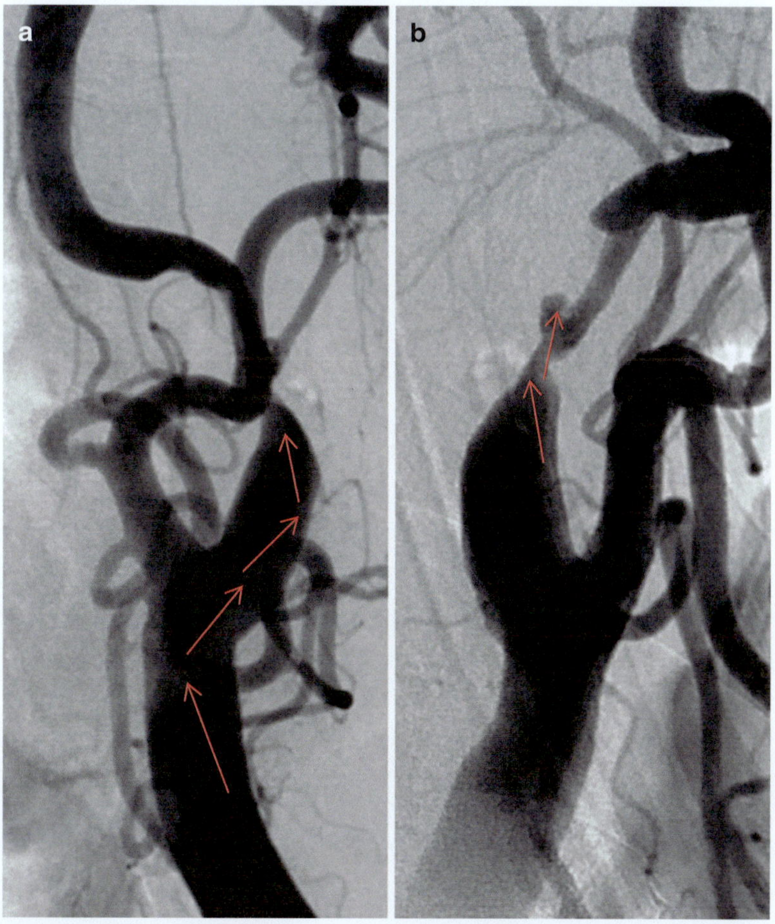

Fig. 96.2 (**a** and **b**) Arrows depicting the course of micro guidewire during the attempt to cross the lesion in oblique (**a**) and lateral (**b**) projections. Due to the curvature in the parent vessel and stenotic segment, the wire repeatedly entered the ulcer and could not be taken across the stenosis

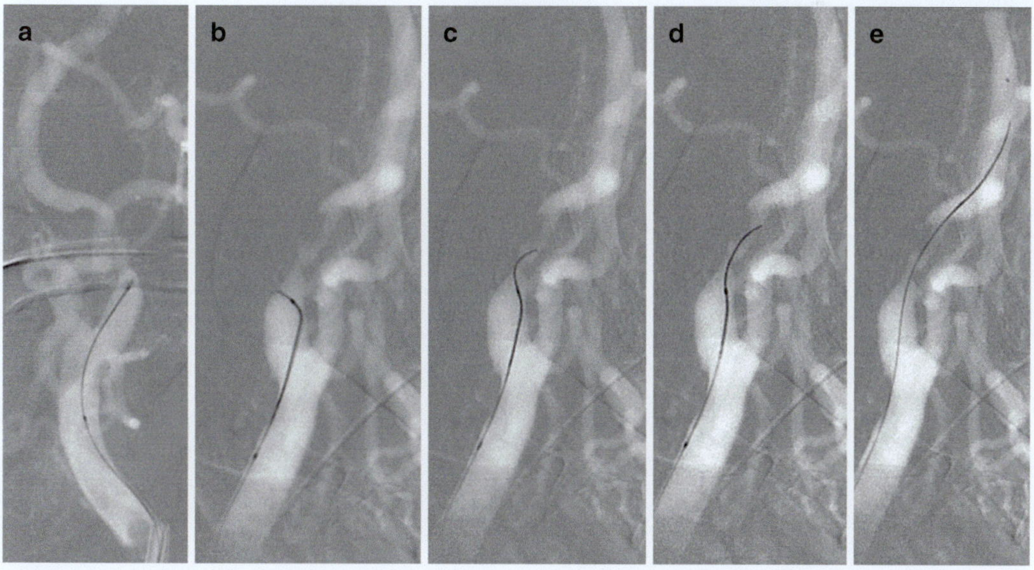

Fig. 96.3 Road map images showing use of microcatheter to cross the ICA stenosis. (**a** and **b**) Road map images in oblique (**a**) and lateral views (**b**) showing microcatheter in lower end of stenosis. (**c** and **d**) Microguidewire being navigated across the stenosis. (**e**) Microcatheter taken over the guidewire to the upper cervical ICA

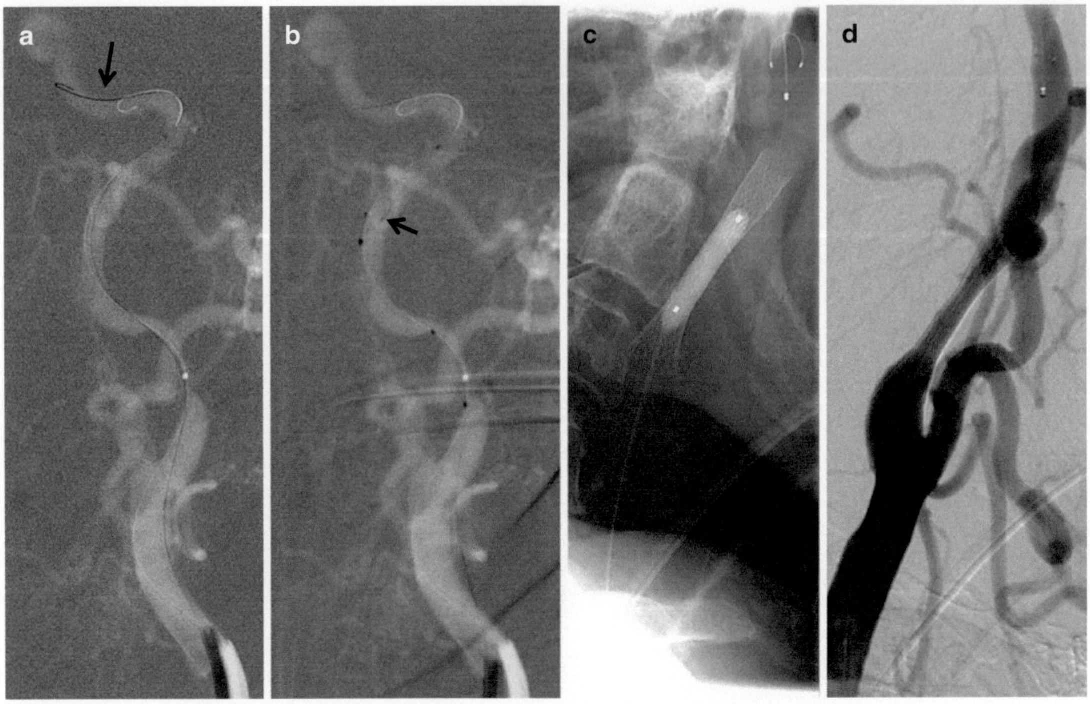

Fig. 96.4 (**a**) Road map image showing exchange wire (arrow) placed through the microcatheter. (**b**) Road map image showing filter device (arrow) in upper cervical ICA. (**c**) Image showing post-stenting angioplasty. (**d**) Final angiogram showing adequate recanalization

Suggested Reading

Parodi FE, Schonholz C, Parodi JC. Minimizing complications of carotid stenting. Persp Vasc Surg Endovasc Ther. 2010;22:117–22.

97 Carotid Stenting with Tortuous Arch

Vipul Gupta

Case

An 82-year-old female presented with transient weakness of the right arm. MRI brain was normal. However, MRA revealed severe stenosis of bilateral ICA (Fig. 97.1a, b). The left CCA was rising at an acute angle from the brachiocephalic artery (Fig. 97.1c). Patient had received radiotherapy in neck region for laryngeal tumor 12 years back. As left ICA stenosis was symptomatic, revascularization was planned, and, in view of previous radiotherapy, endovascular approach was favored over endarterectomy.

Issues

- Difficult catheterization of left CCA to place a stable guiding catheter
- To avoid thromboembolism in an old lady with tortuous anatomy

Management

The procedure was performed under local anesthesia. The plan was to place an 8F guiding catheter in the upper part of the left CCA in a coaxial manner over a long (125 cm) soft tip 5 F Vert catheter (Cook medical, Bloomington, USA). The left CCA could not be hooked because of the acute angle of left CCA (Fig. 97.1c). Thereafter, it was decided to perform an exchange maneuver using a Simmons 2 catheter (Fig. 97.2). The Simmons catheter was given an anticlockwise rotation after hooking the brachiocephalic artery. This helped in placing the wire (Terumo 035) in the left CCA (Fig. 97.2a, b). The catheter was rotated in a clockwise manner and could be navigated into the CCA (Fig. 97.2c, d). Thereafter, an exchange length (260 cm) Amplatz extra stiff wire (Cook medical, Bloomington, USA) was placed in the upper left CCA, and the Simmons catheter was withdrawn (Fig. 97.2e). Following that, the Vert catheter was advanced into the CCA over Amplatz wire (Fig. 97.2f). The guiding catheter was navigated in a coaxial manner over the Vert catheter (Fig. 97.2g). The Vert catheter was placed in the ECA, and the stiff wire was kept in catheter to provide adequate support to navigate the guiding. A filter device (Spider Fx, ev3 Inc., Irvine, California, USA) was placed in upper cervical ICA (Fig. 97.3b). Pre-dilatation was performed with 3-mm coronary angioplasty balloon followed by stent placement (XACT, Abbott Vascular, CA, USA) followed by post-dilatation with 4-mm coronary angioplasty balloon. Thereafter, the filter device was withdrawn. Final angiogram revealed satisfactory outcome (Fig. 97.3c). The guide catheter was withdrawn in a coaxial manner with the Vert catheter. Patient made uneventful recovery.

V. Gupta
Neurointerventional Surgery, Stroke Unit, Artemis Agrim Institute of Neuroscience, Gurgaon, India
e-mail: vipul.gupta@artemishospitals.com

V. Gupta et al. (eds.), *100 Interesting Case Studies in Neurointervention: Tips and Tricks*,
https://doi.org/10.1007/978-981-13-1346-2_97

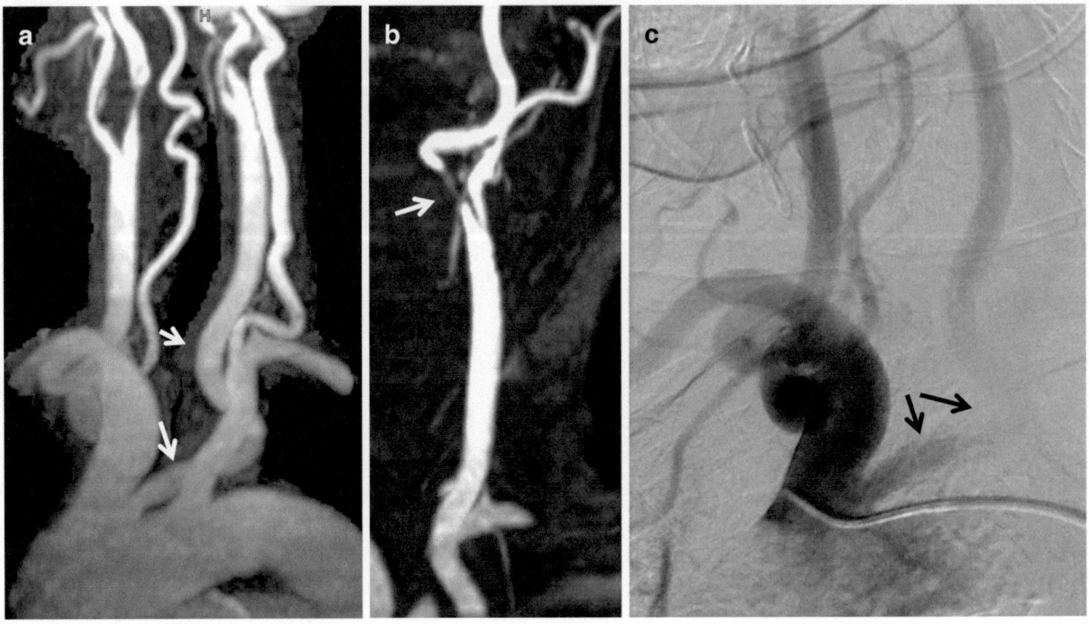

Fig. 97.1 (**a**) MR angiography of aortic arch showing acute angle of origin of left CCA (arrows). Stenosis of bilateral ICA was seen. (**b**) MRA image showing severe stenosis of left ICA (arrow). (**c**) DSA showing the bovine origin along with tortuosity of left CCA

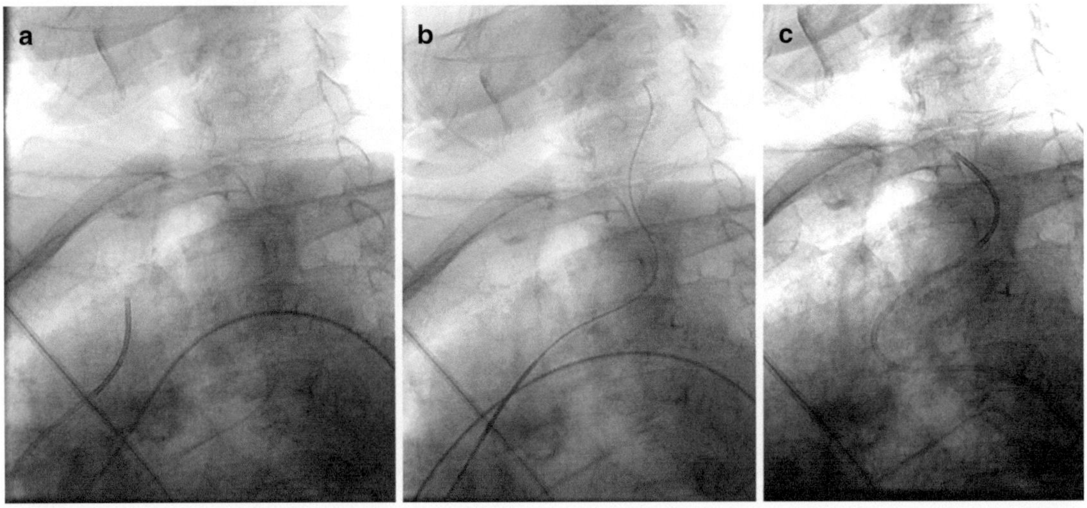

Fig. 97.2 Exchange maneuver with Simmons 2 catheter to place the guiding catheter. (**a**) Fluoroscopic image showing Simmons 2 catheter at the origin of brachiocephalic artery. (**b**) The catheter was rotated to hook the left CCA. (**c**) Catheter in left CCA. (**d**) DSA run of left CCA. (**e**) Exchange length Amplatz extra stiff wire placed in the upper CCA through Simmons catheter. (**f**) Exchange maneuver was performed to place Vert catheter coaxially through the sheath into CCA (the Amplatz wire is still in the catheter to provide support). (**g**) Guiding catheter placed over the Vert catheter and Amplatz wire

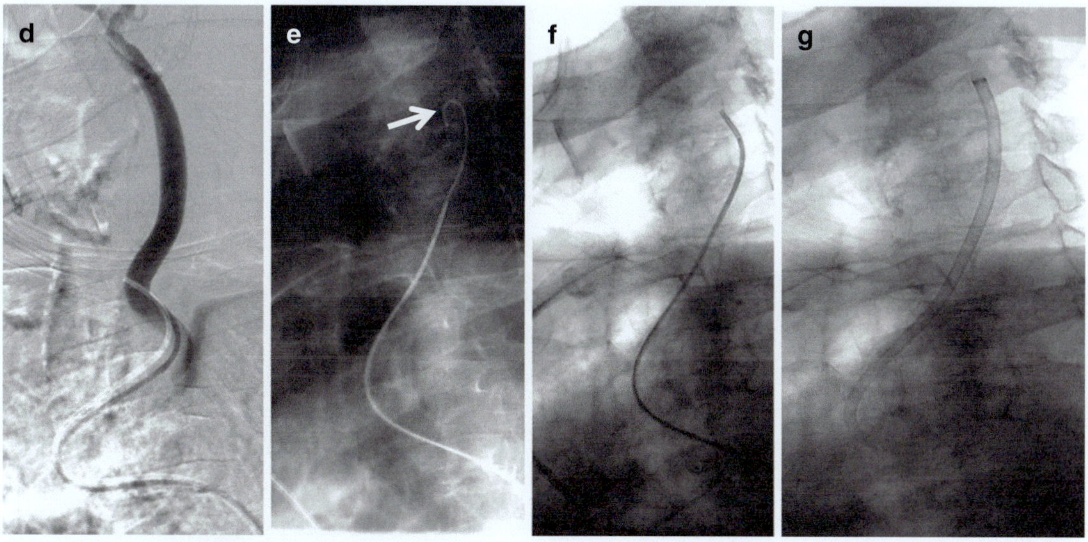

Fig. 97.2 (continued)

Tips and Tricks

1. In patients with extreme tortuosity of the aortic arch, carotid artery stenting is a feasible option, particularly if there are contraindications to endarterectomy.
2. One should have a clear protocol in these cases to catheterize the tortuous vessels and should avoid prolonged struggle in the aortic arch. Manipulations in the arch are major reason for thromboembolism, particularly in old patients.
3. We prefer to perform an exchange maneuver with Simmons and Amplatz extra stiff wire. The Simmons catheter is the most convenient tool to hook difficult to catheterize vessels, and the Amplatz wire provides enough support to place relatively stiff guiding catheter or long sheath to perform the procedure. In our experience, it is relatively difficult to perform exchange with softer wires (such as Terumo 035/038) with Simmons catheter.
4. The loop at the tip of the Amplatz wire may help in avoiding intimal injury.
5. The coaxial use of a long 5F catheter helps in the placement of guiding catheter while avoiding excessive intimal or plaque injury.
6. Care should be taken to avoid wire or catheter manipulation at the site of stenosis. A road map can be used during the exchange maneuver for this purpose.
7. We prefer to give loading dose of heparin (50–75 U/kg) at start of procedure with difficult arch.

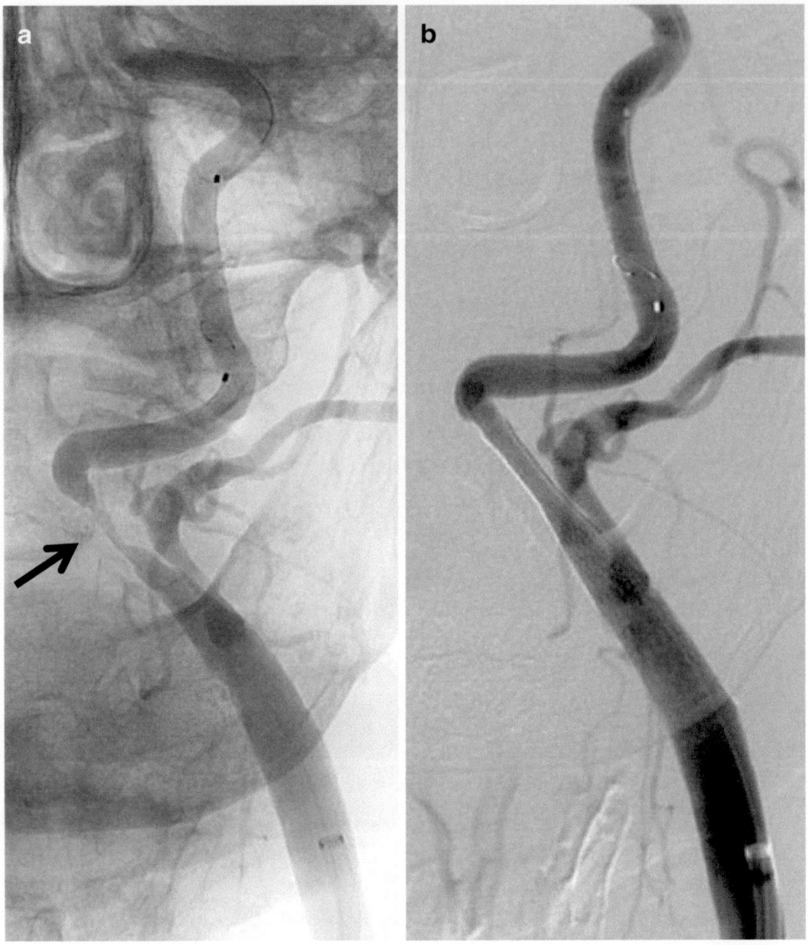

Fig. 97.3 (**a**) DSA image showing severe stenosis of the left ICA (arrow) with filter device placed in the upper cervical ICA. (**b**) Post-procedure angiogram showing recanalization of ICA

Suggested Reading

Choi HM, Hobson RW II, Goldstein J, Chakhtoura E, Lal BK, Haser PB, et al. Technical challenges in a program of carotid artery stenting. J Vasc Surg. 2004;40:746–51.

Verzini F, DeRango P, Parlani G, Panuccio G, Cao P. Carotid artery stenting: technical issues and role of operator's experience. Perspect Vasc Surg Endovasc Ther. 2008;20:247–57.

98 Acute Thrombosis of Carotid Stent

Vipul Gupta

Case

A 63-year-old female, hypertensive and diabetic, presented with transient ischemic attack involving right middle cerebral artery territory. MR revealed severe stenosis at the origin of the right internal carotid artery. Left ICA was blocked at its origin. The patient was planned for stent-assisted revascularization of the right ICA stenosis. Patient was on double antiplatelet therapy (Ecosprin 150 mg/day and Clopidogrel 75 mg/day) for 5 days before the procedure.

Issue

In-stent thrombus formation.

Management

Procedure was performed under local anesthesia. DSA revealed severe (more than 90%) stenosis of the proximal right internal carotid artery (Fig. 98.1a, b). A 6F long sheath was placed in the common carotid artery, and a protection device was placed in the upper cervical ICA. Angioplasty was performed with a 3 mm diameter balloon. After that, stent (Xact, Abbott, US) was placed followed by angioplasty with 4 mm balloon. Soon after the stent placement, irregularity of stent margins was seen (Fig. 98.1c), and additional bolus of heparin (2000 U) was given (as per our protocol, 5000 IU of heparin was given intravenously at the start of the procedure, followed by another 1500 before the stent placement). However, repeat angiogram revealed progression of the suspected clot formation with diffuse haziness of almost the whole length of the stent (Fig. 98.1d). Intra-arterial Abciximab (6 mg) was given through the long sheath over 5–7 min resulting in almost complete resolution of the thrombus (Fig. 98.1e). Protection device was removed. Patient remained stable during the procedure. Post-procedure low molecular weight heparin (Inj. Clexane 0.4 ml twice a day) was given for 24 h. The patient was discharged on twice daily dose of Clopidogrel.

Tips and Tricks

1. It is prudent to perform an angiogram 15–30 min after the procedure to check for any thrombus formation on the stent.
2. This is likely to be due to platelet aggregation, and intra-arterial injection of agents such as GpIIb/IIIa inhibitors usually results in resolution of the clot. One cannot be certain of the reason behind thrombus formation; however,

V. Gupta
Neurointerventional Surgery, Stroke Unit, Artemis Agrim Institute of Neuroscience, Gurgaon, India
e-mail: vipul.gupta@artemishospitals.com

V. Gupta et al. (eds.), *100 Interesting Case Studies in Neurointervention: Tips and Tricks*,
https://doi.org/10.1007/978-981-13-1346-2_98

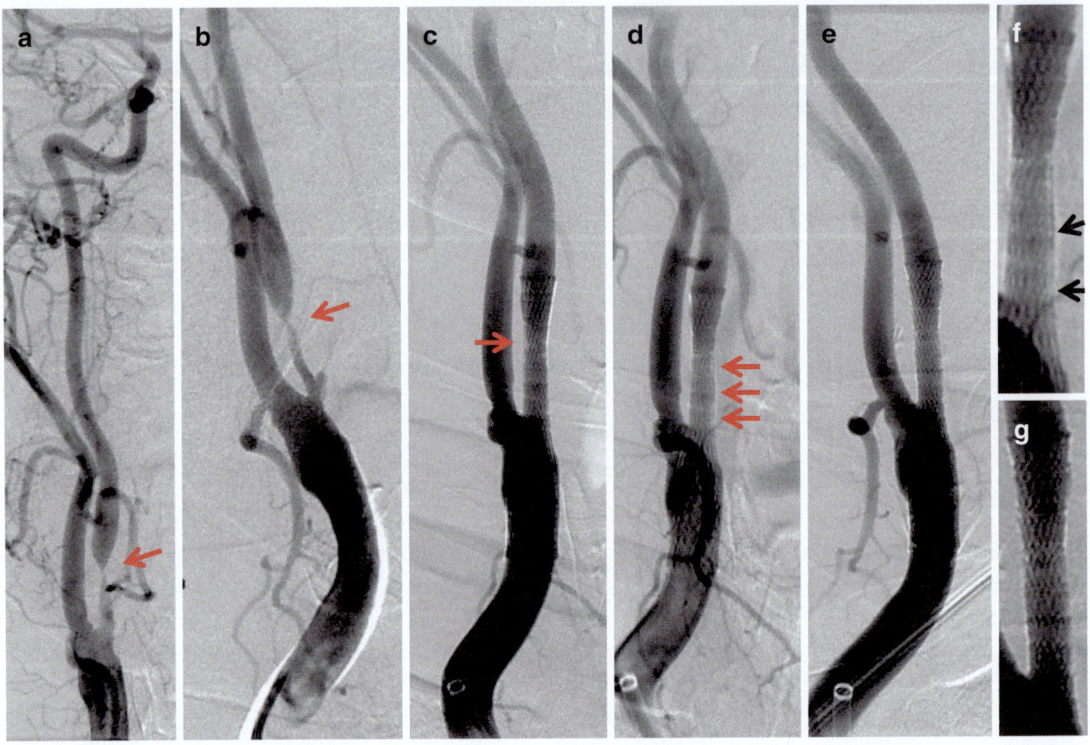

Fig. 98.1 (**a** and **b**) Rt. Carotid angiograms showing severe stenosis at origin of right ICA. (**c**) Carotid artery stenting was performed successfully with help of protection device. Soon after stent placement, small irregular filling defects (arrow) were suspected within the stent, and additional heparin was given. (**d**) Repeat angiogram revealed diffuse haziness within the stent (arrows). (**h**) Abciximab (6 mg) was given through the guiding catheter resulting in almost complete resolution of thrombus. (**e** and **f**) Enlarged images of the stent showing the haziness in the stent (arrows, **f**) which resolved (**g**) after administration of Abciximab

one of the possibilities is resistance to antiplatelet agents especially Clopidogrel.

3. Acute thrombus formation can be one for the reasons for stroke after completion of the procedure.
4. In cases with excessive thrombus formation, one may give intravenous infusion of GpIIb/IIIa inhibitor and may switch to agent such as Ticagrelor which is much less likely to have resistance than Clopidogrel.

Suggested Reading

Bush RL, Bhama JK, Lin PH, Lumsden AB. Transient ischaemic attack due to early carotid stent thrombosis: successful rescue with rheolytic thrombectomy and systemic abciximab. J Endovasc Ther. 2003;10:870–4.

Xiromeritis K, Dalainas I, Stamatakos M, Katsikas V, Martinakis V, Stamatelopoulos K. Acute carotid stent thrombosis after carotid artery stenting. Eur Rev Med Pharmacol Sci. 2012;16(3):355–62.

Carotid Stenosis with Recurrent TIA's: Emergency Stenting

99

Vipul Gupta

Case

A 58-year-old man with history of multiple episodes of left arm weakness and numbness. He was admitted to the emergency room with weakness of the left arm of 1 h duration. Multimodal CT imaging revealed an area of prolonged MTT with preserved blood volume at the right precentral gyrus (Fig. 99.1a–c); CTA revealed tight stenosis at the origin of the right ICA and MRI showed multiple areas of diffusion restriction in thr right ACA-MCA and MCA-PCA watershed territory (Fig. 99.1d–f).

Clinical Course and Management

Patient's symptoms improved after 20 min. In view of the tight stenosis, he was loaded with double antiplatelets. He had two more episodes of transient numbness in the left arm. In view of the multiple repeat attacks despite on medical management, he was taken up for emergency stenting (Figs. 99.2 and 99.3).

Patient had no neurological deficits and was discharged a day after with no new symptoms.

Tips and Tricks

1. The carotid stenosis with ulcerated plaques can be tricky to treat. The risk of distal embolism can be high if appropriate precautions are not taken. Identifying the clot on angiogram is the basic prerequisite and should be carefully assessed in all patients with multiple transient ischemic attacks.
2. Use of filter in these cases is mandatory. The Spider filter is a good choice in such cases so that a soft 014″ or 010″ microguidewire can be used to cross the plaque safely.
3. In cases where pre-angioplasty is required, balloon should be undersized and slowly inflated to avoid clot dislodgement. Use of closed cell stent is advisable in these cases so that the plaque/clot cannot be squeezed through the struts of the stent. Post angioplasty should also be done with gentle inflation.

V. Gupta
Neurointerventional Surgery, Stroke Unit, Artemis Agrim Institute of Neuroscience, Gurgaon, India
e-mail: vipul.gupta@artemishospitals.com

V. Gupta et al. (eds.), *100 Interesting Case Studies in Neurointervention: Tips and Tricks*, https://doi.org/10.1007/978-981-13-1346-2_99

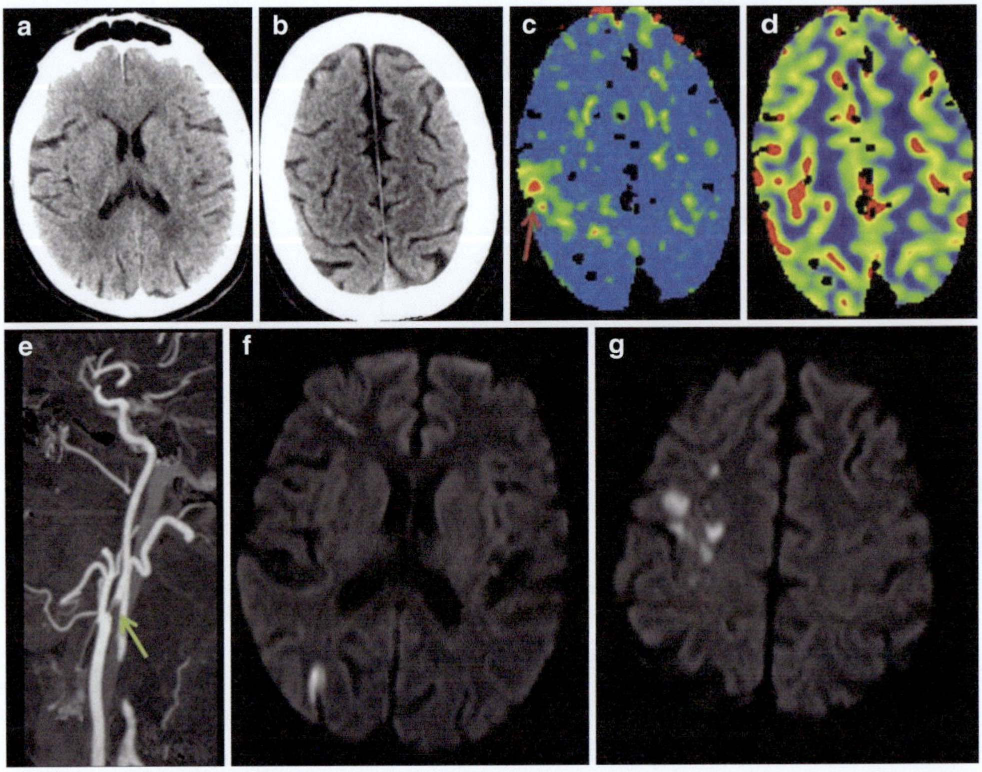

Fig. 99.1 CT head plain (**a** and **b**) No infarct/bleed demonstrated. (**c** and **d**) There is an area of raised MTT in the right precentral gyrus (red arrow) with no defect in the CBV map suggestive of penumbra. (**e**) CT angiography demonstrated 90% stenosis of right ICA at its origin. (**f** and **g**) Multiple areas of diffusion restriction seen in the right ACA-MCA and right MCA-PCA watershed and in the right precentral gyrus

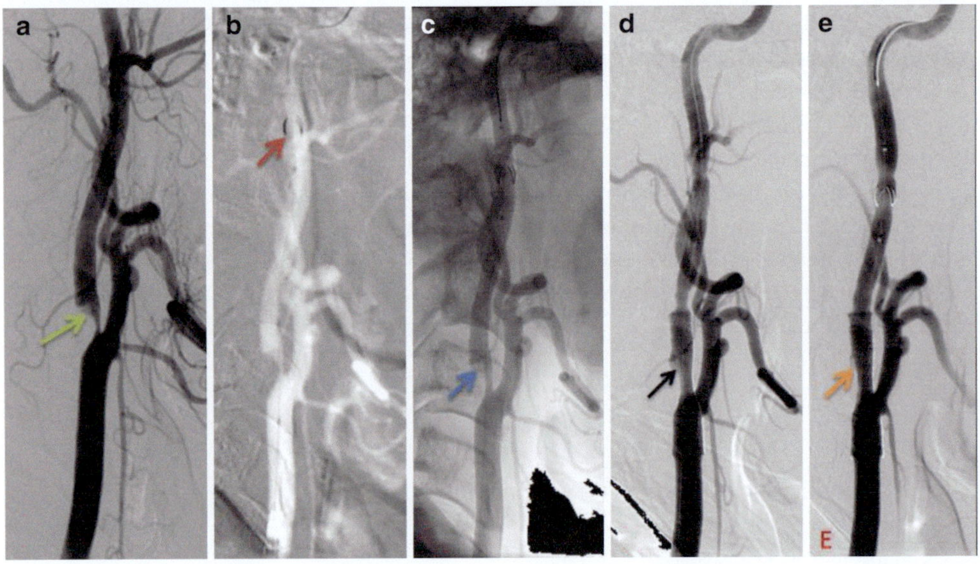

Fig. 99.2 Digital subtraction angiography of the cerebral vessels were performed. (**a**) Selective right common carotid artery injection confirms the 90% stenosis of the right ICA origin with a doubtful clot on the superior aspect of the stenosis (Green arrow). (**b**) The NAV6 filter was taken across the stenosis, taking care that it does not disturb the clot. (**c**) A small balloon 3.00 × 20 mm was used to do a gentle pre-angioplasty. There was no change in the apparent clot (Blue arrow). (**d**) Closed stent Xact 6–8 mm× 30 mm was deployed. Post stenting, the clot is trapped between the wall and stent. (Black arrow). (**e**) Post stenting angioplasty to completely open the stent

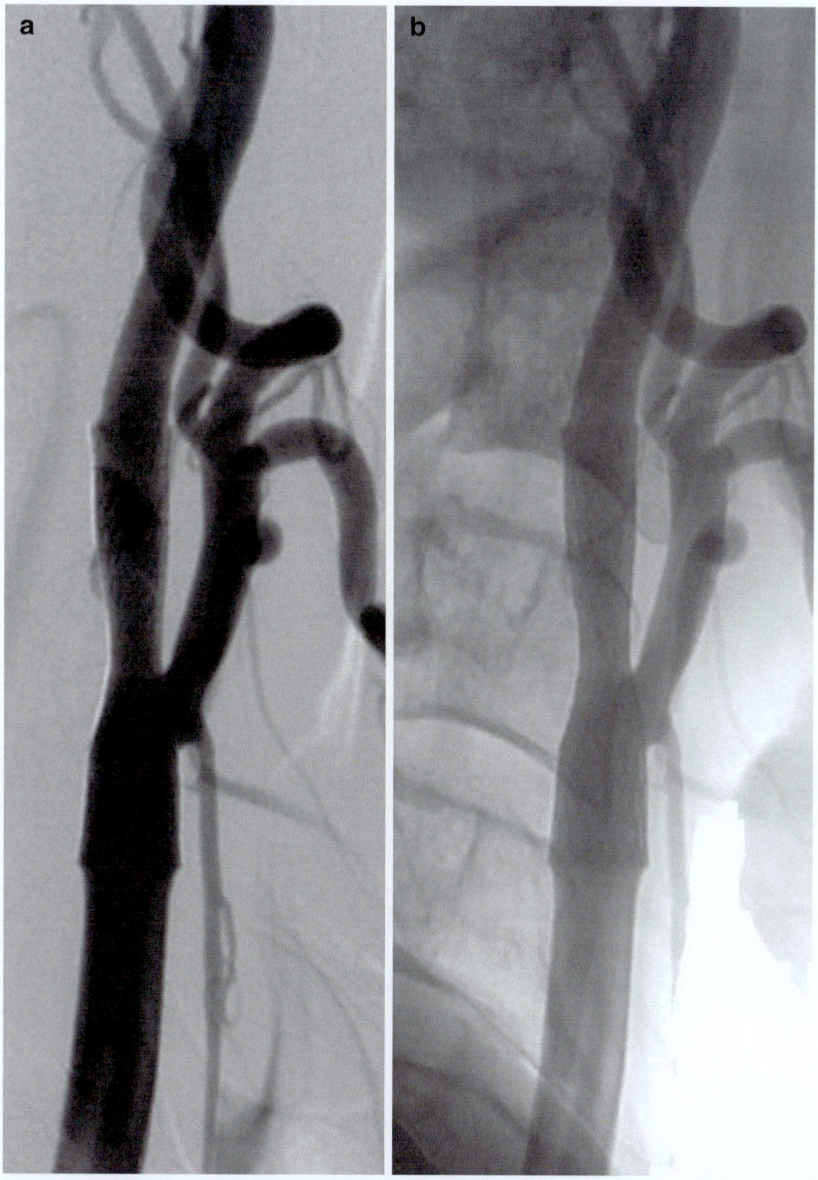

Fig. 99.3 (**a** and **b**) Final result after angioplasty and stenting with near total resolution of the clot

4. Always keep a stent retriever as a backup along with a thrombolytic agent to remove/dissolve the clot if there is distal embolism.

Suggested Reading

Diener HC, Bogousslavsky J, Brass LM, et al. MATCH investigators – aspirin and clopidogrel compared with clopidogrel alone after recent ischaemic stroke or transient ischaemic attack in high-risk patients (MATCH): randomised, double-blind, placebo-controlled trial. Lancet. 2004;364(9431):331–7.

Rothwell PM, Giles MF, Chandratheva A, et al. Early use of existing preventive strategies for stroke (EXPRESS) study effect of urgent treatment of transient ischaemic attack and minor stroke on early recurrent stroke (EXPRESS study): a prospective population-based sequential comparison. Lancet. 2007;370(9596):1432–14.

100 Sub-occlusive Carotid Stenosis with Slow Flow in ICA with Dissection of Cervical ICA During the Procedure

Vipul Gupta

Case

A 70-year-old man with hypertension and coronary artery disease, post CABG, presented with a history of transient left-sided weakness and slurred speech 1 month ago. MRI brain showed small right MCA territory infarcts. CT angiography shows 95% tight stenosis of the right ICA at its origin. DSA confirmed tight ICA origin stenosis with slow flow distally (Fig. 100.1a–e).

Issues

1. Difficult to cross very tight stenosis
2. Avoiding hyperperfusion bleeding
3. Upper cervical dissection during the procedure

Management

A short, 11 cm long 8F sheath (Codman & Shurtleff, Inc., USA) was used to access the right femoral artery. Following this an 8F guiding catheter (Concentric Medical, CA, USA) was positioned in the right CCA over a 125 cm long vertebral curve catheter. The stenosis was crossed using a 0.014 Traxess microguidewire (MicroVention, Tustin, California, USA) (Fig. 100.2a) and a pre-stenting angioplasty was done with a 1.5 × 15 mm balloon (Fig. 100.2b). The Spider filter protection device (ev3 Inc., Irvine, California, USA) was guided across the stenosis and deployed (Fig. 100.2d). Following this a 6–8 mm × 40 cm (Protégé, ev3 Inc., Irvine, California, USA) stent was placed followed by the balloon angioplasty of the stent (Fig. 100.2e).

Post-procedure angiogram revealed good recanalization of the stenosed right ICA with good antegrade flow (Fig. 100.3). However, a segment of the cervical ICA was dissected due to manipulation of the wire across the tortuosity or due to the filter device (Fig. 100.4a). Since significant narrowing of true lumen was seen, it was decided to place a stent at the dissected site. The dissected ICA was crossed with Rebar18 (ev3 Inc., Irvine, California, USA) microcatheter over a 0.014 microguidewire (Fig. 100.4b). To prevent ICA occlusion and thromboembolism, a solitaire (ev3, ev3 Inc., Irvine, California, USA) stent 4 mm × 40 cm was deployed (Fig. 100.4c, d). There were no clinical complications during the procedure. The *patient had no neurological deficits and was discharged a day after.*

V. Gupta
Neurointerventional Surgery, Stroke Unit,
Artemis Agrim Institute of Neuroscience,
Gurgaon, India
e-mail: vipul.gupta@artemishospitals.com

V. Gupta et al. (eds.), *100 Interesting Case Studies in Neurointervention: Tips and Tricks*,
https://doi.org/10.1007/978-981-13-1346-2_100

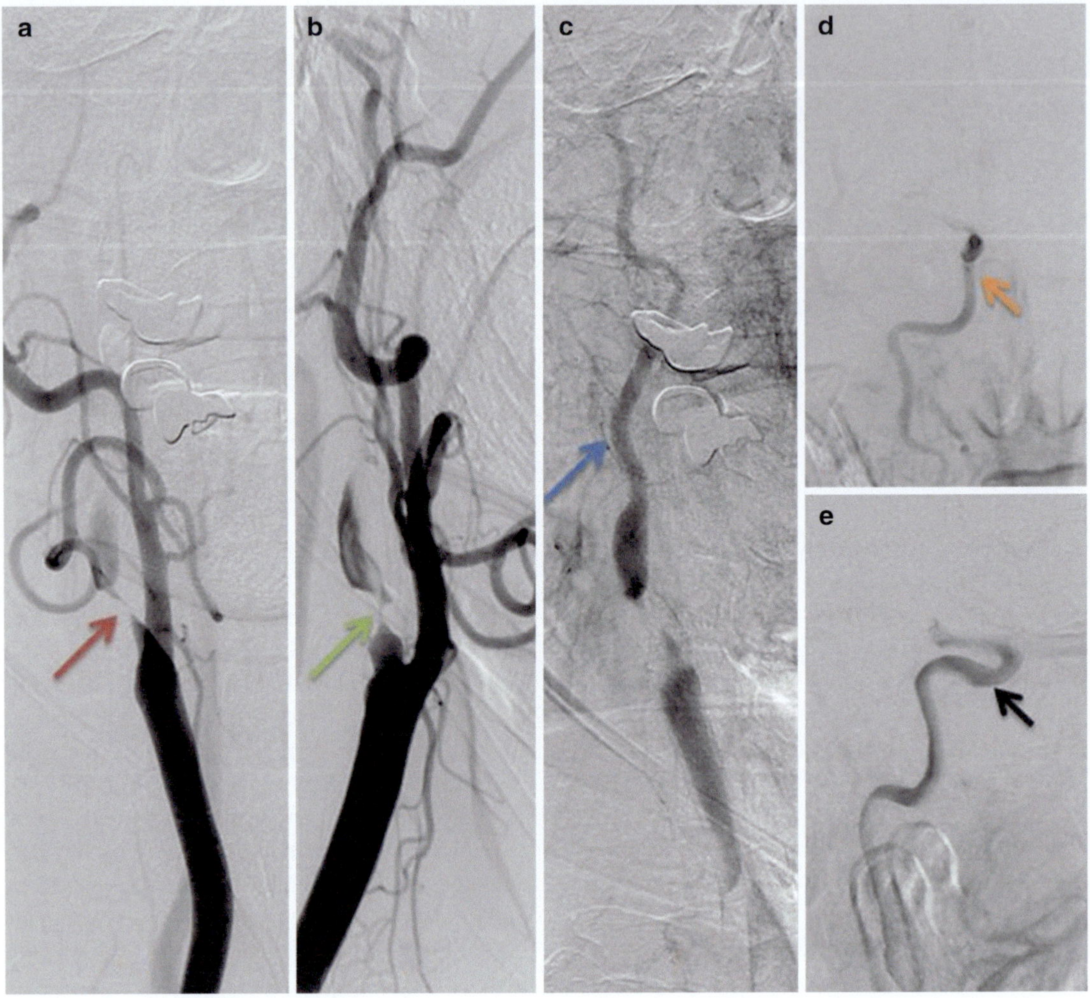

Fig. 100.1 Right CCA injection (**a** and **b**) shows very significant 95% stenosis of the right ICA origin with very slow antegrade flow. (**c**) Stasis of the contrast in the right ICA due to severe stenosis. (**d** and **e**) Very slow antegrade flow in the right ICA intracranially

Tips and Tricks

1. Tight carotid stenosis can be tricky to treat. The use of Spider filter allows us to cross the lesion with a soft 0.014 wire and perform a pre-angioplasty before advancing the filter.
2. The pre-stenting dilation allows us to navigate the filter and stent safely across tight stenosis and establish antegrade flow.
3. The microguidewire itself can be self-occlusive in such tight stenosis. Understanding and anticipation is crucial.
4. Post-procedure angiograms should be carefully assessed for dissection, particularly if there is difficulty in negotiating the systems in tortuous anatomy.
5. Carotid artery dissection is a rare but important complication of CAS. Factors which may predispose to this complication include:
   (a) Severe "bends" or "kinks" in the ICA
   (b) Aggressive hardware (guide wires, balloon catheters, stents) manipulation within the ICA
   (c) Post-dilatation of the distal stent edge within the ICA

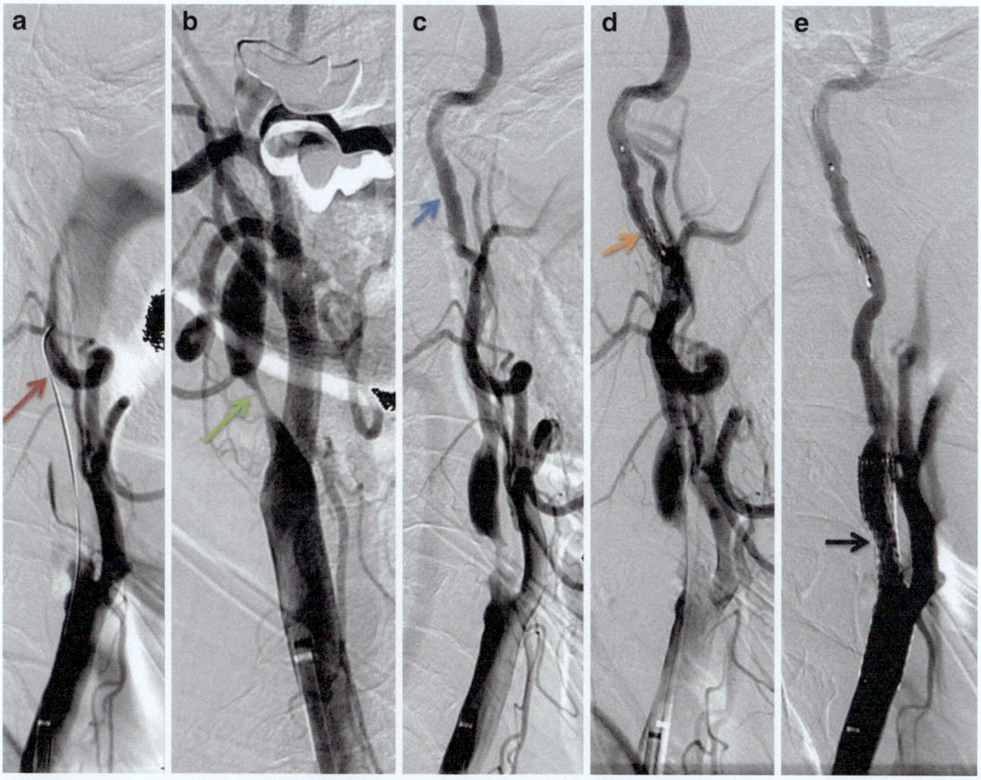

Fig. 100.2 (**a**) The stenosis was crossed using a 014 Traxess microguidewire (MicroVention) and (**b**) a pre-angioplasty was done with a 1.5 × 15 mm balloon. (**c**) Good antegrade flow was established immediately. (**d**) The Spider filter protection device (ev3) was guided across the stenosis and deployed. (**e**) 6–8 mm × 40 cm (Protégé ev3) stent was placed followed by the balloon angioplasty of the stent

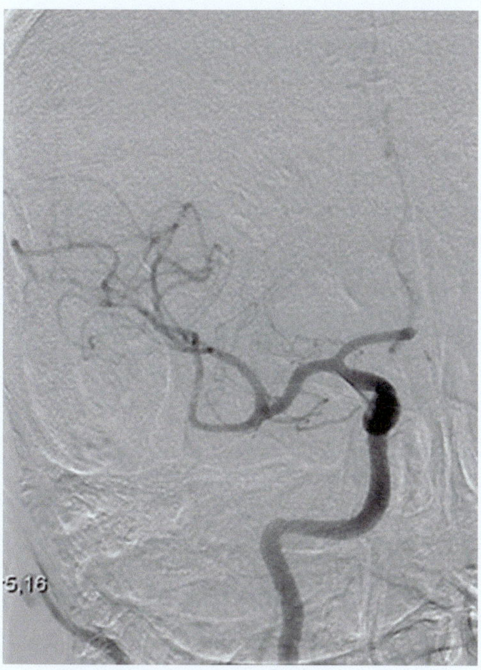

Fig. 100.3 Good recanalization of the stenosed right ICA with good antegrade flow

   (d) Aggressive manipulation of the guiding sheath tip, which is usually located in the common carotid artery
6. Spasms, pseudo-spasms, and distally displaced kinks should be recognized, and stenting of these conditions must be avoided.
7. Generally, dissections are treated by additional stenting prior to removal of the guiding catheter/sheath. When there is suspicion of a carotid dissection, it is mandatory to maintain the guide wire position until the final angiographic assessment has been completed and the presence or absence of dissections has been ascertained.
8. Use of detachable stents is very helpful in these situations. Small dissection with maintained true lumen can be managed medically. However, when there is significant luminal narrowing or sluggish flow in the artery, stent recanalization has to be considered.

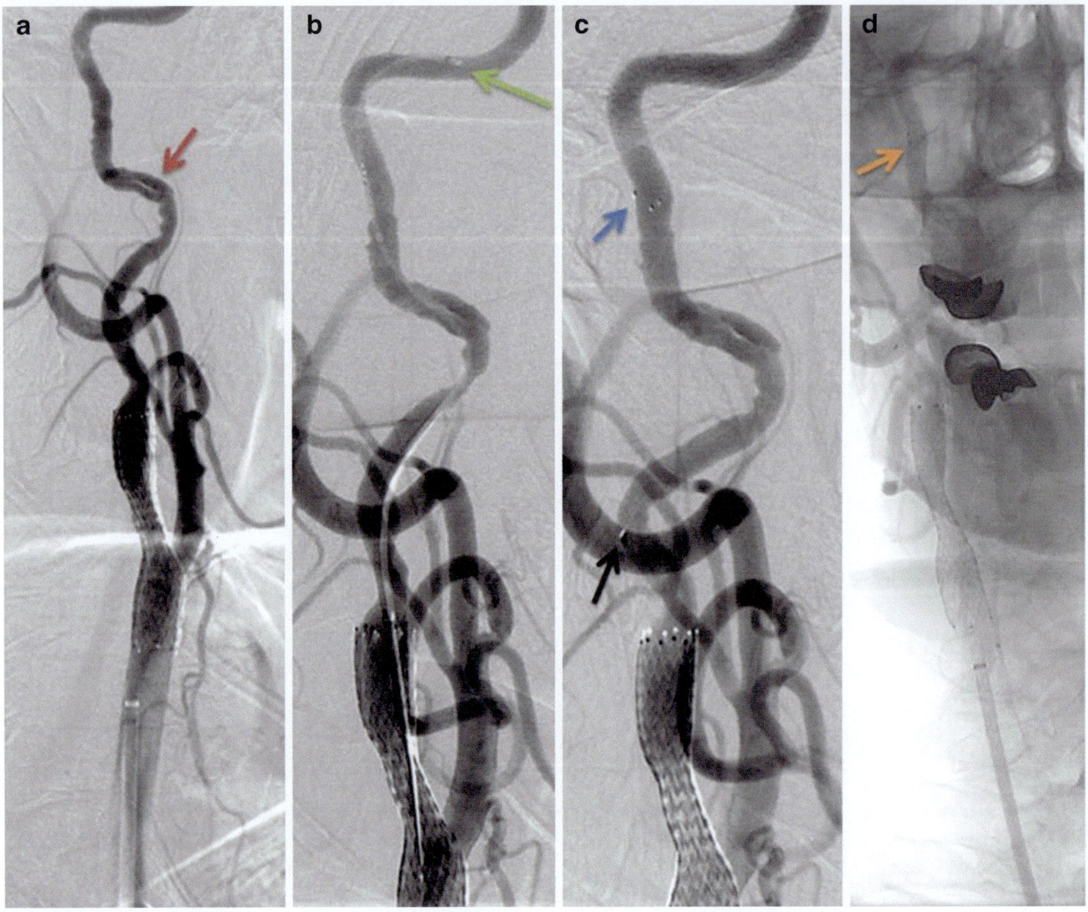

Fig. 100.4 (**a**) Segment of the cervical ICA was dissected due to manipulation of the wire across the tortuosity. (**b**) The dissection was crossed using a Rebar18 microcatheter over a 014 microguidewire. (**c** and **d**) Solitaire (ev3) stent 4 mm × 40 cm was deployed

Suggested Reading

Jauch EC, et al. Guidelines for the early management of patients with acute ischemic stroke: a guideline for healthcare professionals from the American Heart Association/American Stroke Association. Stroke. 2013;44(3):870–947.

Siddiqui AH, Natarajan SK, Hopkins LN, Levy EI. Carotid artery stenting for primary and secondary stroke prevention. World Neurosurg. 2011;76(6 Suppl):S40–59.

MIX
Papier aus verantwortungsvollen Quellen
Paper from responsible sources
FSC® C105338

If you have any concerns about our products,
you can contact us on
ProductSafety@springernature.com

In case Publisher is established outside the EU,
the EU authorized representative is:
Springer Nature Customer Service Center GmbH
Europaplatz 3, 69115 Heidelberg, Germany

Printed by Libri Plureos GmbH
in Hamburg, Germany